DOCTORS

The Illustrated History of Medical Pioneers

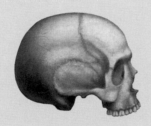

SHERWIN B. NULAND

BLACK DOG
& LEVENTHAL
PUBLISHERS
NEW YORK

PHOTO CREDITS
Cover photograph courtesy of Art Resource
Alan Mason Chesney Medical Archives of The Johns Hopkins Medical Institutions: 366, 370, 408, 418, 426
Art Resource including the following which have additional attributions:
Alineri: 15/Bildarchiv Preussischer Kulturbesitz: 26, 29, 149/Cameraphoto Arte, Venice: 16, 158/DeA Picture Library: 111/Erich Lessing: 18, 22, 24, 31, 35, 45, 51, 61, 91, 102, 103, 106, 123, 146, 152, 235, 239/Giraudon: 63, 79, 98/HIP: 72, 335/Réunion des Musées Nationaux: 32, 442/Scala: 42, 66, 104/Snark: 12, 76
Corbis: 317, 387 including the following which have additional attributions:
Bettman: 238, 303, 308, 319, 384, 394, 432, 433, 445, 447, 448, 451, 453, 458, 459/Michael Maslan Historic Photographs: 312/Miroslav Zajíc: 462
Granger: 49, 64, 69, 73, 74, 82, 85, 86, 88, 92, 94, 101, 109, 112, 115, 116, 121, 127, 129, 131, 134, 136, 140, 163, 167, 170, 177, 189, 198, 210, 211, 216, 225, 227, 228, 232, 233, 242, 248, 252, 255, 257, 258, 259, 261, 263, 264, 266, 267, 269, 271, 272, 274, 277, 288, 298, 304, 310, 314, 350, 375, 378, 379, 381, 383
IstockPhoto: 36
Photo Researchers including the following which have additional attributions:
Bo Veisland: 142/Jean-Loup Charmet: 58/John Watney: 436/Kwangshin Kim: 209/Mary Evans: 137, 150/National Library of Medicine: 160/Science Photo Library: 206/Scott Camazine: 81/Sheila Terry: 46, 124
The Royal College of Surgeons in England: 164, 173, 176, 178, 180, 181, 182, 184, 188, 190
including the following which have additional attributions:
Presented to the Hunterian Museum at The Royal College of Surgeons of England by L.D. Sheard: 213
Science Photo Library including the following which have additional attributions: Dr. Gopal Murti: 311/Humanities and Social Sciences Library/ New York Public Library: 156/John Reader: 295, 307/Library of Congress: 321
The Estate of Yousuf Karsh: 402
United States National Library of Medicine, Bethesda, MD: 154, 198, 204, 250, 415, 416, 420, 423, 429, 454
Wellcome: 38, 54, 57, 118, 132, 192, 196, 200, 218, 221, 231, 245, 246, 278, 281, 285, 292, 301, 324, 328, 329, 332, 337, 338, 340, 343, 344, 347, 349, 357, 358, 361, 365, 374, 389, 393, 397, 407, 411, 439
Yale Medical Historical Library: 36, 60, 113, 439

Published by Black Dog and Leventhal Publishers, Inc.
151 West 19th Street
New York, NY 10011

Distributed by
Workman Publishing Company
708 Broadway
New York, NY 10003

Manufactured in China

Cover and interior design by Lindsay Wolff

ISBN: 978-1-57912-778-7

h g f e d c b a

Library of Congress Cataloging-in-Publication Data available upon request.

The history of medicine is, in fact, the history of humanity itself, with its ups and downs, its brave aspirations after truth and finality, its pathetic failures. The subject may be treated variously as a pageant, an array of books, a procession of characters, a succession of theories, an exposition of human ineptitudes, or as the very bone and marrow of cultural history. As Matthew Arnold said of the Acta Sanctorum, "All human life is there."

—Fielding Garrison, 1913

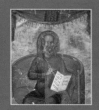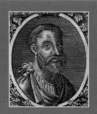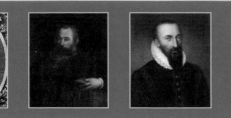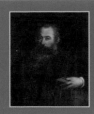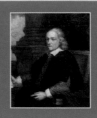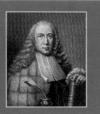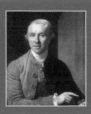

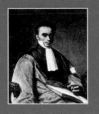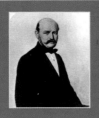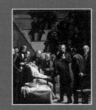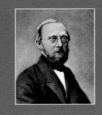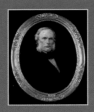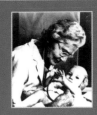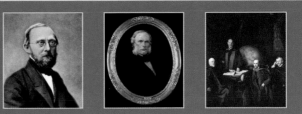

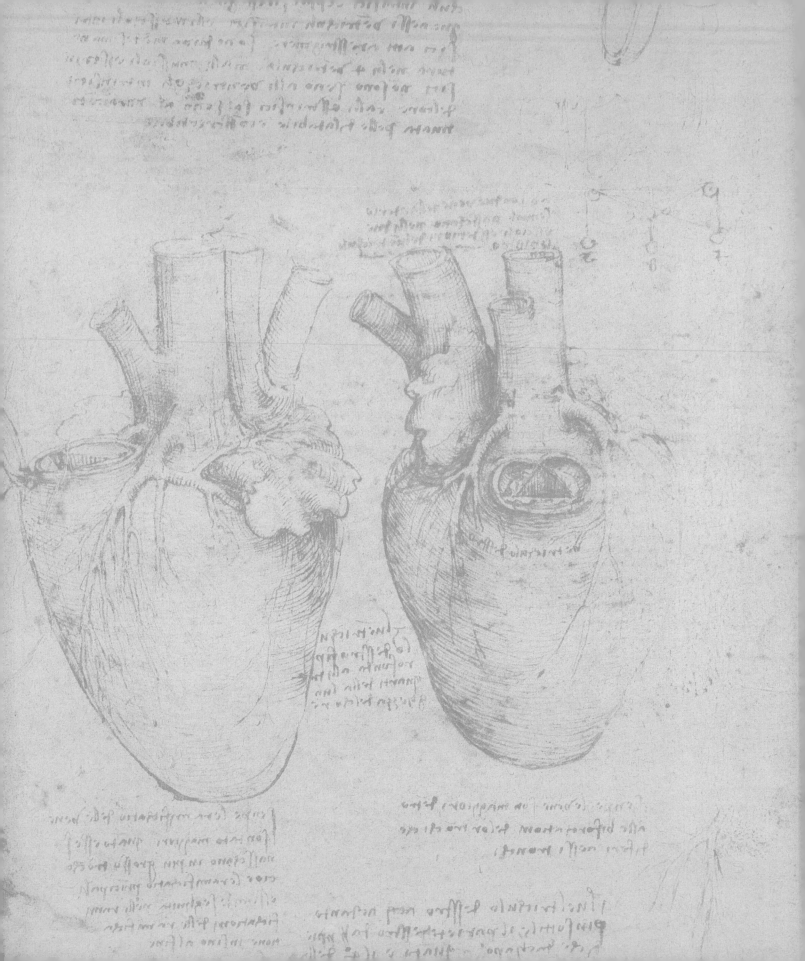

Introduction

The good physician knows his patients through and through, and his knowledge is bought dearly. Time, sympathy, and understanding must be lavishly dispensed, but the reward is to be found in that personal bond which forms the greatest satisfaction of the practice of medicine. One of the essential qualities of the clinician is interest in humanity, for the secret of the care of the patient is in caring for the patient.

—Dr. Francis Weld Peabody,
lecture to Harvard medical students, 1927

This book was written in a library. Of all the libraries in all the educational institutions of our world, there is none quite like this one. I like to think of it as my own personal place, even though it is shared by hundreds of men and women very much like me, who are often overwhelmed by the need to look backward in the midst of trying to go forward. None of us has yet been turned into a pillar of salt.

That large, comfortable book-lined room of mine is a sanctum containing the lore and the collected reminiscences of the art of healing. It is a museum, a portrait gallery, a storehouse of the literature of medicine's past, and a refuge from the hurly-burly of modern scientific technology that surrounds it. For those of us who are privileged to care for the sick or to carry out the research that makes that care possible, the Yale Medical Historical Library has been at once a safehouse from daily disquiets and a nurturing spring for renewal and strengthening of purpose.

There is no laboratory or patient-care area of our medical center that is more than a few minutes' walk from that high-vaulted, balcony-rimmed reading room and its layers of treasured stacks. The library is exactly the length of two football fields away from the operating rooms where I spend much of my day. Three decades ago, I could have covered the distance in twenty-five seconds. Even my present middle-aged shuffle gets me there in something under three minutes, counting the staircases.

That it is so easy to make what one of the library's donors called "voyages to other times and other places" is due to the vision of three ardent bookmen, who banded together in the 1930s to create a bibliophile's paradise in which their extensive personal collections might be joined into one, and domiciled in such a way as to be accessible to everyone wishing to learn about the history of medicine. They were John Fulton, one of America's most productive researchers in neurophysiology, and a human dynamo whose restless stimulus catalyzed many a major project in the science and humanism of medicine; Harvey Cushing, who had recently come to Yale after his retirement as Chief of Surgery at Harvard's Peter Bent Brigham Hospital, where he had established the specialty of neurosurgery; and the Swiss physician-bibliographer Arnold Klebs, who wrote the phrase about voyages. In honor of their communal project, they dubbed themselves the Trinitarians.

Since its opening ceremonies in 1941, the library founded by those three friends has grown at a rate beyond even their most optimistic predictions. The Yale Medical Historical Library has become one of the very few places in the world where medical *littérateurs* can book passage on uninterrupted pilgrimages to yesteryear. Indeed, if we accept Lord Macaulay's criterion that "The perfect historian is he in whose work the character and spirit of an age is exhibited in miniature," then this library that I call my own is the perfect historian for Western medical civilization, in a way that no flesh-and-blood striver can hope to be. There is to be found in it the visible evidence of Macaulay's concept of the writing of history as "a compound of poetry and philosophy."

Over the huge fireplace built into the wall at the far end of the reading room, there is a large plaque on which is engraved an inspirational inscription, addressed to those who would best use the collections for their intended purpose. The visitor has but to wander among those collections, and "listen," in order to appreciate the wisdom of its opening words: "Here, silent, speak the great of other years."

This book is the result of a lot of listening. It was originally subtitled *The Biography of Medicine* because I have chosen to tell healing's history in the form of biographies of some of its landmark contributors. But I have wondered, especially as I came to the writing of the last few chapters, whether I might not have better explained myself by using the word "*Autobiography.*" For what I have tried to do in this book is to describe the evolution of the process by which every doctor of today has come to his or her basic suppositions, and the shared theories by which all of us view the process of disease. The story of medicine is therefore the story of my professional life.

When I sit at the bedside of a patient, trying to reconstruct the sequence of pathological events within his body that has brought him to me, I am applying a method of reasoning that originated in Greece twenty-five hundred years ago. Each time I trace the development of an illness to the point at which it presents itself to me, I trace also the development of the theories upon which modern medicine is based. I begin afresh on every occasion, with the very concept of just what it is that constitutes a departure from health, and I proceed on the principle that a disease can be effectively treated only when I as a doctor understand its causes in that particular patient, its site of origin, the internal havoc it creates, and the course which the process is likely to take whether treated or not. With that knowledge, I can make a diagnosis, prescribe a program of treatment, and predict an outcome.

Greek physicians originated each of those steps in the days of Hippocrates, the Father of Medicine. The history of medicine has been the history of the increasingly successful efforts made by succeeding generations of doctors to find the ingredients that might bring the entire process to a state of perfection. Beginning in the sixteenth century with the first real knowledge of man's internal anatomical structures, and then proceeding in the eighteenth to an understanding of the ways in which those structures are distorted by sickness, the healers went on to develop a method of physical examination by which they could trace symptoms and signs to their organs of origin; they could then evaluate their diagnostic accuracy by following many of their patients to the autopsy table.

The identifying of disease sites became gradually more specific as diagnostic tools, such as the stethoscope, were invented. With the aid of improved technology in the making of lens systems, it came to be appreciated that organs sicken because the microscopic cells within them sicken. Having identified the minute locus in which disease originates, doctors next turned their attention to finding the primary inciting agents that make normal physiology go awry. This is where things stood in the middle of the nineteenth century.

As the decades of that century went by, this entire developmental process of the art of healing became more and more dependent on the objective study of organs, tissues, and cells, and therefore more and more dependent on the ways of science. The result was that doctors, necessarily focusing down in a way that historians call reductionist, sometimes lost sight of the whole patient who had come to be healed. As much as the best of the healers always strove to keep in perspective the entire reality of a patient's life, the demands of science made it ever more difficult to be a "whole-ist."

Of course, there is nothing about "whole-ism" (or holism) that makes it inconsistent with scientific medicine, and the truth is that now, in the last years of the twentieth century, as we gather more information about the processes by which healthy people get sick, we have begun to appreciate more fully the complexity of the factors involved. Much less than before do we now look for single causes; much more do we find ourselves seeking out each one of the plentiful number of elements that take part in the sickness of any individual patient. For someone to be sick, a sequence of things must have gone wrong, and the individual events are probably different for each of us. Though they may both harbor the streptococcus, your sore throat and mine have different antecedents, different ways in which the stage was set for the microbe to do its dirty work.

This emerging new way of looking at disease has been lucidly expressed by W. Jeffrey Fessel, who is both a physician and a prophetic philosopher of medical theory:

> *In most circumstances, disease is not an inevitable outcome of a single event occurring at a point in time but generally a probabilistic result of many events, each impinging on the organism at separate times and each producing its own sequence of biological reactions. The sum total of these events produces sufficient discomfort to the person to be recognized as illness. . . .*
>
> *Although the ultimate tissue reaction that has clinical expression may be the same in different persons, suggesting a uniform illness and, by extension, a disease entity in its own right, each person nevertheless probably has a unique and separate illness by*

virtue of the probability that no one else has the same combination and permutation of antecedents and their time relations. In this sense, every disease consists of multiple diseases; in this sense, too, there are no diseases but only sick people.

It is a statement that Hippocrates and every caring physician since his time could subscribe to. And so Jeffrey Fessel and I, and all physicians who have ever tried to make a diagnosis and then carry out a plan of therapy and attempt a prognosis, are heirs to the same tradition—the beneficiaries of the heritage of the doctors described in the following chapters. For that reason, this book is the autobiography that any one of us might have written.

I present it with a small handful of caveats. The first is almost a necessity for anyone who uses the biographic form to write history. It consists of begging readers' indulgence, that they not quarrel with my choices of eminent contributors. A few other stars shine just as brightly in the medical galaxy and would have been just as appropriate for my purposes. In fact, some of those others are more luminous and perhaps objectively more deserving of tribute than are several of my subjects. I have picked those I have picked because they are the ones who interest me most; that has seemed to be the best way for me to tell my story.

I could also be criticized for inserting into the narrative anecdotes and colorful episodes that may not always be considered of significance by the professional historians who have studied the lives of my heroes. In this I find some justification in Macaulay, who said, "The perfect historian . . . considers no anecdote, no peculiarity of manner, no familiar saying, as too insignificant for his notice which is not too insignificant to illustrate the operation of laws, of religion, and of education, and to mark the progress of the human mind. Men will not merely be described, but will be made intimately known to us." But while I am grateful for those words, and obviously don't hesitate to quote them, they do not totally apply to an imperfect (and quite amateur) historian like myself. Besides, my motives are less pure, and have to do with what is perhaps an idiosyncratic view of historiography, as well as one of my own hidden reasons for pursuing it: I confess to being a voyeur and a gossip to boot. I like to peek in on the lives of famous doctors, and I write about them to tell what I have seen. The perfect historian, the human kind, has not yet been born. Until he or she comes along to shame our pretensions, we can all presume to be tellers of tales.

One final warning. One of the colleagues whose opinions I most value has pointed out what some may perceive to be a very real defect—a tendency toward too much of a "gee whiz!" kind of writing. I seem to be so impressed, says my friend, with the contributions of all but a few of my characters that I cannot have enough of heaping compliments on them. Well, that certainly is an accurate perception. But I do not apologize. I *am* most assuredly not only impressed but quite frankly flabbergasted at the talents, industriousness, and accomplishments of most of these people. They are, after all, among the greatest medical innovators who have ever lived. The distinguished (see what I mean?) medical teacher William Osler once said that it is for what he called "the silent influence of character on character" that we study history, as much as for the events themselves. I have come away from examining the lives of my chosen doctors with a renewed optimism about the future of our civilization.

In these days, when it seems unrealistic to predict a future for mankind that is anything but bleak, I find something in this "procession of characters" of mine that gives me hope. The reverence for life, the zeal for learning Nature's secrets, the willingness to sacrifice for progress that you will read about in these chapters—these are characteristics that I believe are inherent in our species, notwithstanding the mass self-inflicted tragedies to which our century has been witness. I will go even further: I am convinced that there is a biologically determined characteristic that is the human spirit—that there is a gene or genes for it just as surely as there is a gene or genes for the color of our eyes or the length of our fingers. I have no idea whether it was put in place by the power that some call God or the power that some call chance, but it is reproduced within us with the same predictability as the rising and setting of the sun. It is not our intellect or even our physical structure that is the criterion of our human-ness; man is the most fulfilled animal on this planet because there resides in us the motivating and civilizing force of the human spirit. It gives us the ability to think courageous thoughts, do courageous deeds, and give courageous sustenance to our fellows. I predict that it will one day be the subject of scientific research and validating experiment. Though such studies will probably begin in a very soft science like sociology, they will eventually proceed into the realm of quantification and analysis. I don't believe for a minute that minds capable of solving the mysteries of DNA will not, in some distant future, elucidate what are now seen as the miraculous mysteries of human nature. There are, as Goethe tells us, no miracles; there are only those mysteries of nature, and they wait to be solved.

When the biological basis of the human spirit is understood, we will be able to explain such qualities as altruism and the inborn capacity of one person to nurture another back to health. Though similar capabilities have been observed in other species of animals, they are nowhere so highly developed as in our own. They form the underpinnings for many of the relationships we think of as uniquely human. Among them is the eternal foundation of the relationship between doctor and patient.

About this I am also encouraged. Unlike so many pessimistic seers of our time, I have faith in the future of medical caring, even if only because it is an expression of that biological quality I have called the human spirit. I use the word "eternal" advisedly—I do not think it will ever vanish.

More than half a century ago, Dr. Francis Weld Peabody addressed a class of Harvard medical students on the dangers of allowing the *science* of medicine to interfere with the *art* of medicine. "They are not antagonistic," he said, "but supplementary to each other." He concluded his lecture with the three sentences that I have used as the epigraph to this Introduction. They have since been repeated countless times before countless groups of students, because they so clearly identify the greatest key to being a good doctor, and its greatest bounty as well.

S. B. N.
New Haven, January 1988

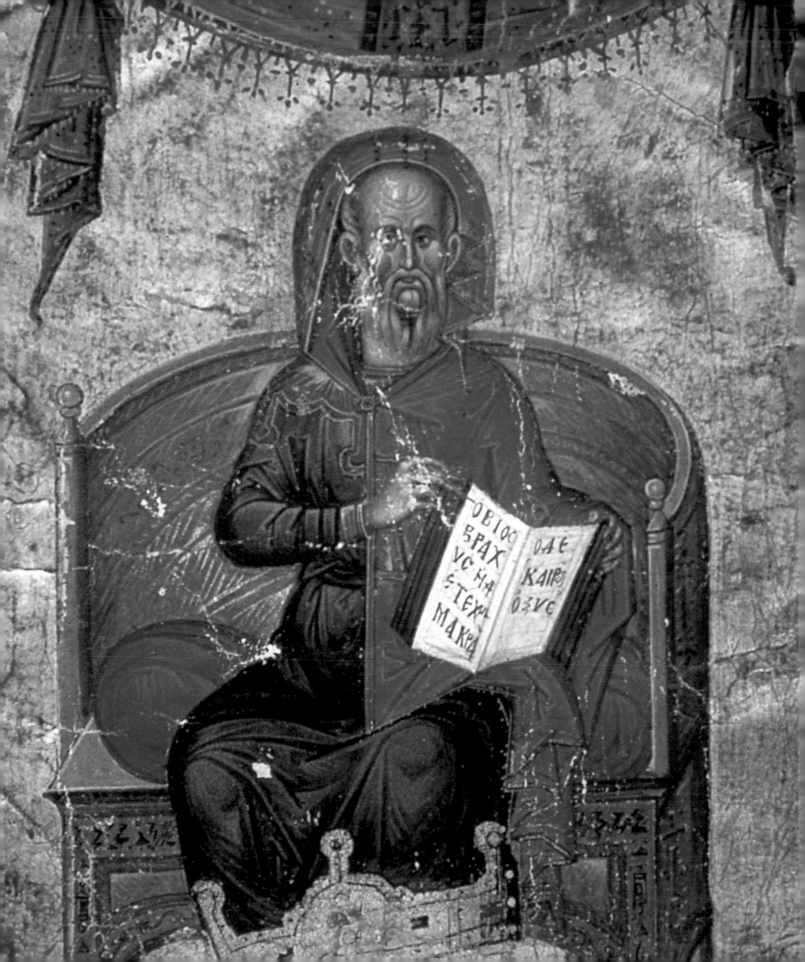

Ὁ βίος βραχὺς ἡ δὲ τέχνη μακρά ὁ δὲ καιρὸς ὀξύς

1

THE TOTEM OF MEDICINE

Hippocrates

There are those who believe that the Jesus of the New Testament never existed. They dispute the deeds attributed to him and doubt that his scriptural words were ever spoken. Similar suspicion has been expressed concerning the founders of many of the other major religions and sects of the world. Even when seemingly solid evidence of sacred lives is available, some thinkers remain unconvinced.

In spite of personal commitments that each of us may have to either rationalism or religion, we possess no indisputable knowledge of where the reality lies. Those with deep traditional faith see a certainty that requires no documentation. History is for them illuminated by the light of God, which shines gloriously over precisely the same area that appears as an obscure emptiness to the skeptics. And so debates will go on as long as our successors survive to inhabit this earth, between those who pursue the truth and those who pursue the Truth.

On a strictly practical level, it makes not an iota of difference which group of pursuers is right. Investigating the shrouded origins of the modern

ethical religions is far less important than understanding what the various groups have grown to be, and what effects each has had upon the history of the world and upon its moral vision. Most meaningful of all may be the question of their collective impact upon the thinking of contemporary man.

It is much the same with Hippocrates, the Greek physician whom we call the Father of Medicine. We think we know a few facts about his life that are separable from legend, and we think also that we have good reason to honor him in the parareligious way that has been taught us by the keepers of our medical lore. But beyond that, there is certainty about nothing except the existence of his scripture. Tradition is a persuasive teacher, even when what it teaches is erroneous. It tells us that all of the Hippocratic writings are the work of one author; it says the same of the Pentateuch of the Old Testament, and yet hard literary evidence denies such a claim as forcefully for the former as it does for the latter.

As with the books of the Bible, different Hippocratic writings seem to have been composed by different scribes at different times, setting down a permanent record of what had previously been an oral tradition of belief and practice. Although to a lesser extent than the Biblical writ with which we make analogy, the Hippocratic Collection (or, as it is often called, the Hippocratic Corpus) contains some eternal truths and some soaring literature. The whole is united by a theology, and it is the theology, rather than the author, which makes it Hippocratic. Both the Bible and the Corpus deal with man's relationship to man and to another power outside himself. In the Greek writings, however, that power is Nature; God and other forces that can be seen only with supernatural sight are excluded.

This injunction to turn a blind eye to the possibility of a deity or mystical influence in the causes and treatment of disease was the greatest contribution made by the school of Hippocrates. The Swiss medical historian Erwin Ackerknecht has called it "Medicine's Declaration of Independence."

There is not, in the entire Corpus, the slightest hint that disease is traceable to causes beyond the powers of the physician to understand. Each set of symptoms has a specific cause or causes, and treatment must be directed toward correcting the circumstances in which they appear and not only the consequences of their presence. Thus, the setting in which the illness takes place should be considered as important a factor as the manifestations of sickness themselves. The Greeks were the first to believe that the universe functions by rational, reasonable rules. They gave us the concept of cause and effect and thereby laid the groundwork for science. Even before Aristotle, there was Hippocrates; what we have in the Corpus is a treasure house containing the earliest extant scientific treatises in any language.

Though our debt is not so much to the Father of Medicine himself as it is to the philosophy and practice that bear his name, Hippocrates nevertheless did live, and he seems to have been a distinguished physician of his day. But before telling what little is known of his life, it is necessary to describe something of his mythical antecedents and contemporary counterparts, and most specifically the system of belief whose practitioners were known collectively as the cult of Aesculapius.

In post-Homeric times, the healing powers originally attributed to several of the principal gods, Apollo, Artemis, and Athena, were gradually transferred in large measure to a lesser deity, Aesculapius, son of Apollo by the nymph Coronis. The Aesculapian myth is polymorphous, arising, as did Greek culture itself, from a confluence of many earlier civilizations and traditions. Legend ascribes numerous miraculous cures to the god, carried out primarily by means of visions attained in dreams which the faithful sick experienced while sleeping in temples dedicated to him.

The sites of Aesculapius' shrines had qualities which all cultures have recognized as ideal for the purpose of restoring health: they were often on breeze-touched hills in the vicinity of clear flowing streams or springs, whose waters were of high mineral content. The salubrious air, the visual comfort of the surrounding forests, the beautifully cultivated gardens, and the spiritually nurturing presence of the robed priests combined to create a reassuring atmosphere in which health could be expected to reenter the body of the suffering pilgrim. Of course, the stricken petitioners had come to beg the help of a divinity, and so there were also prayers, animal sacrifices, and the diligent carving of votive tablets. Sacred serpents anointed injured limbs, licking and slithering their silent restorative way from one raw wound to another. While all of this inspirational theotherapy was in progress, the sonorous voices of the priests could be heard intoning solemn incantations and magical formulas. Surrounded by their eagerly devout supplicants, they recounted the wondrous cures that had been brought about by the power of Aesculapius and his legendary children, among whom were his daughters, Hygeia and Panacea. The god himself was present in effigy bearing a long staff around which was entwined the famous sacred snake; from this otherworldly origin comes the symbol of the modern scientific medical profession.

The focus of the cure was the god-given dream, in which Aesculapius conveyed to the sleeping patient, either directly or in symbols, the means by which recovery might be attained. Having been brought to the proper level of emotional readiness by the mystical ceremonies and the supernal atmosphere of the shrine, the patient spent several nights sleeping in the awesome temple itself, until the oracular vision made its appearance. The spectral message was then interpreted by the priests in ways that were consistent with their system of therapeutics, which meant that they were likely to see in it such treatments as might be obtained through diet, exercise, or what we nowadays call recreational or music therapy. Sometimes the cure required bloodletting or purging, or even an occasional quite fanciful directive that instant restoration of health occur, probably meant to invoke the

power of suggestion. If the priestly treatment was successful, the credit went to Aesculapius and to his agents, who accepted the prayers and the money of their patients with equal piety. If the treatment failed, the petitioner himself was to blame.

In sum, the Aesculapian system—despite the "health-resort" methods to be found in its therapeutic arsenal—was based on a theurgical philosophy of disease: illness was caused by unknow-

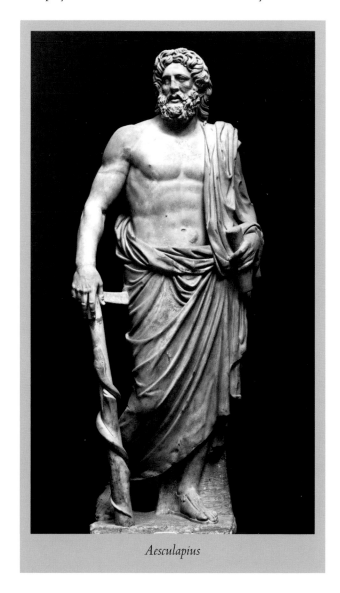

Aesculapius

able supernatural forces, and so the cure had also to come from those same sources.

For many centuries, it was thought by historians that the medicine of the Hippocratic physician grew out of these roots, and that the priests were the forerunners and teachers of Hippocrates and his school. The truth is somewhat different: The teachings of the Hippocratic physicians came about in opposition to the supernaturally-based precepts of the shrines. The new teachings were rational, empirical, and founded on the principle that every disease has a cure which is not only quite natural, but quite discoverable as well.

The historical confusion probably arose from the fact that some of the physicians called themselves Asclepiads, thus giving the mistaken impression to later observers that they were followers of the cult of Aesculapius.

Hippocrates himself was born about 460 B.C. on the island of Cos, near the western coast of Asia Minor. In spite of all subsequent historical and legendary embellishment, this is all truly know from our only contemporary sources, two of the dialogues of Plato, the *Protagoras* and the *Phaedros.* Later writers said of him that he was the son of Heraclides, a hereditary Asclepiad.

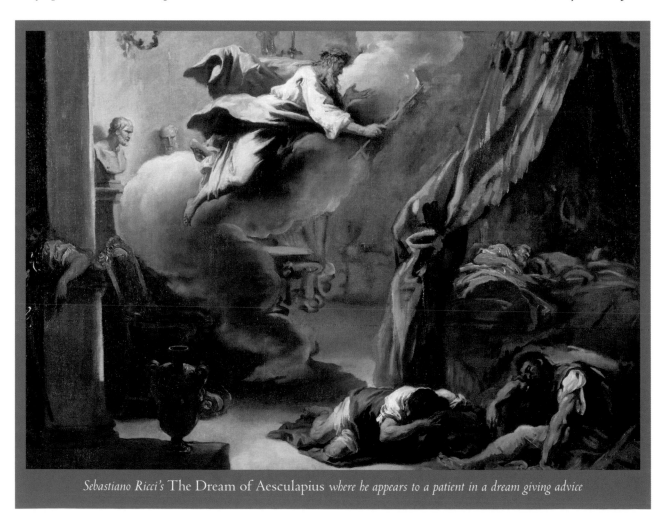

Sebastiano Ricci's The Dream of Aesculapius *where he appears to a patient in a dream giving advice*

Unfortunately, twentieth-century archaeological evidence suggests that the cult of the god Aesculapius settled on Cos after 350 B.C., when the Father of Medicine was no longer living, which casts considerable doubt on the rest of the traditional biographical account. It is easy enough to dismiss the myth that he was the nineteenth lineal descendant of Aesculapius, but much of the rest of the traditional life history is neither provable nor disprovable, so it will be here presented as it is usually recounted. Most of the details come from the adulatory biography written by one Soranus of Ephesus in the second century A.D., when its revered subject had been dead for more than five hundred years. It deserves as much credence as could be given to a modern biography of Joan of Arc that was based only on oral accounts and was written by a leader of the French women's movement who was also a religious mystic. Nevertheless, it appears to be the first written description of the life of the Father of Medicine, and it is the source of our present sketchy outline.

Hippocrates is said to have been taught medicine by his father, Heraclides. Like all physicians of his day, he spent a considerable amount of time traveling, practicing his art throughout the neighboring cities and Aegean islands. He apparently lectured on medicine and surgery during these travels, and was paid fees by both students and patients. As his fame grew, his services came more into demand. Tales were told of various remarkable cures that he was able to effect and of the many honors he received. No one is at all sure what he looked like, but in several pieces of statuary that have been "identified" to the satisfaction of enough authorities he is depicted as an elderly, distinguished-looking sage with a bald head, a

bearded chin, and an intelligent, sensitive face. As a highly respected member of the medical academy centered on the island of Cos, he was one of the most influential physicians of his era. He seems to have lived to a great age, being approximately one hundred years old when he died in Larissa.

In placing Hippocrates temporally, it is helpful to remember that his long life spanned those of Socrates and Plato, and that he died about a decade before the birth of Alexander the Great, when Aristotle was a young man. Pericles, Euripides, Aeschylus, Sophocles, and Aristophanes were his contemporaries. Obviously, it was a time of great intellectual ferment in Greece—a veritable premier Father's Day of the mind, with Hippocrates, Herodotus, and Aristotle in the midst of giving life to medicine, historiography, and literary criticism, respectively. It was the period of one of those great bursts of mental energy which from time to time appear in the culture of Western civilization to thrust it forward into new patterns of thought and deed, and new ways of expression.

With the Hippocratic physicians, medicine as we know it began to develop. Divorced from superstition and necromancy, devoted to systematic observation of disordered life processes, and committed to a set of ethical principles that declared the physician's primary obligation to be to his patient, it formed the trellis upon which subsequent growth of medical thought could be guided.

It is one of the ironies of this history that the academy of Cos, the so-called Coan School, had a rival, situated on the opposite peninsula at Cnidus, which practiced a form of medicine that was in some ways more like our own than that of the physicians of Cos. The Cnidian focus was on the disease, while that of Hippocrates was on the patient. The Cnidian physicians, like those of to-day, were reductionists, fine-tuners who directed their efforts to the classification of the processes of sickness and to exact diagnosis. They sought to know the specific local organ disturbances that caused the symptoms they so assiduously categorized. Why, then, one might ask, is it the Hippocratics whose teachings survived to become the foundation of modern medicine?

In ancient Greece, the Cnidians' approach had an inherent weakness: to succeed, the Cnidians would have required a much more accurate knowledge of anatomy and organ function than was possible at the time. Proscriptions against human dissection existed, arising out of the prevailing religious dicta of the day, which required burial immediately following death. There was, in addition, a culturally-based horror of corpses that was difficult to overcome, even by the more detached physicians. Although some degree of anatomical knowledge was acquired from studies of animals and rare, hurried, partial postmortems of humans, it remained only sketchily supplemented by an occasional lucky look into the slashed body cavity of some wounded combatant. In the entire Hippocratic Collection, there is no conclusive, indisputable evidence of formal dissection of the human body.

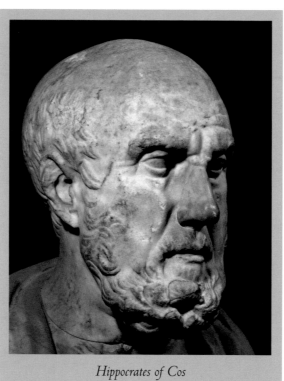

Hippocrates of Cos

Even had the requisite detailed information been available, it would have been necessary to do thousands of meticulous studies of diseased organs in order to understand the ways in which morbid processes cause the symptoms exhibited by patients. And even then, who would be benefited by a physician who understood a pathological process he had no way of treating? Specificity of diagnosis does not help the sufferer unless it can be followed by specificity of treatment, a fruitless fantasy in that scientifically primitive age. The fulfillment of the Cnidian philosophy had to await the coming of modern medicine, with its gradual evolution of understanding of the physical and biochemical bases of the mechanisms of disease, and subsequent strides in the technology of cure. That succession of triumphs would not get under way until the late Renaissance; the Cnidian physician entered the arena long before his time.

Given the limitations of Greek science, the Coan School fared much better. The Hippocratic physicians saw diseases as events that happen within the context of the life of the entire patient, and they oriented their treatment toward restoration of the natural conditions and defenses of the sick person and the reestablishment of his proper relation to his surroundings. To be sure, they suffered the consequences of the major error of their system, which was the grouping of dissimilar clinical conditions under one fused, and therefore *con*fused, heading, a state of affairs that arose out of their propensity to categorize a disease on the basis of its major symptom, such as fever. However, by concentrating their treatment not on the actual diagnosis but on the patient and his environment, and by making him a member of his own therapeutic team, they achieved successes that eluded their rivals; in this can be recognized the seeds of what has come to be called holistic medicine, or at least holistic medicine divorced from some of the crackpot ideas which have encumbered it of late.

(In the preceding paragraph I have used the word "clinical," for the first of what will be many times. Although taken for granted by physicians, "clinical" is a term often confusing to others. It derives, appropriately for its present context, from the Greek *klinē*, a couch or bed, and therefore came to be used in reference to a patient lying down. In fact, one of its philological descendants is "recline." What is clinical is that which deals with sick people and their diseases, as distinct from lectures, laboratories, and pure science—in other words, it is bedside medicine. The healer is a clinician; his expertness is in clinical medicine; his venue is the clinic, whether it is a small outpatient department at the end of a hospital corridor or a complex corporate structure with a famous name like Mayo or Lahey associated with it. Although the people who make their way to such facilities are known as patients—from Latin *patior*, "to suffer"—they might just as well be called clients, another word that has evolved from *klinē*.)

It was, thus, the basically holistic clinical approach of Hippocrates that provided the clear light which led Greek medicine out of the mire of theurgy and witchcraft. Unfortunately, however, its clarity was to endure for only half a millennium. It became misinterpreted and garbled after the fall of the Roman Empire; then its distorted form refused to yield the stage for yet another thousand years thereafter. Having originally cleared the way for progress, Hippocratism was destined to become, in the end, an obstacle to the same kind of inquiring spirit which had given it birth.

Even after the Renaissance, the hoary-minded adherents of the corrupted residues of Hippocratic medicine continued to man the barricades against the gradually strengthening forces of the dissectors and the chemists who sought answers in organs, then in tissues, and finally within the structure of the cell itself. The next baton-passing in the struggle between Coan and Cnidian did not take place until two centuries ago, when the scientific world was ready to take a firm stand in favor of specific organ pathology. When that happened, the micro-

> *It was, thus, the basically holistic clinical approach of Hippocrates that provided the clear light which led Greek medicine out of the mire of theurgy and witchcraft.*

scope replaced the clinician's scrutinizing eye, and the molecule replaced the patient. The reductionists took over, and brought with them the principles of modern medical science.

The Hippocratic Corpus, misunderstood (and for a time lost) though it was, sustained the formulations of the physicians of Cos during the long centuries between Rome and reductionism. It is thought by most authorities to be the remains of a library collected on that island center of medical learning. That such libraries existed is beyond doubt, even though this particular one is their only surviving relic. It is safe to assume that they contained many different types of texts, ranging from the works of the leading Asclepiads to books acquired by chance, and including clinical records, lectures, handbooks and manuals, and essays dealing with medicine or its related philosophy. In other words, the books and papers of any medical library are related to each other by no other criterion than the fact that they all contain material that is of use in the study of disease. That describes the Hippocratic Corpus. It consists of a group of some seventy variegated texts, all written in the Ionic dialect, in a wide assortment of styles, and sometimes contradicting each other on doctrinal points. Very likely, the entire Corpus found its way to one of the other later ancient libraries, perhaps the great one at Alexandria, and was there treated as one great work of one great man whose name was already famous.

By common consent of the foremost scholars of this material, certain of its texts stand out among the rest for the clarity of their thought, the high moral message they transmit, and the scientific objectivity of their approach. Because these qualities result in certain stylistic similarities, this group of treatises was in former years thought, even by those convinced of the mongrel nature of the Corpus as a whole, to have a single author, and therefore to be what are called *The Genuine Works of Hippocrates*. Although the "genuineness" of even this subset is unlikely, the distinction is useful, because it separates out the particular portions of the Corpus that represent the greatest contributions of Greek medical thought. It is chiefly for these specific works that we memorialize the name of Hippocrates and honor him as the Father of Medicine.

The disciples of most great leaders, either of the divine or political sort, cling to the more pithy pronouncements of their patriarchs and make philosophical amulets of them. For the Cos-inspired physicians, these were the *Aphorisms of Hippocrates*. The very first of those medical proverbs is the most-quoted single statement in the entire collection of ancient medicine, perhaps of all medicine, or, as the Greeks were fond of calling it, the Art: Life is short, the Art is long, opportunity fleeting, experience delusive, judgement difficult.

Has there ever been a better description of the obstacles faced by those who would be healers of the sick? That it is too long and too arduous a calling to be mastered in any human lifetime is known by everyone who has ever tried it. But does everyone, do even all doctors, realize how few are the genuine opportunities to study people and their diseases carefully enough to add anything of lasting importance to the sum of man's knowledge? We speak often of the value of experience, but we all know how misleading anyone's accumulated collection of memories can be, even when viewed with all of the clinical objectivity that a mature physician can muster. Remarkably, the quantifying and measurement of the combined disease encounters of many clinicians, which we dignify with such puffed-up names as biometrics and statistics, are also delusive. If they were not, everyone's numbers would always agree—and they often don't. Whether we rely on memory, data, or interpretation, experience too frequently leads us astray.

And finally, there is judgment. We try to teach it to our students, but we wonder if we understand it ourselves. After thirty years in medicine, I don't even know how to define the word, much less recognize its presence in my thoughts at the bedside. I try to do what seems right, but sometimes the course that seems right for this particular patient today is exactly the opposite of what seemed right for someone with what seemed to be exactly the same problem yesterday. If even statistics give fuzzy answers, how much more unsteady must be judgment? Were it infallible, doctors would never disagree. Like statistics, the judgment of one doctor often conflicts with that of another; and like statistics that disagree, there is no guarantee that one course or the other will lead to a successful outcome. The problem thus distills itself down to the first aphorism of Hippocrates: judgment is difficult to learn, to apply, and even to recognize; medicine has few certainties—the ancients correctly called it the Art.

To the Hippocratic physician, the fundamental principle of his Art was the concept that Nature seeks to maintain a condition of stability; its forces are constantly adjusting and readjusting the normal constituents of the body to preserve a balance among them. When this balance exists, we are healthy. Under any of a variety of influences, the equilibrium may be disturbed, resulting in one constituent's appearing in excess. When this happens, sickness develops, the particular disease depending primarily upon which substance has gained the ascendancy. It is the function of the physician to help Nature restore the state of equilibrium. Since each disease has a distinctive natural course of its own, the physician must make himself so familiar with it that he can predict the sequence of events and know whether and precisely when to intervene with treatment that will help Nature to do its work.

The concept of the equilibrated harmony of Nature's forces was not original with the Hippocratics. Long before they came upon the scene, disease was thought by certain groups of physicians to be caused by an imbalance among the four "humors"—blood, yellow bile, black bile, and phlegm. These four primary fluids were said to be constantly renewed by means of the food which is eaten and digested. The blood was thought to originate in the heart, the yellow bile in the liver, the black bile in the spleen, and the phlegm in the brain.

The theory had considerable appeal to the Greeks because it satisfied the requirement of objectivity in their system, in the sense that the humors were visible under various circumstances, so there could be no doubt about their existence. They were tangible substances. Black bile is the only one of them whose observability is a little difficult to explain, but it is thought to have been represented by the black stools of gastrointestinal bleeding or the coffee-grounds vomit frequently seen in a variety of clinical conditions.

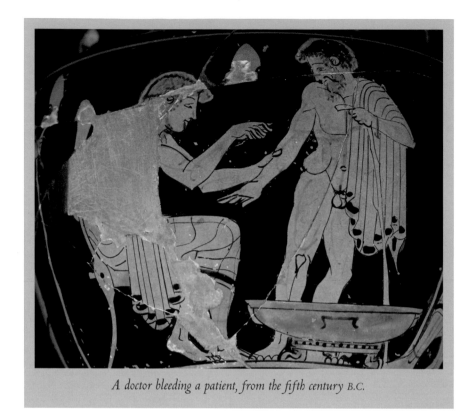

A doctor bleeding a patient, from the fifth century B.C.

It was readily observable that phlegm, the cold-wet humor, increased in the winter. Since the Greek spring was wet and hot, there was thought then to be an increase in blood. Yellow bile was more prevalent during the dry heat of the summer, while the cold, dry autumn encouraged the dominance of black bile. Bilious vomiting, dysentery, nosebleeds, catarrh, jaundice, and fevers of various sorts are frequent in the Hippocratic descriptions of disease, and each of them could be related to one or more of the humors and the season in which it predominated. This was particularly true of those infectious diseases which are most prevalent during certain times of the year. Thus was man's health related not only to the humors within him, but also to the greater universe of which he is a part.

There are other implications of this system. Normal seasonal variations in the humors were thrown awry if the season itself had some abnormal features in any given year. Moreover, inhabitants of certain areas were predisposed to particular diseases depending upon the prevailing winds, the source of the water supply, the angle of the sun, and even such considerations as the direction faced by the town in which they lived. As might be imagined, marked and rapid fluctuations in temperature and humidity were considered to be particularly dangerous because of the sudden

The Greeks believed that the humors were moved and mixed in the body by the driving force of the "innate heat," which was a form of energy generated by the heart, and which in turn generated the humors from the food that was eaten, and tended to keep them in balance. "Innate heat" was thus the essential ingredient of man's composition. It was part of Nature's healing power, the force that acted both to maintain equilibrium and to restore it when it was lost.

The humors bore a direct relationship to the four "elements," fire, air, earth, and water, and therefore to the four "qualities" of hot, dry, cold, and wet. So the blood represented the hot-wet characteristics, the yellow bile the warm-dry, the black bile the cold-dry, and the phlegm the cold-wet. Because of the role of the qualities, the body's equilibrium was influenced by the seasons.

changes in humoral balance they brought with them. Obviously, the ingestion of foods of different sorts and in different amounts would have a significant effect on the quantity of any particular humor.

There were numerous other influences that the Hippocratic physician had to take into account in his attempt to discover the cause of any disease and support Nature in restoring balance. Not the least of them was his patient's fundamental constitution, since the basal state of the humoral interaction affected personality and character. Our language and our literature have been enriched by our ability to describe people's dispositions as sanguine, melancholic, bilious, or phlegmatic.

In order to determine the nature of the humoral imbalance that was at the root of a given disease process, it was necessary to look beyond the obvious symptoms, to seek objective evidence of the effects being produced. To this end, a highly sophisticated type of physical examination was developed, in which the physician, by skillful use of his five senses, sought manifestations of the underlying disorder. It is fascinating to read some of the Hippocratic case reports, with their descriptions of changes in temperature, color, facial expression, breathing pattern, body position, skin, hair, nails, abdominal contour, and a host of other clues that today's best diagnosticians still seek out during the course of a careful consultation. Anticipating the laboratory tests that would only come into being twenty-five hundred years later, the Hippocratics tasted the blood and the urine, and did not hesitate to do the same for skin secretions, ear wax, nasal mucus, tears, sputum, and pus. They smelled the stool, and they took due note of the degree of stickiness of the sweat. No discharge

or product of their patients' bodily functioning escaped their keen analytical scrutiny.

What must be emphasized here is the empirical quality of the process of diagnosis. It depended, as did the entire humoral theory, on phenomena that were observable. This was something new in medicine. Previously, either diseases had been diagnosed without regard to any but the most overt major symptoms or no attempt whatsoever had been made to discover primary causes, since treatment depended upon supernatural intervention. There was an amazing consistency to the Hippocratic method, and once it had been accepted by a student being introduced to it, everything followed appropriately from the basic theory. Obviously, that theory was formulated on erroneous interpretation of the original observed events, but within its own set of premises it remained a rational system that appealed to logical thinkers. Not only that, it encouraged the making of observations, and thereby paved the way for the introduction of the scientific method into medicine. The Hippocratic approach was experiential, the forerunner of the experimental. The careful recording of data, with inferences being made only from phenomena that could be identified, was its hallmark. It was taught as scientific medicine would one day be taught, with case records, bedside teaching, and clinical lectures and demonstrations.

Its basic philosophy was the same as the basic philosophy underlying the rational understanding with which today's scientifically trained physicians approach the problems of sick people. In this view, disease should be looked upon as a combat between Nature and what may be called morbid causes. The role of the physician is to observe the struggle closely enough to know the pro-

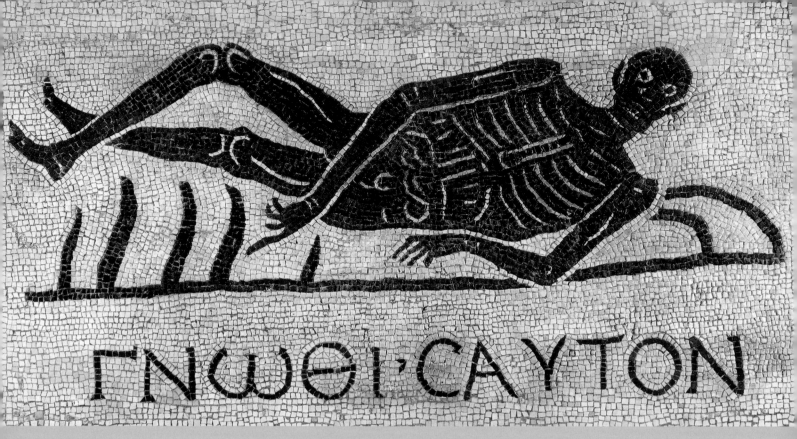

Inscription from first century A.D. Greek mosaic: Know thyself.

pitious moment at which to intervene, as well as to recognize that in most cases the intervention is best kept minimal, if indeed it is required at all. Sickness, it must be remembered, runs the gamut from colds to cancer.

The Hippocratic physician understood that the power which he called Nature is a formative, constructive, and curative power; the human body tends to heal itself. It is only in unusual circumstances that the morbid causes can overwhelm the natural inclination of the organism, which is to reestablish the equilibrating rhythms of health. The guiding principle that governs the therapeutic efforts of the physician of today remains the one that was placed in trust for him by the sages of Greek medicine. Although expressed in different ways throughout the Corpus, it is most directly stated in the text of the book *Epidemics* (I, II):

"To help, or at least to do no harm." For reasons that will become apparent in the next chapters, that fundamental teaching has been carried down to us in its Latin translation: *Primum non nocere*— First, do no harm.

A sage of our own times has said the same thing about the healing powers of Nature in words that are less resounding, but no less profound for their lighter tone. Some fifteen years ago, in the august surroundings of the Yale Corporation Room, that greatest of all Biology Watchers, Lewis Thomas, told several of us something that encapsulated the experience of my own clinical lifetime, and no doubt of his. I don't remember the exact words he used, but they are easily rediscovered. Because his conversational patterns are adorned by the same lovely lyricism and aphoristic accuracy found in his writings, he probably said it much as it appeared in his essay "Your Very Good Health":

The great secret, known to internists and learned very early in marriage by their wives [and nowadays by their husbands too], but still hidden from the general public, is that most things get better by themselves. Most things, in fact, are better by morning.

How does Nature accomplish her cure, and how can she be helped by the physician? Having become sick because one of his four humors has achieved dominance over the others, the Hippocratic patient could not recover unless the excess material was driven out of his body. In order for this to happen, the body was thought to use its innate heat in an attempt to ripen, or cook, the raw noxious excess humor into a form that could be expelled. The process was called pepsis, or coction, and it resulted in the production of such recognizable effluvia as phlegm, pus, diarrhea, intestinal bleeding, nasal discharges, and foul coughed-up plugs of mucus. If the coction succeeded and the morbid material was properly discharged, the patient recovered; if not, he died. The expulsion of the end-product might be rapid and dramatic, in which case the cure was said to occur by crisis, or it might be quite gradual, coming about by what was called lysis. The entire process was a war, between the disease and the defensive powers of the patient's intrinsic constitution.

The Greek physician did not have vast pharmaceutical or physical resources with which to help Nature do its work. He sought signs of coction by examining the various effluvia of the body, and he watched carefully for evidence of lysis, crisis, or impending death. He was called upon by one of the most basic doctrines of Hippocratic medicine to be a master of the art of prognosis. There were good reasons for this, which had to do with the conditions under which he worked. In a society where there was no licensing and no certain way of proving one's qualifications, the trained physician needed some method of distinguishing himself from anyone else who might claim to have powers of healing. Most of the doctors of the day were itinerants, traveling from place to place, offering their services in much the same way as did wandering craftsmen. If things went well in a particular community, the healer might stay for a while, until the need for his doctoring lessened. In such a situation it was necessary to acquire a reputation quickly, in order that patients might know that they were dealing with a well-trained master of the healing art. What better way could there have been to build up confidence than by making an accurate prognosis?

The Hippocratic physician was trained in a school in which the study of the course of the disease process was a paramount consideration. Insofar as the level of contemporary science allowed it, he was an expert on the evolution of clinical syndromes. He understood how certain symptoms often come together in specific groupings, and how some conditions of sickness frequently follow predictably after others have made their appearance. Thus, he was well equipped to prognosticate, and he was encouraged by the ethos of his school to do so. As is well-recognized today, a physician in whom one has confidence serves not only himself, but his patient as well. It comes as no earthshaking revelation that the confidence of the patient in his physician is one of the cardinal factors in the art of healing. In the words of our ancient author:

Some patients, though conscious that their condition is perilous, recover their health simply through their contentment with the goodness of the physician.

The validity of that Hippocratic aphorism is well illustrated by the following case history. It is not a unique tale that you are about to read—any experienced clinician would be able to tell several like it.

Twenty-five years ago, I was one of several physicians involved in the care of the then chaplain of Yale, the charismatic (a word much in use during those heady days of the Kennedy Camelot) William Sloane Coffin. Following a particularly bitter civil-rights campaign, Bill Coffin had returned to New Haven feverish, coughing, and exhausted from a sojourn in a filthy Mississippi jailhouse. The chaplain was known for his remarkable physical and moral resilience, but after a few days of worsening symptoms, even that good-natured toughness that we so much admired gave way, and he reluctantly allowed himself to be admitted to the Yale-New Haven Hospital.

His disabling symptoms were found to be due to a severe form of pneumonia, with a large collection of staphylococcal pus in the chest. The outcome remained uncertain for days, as his temperature hovered in the 102° range and his "morbid cause" resisted the combined efforts of the infectious-disease specialists with their antibiotics, and me with my pus-draining needles and tubes. Finally, it became apparent that only an operation of considerable magnitude and risk would save his life. The difficult decision having been made, and discussed with the patient, I scheduled the surgery to take place on the following morning, a Wednesday. On Tuesday evening, the enervating fever suddenly broke, exactly as though some miraculous coction and crisis had taken place at the penultimate moment before the perilous surgical journey. The operation was canceled, and the chaplain went on to recover rapidly over the course of the succeeding days. None of us would ever be able to explain what invigorating event had occurred in the immune system of our critically ill patient, or so we thought.

Some five years later, I found myself at a faculty wedding at which the robustly healthy Reverend Mr. Coffin was officiating. Although ours is a small city, our paths had

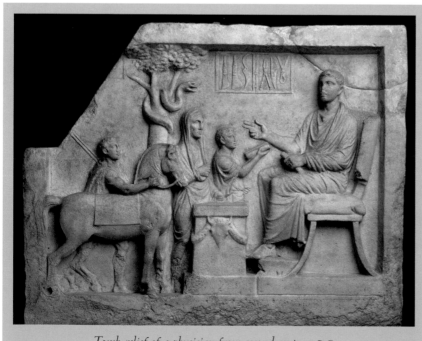

Tomb relief of a physician from second century B.C.

not crossed since his recovery. At the reception, I cornered him, and asked what he thought had happened on that dramatic evening to account for his sudden and, to my mind, almost preternatural cure. Expecting to hear a recounting of some personal religious insight, I was quite unprepared for his answer. "I did it," he said with absolute conviction, "for Bizzozero."

Had I heard wrong? Had he said "Beelzebub"? Was it possible that Yale's leading divine, in a fit of fever, had actually believed that he had made a contract with the devil just to avoid the hazards of spending a few hours with me in the operating room? Having as little tolerance for such magical ministries as did the Hippocratics, and knowing also that a healthy William Coffin was the most rational of men, I dismissed the possibility. Cupping my hand behind my ear to trap the sound waves that were being lost in that noisy room, I half-shouted, quite ungrammatically I fear, "For who?" This time I heard the name distinctly—Bizzozero.

Who was this inspirational afflatus, this mahatma Bizzozero who had so aroused the chaplain's natural forces as to enable him to expel the lethal humor from his fever-racked body? Gurus then having recently come into vogue, it flashed across my consciousness that what I was hearing was the unconventional Coffin's personal pronunciation of some Hindu title. Then I remembered. Bizzozero was no guru—he was the intern

The Hippocratic physicians understood things that we are only now, millennia later, beginning to study and quantify.

on the case, a dedicated, talented, and extremely compassionate young man who had spent countless hours at his patient's bedside, now adjusting this therapeutic modality, now titrating that one, and modifying the others as needed; in short, doing everything that a devoted physician could to bring his patient out of the valley of the shadow. Most evenings, when things quieted down a bit, they had long talks, this embryonic doctor and his dreadfully sick charge. In time the talks and Dr. Bizzozero's scrupulous care (and caring) began to fill Bill Coffin's chest with the medicine it needed most, the radiant insight that, to at least one of his medical attendants, the real challenge was to restore health to a human being, and not merely to cure an interesting disease that happened to reside in someone's body. To die would have been unfair to a doctor who gave so much of himself. And so Joe Bizzozero brought about a miracle where the rest of us were failing. He was able to do it because he knew, better than his teachers did, what it means to be a healer. As his now vibrantly healthy patient said to me on that celebratory evening, "I did it for Bizzozero; I couldn't let him down."

The marriage that had occasioned my reunion with Bill Coffin lasted only a few years. The lesson I learned during the reception will be with me all of my life. The Hippocratic physicians understood things that we are only now, millennia later, beginning to study and quantify. After a century of pursuing single causes to explain single diseases, even the laboratory scientists are beginning to reach for new explanations and new factors. We will discover that it takes more than the pneumococcus to produce pneumonia, and more than cigarettes to make a lung cancer. When we have learned how to frame the ultimate questions, their answers will be found in a model of disease that requires not one but many conditions to be fulfilled before sickness can occur. Most of the chapters of this book tell the story of medicine's search for specificity of diagnosis and of treatment, of the coning-down on causes that was an essential step in the conquest of medical ignorance. The chapter that cannot yet be written will tell of the next step. That achievement will prove to be the formulation of a construct that philosophers of science are beginning to call a new paradigm, in which disease is recognized as being due to the combination of entire sets of disordered function, and it is well within the range of probability that some of them will be found in the mind.

Thus, now near the end of the twentieth century, we seem to be readying ourselves for yet another phase in the old struggle between Cnidian and Coan, a phase of rapprochement in which the two systems may prove to be quite compatible. Both in the maintenance of health and in the treatment of disease, the ancient antagonists are proving to be mutually supportive. More and more, there is less and less to fight about. The whole patient, and every one of his cells, will be the better for it.

Doctors who have been accused of not paying enough attention to the emotional needs of their patients can take heart from the knowledge that this particular charge has been leveled at members of their profession since the days of Hippocrates. Perhaps professional impersonal-ity is particularly characteristic of the technological era in which we now live, but the coolness of some doctors was as much discussed on the pathways near Cos as it is in the condominiums of New York. It was his emphasis on prognostication that was the main basis for criticism of the Greek physician. Even in retrospect today, he is seen by some, usually nonmedical, historians as being not much more than an observer and a minute-taker of Nature's behavior. Critics of this persuasion claim that he was more interested in the progress of the disease than he was in the recovery of his patient. That accusation implies a certain callousness to the plight of a suffering fellow creature. That there is no justification for such a charge is easily demonstrated by a careful reading of the major treatises in the Corpus, and by even the most superficial acquaintance with the famous Oath of Hippocrates.

The fact remains, nonetheless, that for many of his patients the Hippocratic physician had but little therapy to offer beyond searching for hopeful signs or confirming the reality that they must make their peace with the gods and their earthly intimates. The healer's ability to make reasonably accurate predictions by recognizing prognostic factors arose out of his highly developed knowledge of the course of disease. The more he observed and the more he recorded, the greater grew his understanding, and the greater became his ability to intervene in those situations in which he could be of some help. The help that can be given by a physician comes in many forms, ranging from the placebo of psychological support to the actual intervention of physical methods. Of the latter, the doctors of ancient Greece had a few that they depended upon.

Some of those Hippocratic remedies became staples in the medical storehouse that would not be replaced for almost twenty-five hundred years. They included purgatives, emetics, baths, fomentations, bloodletting, wine, bland drinks, and a calm atmosphere. Obviously, the purpose of much of this battery of available treatments was to aid Nature in her attempts to rid the body of excessive humors. Except for the addition of botanicals and a few drugs, the authors of the Corpus could easily have been describing the medical arsenal of an early-nineteenth-century physician in Paris or Philadelphia—which says as much about the great and lasting contributions of the Greek physicians as it does about the inhibiting effect the misinterpretations of their successors exerted on the advancement of true science until relatively recent times.

The Hippocratic philosophy of objective evidence had its greatest test in the realm of surgery. Theories are fine so long as diseases arise in invisible internal organs and exert their major influences through the silent streaming of the circulation. When the problem is right there on the outside of the body where everyone can see it, the situation demands a cure that is equally visible and unquestionably successful. Surgical methods have to work, or their failings, as well as those of their proponents, are quickly discovered. Particularly was this true in ancient times, when all operations were done on the body's surface. It is in the area of surgery that the Hippocratic physicians left the tranquil meadows of philosophy and entered the harsh arena of direct confrontation.

They often won. Above all else, the Greeks were practitioners who knew the value of what could be learned from experience, and they did

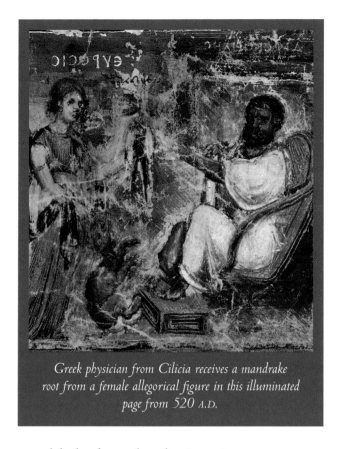

Greek physician from Cilicia receives a mandrake root from a female allegorical figure in this illuminated page from 520 A.D.

not delude themselves by ignoring a poor outcome. They developed a useful body of technical expertise that was much less subject to distortion by later generations than was their strictly medical treatment. To the modern reader there is nothing recondite to be found in any of the Hippocratic surgical teachings. The recommendations, clear and useful, were obviously made by practitioners of considerable skill and wisdom.

As may be imagined, the Greeks treated a great deal of trauma. They understood the principles of setting and splinting fractures, and they knew the necessity of sawing off the projecting bone ends when the fractures were compound. They drained blood and pus from the chest, and they were skillful at the removal of fluid from the abdomen. Liver and kidney abscesses were vented, and rectal diseases like hemorrhoids and fistula had a high rate of cure, through the use of principles that to this day underlie the successful treatment of two ailments whose miseries are only fully appreciated by those unfortunates who have been afflicted with them. Who knows—it may have been the successful Hippocratic treatment of his sore anus that motivated a grateful Soranus to write that adulatory biography.

The Hippocratics were particularly successful in the treatment of head wounds. They had sensible rules to determine which sorts of injuries required trepanning, or perforation of the skull. They well understood the implications of pressure on the brain if it was allowed to go unrelieved, and, unlike the Egyptians who preceded them, they favored early operation on the skull when closed head wounds seemed serious. Here again, they knew how to predict outcome.

The surgical writings are sprinkled throughout with sound advice about the necessity for developing great skill in the use of the hands. The modern surgeon, who is certain that meticulous operating-room technique is a phenomenon of the twentieth century, does well to note the value placed by his Hippocratic forebears on craftsmanship and manual dexterity. They recognized, as does every intern, that these are not God-given gifts, but can only be acquired by diligent practice and endless striving toward the ultimately unattainable goal of perfection. A director of surgical training in one of our great university hospitals would be hard put to improve on the counsel offered by Hippocrates two and a half millennia ago:

Practice all the operations, performing them with each hand and both together—for they are both alike—your object being to attain ability, grace, speed, painlessness, elegance, and readiness.

There are certain characteristics, even in the clinical writings, that elucidate a great deal of the Hippocratic philosophy. Scattered through some of the treatises, and densely interlarded into others, are the ethical *principia* of the Greek physician. We are dealing here with the real origins of Western medical ethics, which in our own day have emerged primarily from a mix of Judeo-Christian precepts, the teachings of the moral philosophers, and the heritage of the Hippocratic school. Each has given to the others and blended with them to the point where it is difficult to distinguish the primary sources of specific principles.

It is appropriate to question the basis of the Greek contribution. With the other two tributaries to the ethical stream there are such operative factors as the influence of monotheism, whose adherents strive to identify with an all-virtuous and loving God; there are the viewpoints of the philosophers, telling us, for example, that we exist as part of a whole, to each of whose constituents we owe the obligations of caring and charity. There do, therefore, seem to exist numerous examples of the ways in which religious and philosophical principles have entered the consciousness of the healers. But, with all due respect to those who believe in the innate goodness of man, the "why" of Greek medical ethics remains obscure. Why, exactly, did the Hippocratic physicians practice their art in a manner that not only was on an ethical level beyond reproach, but also served as a model for almost a hundred generations after them? What motivated their medical morality, and what motivated their concern for patients as individual fellow human beings? Why, when so many of the non-Hippocratics were self-serving charlatans, did the physicians of Cos preach the doctrine that one's duty to a patient transcends all other considerations? With no outside authorities to regulate them, why did they, in the pagan communities in which they traveled, comport themselves in a manner which we moderns associate with the highest levels of our own religious and philosophical beliefs? Looked at with the jaded eye of behavioral *Realpolitik*, what was the payoff?

There were really no societal or legal restraints on physicians during this period, nor any method of certification. The Greeks themselves were uncertain about how such a situation had come to pass, in which the doctors were beyond the authority of the greater society to penalize or punish. The Corpus describes this state of affairs in the short treatise called the *Law*, here presented in the Jones translation of the Loeb Classics:

> *Medicine is the most distinguished of all the arts, but through the ignorance of those who practise it, and of those who casually judge such practitioners, it is now of all the arts by far the least esteemed. The chief reason for this error seems to me to be this: medicine is the only art which our states have made subject to no penalty save that of dishonour, and dishonour does not wound those who are compacted of it. Such men in fact are very like the supernumeraries in tragedies. Just as these have the appearance, dress, and mask*

of an actor without being actors, so too with physicians; many are physicians by repute, very few are such in reality.

The classicist Ludwig Edelstein has put forth the proposition that the catalytic factor in the development of Greek medical ethics was a thoroughly practical one: a system of ethics set the Hippocratic physicians apart from those aforementioned charlatans with whom they were in competition. Thus their ethical code served the same function as the injunction to prognosticate. It was a proof to patients and families that this

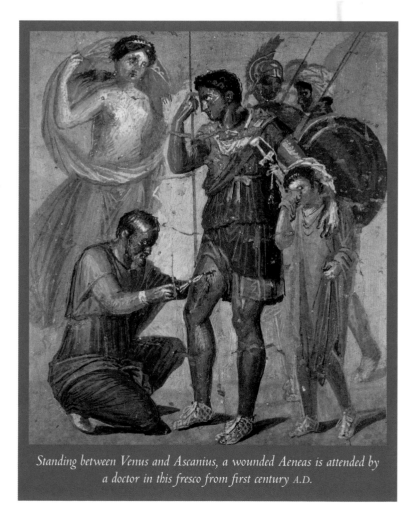

Standing between Venus and Ascanius, a wounded Aeneas is attended by a doctor in this fresco from first century A.D.

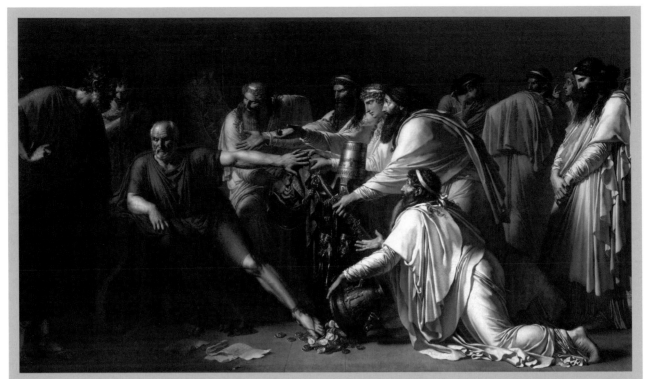

Hippocrates refusing the presents offered by the ruler Artaxerxes, because he was the enemy of the Greeks

doctor and his school typified a different order of healer than did the impostors who roamed the land in pursuit of the purses of the sick. In Edelstein's view, it was "an ethic of outward achievement rather than of inner intention."

Even accepting Edelstein's opinion that it was reputation and the enhancement of practice that were being sought, we can nevertheless note a magnificent by-product of the quest: the practitioners of Cos became careful observers and recorders of the processes of disease, sensitive therapeutists, accurate prognosticators, and the founders of a system of ethics that has been the hallmark of the art of healing ever since it first emerged from its pragmatic sources. This point is well put by the German historian Markwart Michler:

As much as this ethic may, in a strictly philosophical sense, still be far removed from a theoretical system of medical moral principles, it might yet be compared with that arete *which Aristotle later on assigns to the morally noble actions of the statesman. Such a* praxis kale *in a specifically medical guise increases its "help" and equates it with the words of the Oath, according to which the physician should order what is to the advantage of the patient; it makes it the nucleus of a moral philosophy which later on helped to establish the* humanitas *of the Greek physician.*

These are persuasive arguments, and no doubt valid ones. But the reality that Greek medical ethics arose against a background of pragmatic necessity does not in any way vitiate the proposition that high principles of morality were just as important a motivating force. One cannot read either the Hippocratic texts that concern therapy or those that deal with the conduct expected of the physician without recognizing a sense of justice, a sense of obligation, and a sense of personal decorum that is transmitted throughout. These writings deal with what are called deontological concepts, concepts that arise from a sense of duty and the obligatory doing of things because they are, quite simply, the right things to do. There is a moral law which is universally valid, and it is this moral law that pervades the philosophies of the Hippocratics.

Hippocrates thus becomes the ideal physician, and therefore the idealized physician. In every age, his principles have been looked to as the highest fulfillment of ethical medical behavior and intellectual purity. In western society he has taken on the aspect of an icon. Through him, healing is equated on the one hand with religion, and on the other with humanism—in his *Precepts* we read, "Where love of mankind is, there is also love of the Art."

Hippocratic ethics finds its fullest affirmation in the Oath. Laymen who have never heard the words of the Oath and doctors who have long since forgotten them are united in their certainty that all of the ills of modern medicine would undergo coction and lysis if only we would return to what they conceive to be its unambiguous code of virtue. Undeterred by their total ignorance of the contents of the acclaimed document, some of medicine's critics are nevertheless convinced that its lofty title must mean that it contains some all-embracing statement of ethical impeccability. Like all seekers after a lost perfection, they yearn for something that never was; the moral purity of

the ancient Oath-takers is about as lost, and as irretrievable, as the continent of Atlantis.

Nevertheless, the fact that this particular retrospectroscope is equipped with rose-colored lenses should not be taken to mean that there is no value in looking back at, and perhaps trying to reexamine, some of the simpler virtues of a simpler time. Consistent moral decency is not a goal any less worth pursuing merely for being beyond the reach of ordinary human behavior. The Greeks understood this, and they tried, as we try, to do what was expected of them. I suspect that in their everyday practices, they were neither more nor less successful at it than we are.

The Oath divides itself into two sections, one of which may be called the covenant and the other the ethical code. As with all ancient writings, scholars have debated the origins, interpretations, and intentions of each of the parts, and will probably continue to do so until civilization's last classicist shuffles off this mortal coil. Some view it as a product of the ascetic moralism of the Pythagorean sect, while others credit that group with much less influence, or even none at all. An element of confusion is added also by the fact that certain of the Oath's prohibitions, such as those against abortion, cutting for stone, and aiding a suicide, fly in the face not only of the usual medical practices of the time, but specifically of those in which some of the Hippocratics are known to have engaged. In addition, the Oath contradicts, in the area of surgery, certain passages that appear in other sections of the Corpus. The only way to deal with the disputes in a work of the present kind is to avoid them, which I will try to accomplish by the simple stratagem of taking the text at face value. Since none of the authorities seem to have irrefutable proof concerning a single one of the disputed issues, what follows is less a digest than an attempt to present a point of view.

The first section of the Oath deals with the ground rules of a professional society. There is nothing so awe-inspiring to the beginning medical student of today as the realization that, from the very first day of classes, his senior professors have begun to look on him as a colleague with whom is to be shared a huge mass of knowledge that is technological and scientific at the same time that it is philosophical and subjective. The opening paragraph of the Oath is a statement of the obligation, willingly accepted by all members of the profession, to share that knowledge with one another and to impart it to succeeding generations of those most qualified to receive it. The teaching of medicine was, and is, considered to be a principal duty of the physician.

THE OATH OF HIPPOCRATES

I swear by Apollo the physician, and Aesculapius, Hygeia and Panacea and all the gods and goddesses, that, according to my ability and judgement, I will keep this Oath and this covenant:

To reckon him who taught me this Art equally dear to me as my parents, to share my substance with him, and relieve his necessities if required; to look upon his offspring on the same footing as my own brothers, and to teach them this Art, if they shall wish to learn it, without fee or stipulation; and that by precept, lecture, and every other mode of instruction, I will impart a knowledge of the Art to my own sons, and those of my teachers, and to disciples who have signed the covenant and have taken an oath according to the law of medicine, but no one else.

I will follow that system of regimen which, according to my ability and judgment, I consider for the benefit of my patients, and abstain from whatever is deleterious and mischievous.

I will give no deadly medicine to anyone if asked, nor suggest any such counsel; and in like manner I will not give to a woman an abortive remedy. With purity and with holiness I will pass my life and practise my Art.

I will not cut persons labouring under the stone, but will leave this to be done by such men as are practitioners of this work.

Into whatever houses I enter, I will go into them for the benefit of the sick, and will abstain from every voluntary act of mischief and corruption; and, further, from the seduction of females or males, of freemen and slaves.

Whatever, in connection with my professional practice, or not in connection with it, I see or hear, in the life of men, which ought not to be spoken of abroad, I will not divulge, as reckoning that all such should be kept secret.

While I continue to keep this Oath unviolated, may it be granted to me to enjoy life and practice of the Art, respected by all men, in all times. But should I trespass and violate this Oath, may the reverse be my lot.

The second portion of the Oath is actually no more than a capsulized form of the ethical doctrines that permeate the entire Corpus. Although the Hippocratic works contain several treatises devoted specifically to the behavior expected of a physician (*The Law, On Decorum, The Physician,* and *Precepts*), students were required to take the Hippocratic Oath as an avowal of the entire credo that was elsewhere sprinkled throughout the textual material. Whether this took place at the beginning of medical education or at the time of completion of formal studies is debated, but what is important is that one was not permitted to treat patients until Apollo had heard the promise sworn to him.

It is important to note that though it invokes Apollo and the Aesculapian family, the Oath is not a religious statement; it is meant specifically to be a pledge of trust rather than a priestly document. Although the first and last sentences are the product of Greek religious or mystical belief, the gods are not invoked as agents of disease etiology or treatment, either here or anywhere else in the Corpus. The separation of science from religion is complete.

The Oath's prohibition against abortion has given rise to much scholarly speculation. It is well known that abortion was common among the Greeks, and was in fact viewed by some, including Plato and Aristotle, as a desirable option in an ideal state. Given this attitude, there still remained the question of how late in pregnancy the procedure could safely be accomplished and still avoid the possibility of killing a conceptus that was already a human being.

Those who expect that such a perpetual moral dilemma will be solved by late twentieth-century philosophy, science, or goodwill are well advised to review the social history of ancient Greece. The arguments will be familiar. Aristotle favored abortion before animal life commences, but even modern neonatologists have been unable to resolve that sticky issue, with respect to either the word "animal" or the word "life." The Platonists and the Stoics held that the auspicious instant was the moment of birth, but the Pythagoreans placed it at the moment of conception. Given the Pythagorean viewpoint, all abortion should be forbidden, which is the doctrine expressed in the Oath. That doctrine placed the Hippocratics in the minority of informed opinion. Why, in view of their general sense of obligation to the well-being of those who came to them for help, would Hippocratic physicians refuse to terminate a pregnancy?

The reason, I think, is to be found in the implied general principle of *Primum non nocere* which guided their treatment. They were not interventionists, but rather facilitators of the will of Nature. Abortion, in those pre-antisepsis days, must surely have had an unacceptable rate of complications and a significant mortality. Risking injury to a healthy person was not the Hippocratic

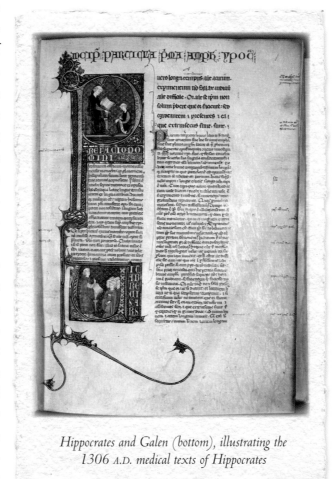

Hippocrates and Galen (bottom), illustrating the 1306 A.D. medical texts of Hippocrates

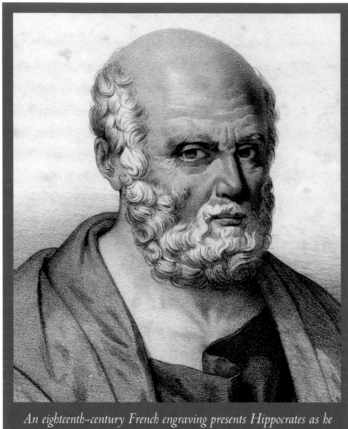

An eighteenth-century French engraving presents Hippocrates as he has traditionally been portrayed through the ages. Though based on scant evidence, this is the universally accepted image.

suffering. Why, then, did the Hippocratic physician dissociate himself from it? Very likely, the answer is again to be found in the same two basic considerations. From the pragmatic viewpoint, suicide meant a failure of treatment, and from the moral viewpoint, it meant a deliberate destruction of human life. Neither was considered an appropriate basis of action, regardless of the agony and despair endured by the suffering patient.

These arguments apply equally well to the proscription against "cutting for stone." Later commentators have recorded horrifying descriptions of the brutal methods required in those far-off times to extract bladder stones through holes cut and torn between the spread legs of shrieking sufferers, their torments diminished but barely by the ingestion of poppy or mandrake. Many patients died, some postoperatively and some during the most agonizing moments of those savage surgical assaults.

Others were left with permanent draining fistulas that constantly leaked infected and foul-smelling urine. These were not operations that fell within the ethical province of the Hippocratic physician. They were best left to "such men as are practitioners of this work," a group of itinerant craftsmen who were specialists in this particular form of necessary medical mayhem.

The disciples of Hippocrates were not reticent about calling for help when it was needed, either from such surgical artisans as the stone-cutters or from their fellow physicians. In fact, the very nature of the professional brotherhood celebrated by the Oath encouraged consultation and fra-

way. A woman who died as the result of an abortion was a woman who had been killed; such an outcome not only was morally reprehensible but devastated the reputation that meant so much to the Hippocratic physician. Abortion was a form of risk-taking that violated his principles of morality and his principles of pragmatism both, the two predominant concerns of the Father of Medicine.

It is difficult to know why the Hippocratics would not help patients take their own lives. Here again, the general attitude of Greek society was a liberal one; suicide, usually by poison, was an accepted solution to painful illness and desperate

ternal discussion of cases, as did the words of the Corpus: "When a physician is uncertain as to the condition of a patient and is disturbed by the novelty of an affection that he has never seen before, he should never be ashamed to call in other physicians to examine the patient with him."

The Oath reaches the pinnacle of its philosophy of personal medical morality in the paragraphs dealing with the obligations of physicians not to take advantage of the privileged position in which their calling places them. Sexual restraint and the maintenance of patient confidentiality are enjoined as forcefully upon the novitiates as are the responsibilities to treat and to teach. A corollary statement about demeanor is to be found in the text of *The Physician:*

Touching his state of mind, he must be heedful of the following. He must not only know how to be silent at the right time, but must lead a well-ordered life, for this adds much to his good repute. Let his disposition be that of a man of honour and as such let him behave to all honourable men in a friendly and easy spirit. Precipitation and impetuosity are not liked even though they be of use. As to his bearing, let him wear an expression of sympathy and not show vexation, which would indicate presumption and misanthropy. Who, on the other hand, laughs readily and is at all times merry, becomes a burden, whence this is particularly to be avoided.

The cultural theorists of psychoanalysis tell us that the origins of religious beliefs are intertwined with the practice of totemism. The members of a primitive society, according to this formulation, find an inspiring figure to lead them out of the morass of ignorance, or slavery, or fear. The tribesmen then invest this leader with the qualities of a god-king. Once he is thus enshrined or enthroned, some (usually young) members of the society do their best to destroy him, in order to succeed to his power. The destruction having been accomplished, the dead leader is elevated to the position of supreme deity of the cult. Myths are created concerning his life, a scripture may be attributed to him, and the glow of immortality surrounds his memory. He is worshipped as the epitome of tribal values. The tradition of the totem may become so shrouded in legend that the original man may not have been a leader at all, but only a chance figure upon whom the entire mythology is focused. The followers of Moses and Jesus, no less than the pagan members of wilderness cults, are said by the Freudian formulators to have passed through these steps in the early stages of the evolution of their religions.

In certain ways, this is reminiscent of the way in which Hippocrates has been treated by the ages. The only major ingredient missing is the murder. Hippocrates is our medical totem. As has been said of the founders of other religions, it makes little difference, from the practical point of view, whether or not he ever lived; it is of scant consequence whether the doings and the writings attributed to him are authentically his. We worship not the man, but the quality of his heritage and the philosophical influence it has had upon succeeding generations. A culture that sets its moral course by the Ten Commandments is thus at one with a culture that lives by the words of the Father of Medicine:

With purity and with holiness I will pass my life and practise my Art.

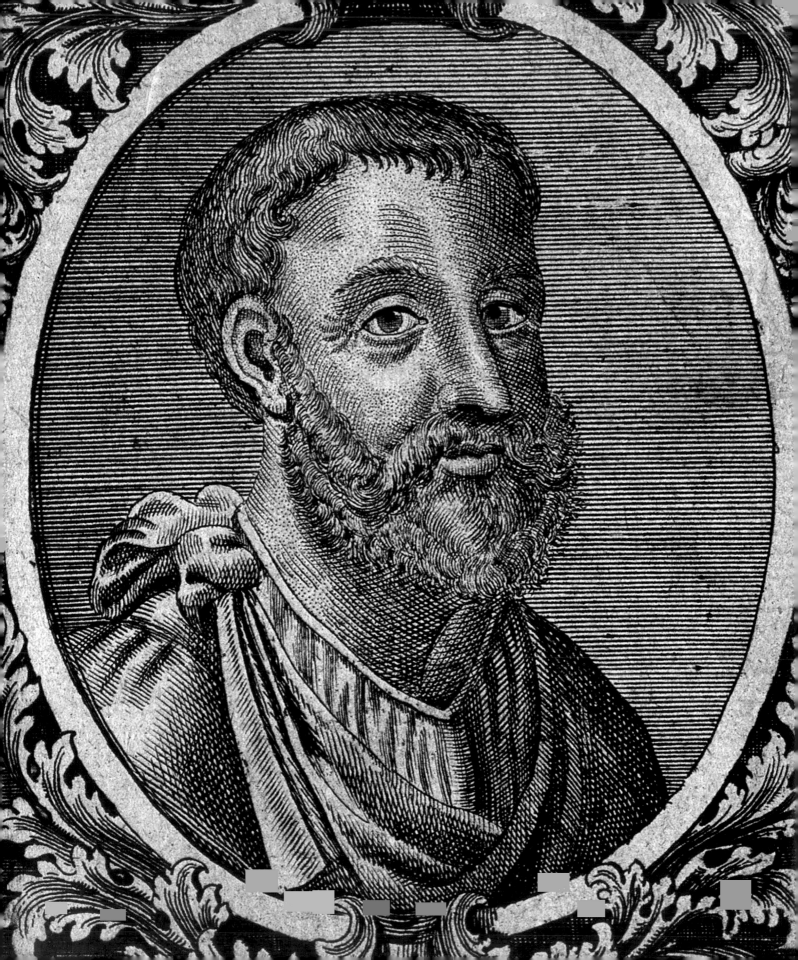

2

THE PARADOX OF PERGAMON

Galen

All nature is but art, unknown to thee;
All chance, direction, which thou canst not see;
All discord, harmony not understood;
All partial evil, universal good;
And, spite of pride, in erring reason's spite,
One truth is clear: Whatever IS, is RIGHT.

—Alexander Pope, *Essay on Man*

When he wrote these couplets in 1734, Alexander Pope was giving voice to the doctrine of predeterminism, which had formed the basis of medical thinking for fifteen hundred years. To the skeptical mind of the modern scientist, the belief that all is preordained to serve some greater good is an unthinkable proposition. That it should have endured so long without being overthrown by the forces of rationalism seems, in retrospect, beyond comprehension. And yet, at the very time when the English poet was composing his masterpiece, the mighty struggle which would separate medicine once and for all from the master-plan philosophy that had been its keystone since the days of the Roman Empire had barely begun. That

the doctors of the Middle Ages and Renaissance were educated to affirm a dogma so inimical to scientific progress was the intellectual heritage of one man: the second-century Greek physician Galen of Pergamon.

Galen's theology-biology was made up of a series of contradictions, and so was his life. His career was one long exercise in inconsistency: his trust in a supernatural Creator belied his unbiased contributions as a researcher; his often odious personal deportment made a mockery of his self-proclaimed philosophic serenity; he was at once the originator of the experimental method in medical investigation and the obstructing force that inhibited its further development for a millennium and a half after his death; to him we owe the origin of modern medicine's appreciation of anatomical accuracy as the foundation for the understanding of disease, and upon his abiding influence must be cast the onus of impeding research in anatomy until the sixteenth century; he was the ancient world's most eloquent proponent of direct observation and planned experiment, and yet he allowed philosophical and theological conjecture to influence his interpretation of what he saw. He was medicine's best influence, and he was its worst.

Students of ancient science and philosophy will recognize in this description of Galen some of the elements of the thinking of the classical period. Like Aristotle, to whose investigative reasoning methods his have been compared, Galen sometimes made brilliant observations only to draw faulty conclusions from them. But in the case of Galen, the problem was more disabling. His inconsistencies loom so large that he emerges not only as the strongest of the many physician influences on medical history in its twenty-five-hundred-year evolution, but as its greatest paradox as well.

Because the words "God," "Creator," and "Nature" occur so often in Galen's writings, it is necessary to understand what he meant by them. He did, after all, live during the earliest period of Christianity's development, and he was familiar enough with the new religion to know the charac-

Like Aristotle, to whose investigative reasoning methods his have been compared, Galen sometimes made brilliant observations only to draw faulty conclusions from them.

teristics with which both it and Judaism endowed the Supreme Being they mutually worshipped; in several of his books he took great pains to distinguish his own beliefs from those of the Judeo-Christian formulation. His theistic concepts arose out of a different tradition, one in which uncritical faith was seen as a hindrance to the discovery of truth. His was the tradition of Socrates, of Plato, and of Aristotle. It was the same tradition that had enabled the Hippocratic physicians to break away from the mystical theories and cures of the cult of Aesculapius and to abandon a pagan trust in deities-by-the-dozen. It was a tradition that cherished no belief in miracles or in divine revelation. It was therefore a tradition which, in its very nature, stood opposed to Jewish and Christian theology.

The one doctrine held in common by all three heritages was the belief in a Supreme Being. It was in their differing conceptions of the characteristics of that Being that they parted theological company. To the Jews and Christians of the second century, God created the world, its botany, and its zoology out of nothing. Having done so, He continued to make fine adjustments to the product of His creativity by performing periodic miracles of various magnitudes. He spoke to His creatures, He parted waters, He cured the incurable, He inflicted scourges on those who rejected His Word or harmed His Chosen, and He sent a Messiah to heal the moral ills of mankind or, according to the Jews, at least promised that He would one day do so. That these events had taken or would take place was not to be questioned, was accepted through a purity of faith that rejected any possibility of the facts being eventually proved to be not facts at all but simply misunderstandings or myths. Accepted also by the faithful was the certainty of the resurrection of the dead from the putrefaction and dust of the grave.

This last was, of all the attributes of Judeo-Christian belief, the one least palatable to the Greek—and therefore Roman—mind. Aulus Cornelius Celsus, a first-century Roman medical compiler, summarizes the classical pagan opinion of this sort of thing:

> For what sort of body, having once been completely destroyed, can return to its previous nature and to that very structure from which it has been released? Having no reply to offer, they take refuge in the ridiculous position that everything is possible for God. But God is not capable of anything ignoble nor does He will things contrary to nature; nor, if one in his wickedness desires what is disgusting, will God be able to produce it, and one ought not to believe that it will happen instantly.

It is the "everything is possible for God" that the Greeks disputed. Their philosophers had to a great extent replaced the primacy of the multiple gods of an earlier time with that of a single Supreme Being, but not one with the unlimited power of a Jehovah. He could not create matter from nothingness, nor could He act contrary to the never-changing laws of Nature. The world of Aristotle and Galen was a world in which events are determined by natural laws unbreakable even by the Deity. It became, in this view, the duty of

the pious to discover those laws by use of their own critical faculties, and to accept nothing on faith. Uncritical faith, the basis of Jewish and Christian orthodoxy, was to Galen the enemy of true knowledge; a belief in divine revelation was seen as an opacity between intellect and truth. The proper way to worship the Creator was therefore not with prayer and sacrifice but with experiment and observation, in order to know His ways and to bring His perfection to all things. In his greatest extant anatomical work, *De Usu Partium*, Galen described his text as "the sacred discourse which I am composing as a true hymn of praise to our Creator." He continued:

> And I consider that I am really showing Him reverence, not when I offer Him unnumbered hecatombs of bulls and burn incense of cassia worth ten thousand talents, but when I myself first learn to know His wisdom, power, and goodness and then make them known to others. . . . To have discovered how everything should best be ordered is the height of wisdom, and to have accomplished His will in all things is proof of His invincible power.

The Hippocratic physicians had rejected supernatural forces in order to learn the ways of Nature; Galen studied Nature in order to learn the great and perfect ways of his Creator. Neither metaphysics nor miracles had any role to play. It was a credo worthy of a modern scientist.

Obviously, Galen's thesis did not go unchallenged. Jewish writers in particular attempted to refute him, especially since several of his statements are attacks on the Creation story and the Pentateuch of Moses, according to which God's power is limitless. His most eloquent critic, however, was not to be heard from until a thousand years later, when the greatest of Judaic physician-philosophers,

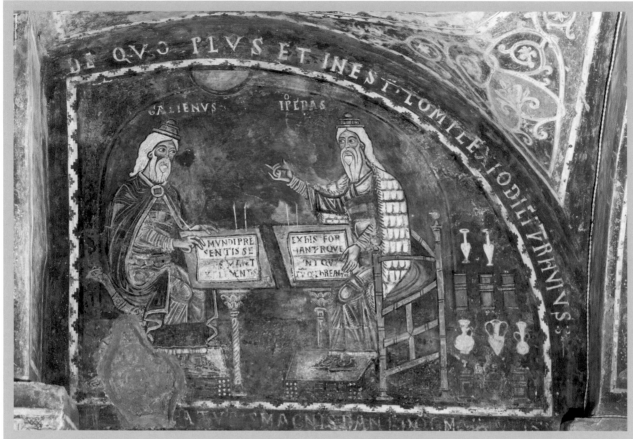

Hippocrates and Galen in thirteenth-century fresco

Maimonides, who revered Galen as his principal source of medical knowledge even as he deplored his theology, addressed the problem in his *Aphorisms in Medicine.* Declaring that God *is* almighty—that is, able to act against the laws of Nature—Maimonides asked only that any perplexed doubter accept but a single miracle that he has witnessed, for if even one such has occurred, it must follow that God can perform every kind. In the words of the Hebrew sage, "The perception of one miracle on the part of him who perceives it is a stringent proof of the creation of the world."

According to Maimonides, God's power is limited only by His inability to do evil. Here the two theologies meet. The Greeks used the Platonic word "Demiurge," or "Craftsman," which we find in earlier English translations; but in this one sense the Supreme Being of Greeks, Christians, and Jews embodies that single characteristic which is the foundation stone of monotheism: God is goodness; we must learn His ways that we may be like Him. As pointed out by the Oxford medievalist Richard Walzer in his brief monograph *Galen on Jews and Christians,* this idea among the Greeks is traceable to Plato's *Timaeus,* in which the philosopher writes, "The Demiurge was good, and in the good no jealousy in any matter can ever arise. So being without jealousy He desires that all things should approach as much as possible to being like Himself." This was the God of Galen: on the one hand He was a stimulus to research that might demonstrate the perfection of His work, while on the other the belief that structure and function were created in perfection made further investigation unnecessary once the basic facts had been identified.

The first, the most lasting, and the most pervasive of Galen's contradictory contributions, then, was this: he used experiment and observation to learn about Nature, but he left a body of knowledge that he and his successors treated as a form of writ so conclusive that it inhibited further research for fifteen hundred years. For that period of time, to study medicine was to study Galen. His reverence for the dispassionate observational methods of Hippocrates served not only his methodology but his image as well. He sought to appear as the prime interpreter of the venerated Hippocratic writings, and in this he succeeded. He proudly boasted that he was the first of Hippocrates' successors to clarify the teachings of the Father of Medicine so that they could be made useful. He invoked the analogy of Trajan's paving of the military roads of the Roman Empire, which had originally been cut by the ancients: by improving the rough roads of the Hippocratic Corpus, he made them passable. That he was considered the intellectual heir to the physicians of Cos was due not only to a careful attention to objectivity in his studies, but to a self-promotion at which he was very skilled. He was legitimized by the value of his contributions, but also by the general acknowledgment of succeeding generations that he was the vector of the Hippocratic philosophy.

After the golden period of Greece, the solid body of Hippocratic teachings had begun to diverge in several different directions, each based upon one form or another of speculative thinking. The result was the gradual emergence of a group of medical-philosophical sects in a continuous state of conflict with each other. Except that each group retained the rejection of mysticism, the rational tradition of Cos began to fade even as the reputation of Hippocrates as a healer increased with the passage of time. The various sects created systems based more on conjecture than reality. Theory replaced experience; with a few notable exceptions, the accurate descriptions of the Hippocratics gave way to surmise, guesswork, and unsupported inference. In time, the only dictum of Hippocrates that continued to be honored by other than lip service was the injunction against supernatural causes, but even those ancient crutches eventually reclaimed some of their old fantastical fascination.

As the Roman Empire grew, so did the theoretical edifices of the various schools. By the middle of the second century A.D., any young man starting out on his medical education was confronted by a bewildering array of doctrines. Perhaps the example of the diversified Greek philosophies—Stoic, Neoplatonic, Pythagorean, Peripatetic, Epicurean—served as a model for the variegated schools of physicians—Dogmatic, Methodist, Empiric, Pneumatic, and Eclectic. Their internecine and quite public disputes were magnified by the increasingly labyrinthine constructs they formulated to bolster their respective positions. The stage was set for the entrance of a logical thinker, to extract what was true from each system so that he might lead medicine back to the path of direct observation. That was to be the role played by Galen.

There is no better summation of Galen's contribution to the history of medicine than the one given to me in the offhand remark made by a colleague shortly before this book began to take form. "Galen," he said, "really started the whole thing, didn't he?" Galen introduced physicians to the anatomical concept of disease, the intellectual system guided by the doctrine that a detailed knowledge of the body's structure is the foundation upon which understanding of disease must be based. Until very recently all progress made in medical science has been the result of an increasingly clear comprehension of man's structure and the manner in which each part functions in health and disease.

The appeal of capsulizing Galen's contribution by the expression "he really started the whole thing" rests on a consideration of just what it was that he started. It is this principle: the sick can be properly treated only if physicians understand how the body works and the ways in which disease disturbs it. To know those normal workings physicians require a detailed knowledge of structure, which we call anatomy, and of the function of all parts, which we call physiology.

To moderns, such principles are so self-evident that it seems inconceivable that they have not always been understood and accepted. The same may be said of the circulation of the blood, the pumping action of the heart, and the fact that we think with our brains. These too are so easily proved that we cannot imagine a time when intelligent men and women did not know about them. But the way in which disease is understood in any society is an expression of that society's culture,

and not its intelligence. Modern western man prefers to explain natural phenomena by the method of science, which involves not only observation but experiment, recording of data, and a devout refusal to admit any evidence not verifiable by the five senses. The development of the scientific method has been a process of twenty-five hundred years, and medicine entered it full-force only when Galen began to write.

To the medicine of Galen's predecessors, a knowledge of anatomy, except in the most general sense, was superfluous. He recognized the absurdity of persisting in such a misguided state of ignorance, and he devoted his life to dissecting, experimenting, and demonstrating the form and function that he considered to be the perfection of God's work. Believing, like Aristotle, that "Nature makes nothing in vain," he desired to prove that each structure has a specific function, the need for which is the reason the structure exists. Thus, of all of his many writings, the most renowned is the book *De Usu Partium,* or *The Uses of the Parts of the Body*. Conceived to demonstrate how God, in the words of *De Usu Partium,* "has shown His goodness in providing wisely for the happiness of all His creatures," Galen's researches into anatomy and physiology pointed the way to a new understanding of the body and how it gets sick. Perhaps it is he, and not Hippocrates, who deserves to be called the Father of Medicine.

In the extreme northwest corner of Asia Minor, fifteen miles inland from the Aegean along the verdant valley of the Caicus River, lay the thriving city of Pergamon, a bustling little community of Greek culture and Roman law. At an earlier time Pergamon's library had so rivaled that of Alexandria that one of the Ptolemies had tried to hinder its growth by forbidding the export of papyrus. Deprived of it, the Pergamene scholars had turned instead to animal skin, which became known as *charta pergamena*, or *pergamentum*, from which derives our word "parchment." Although parchment was less suitable than papyrus for use in scrolls, it was found to be more adaptable to the structure of a codex, or book, a characteristic that led eventually to the development of that form. So, in the city of Pergamon, now a vestige in the Turkish town of Bergama, were born parchment, the book, and, in A.D. 130, Galen.

Although Pergamon itself was a particularly good example of a Hellenized community, the entire Roman world had by this time become so like it in that regard that a thorough familiarity with the Greek language, literature, and philosophy was indispensable to scholars and people of culture. It was customary to write all scientific works in Greek, for the practical reason that all science of the time was based on Hellenic thought, and Rome was permeated with an atmosphere of Hellenic cultural superiority, which Galen affirmed his whole life long. In later years he wrote, with his usual directness:

> *Would you then neglect the Grecian language, so very pleasant and so expressive of man's deepest feelings, a language, too, in which so much grace and beauty abound? Would you prefer to acquire your medium of expression from methods of speech that are as unsuitable as they are ugly? It were much better to learn one language, and that one the most perfect of all, than to acquire six hundred debased tongues. . . . You do not wish, Sir, to learn the language of the Hellenes, well, be a barbarian if you will!*

And so it was into a totally Grecian atmosphere that Galen was born on September 22, A.D. 130, the son of Nikon, a cultivated and highly successful architect and landowner. The boy's name was derived from the Greek word *galenos*, meaning calm and serene, qualities that, according to Galen himself, very well describe his father, but not his mother: "It was my good fortune to have a father who was perfectly calm, just, gallant, and devoted; my mother on the other hand was so irascible that she sometimes bit her maids. She was always babbling and quarreling with my

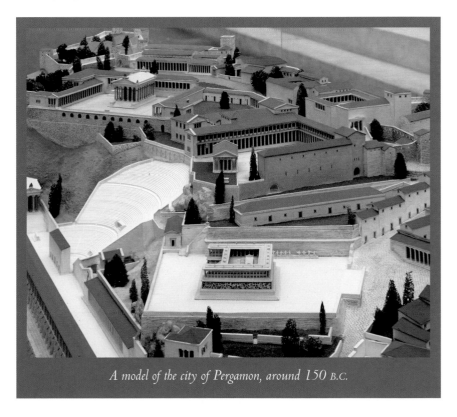

A model of the city of Pergamon, around 150 B.C.

father, as did Xanthippe with Socrates . . . and while he was not affected by the most serious, she choked with anger over the pettiest inconvenience." Sad to tell, it was not for the personality traits inherited from his father that Galen was to become known among his contemporaries, but rather for those that were the most obnoxious legacies of his mother.

Until his fourteenth year, Galen was educated in literature, grammar, arithmetic, geometry, and the rudiments of philosophy by Nikon, who taught him also the skills necessary for running the family's large and profitable farm. From age fifteen to eighteen he was sent by his father to study the separate philosophies of all the leading systems of the time. It was not Nikon's intention that his son choose one of the sects, but rather quite the opposite: he sought by this means to impress the boy with the importance of maintaining his independence from all of them. His father's advice was often quoted and never forgotten. Throughout his life, Galen avoided being identi-

fied with any one school of philosophy or medicine, choosing to go his own way and develop his own patterns.

Another lifelong practice also made its first appearance at this time, but this one was of a far less rational nature. Nikon, who had provided his son with such a superior education in order to prepare him for a career in the service of the empire, had an Aesculapius-inspired dream telling him to guide the boy into the study of medicine. He and Galen accepted the revelatory message, with the result that the youth shortly thereafter started his professional education. Thus begins a chronicle of the contradictions that were to mark Galen's life. When he was twenty-seven years old, a dream told him to open an artery in his hand to cure himself of an abdominal abscess; when he was thirty-eight, a dream told him not to go off to war with the Emperor Marcus Aurelius; when he was forty-three, a dream told him to complete an unfinished treatise on the structure and function of the eye. Throughout his career he would from

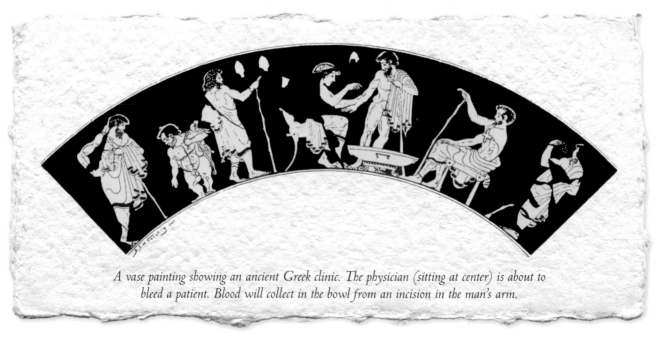

A vase painting showing an ancient Greek clinic. The physician (sitting at center) is about to bleed a patient. Blood will collect in the bowl from an incision in the man's arm.

time to time use treatments revealed to him during sleep. The repudiator of miracles never lost a childlike faith in the power of Aesculapius.

Pergamon was the site of one of the greatest of the god's shrines; perhaps neither Galen nor Nikon could have failed to become taken with its mysteries, despite Hippocrates' denial of them. There is evidence, in fact, that Galen looked upon the physician of Cos as himself having been elevated to the position of a god, whom he might one day meet in the eternal home of the immortals. This reverence probably never struck him as incompatible with his rejection of miracles. If he had thought he was being inconsistent, he would surely never have written so openly on both sides of the issue. Perhaps it is only post-Enlightenment westerners who are troubled by such incongruities, insisting upon a purity of allegiance to either atheism or faith, at least in others. Somehow it seems to be a standard to which most of us can only aspire.

Galen commenced his training in medicine at the age of seventeen. After he had studied four years in Pergamon, his father died, and he left home, perhaps to get away from his mother. He then attended lectures and demonstrations at other centers of medical learning, chiefly Smyrna and Corinth. In the year 152, he arrived at the great city of Alexandria, where he spent five especially valuable years.

Although in his experimental work Galen stands alone, his ability to discover and describe previously unknown anatomical structures put him in a tradition begun by Greek investigators during the golden years of Alexandria. Herophilus and Erasistratus, for example, had actually managed to dissect human cadavers in the third century B.C., and perhaps even some living condemned criminals. Unfortunately for the advancement of knowledge, the period of investigative freedom during which they were allowed to open dead bodies was all too brief, Roman law finally putting a premature end to it and forcing the few serious anatomists to return to the study of animals, with all of its inherent potential for error. Still, the results of those earlier researches were available at Alexandria, and Galen doubtless learned a great deal about human structure from them. Also available to him was the first full-scale anatomy text, a work in twenty books written in the first century by the Roman Marinus and now lost, to which Galen later made considerable reference, much of it surprisingly respectful.

After his first period at Pergamon, Galen had become very much the equivalent of the modern graduate student, attending courses even as he pursued his own beginning research and writing. He had worked with some of the leading physicians of his day, and benefited from the best medical education available, not only learning what little was then known of anatomy and physiology, but becoming expert in the theory and practice of the Hippocratic medical legacy, splintered though it was.

In the second century, theories of disease causation were still based, as they would be for centuries to come, upon the Coan factors of climate, diet, geographical location, occupation, temperament, and the effects of each on the balance of the four humors. The body of the patient was carefully inspected, as the Hippocratics had taught, and its various effluvia scrutinized. Therapies were somewhat more aggressive than they had been five centuries earlier, though there is no evidence that they were any more successful, and a large number of botanical and animal products had entered upon the therapeutic scene, which seem to have been prescribed with an enthusiasm that was not justified by any demonstration of their efficacy.

As to theory, the Greeks were vitalists—they believed that living creatures differ from inanimate objects because they are endowed with a spiritual essence that is the life principle. In various forms the concept of vitalism has persisted throughout the course of history, and even modern molecular biology is not yet completely done with it. In the Greek belief, there was an undefined, undescribed spirit in the world, having neither substance nor texture, to which was given the name *pneuma*. According to this system, we are surrounded by a world-pneuma, which, while it is not exactly air, is drawn into the lungs by breathing, whence it enters the left side of the heart and then passes into the arteries, whose pulsations are caused by its rhythmic dilatation; the arteries, being filled with the pneuma, were thought to be bloodless. Thus was life brought to the flesh of man. The blood, on the other hand, was believed to be carried only in the veins, to give nourishment of a more physical sort to all parts of the body. In the Greek formulation, the essential elements of the human body were the four humors created by the process of digestion, the innate heat produced in the heart, and the pneuma introduced from without.

By the time Galen returned to Pergamon in 158 he was not only a physician fully trained in this system but was already celebrated for a series of treatises he had written on anatomy and physiology. He was also, like the Hippocratics, equipped to practice surgery.

During his twelve years of training he had learned to treat fractures and dislocations, and to deal with head injuries by the technique of trephination, or venting, of the skull. Lacerations were stitched or strapped, torn vessels were tied with a ligature, and external cancers, cysts, and polyps were removed with the knife or the hot iron. Fluid was drained from the chest and abdomen, and various types of hernia incised and stitched; even bladder stones were commonly operated upon, the Hippocratic Oath and the screams of the victims notwithstanding.

Galen's skills and his good relations with the local Aesculapian cult served him well, for the high priest was authorized to select the surgeon to care for the gladiators of the city's coliseum, and he awarded the position to Galen, who carried out his duties so effectively that the appointment was renewed each year during the period he resided in the city. The post afforded the young physician an unmatched opportunity to study living anatomy and the ways in which function is altered by various types of injuries. As may be imagined, the ghastly open wounds sustained by some of the contestants provided a kind of human vivisection that would have been impossible under any other circumstances. The beating of the heart, the forceful pulsations of the major internal blood vessels, and the snaky undulations of the gut could be observed in animals, but to a physician trying to discover the secrets of man's body, there is no substitute for the real thing.

By the year 162, however, Galen had decided that he had accomplished all that he could in Pergamon; filled with a driving ambition and conscious, to a fault, of his considerable abilities, he yearned for a more suitable arena in which to expand his activities. When a war broke out between the Pergamenes and the neighboring Ga-

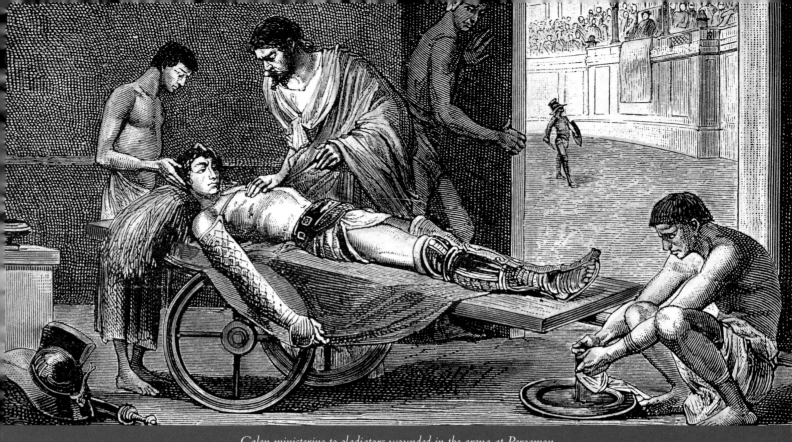

Galen ministering to gladiators wounded in the arena at Pergamon

latians, he pulled up stakes and moved to Rome. He began his career in the imperial city at the age of thirty-two.

Rome at that time was a magnificently prosperous metropolis of a million souls, whose medical needs were served by some two thousand healers of various persuasions. In addition to the five major sects—Dogmatic, Methodist, Empiric, Pneumatic, and Eclectic—there were subsidiary groups and mixtures of doctrine, some with unwieldy names such as Thessalon Methodists, Erasistratean Pneumatists, and Pneumatist Eclectics. There were also approximately 150 midwives, who not only delivered babies but functioned as physicians to women. Besides these, one hundred religious healers lived in the city. It is estimated that there were at least another hundred slave practitioners, who treated the minor illnesses of members of their owners' families. Interestingly, many of these were Jews captured after the unsuccessful Judean revolt led by Bar Kochba in 132.

Fortune smiled on Galen from the beginning. By a combination of circumstance and skill, he swiftly accomplished a few impressive diagnostic feats and soon found favor with members of the upper echelons of Roman society. His excellent education in literature and philosophy attracted the friendship of some of the leaders of those circles. The philosophers in particular welcomed him as one of their own. During his first two years in the city he gave public demonstrations in anatomy that proved popular beyond his expectation. These and his newly made connections brought him celebrity among both patients and those impressed by his research and pedagogical talents. But jealousy followed not far behind.

The medical community was divided not only by its sects, but also by widely different levels of learning and ability within each group. The competing physicians perpetrated vicious verbal assaults on each other, publicly ridiculing opponents in the most insulting terms. Galen made the double mistake of being both talented and arrogant about it. The greater his achievements, the more shrill became the derogations, and the more forceful in turn became his own denunciations of his adversaries and the sects to which they belonged. He boasted shamelessly of his successes and poured scorn, albeit often justified, on the heads of lesser men. It was a tasteless display, mitigated not at all by the inferior quality of many of his rivals.

Enemies appeared everywhere. Although Galen was lionized in the literary circles of Rome and adored by the moneyed elite who paid him high fees, his attacks on the various sects and their individual members eventually put him in some physical danger. In time, it became unsafe for him to remain in Rome. He left the city in haste and in secrecy, making his way back to Pergamon. It has been charged that Galen feared more than assassination—that the real reason for his flight was the rapid approach of a major epidemic of plague that was overrunning the eastern part of the empire. The charge is difficult to prove, since the disease seems already to have been well established by the time of Galen's departure. One thing, however, is certain. No honor accrues to the physician who deserts his post when epidemic is rampant. History has never forgiven Galen his getaway, even though his Roman patrons welcomed him with enthusiasm when he came back to the city a year later.

His return was occasioned by the invitation of the emperor himself, Marcus Aurelius. A campaign was being prepared against the hordes of the Marcomanni, who were threatening from the north, and the emperor "requested" the renowned physician to accompany his army. Galen, having no real choice in the matter, journeyed to meet the expedition in Aquileia during the winter of 168–69. However, the plague broke out anew and Marcus Aurelius was forced to return to Rome, taking Galen with him. It was during the time that the campaign was being reorganized that the physician had the Aesculapian dream mentioned earlier, it being revealed to him that he should stay behind. He managed to do this by taking on the care of the young heir apparent, Commodus, and on the death of the court physician shortly thereafter, he was appointed to that honored post.

Under the protection of the emperor, Galen no longer had need to fear the vendettas of his rivals, and from 169 until Marcus Aurelius died in 180, he accomplished some of the most significant of his researches. He had the freedom to pursue his scientific investigations and plenty of help in the preparation of his manuscripts. It is uncertain what relationships he had with subsequent emperors, but in each case it appears to have been one of trust. Although it has been verified that he lived until the year 201, the place of his death is unknown, as is the location, whether Rome or Pergamon, in which he spent his last years.

All through his long career, Galen played two quite different public roles. At times he spoke like a Socratic sage, describing the sublime selflessness of medicine and his ideal that the best physician is also a philosopher, a phrase which he used as the title of one of his short papers. His writings often refer to the wise guidance of his father, who told him, as did the dialogues of Plato, that "as desirable as are all the sciences, more desirable still are the virtues of wisdom, justice, fortitude, and temperance, virtues extolled by everyone, even those who have them not."

First among "those who have them not," however, was Galen himself. He was vain, petulant, contentious, impatient, and quick to take offense. Proclaiming the wisdom of emulating God, who is without jealousy, he was the most jealous of men.

In the uses of money and the pursuit of fame, he seems also to have used two standards, one expressed in his writings and another in his doings. Late in life he wrote:

The precepts learned from my father I have followed to this day. I profess no sect though I have studied all with the same industry and ardor, and like my father I dwell without fear as to the daily happenings of life. My father taught me to despise the opinion and esteem of others and to seek only the truth. . . . He insisted further that the primary end of personal possessions is to relieve hunger, thirst, and nakedness, and if more than sufficient remains it should be transmuted into good works.

He describes "sharing clothes with this one, giving nourishment and free medical care to another, and paying the debts of a third." In all, he presents the image of one who does not cultivate riches, preferring to live a scholarly variation of shabby gentility.

That a great deal of Galen's income went to pay copyists for the publication of his writings is undoubted, as is the fact that he spent considerable money on the purchase of books. Less is known of his charities, but there is no reason to doubt the statements he makes about them. However, it must be pointed out that Galen had throughout his life a quite substantial income, even if he did choose to lead a simple bachelor existence. High-

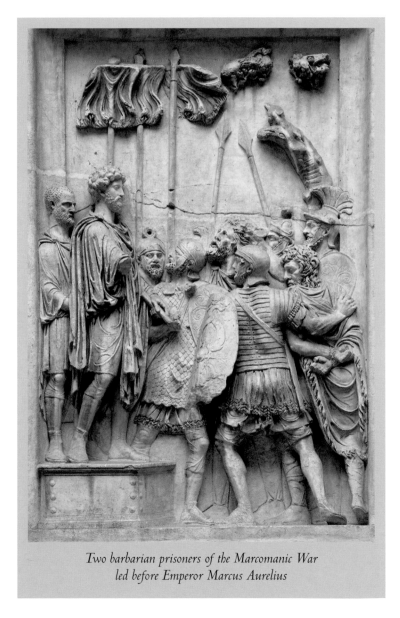

Two barbarian prisoners of the Marcomanic War led before Emperor Marcus Aurelius

flown declarations about the meaninglessness of money are easy to make when one has inherited from his father a sizable and productive farm, which yields lifelong revenue. Galen wrote that "It is impossible at the same time to engage in business, and to practice so great an Art" and criticized those who did so, but he enjoyed an inheritance, and in addition his practice was conducted largely among the grateful wealthy. Through the ages it has been observed by more than one cynic that the life of a philosopher is made less difficult by the assurance of a full belly.

As for being a man to "despise the opinion and esteem of others," the claim is outrageous. There is hardly a figure in the history of science whose writings are so filled with verbose self-promotion, self-righteousness, self-importance, self-congratulation, and just plain self as are Galen's. He was neither modest nor reticent in proclaiming his superiority over all rivals, in spite of his attempt to convey at some times a lofty disdain for honors and acclaim, and at others a philosophical detachment from such human frailties as the need for recognition.

Such criticisms, valid as they are, should not detract from the magnitude of Galen's accomplishments; after all, there is nothing about a deplorable personality that hinders the development alongside it of a beautiful clarity of intellect. This was the case with Galen of Pergamon. Competitive, arrogant, contentious, and often a hypocrite, he was gifted with an intellectual vision that enabled him to look directly at the phenomena of Nature and see truth where others constructed fantasy. By rejecting the dogmatic notions of the various sects of his day, he approached his observations unburdened by preconceptions. When his

doctrine emerged, it was one that would transform the heretofore philosophical approach to disease into the experimental. Hippocrates had introduced the healers to the concept that medicine is an art; Galen now taught them that it can be an art that is based upon the truths of science. The Hippocratic physicians had established dispassionate observation as the first rule of clinical medicine; Galen now applied it to research. That the rule was ignored after his death is perhaps the greatest of the Galenic paradoxes, in the sense that it was precisely because of his enduring posthumous influence over medical matters that free thinking and experimentation were inhibited for almost fifteen hundred years. When research was resuscitated in the sixteenth and seventeenth centuries, it was by those who forgot from whose gospel it had come.

The system that Galen developed was founded on the basis of dissections in anatomy, experiments in physiology, and clinical observation of patients. When he went wrong, he did so because he was a man of his time—a Greek to whom philosophical speculations and the application of logic were just as valid as unbiased observation. A scientist who believes that all structure and function are predetermined by a Supreme Intellect will not feel that he prejudices his conclusions by assuming a teleology—that is, by interpreting his observations as proof of a grand design in Nature. He does not consider himself inconsistent when he fills in the gaps between things which are known with things which are not, provided that the outcome reveals the reasoned plan of God. Nevertheless, paying homage to that plan, which Galen thought to be his great strength, proved to be his great weakness.

Galen was simply unable to recognize that when it came to explicating the structure and function of the human body, his reasoning powers were no replacement for his sense organs. To him, hypothesis was as valid as hard fact, conjecture as convincing as experiment. What he could not see, he imagined, and then wove his imaginings around the thesis of the superlative work of the Craftsman, whose every creation is perfect and whose creatures are endowed with life by the entrance of pneuma into their bodies.

Perhaps we should not criticize Galen too harshly for relying so heavily on speculation. Speculation is part of all science, particularly that endlessly fascinating compound of science and art we call medicine, in which our need to treat is often in advance of our ability to see. In modern research, we dignify speculation by calling it theory. In justice to our scientific colleagues, we should hasten to add that their theories are constructed on strong evidence, but that is only because eighteen hundred years have passed since Galen's day, and today's investigators have better ways of getting their evidence and more people to search for it. Viewed as theories based on the few facts that were then known, Galen's speculations become more forgivable. That does not, however, excuse such a gifted experimenter for wasting so much potential research effort by

> *Galen's greatness lay in the beautifully designed experiments that provided the data for each point; his failure lay in the scarcity of the points, the ways he joined them, and the ways he extrapolated from them.*

philosophizing. It is here that Galen and modern science take divergent paths. The investigator of today is in the main an experimenter and observer; a theory must force itself on him by an abundance of data. Galen was primarily a theoretician, whose scientific method erred in two ways. First, he approached his observations teleologically—that is, he invoked on them a sense that they fulfilled some grand purpose. Secondly, by making good observations but not enough of them, he often drifted off course, veering from the direction in which more experiments might have taken him. His process is comparable to attempting to draw a graph with too few proven points scattered diffusely along it, and with the further handicap of having decided beforehand what the graph is to look like. Galen's greatness lay in the beautifully designed experiments that provided the data for each point; his failure lay in the scarcity of the points, the ways he joined them, and the ways he extrapolated from them.

Stated another way, the modern scientist is fascinated by the minute details of his daily research findings, which eventually form a pattern that directs him inexorably toward a theory that he has reason to believe can be proved true. Galen, on the other hand, proceeded from a certainty that he already knew the final Truth—his research, no matter how objective-

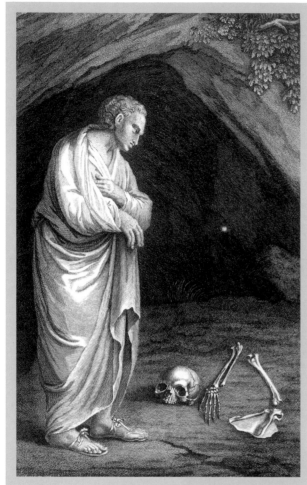

Galen studies a group of bones lying on the ground.

rotting remains taught him nothing. Of course, he did know a great deal about the human skeleton from his days in Alexandria, but beyond this, everything he learned came from his careful dissection of animals of all kinds, both living and dead. His favorite subject was the macaque monkey, very like a human being in appearance and just the right size to enable the studies to be completed before the corpse began to decompose in the often hot climate of southern Europe. He commonly killed his subjects by drowning, in order that the structures might remain undisturbed. Rather than leaving the skinning to an assistant, he did it himself, a practice which paid dividends when he discovered the flat platysmal muscles of the skin, which had eluded the few other dissectors of antiquity.

Galen proclaimed his credo in the second book of *De Usu Partium*, interlarded with his usual boasting:

> *Now let me once and for all make this general statement to apply to my whole treatise so as not to be forced to say the same thing repeatedly: I am now explaining the structures actually to be seen in dissection, and no one before me has done this with any accuracy. Hence, if anyone wishes to observe the works of Nature, he should put his trust not in books on anatomy but in his own eyes and either come to me, or consult one of my associates, or alone by himself industriously practice exercises in dissection; but so long as he only reads, he will be more likely to believe all the earlier anatomists because there are many of them.*

Ironically, when Galen's errors were exposed by Andreas Vesalius in 1543 and William Harvey in 1628, it was because they put their trust not in his books but in their own eyes. Each, "alone

ly each experiment was devised, was carried out in the service of that Truth, and its results were interpreted to confirm it.

Galen's work had another great weakness, but this was one of which he was to some extent aware—his anatomy was the anatomy of animals. Galen never saw a human dissection. On one occasion he came upon the corpse of a robber by the side of the road, most of the flesh stripped away by birds. Another time, he found a moldering body thrown up on a riverbank after a flood. The unsatisfactory viewing of those

by himself," industriously practiced exercises in dissection and experimentation until much of the edifice of Galenic medicine began to crumble.

But not all of it came down, not then or ever. When Galen followed his credo, he was an incomparable investigator; by precept and by example he might have been a fit mentor for young scientists of any era. Representative is his proof that the arteries contain blood, generally agreed to be the most important of his contributions to medical science. His predecessors believed that arteries served as the conduits only for the pneuma, which reached them from the left ventricle, having been inhaled and passed into that chamber by the large vessels entering the heart from the lungs, the pulmonary veins. The fact that a cut artery did indeed bleed was explained away by invoking a series of presumed but imaginary connections, or anastomoses, between venous and arterial vessels by which the blood poured into the latter from the former as soon as they were cut. Galen grounded this flight of fancy by an experiment in which he placed two ties around the artery of a living animal, isolating a segment of the vessel short enough that it could be shown to include no anastomoses from veins. When the artery was cut, the blood that was predictably found in it could only have been there before the incision was made.

He used ligatures also to show that arterial pulsations originate in the heart and are not, as his contemporaries thought, caused by rhythmic dilatations of the pneuma within them. By tying off a major artery in the leg of a dog he obliterated the pulse beyond it, even though the distant portion of the vessel was still filled with blood. When the ligature was removed, the pulse returned, which allowed him to reach the proper conclusion that arterial pulsation is transmitted from above, specifically from the heart.

To demonstrate that the heart, like the arteries, also contained more than pneuma, Galen inserted a fine-bore rigid tube through the wall of an animal's beating left ventricle and into its chamber, resulting in a pulsating spurt of red blood. At this point, however, the Greek philosopher in him could not resist the accustomed cogitations, which resulted in his thesis that the seemingly thinner brighter red substance in the left side of the heart and arteries is blood into which has been mixed the inhaled, life-giving pneuma. Noting that the wall of the left ventricle of the heart is always thicker than the right, he argued that this was necessary in order to maintain the central balance and vertical position of the organ, since the pneuma-filled contents of the left side are not as heavy as the dark, apparently more viscid blood of the right.

Galen's knowledge of the heartbeat came from his animal vivisections and from at least one experience he had in which the diseased breastbone of a child decayed away, allowing him a direct view of the heart's action. His conception of the circulation of the blood is too complex to discuss in a work of this nature, but essentially he thought of it as a soaking to-and-fro system of irrigation rather than a circular series of events in which the same liquid is purified, aerated, fortified, and repumped again and again. Since his theoretics required that the pneuma somehow find its way into the veins, he presupposed that there are po in the septum between the left and right ventri which allow the spiritual essence to pass int part of the bloodstream that brings nutriti the periphery of the body while blood pa the opposite direction, from right to left ventricle. William Harvey's proof, in 1628, that these pores do not exist became one of the most devastating brickbats thrown at the Greek physician's reputation by the researchers of the seventeenth and eighteenth centuries.

Galen's study of the role of the diaphragm and chest wall in respiration, however, was another masterful investigation: a series of ingenious experiments involving the cutting of various specific nerves and muscles, in order to discover the ways in which the movement of air was affected. As a result, Galen was the first to propose that it is the expansion of the cavity of the chest by the diaphragm and thoracic muscles that fills the lungs, rather than vice versa. An experiment he did to prove his thesis is illustrative of the sophistication of his methods, which were so in advance of their time as to match those of laboratory investigators of a much later period. He made a small incision between two ribs of an animal, around which he then snugly stitched the mouth of a bag or animal bladder after a bit of air had been allowed to enter the cavity of the chest. The bag could then be observed to fill and empty during expiration and inspiration respectively, demonstrating the partial vacuum created by expanding the chest cavity. It is this partial vacuum that sucks the outside air into the windpipe and lungs; that Galen was able to prove it speaks volumes for the clarity of his thinking in those situations when he chose not to obscure his interpretations with the obfuscating fog of philosophy.

In yet another brilliant experiment Galen refuted the commonly held belief that urine is produced not in the kidneys but in the bladder. Here too, he used the ligature wisely. He tied off the conduit between the two organs, the ureter, and pointed out that no matter where along its length he did so, the column of urine never could be shown to pass beyond the ligature. If he tied each ureter at its exit point from its kidney, both of them and the bladder remained empty, a plain confirmation that it is the kidney, and not the bladder, in which urine is made. Sometimes the simplest proofs are the most elegant.

There are many more such experimental examples in Galen's writings, cleverly designed and properly interpreted. Rather than attempt to catalogue his discoveries, I will confine the remaining discussion of them to his exemplary studies of the nervous system.

Here Galen's physiological experiments are models of precision and accuracy. Mention has already been made of his study of the mechanism of breathing: by cutting the phrenic nerve, which passes down from the neck to supply the diaphragm, he demonstrated the role of this structure in respiration; by destroying the nerve distribution to the muscles of the chest wall, he was able to identify the role played by those structures as well; by cutting the spinal cord at various levels in the upper back, he disabled successive segments of muscle, in order to investigate the coordinated effort required to expand the cavity of the thorax.

He noted that when an up-and-down incision is made along the central axis of the spinal cord, no paralysis ensues, since each side sends out its nerves independently of the other. On the other hand, cutting the cord transversely at any level results in paralysis of all muscles supplied by the nerves below the incision. If only one side is cut, the palsy is restricted to either left- or right-sided muscles.

Galen's experimental studies of the spinal cord were confirmed by clinical observations of injuries he treated in his practice. Since the nerve supply to the arms arises in the neck, trauma to cervical vertebrae served as an opportunity to learn about the effects of cord compression on the function of the arm as well as the diaphragm and the muscles below the injury.

None of these matters had been understood before Galen, nor had any such experimental methods been used. With similar techniques, he demonstrated again and again to any who responded to his oft-repeated invitation to "come and see for yourselves" that the voice originates not from the heart, as his contemporaries had been taught by studying Aristotle, but from the larynx, which is the uppermost portion of the trachea, or windpipe. He explained that the recurrent laryngeal nerves, which he discovered, activate the larynx to make it modify the rush of air expelled from the lungs in such a way as to cause its vocal cords to vibrate. Since the nerves originate in the brain, it is therefore the brain that controls speech, and not the heart, as tempting as that more romantic proposition might seem. "The voice," Galen tells his reader, "re-

ports the thoughts of the mind." In his exposition of this process, Galen warns of the dangers of using simple assertion instead of observed facts to explicate the workings of the body, never quite appreciating that he himself was given to the same failing each time he took leave of the principles enunciated in his credo, by indulging in theology and surmise. Here is Galen, inveighing against those who have eyes but will not see the truths he brings to them:

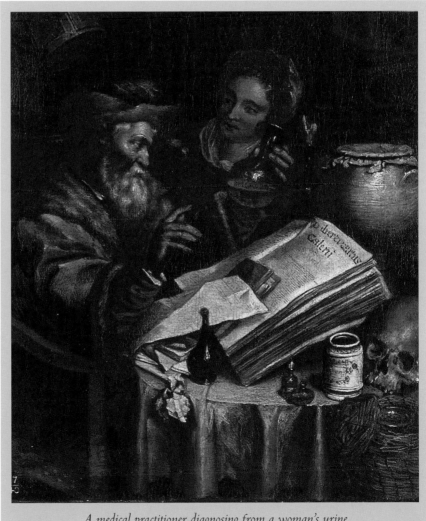

A medical practitioner diagnosing from a woman's urine with the aid of a book by Galen

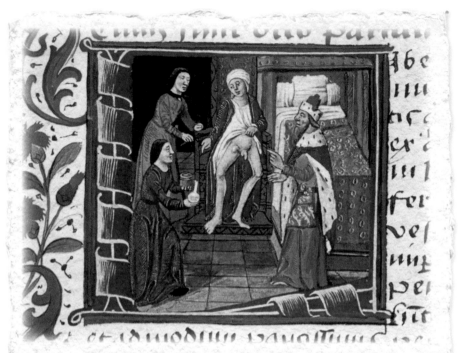

Historical artwork from a fifteenth-century German edition of the writings of Galen of a patient suffering from a fistula, an abnormal channel connecting parts of the body, or an internal organ with the exterior

shall see clearly in the animals themselves that free or normal inspiration is caused by certain organs, muscles, and nerves. . . . Also I will show you the organ of voice, the larynx, its motor muscles and the nerves of those muscles coming from the brain; and similarly with the tongue, the organ of speech. I will prepare several animals, and show that sometimes one, sometimes another, of these activities is abolished when the several nerves are divided.

When I tell them this, and add that all voluntary movement is produced by muscles controlled by nerves coming from the brain, they call me "a teller of marvelous tales," and have no argument beyond the simple assertion that the trachea is near the heart. But what I say I can demonstrate by dissection. They have chosen the short and easy way instead of the long and arduous way which alone leads to the desired end; but the short and easy way fails to attain the truth. . . . No one has ever been able to withstand me when I have demonstrated the muscles of respiration and voice. The muscles move certain organs, but they themselves require, in order to be moved, certain nerves from the brain, and if you intercept one of these with a ligature, immediately the muscle in which the nerve is inserted and the organ moved are rendered motionless. Whoever is really a lover of truth, let him come to me, and if only his senses are unimpaired he

Galen's new anatomical discoveries were important, but were not as valuable a contribution as the detailed precision of description he brought to the understanding of the relationships between already known structures. His anatomical narratives provided a three-dimensional image that clarified perception of just where it is that various organs, tissues, and vessels really lie in the living patient. Like all good teachers of clinical medicine today, he stressed the importance of topographical anatomy, so that the properly trained physician might know exactly what lies underneath every small area of skin surface; without such knowledge, physical examination is a useless exercise.

Galen built upon the ideas of his predecessors to construct a conceptual scheme of the body's mechanics. By his formulation, the three fundamental organs of the body are the heart, the brain, and the liver; the pneuma, the innate heat, and the four humors are, as before, the essential ingredients. From its source in the inspired air, the pneuma enters the left ventricle of the heart, where it is acted upon to undergo a change into what is called "vital pneuma." The heart being the source of the innate heat, the substance that is transmitted from the left ventricle into the arteries is blood that contains life itself, since it is mixed with the vital pneuma and warmed by the innate heat. The pneuma that ascends to the brain is there converted to the "psychic pneuma," in a way that depends for its consummation on one of Galen's anatomical leaps of faith: because he found a coiled network of blood vessels, called the *rete mirabile*, at the base of the skull of his animals, he decided that in passing through its convolutions the pneuma was delayed long enough to permit the start of its conversion from vital pneuma to psychic pneuma, the product of the brain. The brain being the regulator of thinking, feeling, and movement, the psychic pneuma is sent out in the nerves, which are of necessity therefore hollow, to reach their ending points throughout the body.

The role of the liver, according to the Galenic formulation, is to take in digested food at its bottom and change it into blood, which leaves by going out the large vein at the top. In this organ also, the vital spirit which was originally inhaled is converted to "vegetative pneuma," the source of nourishment of the animal. The vegetative pneuma, mixed with the blood, enters that large vein, the vena cava, which immediately branches and becomes the source of all the other veins of the body.

The scheme thus becomes clear. The veins are the conduits for the nourishing blood, the arteries for the life-giving vital pneuma, and the nerves for the psychic pneuma which brings movement and sensibility to the tissues. The periphery is united with the center of life and innate heat. In the second century, and even in the seventeenth, there seemed to be a kind of reassuring coherence to the whole thing.

Unfortunately for Galen's modern reputation, however, the human body has no pneuma, no humors, and no innate heat, just as surely as it has no *rete mirabile*. In the very paragraph in *De Usu Partium* in which he describes how he knows the function of the *rete mirabile* even though he has no experimental proof of it, he reveals, and proudly at that, the teleological hand of the theology that guides his dissections even more than does the hand of science:

> And I shall now say again what I said at the beginning of the whole work, namely, that it is impossible for anyone to find the correct function of any part unless he is perfectly acquainted with the action of the whole instrument.

To Galen, the "action of the whole instrument" is to demonstrate the perfection of God's work.

This has perhaps been an oversimplified summary of a series of ideas that in the original are far more complex and often contradictory. It is presented only to demonstrate how far afield Galen was taken by his speculation and theology. It was just this kind of thinking that was the despair of scholars of medicine when the Renaissance revival of learning took place. They tended to become exasperated by his errors, forgetting his real contributions and forgetting also that it was with him that their own experimental methods had originated.

Galen placed diseases into three categories: those of the humors, those of the tissues, and those of the organs. His therapeutics, not surprisingly, are similar to those of the Hippocratics. Noxious substances such as an excessive humor were to be evacuated by the appropriate measures. Symptoms were to be combated by methods that exerted a counteracting influence. Thus, cold was treated by the application of warmth, and bleeding was used to decrease plethora. Bleeding was also considered to be beneficial in the treatment of fever, acute inflammation, and severe pain. Because treatment must be not only specific but general as well, considerable use was made of changes of diet, location, and what we call today the life-style. Patients were given massages, bodily exercises, and a variety of baths, from sun to mud.

Galen inherited from his teachers a great faith in the efficacy of pharmaceutical preparations, which were prescribed singly and in combination. He himself became quite extravagant in the use of drugs, particularly botanical preparations. Such a polypharmacy was much in keeping with the custom of the time, but Galen seems to have exceeded himself in trying to please his patients, a temptation which some physicians to this day have not been able to resist. The historian of science George Sarton points out that Galen's drugs were imported from all parts of the Roman Empire and beyond. His ingredients came from as far away as Syria,

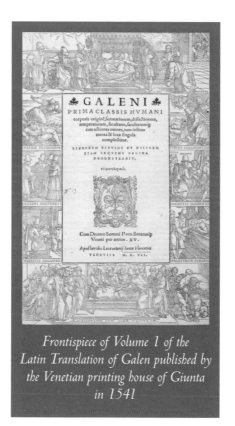

Frontispiece of Volume 1 of the Latin Translation of Galen published by the Venetian printing house of Giunta in 1541

Egypt, Asia Minor, India, Macedonia, North Africa, Spain, and Gaul. His writings contain many highly complicated prescriptions, including one with approximately a hundred constituents. The word "galenical" remains still in the pharmaceutical vocabulary, signifying a class of drugs that are not chemical in nature.

Long after the theories on which they were based had been debunked, Galen's concepts of sickness and its treatment continued to have a pervasive influence on the daily practice of medicine. Indeed, it is a measure of medicine's progress over the past fifty years that a goodly number of his remedies were still being used until well into the twentieth century. They are listed in a 1934 publication by the Galen scholar Joseph Walsh as follows:

Opium, hyoscyamus, tannic acid, chalk, ginger, aloes, scammony, colocynth, cassia, rhubarb, castor oil, olive oil, barley water, licorice, turpentine, squills, ammonium chloride, sulphur, zinc oxide, copper sulphate, valerian, gentian, cardamon, cinnamon, and various balsas and gums. They [ancient physicians] had supposed hydragogues [substances that cause watery evacuations, such as urine or loose stool], cholagogues [medicines that increase the flow of bile] like scammony, expectorants and analogous preparations without number. They had more highly recommended remedies for baldness than a dozen modern barbers and more depilatories than are advertised in our daily newspapers. In addition we still employ, though not to the same extent, massage, ointments, baths, mustard plasters, cupping and bloodletting.

No wonder that Oliver Wendell Holmes told the Massachusetts Medical Society in 1860: "I firmly believe that if the whole *materia medica* as now used could be sunk to the bottom of the sea, it would be all the better for mankind—and all the worse for the fishes."

Of all the principles of Hippocrates honored by Galen, none held a higher position than the importance of prognosis. It is clear from his writings that he considered it not only a great help in determining proper treatment, but of incalculable value in practice-building, a merit not underestimated by the physicians of Cos, or of New York and Boston, for that matter. It seems to have been the most important of the ingredients of the treatment by which Galen, in 176, cured Marcus Aurelius of an affliction he correctly diagnosed as overindulgence. The impression made on the emperor by the diagnosis, prognosis, and therapy must have gone a long way toward ensuring the doctor of the high place in the esteem of his distinguished patient which he was to hold for so many years. Galen describes the event in graphic and immodest detail, concluding with Marcus' statement of gratitude:

He said to Peitholaos that now at last he had a physician and a courageous one, repeating that I was the first of

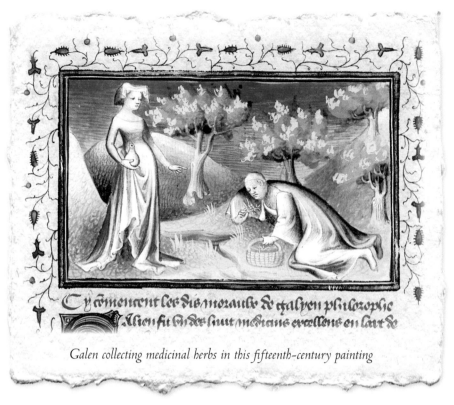

Galen collecting medicinal herbs in this fifteenth-century painting

physicians and the only philosopher; he had tried many, not only the covetous but those greedy of fame and honour and those filled with envy and malice. As I have just stated, this is the most remarkable diagnosis I have made.

In his studies, Galen recorded everything. He employed research assistants, scribes, and all the human impedimenta of what would today be the equivalent of the laboratory of a senior investigator with attached publishing house and printer. The sheer volume of his life's output is staggering. He began writing in his teens and continued until he died at the age of seventy, leaving a body of surviving works which form half of all of the ancient Greek medical writings remaining to us; if the Hippocratic Corpus is omitted, the fraction becomes five-sixths. They occupy twenty-two thick octavo volumes of closely printed material, in the standard edition produced by Karl Kuhn between

1821 and 1833. There were doubtless many other Greek physicians who published a great deal, both before and after the master, but it says much about the esteem in which Galen was held that very little of their work was considered important enough to be preserved.

There are unexpected pleasures in reading those few of Galen's treatises that have been translated into English. Beyond what has been described in the foregoing account, his autobiographical comments and those on ethics, philosophy, religion, and contemporary life are spread throughout the writings in such an unplanned way that the reader never knows when a particularly timeless gem will light up a page. Among my favorites is one that applies even more to the world of today than it does to the period in which it was written. It deals with the verbal superabundance which the medical writers of every age have left as their literary monuments. According to Kenneth Warren, who at the time was Director for Health Sciences at the Rockefeller University in New York, there were twenty thousand biomedical journals in the world in 1981. The present number can only be estimated by using the figures provided by the Yale science historian Derek de Solla Price, who tells us, "For more than 300 years, the pace of growth in quantity of all learned literature has been maintained at a compound interest, with an exponential increase of about 6 to 7 percent each year, a doubling in size every 10 to 15 years, and a tenfold increase in every generation of 35 to 50 years." Statistics like these support the validity of the comment made by a 1985 correspondent to the *New England Journal of Medicine*, who pointed out that the multitude of available outlets

assures "that all high-quality and important papers will be published, as will almost all mediocre papers and the great majority of poor or trivial ones." Anyone who reads even a few of the basic journals of his own specialty knows well that today's medical literature contains far more duplication than is required to confirm findings, far more verbiage than is needed to make clear statements, and far more poor writing than readers should have to tolerate. Although things are certainly worse than they have ever been, the disease has ancient roots, traceable at least as far back as the civilization of Egypt. Galen, who would have hotly denied it if told that he was as guilty of such charges as anyone who has ever thrilled to the sight of his own name in print, had a solution:

> It was a law in old Egypt that all inventions in the handicrafts had to be judged by an assembly of educated men and be written on pillars in a sacred place. Likewise we should have an assembly of just and equally well-educated men. They should scrutinize all that has been written, and deposit in a public place only what appears worthwhile but destroy what is worthless. It would be even better if the names of the authors would not be preserved, as they used to do in ancient Egypt. This would curb at least the excessive zeal for fame.

Galen was convinced that he had provided definitive answers to many of the mysteries of Nature, answers which would forever be venerated as truth. His message to posterity was that further investigation was superfluous: "Whoever seeks fame by deeds, not alone by learned speech, need only become familiar, at small cost of trouble, with all that I have achieved by active research during the course of my entire life."

Throughout the Dark Ages and well into the sixteenth century, men took him at his word: instead of recognizing that he had laid down the principles of scientific investigation, they ignored those parts of his treatises that described the experimental method, looking only at the absolute finality of his answers and not at the questions he posed; instead of rejecting his irrationalities and conjectures, they clung to them as though they had been composed by an oracle; instead of thinking for themselves, they enslaved their minds to the memory of Galen.

We do not have much information about the century and a half that followed Galen's death. We know only that by the middle of the fourth century he had become established as medicine's leading authority. From this point onward, he was everyone's source of reference; he became the real physician who once walked this earth to interpret and disseminate the teachings of Father Hippocrates, that by then mythical figure he had succeeded in elevating to the stature of a god. As the glory of Rome faded, the rising force of Galenism began to flood Byzantium and the East with the peculiar flickering light of half-science. Made even eerier by being refracted through prisms of selectivity and translation, its spectral glow illuminated less than was obscured by the shadows it created.

When the power of Rome declined late in the fourth century, it gave way to the Eastern Empire centered in Constantinople, which lasted over a thousand years. During that millennium, science went nowhere, along with the rest of scholarly activity, as the energies of the empire were given over to religious conflicts and the kinds of connivance that have been called "byzantine" ever since those dark days. Fortunately, the birth of the Moslem nation in the eighth century created a culture eager for learning, and the scientific treatises of the Greeks were soon translated into Arabic. Not alone Galen and Hippocrates, but Euclid, Ptolemy, and Aristotle became lodestars to the Arabs, whose subsequent medical and scientific writings were to a great extent variations, interpretations, and expansions of Greek teachings. Arabic texts became the repository of Greek science.

But there were problems, of the sort that are inherent in the transfer of knowledge from language to language and society to society. The first difficulty lay in the very act of transla-

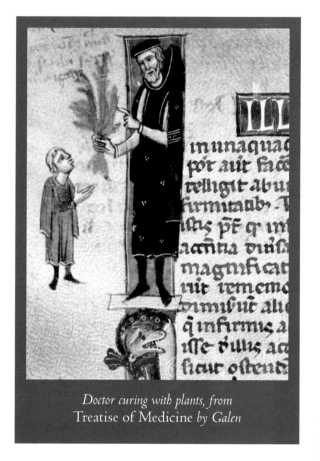

Doctor curing with plants, from
Treatise of Medicine *by Galen*

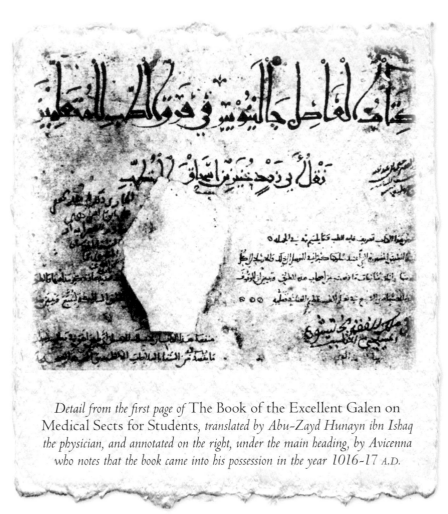

Detail from the first page of The Book of the Excellent Galen on Medical Sects for Students, *translated by Abu-Zayd Hunayn ibn Ishaq the physician, and annotated on the right, under the main heading, by Avicenna who notes that the book came into his possession in the year 1016-17* A.D.

tury, Aetius and Alexander of Tralles in the sixth century, and particularly Paul of Aegina in the seventh century. Paul's *Seven Books,* based largely on Galenic writings, formed the foundation of medicine during the entire period when Moslem physicians were at the height of their repute. He was the greatest of the safekeepers of Greek medicine, but its most prominent revisionist as well, despite his praiseworthy intentions. Two hundred years after it was written, his canon was translated by the Arabs, to become the basis for the medicine practiced by both Moslem and Arabic-speaking Jewish physicians of the period. There were many of them—Rhazes, Haly Abbas, Albucasis, Isaac Judaeus, Maimonides—but the greatest was Avicenna, whose eleventh-century *Canon* became, in the words of Fielding Garrison, "the fountainhead of authority in the Middle Ages." That some critics resented his revisionism is indicated by a remark made two and a half centuries later by the physician-philosopher Arnold of Villanova, who saw him as "a professional scribbler who had stupefied European physicians by his misinterpretation of Galen."

It was these Arabic materials then that finally found their way into Latin in the eleventh and twelfth centuries. The process began at the Benedictine abbey of Monte Cassino in the eleventh century. There, a Carthaginian-born

tion, which in itself distorts greatly even when thoughts are transmitted between cultures far less dissimilar than the Hellenic and Moslem. Were this not enough, the form in which many of the ancient writings came to the translators had been already warped by several generations of compilers and epitomizers. When an Arab physician pored over Galen, he was likely to be studying not a translation from the original but the teachings as they had been interpreted by one of the small herd of self-appointed commentators who appeared in Byzantium after the master's death. Among the most prolific of these literary jackals were Oribasius in the fourth cen-

monk known as Constantine the African, the "Magister Orientis et Occidentis," translated large numbers of Arabic medical texts into Latin. His work has been referred to by the German medical historian Karl Sudhoff as "a symptom of a great historical process," the entry of Moslem and Jewish thinking into western medicine, with the return to its origins of the prodigal art of healing. But although the translation of Hellenic scientific texts into Latin exerted a great energizing effect on European thought, what the Europeans were studying was Galen by way of compilers like Paul, and translations from Greek to Arabic to Latin. When to the problem of multiple translations is added the potential for error introduced by medically untutored scribes laboriously handprinting each manuscript, it becomes obvious that it would have taken a series of miracles to prevent major distortions from appearing. Alas, no such miracles occurred, and the true revival of Greek learning had to wait until after the conquest of Constantinople by the Turks in 1453, when Greek scholars migrated to Italy, bringing with them the actual books and manuscripts of the ancients. Europeans thereupon began to learn Greek, to read Galen and Hippocrates in the original, and to translate them directly into Latin. Only then could real medical science begin again, where Galen had left it thirteen hundred years before. It is a sad irony that his new intellectual heirs would use his experimental method to trample his reputation into the dust, his errors and the centuries of corruption of his teachings blinding them to the fact that it was he who had constructed the framework upon which they would now build.

In 1896, in the Harveian Oration to the Royal College of Physicians, Galen's ill-deserved fate was lamented by Dr. Joseph Payne, Physician to St. Thomas's Hospital:

Harvey's discovery of the circulation [1628] was the climax of that movement which began a century and a half before with the revival of the Greek medical classics and especially of Galen; for without Galen's insistence on the all-importance of anatomy in every branch of medicine and surgery the anatomical revival would probably never have taken place. What honour or gratitude has Galen received for this signal service? In modern times scanty praise or none. . . . In some modern works, nay, sometimes even in a Harveian Oration, we hear only of the astounding errors of Galen. There is, perhaps, no other instance of a man of equal intellectual rank who has been so persistently misunderstood and even misrepresented—a reaction doubtless from the extravagant homage formerly paid him.

Finally, it is to Marcus Aurelius that we must turn to find the words by which Galen himself would have chosen to be described. A dozen generations of European schoolboys have improved their Greek through reading the philosopher-emperor's *Meditations,* called by classicists the highest ethical product of the ancient mind. At every instant of its gentle author's life, but only at the best moments of Galen's, these two great thinkers of the second century affirmed and exemplified one of the most often quoted of the majestic pronouncements to be found in that sublime testament:

I search after truth, by which man never yet was harmed.

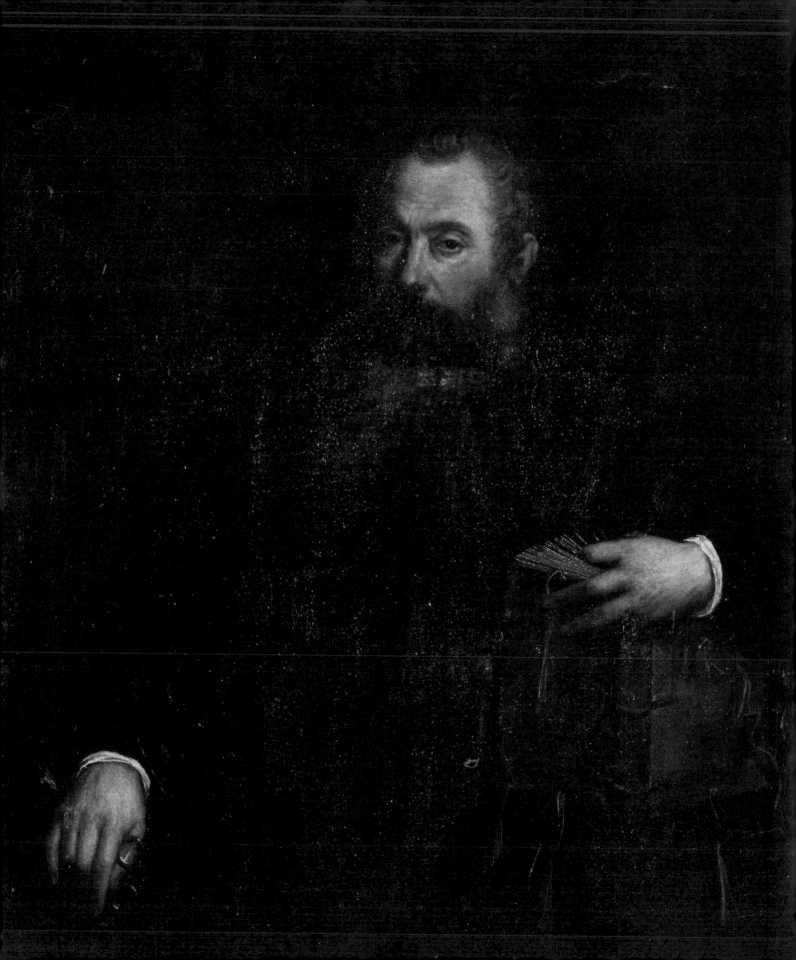

3

THE REAWAKENING

Andreas Vesalius and the Renaissance of Medicine

A certain few writings have marked such profound turning points in the development of science that their subject matters, or at least their authors, are familiar even to people without much knowledge of the field. Perhaps the best example is Charles Darwin's *Origin of Species*. There are not a lot of others—only a small number of works are perceived as being truly monumental, the products of the genius of such easily recognizable figures as Galileo, Newton, Freud, and Einstein. This perception of extreme rarity is, however, myopic. It does not take into account a fact that is but poorly recognized: other branches of scientific learning that are not as well celebrated as, for example, physics and psychology have taken just as startlingly new courses following the appearance of a single publication less well known and of a significance less universal than the contributions of those ascendant figures.

There exists another defect of popular perception as well, this one due less to shortsightedness than to a blurred image of just how scientific

progress is actually made. This particular form of intellectual astigmatism results from the belief that any given major advance appears in a lightning bolt of inspiration, creating knowledge where none had previously existed. But in fact, no great scientific discovery comes about in this instantaneous way; valuable concepts arise only from valuable precedents. The operative verb chosen for the first sentence of this chapter is "marked," not the more dramatic "created." For in truth the great scientists have always presented their gifts to a world made ready to receive them (albeit sometimes kicking and screaming) by cultural changes which have brought mankind to that point and prepared the milieu out of which the insights of notable individuals can emerge. Every giant of science has had his coming presaged, indeed made inevitable, by predecessors whose own work attested that a new way was arising of finding and interpreting information. And so the famous texts *mark* rather than *create* the moment at which one individual boldly announces that it is time to acknowledge openly what others have begun to suspect. A new vision of truth then appears, which finds its form because a particular investigator has had the courage to stick his neck out and take matters one critical step beyond his fellows.

Even the less-known turning points in science, although not as rare as is commonly thought, are nevertheless few and separated by long gaps in time. But, wondrous to tell, two of them occurred in a single year, one in astronomy and the other in medicine. Making the coincidence all the more remarkable are two circumstances: first, that the contribution in astronomy was made by one of the oldest workers who ever advanced science, while that in medicine came about through the efforts of one of the youngest; second, that both men had been trained as physicians at the same school, the University of Padua. The graybeard was the seventy-year-old Nicolaus Copernicus, who in 1543 received, probably on his deathbed, the first printed copy of his *De Revolutionibus Orbium Coelestium*, which showed that it is the sun, and not the earth, that is the center of our solar system. The youth was the twenty-eight-year-old Andreas Vesalius, whose *De Humani Corporis Fabrica* paved the way for modern scientific medicine by presenting to the world the first accurate knowledge of human anatomy and a method by which it might be studied.

The book of Vesalius is an exemplar. It epitomizes the confluence of science, technology, and culture in a way that few, perhaps no, other books have ever done. It was an outgrowth of the vigorous spirit of the Renaissance, and in some ways is the highest expression of the Renaissance mode of thought: while it celebrates a return to the logical thought and observational methods of the Greeks, it eschews their tendency toward conjecture and philosophical speculation. The best of antiquity

is revived, and its errors discarded. This is particularly discernible in the language of the text, an erudite form of Latin that is reminiscent of the finest of Roman rhetoric. With the publication of the *Fabrica*, as it is commonly called, medicine was finally lifted out of the medieval murkiness into which it had been immersed by the compilers, interpreters, and mistranslators of Galen. The sounds of sweet reason and scientific detachment are heard in the voice of a writer educated in the classics, skilled in the language and literature of the two ancient cultures, and imbued with those rediscovered values of antiquity that gave Europe its Revival of Learning.

While representing a return to the Greek emphasis on the direct study of nature, the *Fabrica* also provided for the first time in history a vehicle—the technically accurate, magnificently annotated illustrations—by which nature's secrets might be learned. For, despite its literary virtues, it was not the text proper that made the project succeed; indeed, the text of the *Fabrica* remains the least-read of the great books of medicine, and to this day only fragments of it have been translated into English. The great glory of the Vesalian masterpiece lies in its illustrations. Executed by one of Titian's ablest pupils, they brought anatomy to life on the printed page.

The artists of the Renaissance were intrigued not only by perspective, but also by motion—the how and why of movement and action. One need only glance at the drawings of Leonardo da Vinci to appreciate that his studies of the human form were the outgrowth of his lifelong pursuit of the mysteries of mobility, whether living or mechanical. Modern medicine owes much to the dissections of Andreas Vesalius, but perhaps even more to Leonardo, to Michelangelo, to Titian, to Raphael, and to all the others who recognized, in their artistic humanism, that the depiction of the functioning human body was worthy of their most devoted labors. For the very title of the Vesalian volume expresses the fact that the anatomy it describes is not static. The writer and the artist go beyond form—they are teaching function. Like Galen before him, Vesalius writes of the *uses* of the parts. The meaning of the word *fabrica* was discussed by the English medical historian Charles Singer in an article he wrote for the *Times Literary Supplement*, published on the four hundredth anniversary of the events of 1543.

> *It must not be translated " fabric," nor does "mechanism" quite render it. In classical usage it means "an artisan's workshop" where something is going on and, by transference, the art or trade itself. This is reflected in modern German,* Fabrik *(factory), and rather better in French,* fabrique, *which means both the process of making and the place where things are made. In Renaissance Latin the word has kinetic associations. A good—if unliterary—rendering would be "works" or "workings."* De Humani Corporis Fabrica, *"On Man's Bodily Works." It was always "works" in action, living anatomy, that Vesalius was trying to describe and, as a corollary, he had always in mind the body as a whole—the living body.*

It must, accordingly, be recognized that the pages of the *Fabrica* are in many ways the culmination of the work of the artists. It would have been impossible had not the artists of the time been observers and doers of dissection, just as the artistic triumphs of the Italian school would never have been created were it not for the anatomists.

There are several other varieties of artist whose work is displayed in the *Fabrica*. These are the printers with their newly developed techniques of typography, and the fashioners of the wonderful wooden blocks to which the drawn pictures were transferred by a technique that had been developed only during the previous halfcentury. To many observers whose interest in the history of science is peripheral, the significance of the *Fabrica* is that it represents a triumph of the art of making

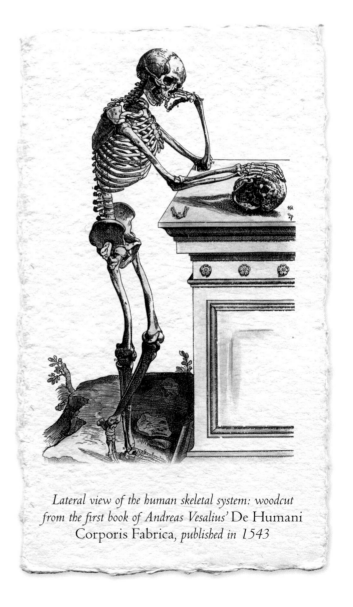

Lateral view of the human skeletal system: woodcut from the first book of Andreas Vesalius' De Humani Corporis Fabrica, *published in 1543*

books. The typography, the illustrations, the correlation of the text with the pictorial material—all of these factors made its publication a turning point not only in medicine, but in the history of education and the history of the printed book as well. Some contemporary publications had approached its qualities, but nothing exactly like it had ever before been published; it became the prototype of a volume for the teaching of science. It went just far enough beyond its closest predecessor to turn the remarkable corner toward the modern textbook.

So the way for the *Fabrica*'s publication had been prepared by the development of the technology of book production and by the humanistic philosophies that accompanied the Revival of Learning. Another vital element was the rise of the universities, especially in Italy.

"University" is a word not easily defined. It refers, in its primary sense, to a community, more or less organized, of scholars and teachers. The beginnings of the concept are usually traced to Plato's Academy, so named for the olive grove of Academe in which the philosopher taught. The great library of Alexandria, founded in the third century B.C., was the nucleus of a similar intellectual unit for study and teaching, but far more extensive. A closely related phenomenon was the development of the rabbinical academies of the first few centuries A.D., out of which came the principles of Talmudic Judaism, and which gave rise to the *yeshivoth*, or seminaries. In fact, these may have had a more direct effect on the genesis of the European universities than did the earlier institutions, since the *yeshivoth*, unlike the Greek establishments, continued to flourish throughout the Middle Ages.

In any case, the school founded at Salerno in the ninth century, primarily for the study of medicine, is generally considered to be the first university. Circumstantial evidence of the influence of the Judaic academies is to be found in the fact that, notwithstanding the rampant religious persecution of the time, Salerno provided a safe intellectual haven for Jewish teachers and students—although, in truth, so many of the custodians of the old Galenic medicine were Arabic-speaking Jews that the university authorities had little choice in the matter, even had they wished it otherwise.

In the eleventh and twelfth centuries, when Arabic manuscripts began to be translated into Latin, and Europe rediscovered Greek learning, scholars congregated in various cities, so that one by one the great universities of the Renaissance made their appearance. Although organized in different ways and founded in response to different needs, the basic function of each was study, investigation, and discussion carried out by faculty and students coming together from various parts of the land, or, in some notable instances, from the entire continent of Europe.

The foregoing implies the existence of a certain freedom of thought and universality of citizenship, but this was not generally the case. For one thing, university teaching was usually under the control of the ecclesiastical authorities; it was further hampered by the various religious wars and intolerances of the time, as well as by territorial conflicts. But the situation was different in Italy. There, the Venetian Republic, recognizing that its economic power rested on free trade and easy access, saw its best interests served by its protection of the foreigners in its midst and the encouragement of their enterprises. The intellectual freedom that was the outcome of this enlightened attitude reaped rewards that have benefited western civilization ever since. Not the least of them was the heady academic atmosphere at the University of Padua, which, under the wise rule of Venice, drew students from all of Europe. The nourishing and flourishing of Renaissance science began in that place. The medical historian Arturo Castiglioni has described its role:

At a time in which a great passion for studies, a great love of beauty, and an inexhaustible desire for glory vivified all the works of the Italian artists and scholars, students and teachers from all parts of Europe came to Padua, which had become the center of scientific research. Here astronomers sought the secret of the stars, physicians the mystery of life, mathematicians the answers to the most difficult problems of geometry and of algebra. Copernicus, the Pole, prepared the way for Galileo; Vesalius, the Fleming, was the forerunner of Harvey and Malpighi; Fracastorius, the Italian, marked the road to modern pathology.

> Of all the manifestations of Renaissance humanism, the most direct must have been the renewed interest in the study of man's body.

Of all the manifestations of Renaissance humanism, the most direct must have been the renewed interest in the study of man's body. Christianity had exerted an inhibiting influence on such investigations. Its doctrines diminished the importance of man's corporeal being as compared to that of his soul, and its authorities were quite satisfied with the teleological precepts of Galen. Although his Creator was quite different from the Judeo-Christian God, the church and the synagogue were united in the belief that the Galenic construct accorded with their dogma far better than did any intrusive efforts of objective research.

Nevertheless, none of this should be construed to mean that the church officially prohibited dissection, because it most assuredly did not. When the medical school at Bologna added to its curriculum the opening of the human body for anatomical demonstrations in 1405, and Padua followed suit in 1429, the bishops uttered no protest. As early as 1345, in fact, a physician named Guido de Vigevano had published in France a text showing the process of dissection. And in 1482 Pope Sixtus IV, who had been a student at both of the Italian universities, came to the aid of the University of Tübingen with a papal bull permitting human dissection provided that local clerical permission was granted.

That the clergy were often cooperative probably had less to do with their appreciation of medical science than with the role of the artists in the beautification of the churches, and the beautification of clerical reputations along with them. In the Renaissance, houses of worship were built to honor not only God, but also the officials who led in glorifying Him; scarcely a decade after the Bull of Sixtus, the prior of the Church of San

Spirito in Florence gave a young painter named Michelangelo Buonarroti permission to perform dissections.

And so the artists gathered around the tables of the anatomists, sometimes themselves picking up the instruments to dissect. The bodies dissected were usually those of executed criminals. They were used by professors to demonstrate the anatomical facts described in the most common texts. The method of instruction is portrayed in an illustration to be found in the *Fasciculus Medicinae* of Johannes de Ketham, published in Venice in 1491. The professor sits perched high on what is quite literally his chair, droning along in his recitation of the Latin Galenic text while an ignorant barber-surgeon dissects the cadaver below and a barely better-schooled demonstrator shows the body parts to the only mildly interested students. The dissections, or anatomies, as they were called, were done once or twice each year with the purpose of proving the truth of Galen's statements. Since the professor never descended from his magisterial throne to actually look at the structures being displayed, and neither the surgeon nor the demonstrator really knew what he was doing, the several days devoted to the exercise each year were

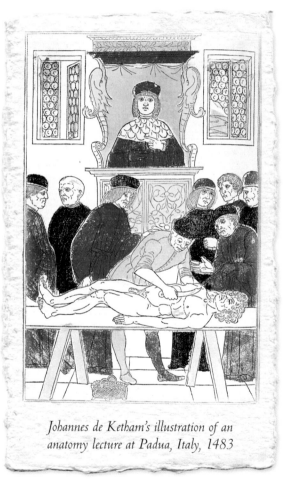

Johannes de Ketham's illustration of an anatomy lecture at Padua, Italy, 1483

little more than a walk-through to satisfy a curricular requirement whose advantages were more theoretical than real. Only the artists really needed to know anatomy. The physicians had no use for it except in the most general sense—everything they required was available to them in the writings of Galen.

And yet, there were isolated individuals whose curiosity led them beyond the mere rote confirmation of the ancient authorities. A small number of anatomists were beginning to dissect the human body in order to learn its structure firsthand. Although they continued to distort their vision by twisting their findings into forms that would fit the Galenic teachings, such warpings were becoming more and more difficult to justify. And then, to say it once again, there were the artists. They cared not a whit about Galen—they sought only the *forma divina* of their fellow man. Andrea Verrochio, who died in 1448, was probably the first of them, followed by such secondary figures as Andrea Mantegna and Luca Signorelli, and then the giants: Leonardo da Vinci, Albrecht Dürer, Michelangelo, and Raphael.

Leonardo has been described by Sigmund Freud as a man who awoke too early in the darkness, while the others were all still asleep. That they continued to slumber was at least as much Leonardo's fault as their own, for he did not succeed in spreading his knowledge or sharing his vision. Though so much of the material from his notebooks has now been deciphered, it was largely inaccessible to his contemporaries except in his art itself and in his one publication, the *Treatise on Painting*. Even this was not published until long after his death, circulating in manuscript to only a few of his contemporaries. Not enough that he wrote his notes backward from right to left, but he was as likely to run words together as he was to divide them arbitrarily at points of his inconsistent choosing. He used no punctuation, formed some of the letters of the alphabet in ways of his own devising, and had a unique personal shorthand. When there is added to these problems his habit of picking up a thought in one corner of a page after having left it in another, or on a different sheet entirely, we are faced with a medium whose message was seen as a hieroglyph in search of a Rosetta Stone. The problem was complicated by one of the characteristics of his extraordinary mind that some consider a facet of his genius and others call a disability—his visualization of thoughts in the form of pictures rather than words. Picture sequences running from right to left adorn some of the most significant of his pages.

The result of the Vincian mystery-writing and reticence was that the impetus he gave to the study of anatomy was felt by very few of his fellows. In the *Treatise on Painting* he makes it clear that he was planning a great anatomical publication, but it was never written. He worked during the winter of 1510 with the young anatomist Marcantonio della Torre, but that project ended with the latter's death the following year. Giorgio Vasari, in his *Lives of the Artists*, tells us that della Torre "threw light on anatomy, which up to that time had been plunged in the almost total darkness of ignorance. . . . In this, he was wonderfully aided by the talent and labour of Leonardo, who made a book drawn with red chalk and annotated with the pen, of the subjects which he dissected with his own hand and drew with the greatest diligence." Elsewhere Vasari writes, "Whoever succeeds in reading these notes of Leonardo will be amazed to find how well that divine spirit has reasoned of the arts, the muscles, the nerves and veins, with the greatest diligence in all things."

The only physician of the time who seems to have written of da Vinci's work in anatomy was

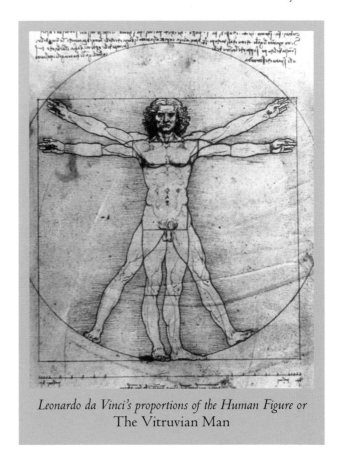

Leonardo da Vinci's proportions of the Human Figure or The Vitruvian Man

Paolo Giovio, who had been a pupil of della Torre. In 1527 he wrote:

In order that he might be able to paint the various joints and muscles as they bend and extend according to the laws of nature, he [Leonardo] dissected in medical schools the corpses of criminals, indifferent to this inhuman and nauseating work. He then tabulated with extreme accuracy all the different parts down to the smallest veins and the composition of the bones, in order that his work, on which he had spent so many years, should be published from copper engravings for the benefit of art.

It is difficult to know how much Leonardo's work directly influenced physicians, for though they may have stirred in their sleep, they surely did not awaken in any great numbers until Andreas Vesalius dragged them out of bed in 1543. My much-admired friend the late Kenneth Keele, who was surely the greatest of the scholars of anatomical Vinciana, accords him more credit than most, calling him "the spearhead of the new creative anatomy," and writing:

Death barred his experiment with della Torre from success. But the movement went on, particularly in Florence. Through Andrea del Sarto, Leonardo's anatomy reached his pupil Rosso Fiorentino, who himself planned an anatomical treatise. . . . Once more the fusion arose in the projected work on anatomy in which Michelangelo contemplated collaboration with Realdo Colombo. These examples reveal how Leonardo had broken the hard ground of bigotry and prejudice which had buried anatomy for so many centuries; how he had stimulated the fusion of art and science in anatomical representation; and how he had prepared the tilth to receive the masterpiece of Vesalius and Calcar. In

1543, when this was published, it was neither lost nor damned.

Whoever deserves the credit, the professors and the artists, stimulated by the invention of movable type around 1450, had begun to collaborate on the production of anatomical texts. The first example was the Ketham *Fasciculus Medicinae* to which I referred earlier, containing some excellent woodcuts. Several such books appeared in the subsequent decades, leading up to two publications by a young Belgian, having illustrations that were much superior to those of his predecessors, although the text was still Galenic anatomy. The Belgian was Andreas Vesalius, the hero of our story.

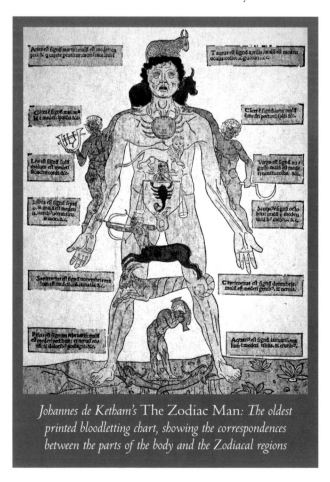

Johannes de Ketham's The Zodiac Man: *The oldest printed bloodletting chart, showing the correspondences between the parts of the body and the Zodiacal regions*

If ever there was a man who embodied both the backward and the forward leanings of the Renaissance, it was surely Andreas Vesalius. He was by early education a classicist and by intellectual persuasion a passionate activist in the cause of scientific exploration. The same fresh winds of change that were carrying the great European navigators to the newly discovered lands of the earth were beginning to flutter the banners of a still small troop of scientists. The Magellans and Da Gamas looked eastward and westward across the seas; the scientists looked outward to the skies and inward to the fabric of the human body.

Born on December 31, 1514, Vesalius was to become the fifth in his family's line of distinguished medical men, all of whom had been either scholars or physicians to royalty. Andreas was named after his father, who was apothecary to members of the Hapsburg family, first to Margaret of Austria and then to her nephew the Holy Roman Emperor Charles V. Although the family resided in Brussels, their ancestral home was the town of Wesel in Cleves, whence they derived the name Vesalius.

Subtle influences were at work from the moment of the boy's birth. The rear of the family's house looked out on an uninhabited, partially wooded stretch of land that was called Gallows Hill, for the presence at its farthermost end of a small area where criminals were executed. The bodies of the dispatched malefactors were left to be picked away by foraging birds and the forces of the elements, so it is apparent that Andreas had plenty of opportunity, grisly though it may have been, to become acquainted with the sight of laid-out human organs and bones. Whether it was in response to these natural anatomy demonstra-

tions we do not know, but in later years he wrote that while still quite young he began to dissect such small field animals as rats, moles, and dormice, along with the occasional stray cat or dog unfortunate enough to come his way.

Pity the luckless animals, but pity also Andreas Vesalius for the use which has been made of this particular morsel of his memoirs. That early exponent of psychohistory, Gregory Zilboorg, wrote in 1943 of Vesalius: "His early interest in dismembering and cutting animals open represents a rather complex set of primitive destructive drives which if sufficiently strong, even if on occasion utilized for purposes of higher pursuits, do ultimately produce depressive states which may in turn become severe enough to be recognized as pathological." Zilboorg proceeded in this way with the rest of Vesalius' life story, eventually extrapolating beyond the borders of reasonable discussion into the giggly land of unsubstantiated silliness. There is more of this sort of thing to come, before its author finally will be seen to redeem himself with one brilliantly perceptive summation.

Having completed the usual forms of elementary education, the fifteen-year-old Andreas left Brussels to study at the University of Louvain. Though fifteen may seem somewhat young to us, this was the age at which college studies usually began in those simpler days. The Louvain course led toward the equivalent of the bachelor's degree, which was called Master of Arts, the prerequisite for entrance into a graduate school. Much of the curriculum was devoted to Latin and Greek studies, as well as philosophy and rhetoric. To this period, and to an earlier time under his mother's tutelage, may be traced Vesalius' lifelong fascination with classical culture. (It was probably also at Louvain that he acquired his small knowledge of Hebrew.) By the close of his course at the university, the eighteen-year-old scholar had determined to follow his heritage by pursuing a career in medicine. Since Louvain did not have an outstanding medical school, he traveled to Paris in August 1533.

Unlike the universities of Italy, that of Paris was a stronghold of the most conservative of medical doctrines and teaching. As a candidate for the Baccalaureate in Medicine, Andreas spent his first year studying the works of Hippocrates, Galen, the compiler Paul of Aegina, and some of the Arab writers. The second year was devoted entirely to Galen's anatomy, taught in the standard way by a "chaired" professor intoning the Latin text in the traditional soporific manner; in the course offered by Jacques Dubois, called Jacobus Sylvius, truth

was further distanced by the professor's use of dog dissections to illustrate the Galenic writings.

In later years Vesalius would write that he learned virtually nothing of human anatomy during his years in Paris. In his own words: "Except for eight muscles of the abdomen, disgracefully mangled and in the wrong order, no one . . . ever demonstrated to me any single muscle, or any single bone, much less the network of nerves, veins, and arteries."

But the young striver refused either to waste his time or to hide his talents. He was impatient and impulsive enough to let it be known that he had some experience of dissecting. Urged on by his fellow students, he took up the barber-surgeon's knife at the third dissection he attended, and carried out a more skillful bit of anatomizing than any of his young colleagues, or indeed their

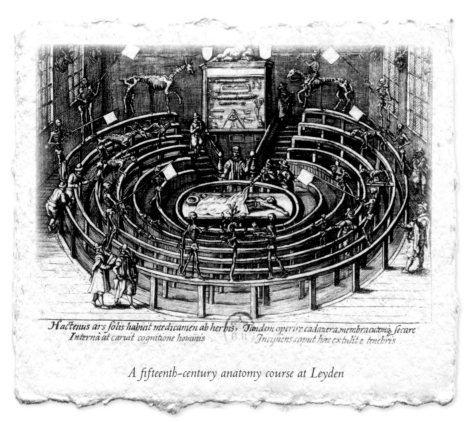

Hactenus ars solis habuit medicamen ab herbis, Tandem operiæ cadauera, membra ciatimq, secare
Interna at caruit cognitione hominis   Incipiens, caput hæc extulit e tenebris

A fifteenth-century anatomy course at Leyden

professors, had ever before witnessed. His self-taught expertise did not go unappreciated. When one of his teachers, Guinter of Andernach, prepared to compile from Galen a small unillustrated book of anatomy, he asked his obviously gifted student for help. In the publication that came out of the ensuing labors, Guinter correctly described his assistant as "a youth of great promise with a remarkable knowledge of medicine and of Greek and Latin, and great dexterity in dissection." Vesalius, never one to praise the undeserving or to understate his own contributions, was less respectful to his mentor, writing some years later:

I reverence him on many counts, and in my published writings I have honored him as my teacher; but I wish there may be inflicted on my body, one for one, as many strokes as I have ever seen him attempt to make incisions in the bodies of men or beasts, except at the dinner table. Nor do I think he will take offense if I say of him, as of not a few others, that he is largely indebted to me for whatever he knows of anatomy apart from what is in the books of Galen, which are common property.

Vesalius was not content with the sparse material made available to him by his occasional opportunities to dissect corpses. He collected bones from the old collapsed graves in the Cemetery of the Innocents of Paris, and made, with some of his classmates, a series of foraging expeditions to the hideous mound at Monfaucon. This grim tumescence was a low hill beyond the northern wall of the city, on which stood what one writer has called "the finest gallows in the kingdom." A large charnel house had been built there, with a colonnade above it of sixteen stone pillars thirty feet high, connected by wooden beams. The corpses of criminals executed in various parts of Paris were brought to this central location to be suspended from the beams until they had disintegrated enough to be put into the vault. It was not a pretty place. The modern junkyard dog is a simpering lap-Fido compared to the vicious marauding canines that roamed those haunted precincts, and many a perilous contest did the students wage with them and the ever-present crows, over the remains of a decaying spleen or a bit of kidney.

Here too, Zilboorg gets in some good licks. Discussing Vesalius' participation, indeed his leadership, in these macabre adventures, his biographer finds in them indications that he was "the captive of his necro- and coprophilic drives," as well as "taciturn, melancholic, unpredictable, spiritually sick, and morose."

Conceivably, all of this may be true; but serious study of the evidence of Vesalius' life provides not a whit of reliable documentation on which to base such determinations. Easier to reconstruct a stained-glass window from a few shards than to evaluate a man's entire personality from his methods of pursuing scientific material, especially given the substantial gaps in our information after the passing of centuries.

In spite of all his psychohistorical babble, however, Zilboorg, when he stayed with the verifiable facts, was able to provide some very telling insights and an image of Andreas Vesalius which, in a few sentences, epitomizes everything that the man represented to the emerging world of medical science:

His fascination with [anatomy] went beyond that of his teachers Sylvius and Guinterius. At the age of fourteen these drives made him cut up rats and cats, but at seventeen and eighteen they made him leave his student bench, discard the dull recitations of Galen's text, stand up before his professors and several hundred students, snatch the knife from the hand of the barber, and undertake himself to dissect the cadaver in his own bold and searching way. During a period of some eleven or twelve years Vesalius worked under the spell of this intense drive for which he found such a happy outlet, almost completely converting the primitive, infantile, sadistic drives into highest endeavors; neither the skepticism of his friends nor the open hostility of his colleagues and teachers seemed to deter him from his purpose. He stood before life as if the conqueror of death itself, because it was out of the dead and decomposing body that he read the mysteries of living human functioning. He seems to have been truly inspired during that period, as if possessed by a single impulse, bent on the achievement of a single ambition.

This is the historical Vesalius. Here, a psychiatrist who in most other respects overstepped the bounds of the available evidence has managed to capture the essence of the man. Vesalius was a dramatic figure about whom legends arose even during his lifetime, and whose every known biographical datum has been subjected to scrutiny. His contributions have been praised by many as an incomparable achievement—and derogated by a few as plagiarism. His single-mindedness has been given as much scholarly attention as have his vacillations, and the number of pages devoted to his Galen-like contentiousness is almost matched by those describing his deferential treatment of contemporaries he might justifiably have scourged as incompetents. But overall, enough is known to produce a picture of Andreas Vesalius that is clear of everything but the magnitude of his contribution and the dedication of the man who made it. And this is the image that is venerated in the annals of medicine.

Vesalius was destined not to remain long enough in Paris to be granted his medical degree. After he had studied for three years, war broke out between France and the Holy Roman Emperor Charles V, and he was forced to return to his homeland within the Empire; in 1536 he enrolled in the medical school of the University of Louvain with what we would today call advanced standing, and in the spring of 1537 he obtained the degree of Bachelor of Medicine. His interest in anatomy remained unabated, as did his zeal in obtaining specimens to study. His enthusiasm and the risks he was willing to take to satisfy it are vividly portrayed in this description he later wrote of the means by which he came to own his first articulated skeleton, a treasure which he glibly told the local authorities he had brought home from Paris. The Gemma of the story is Gemma Frisius, later to become a renowned mathematician and astronomer:

While out walking, looking for bones in the place where on the country highways eventually, to the great convenience of students, all those who have been executed are customarily placed, I happened upon a dried cadaver. . . . The bones were entirely bare, held together by the ligaments alone, and only the origin and insertion of the muscles were preserved. . . . With the help of Gemma, I climbed the stake and pulled off the femur from the hip bone. While tugging at the specimen, the scapulae together with the arms and hands also followed, although the fingers of one hand, both patellae and one foot were missing. After I had brought the legs and arms home in secret and successive trips (leaving the head behind with the entire trunk of the body), I allowed myself to be shut out of the city in the evening in order to obtain the thorax which was firmly held by a chain. I was burning with so great a desire . . . that I was not afraid to snatch in the middle of the night what I so longed for. . . . The next day I transported the bones home piecemeal through another gate of the city . . . and constructed that skeleton which is preserved at Louvain in the home of my very dear old friend Gisbertus Carbo.

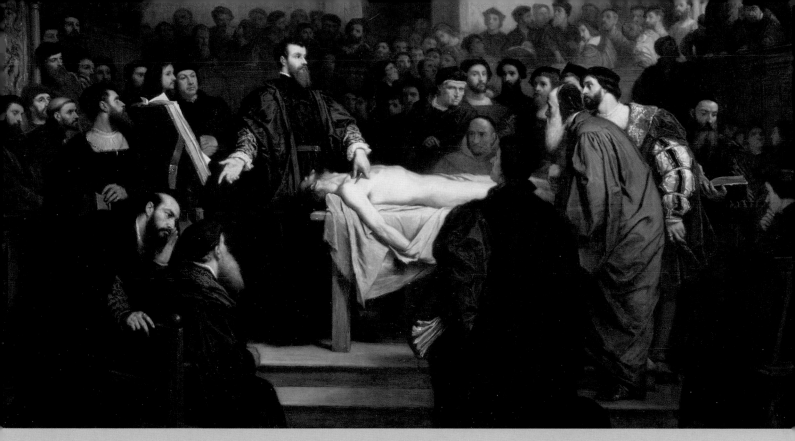

Edouard Jean Conrad Hamman's painting of Andreas Vesalius teaching at Padua

Some time afterward, Vesalius found out that he had exposed himself to danger unnecessarily. The burgomaster of the town, in fact, came to his assistance when he wanted to obtain a cadaver for dissection, something that had not been done in Louvain for eighteen years.

We may assume that up to this point, Vesalius' dissections were being done for the usual purposes of the period—to confirm in his own mind the teachings of Galen, a probability supported by the fact that his baccalaureate thesis was a paraphrase of a book by the Arab physician Rhazes.

The events of Vesalius' life after he completed the requirements for the degree are somewhat obscure. We know that he traveled to Basel, where a second edition of his *Paraphrase of Rhazes* was published by the firm of Ruprecht Winter. He must have been influenced more than a little by his stay in the Swiss city, which was at that time a leading European center of publishing. There is, accordingly, good reason to believe that he may have begun at this time to form in his mind the outlines of the great undertaking which would result in his masterpiece of 1543.

After seeing the second edition of his *Paraphrase* through the press, the new Bachelor of Medicine traveled on to Venice, where he began searching for an artist who might help him to do drawings for the woodcuts of a series of dissections he planned to carry out. He was soon put in touch, perhaps by Titian, with his fellow Belgian Jan Stephan van Calcar. Meantime, he was studying clinical medicine in order to obtain a doctoral degree at Padua. The university being only twenty miles from Venice, Vesalius did his bedside training in the latter city, presenting himself for examination in December 1537. The faculty of Padua not only granted him the degree of Doctor of Medicine with highest distinction, but on the following day appointed him professor of surgery and anatomy, at a salary of forty florins per annum. Although the duties of the new professor included lecturing on anatomy, the chair was not considered an important one compared to those of other medical faculty members, whose salaries were several times that of the twenty-three-year-old novice.

Among the enlightened educational policies of the University of Padua was that members of the faculty were permitted to make reasonable innovations in the school's teaching methods. Vesalius took immediate advantage of this privilege. On December 6, the very day of his appointment, he began a series of cadaver dissections in which he filled all three roles of surgeon, demonstrator, and lecturer. From this running start, he quickly developed the pedagogical style for which he soon became popular among the students—direct personal dissection by the professor himself, with clarifications being made on a skeleton hung alongside the cadaver table. As a means of orientation, he would sketch the outlines of the bones on the skin surface before incising the corpse. He prepared large charts showing the anatomy and what was known of function. The teaching was further illustrated by dissections and sometimes vivisections of small animals to demonstrate living organs or comparative anatomy. The teaching was thus multidimensional, tied in with an explication of physiology, and correlated within the framework of the skeleton, the whole image fixed in memory by the pictorial charts.

Based upon these dissections, and with Calcar's collaboration, six anatomical plates were produced during the course of those first few months. Each consisted of a central drawing with accompanying text along the side of the page, keyed to reference letters marked on the illustration. Printed in April 1538 under the title *Tabulae Anatomicae Sex,* these six charts were the first of the publications that presaged the *Fabrica.*

The *Tabulae* are woodcut plates 19 by 13½ inches in size. Three of them are drawings of the skeleton by Calcar, and the others are Vesalius' own illustrations of the three major circulations, arterial, venous, and portal. Although he was still distorting his own observations so they might fit into a text that is almost wholly Galenic, there are already a few signs that Vesalius was becoming aware of some of his predecessor's errors; for example, he points out discrepancies between Galen's description of certain bones and his own findings. But the extent of his continuing confidence in the old descriptions may be judged from his inclusion in one of the plates of the nonexistent *rete mirabile,* those coiled vessels that Galen claimed to have found at the base of the brain.

The *Tabulae* was a transitional work. Although it was, in all essential points, an exposition of Galen's anatomy and physiology, it was the first attempt ever made by a teacher of medicine to produce learning guides of such detail and quality. More important, in the *Tabulae Anatomicae Sex* can be found the first glimmering hints of its author's most significant contribution to medicine—the liberation of anatomy from authority's yoke. The next inching forward took place a month later, when Vesalius published a revised edition of the text he had helped Guinter of Andernach prepare only two years before. In this new book a few more relatively minor Galenic concepts were amended.

The two Vesalian publications were received with enthusiasm, but even more popular than his writings were the young professor's lectures. Students thronged the amphitheater to witness the new way of learning anatomy and carried word of his teaching techniques to other Italian cities. It was at the invitation of the Bologna student body that he visited that city in January 1540 to give a series of anatomical demonstrations. During a stay of several weeks he justified the excitement of his hosts by a display of the kind of pedagogical incandescence for which he was becoming famous.

There comes a moment in the lives of many revolutionaries when it is necessary to make a daring public statement. Whether by word or deed, whether by design or quickening momentum, a new principle which was until then a formless rudiment, abruptly makes its appearance. From that point on, the gathering force of the thing carries its creator forward, sometimes at a rate of acceleration beyond his control. If the right events and adherents appear in happy consequence, the newly enunciated principle becomes a movement and a doctrine and takes on a vigorous life of its own. In

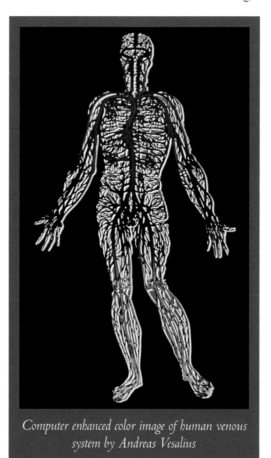

Computer enhanced color image of human venous system by Andreas Vesalius

politics, such lives are often short and ultimately inconsequential; in science, they usually herald a new vision in the history of ideas.

The moment of commitment for Andreas Vesalius came during that brief sojourn in Bologna. The local arrangements called for him to present a series of anatomical demonstrations in conjunction with lectures by one Matteo Corti, a devout Galenist. Their respective attitudes toward dissection epitomized the philosophical differences between the two men, indeed between the medieval world and the Renaissance. The Bolognese professor saw no value in probing the dead human body, since the only purpose to be served by such distasteful investigations was to confirm what was already available in Galen's books. His visitor, on the other hand, had already made it clear in his teaching and in the *Tabulae* that the only true text was the one he called "the book of the human body that cannot lie." In his most recent lectures at Padua, Vesalius had commented on the need for intellectual independence in studying anatomy, and he was by then freely pointing out several Galenic errors that could be shown in the classroom. He had made a few soft sounds that revealed his developing skeptical attitude toward Galen's teachings and his hope, as he put it later in the *Fabrica*, that some of his more open-minded disciples, "drawn by the love of truth, [would] gradually abandon that [backward] attitude and, growing less emphatic, begin to put faith in their own not ineffectual sight and powers of reason rather than in the writings of Galen. These true paradoxes, won not by slavish reliance on the efforts of others, nor supported merely by masses of authorities, they [would] eagerly communicate . . . to their friends." In his questioning and skepticism, he was reasserting the highest principle that Galen himself and the Hippocratics had given to science: the evidence of one's own sensate faculties is the surest path to truth. In the elevation of the Greeks to the status of pedagogical gods, their most important message, intellectual freedom, had long gone unheard. Vesalius, like Copernicus, was about to proclaim it again. The true humanists were those who honored the Greeks best not by slavish devotion, but by understanding the real content of their heritage.

The demonstrations in Bologna, being sanctioned by the clergy, were held in the Church of San Francesco. Four tiers of seats surrounded the dissecting table so that every one of the two hundred spectators might have an unobstructed view.

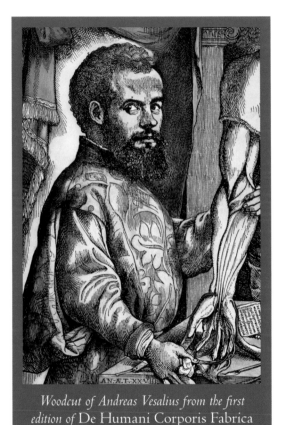

Woodcut of Andreas Vesalius from the first edition of De Humani Corporis Fabrica

The Vesalian dissections began on the morning of January 15, following the completion of five lectures by Corti, during which he used a medieval text, corrected when necessary by reference to Galen. Those, like Corti himself, who believed that Vesalius would utilize his dissections to verify the lecture material were unprepared for what ensued. The students, of course, well knew what maverick rumblings they might expect—this was indeed the reason they had invited their guest anatomist—and the buzz of their anticipation was palpable, though apparently not shared by the professors sitting on the benches beside them.

They were not disappointed. Over the course of the next several weeks, Vesalius found new discrepancies between man and ancient text and for the first time began to wonder whether they had been caused by something more than mere dissecting error or misinterpretation. It was while comparing the skeleton of a human with that of an ape that he noted a bony structure in the anthropoid's backbone that was not to be found in the human's; this structure being a well-known staple of Galenic anatomy, it occurred to him for the first time that the Greek might never have dissected a human body. Since six dogs and other small creatures had been provided for the dissections, he was able to identify certain other parts that are present only in animals. Thus did the truth dawn on him. He who had previously been so reverential of Galen that he had on occasion withheld his own opposed findings from his students decided that all such deceptions must now stop. When Vesalius one morning showed his Bolognese audience the correct insertion of an abdominal muscle, the indignant Corti, piqued by the younger man's presumption, rose to invoke the irreproachable Galenic authority to disprove him. Vesalius did not hesitate. Boldly and without equivocation he stated that whenever he disagreed with the text, he—Andreas Vesalius—could prove that he was right and Galen wrong. The students loved it. Some of the older faculty, however, marched out of the hall like a group of protesting UN delegates. They had turned their backs on the future.

But the facts were there for all to see who would only focus on them. The admiring students, even the less convinced among them, could no longer turn their backs on, or turn back from, the truths that had been exposed to them by a few dexterous maneuvers with the knife.

With the revelation that Galen had learned his anatomy from animals, a fact with still greater implications became apparent: other than Giacomo Berengario da Carpi, a professor of anatomy at Bologna who claimed to have dissected hundreds of bodies but whose 1521 publication was characterized by illustrations more diagrammatic than detailed, *no one* had ever written a treatise based on dissections of the human body; except as derived from studies on dogs, apes, and who knew what else, human anatomy was uncharted territory, waiting to disclose its secrets to the explorer who

knew how to use his blade and his eyes. Moreover, the Art, as the Greeks had called it, could progress not a step further until the mysteries of man's structure had been solved. Vesalius' elders still lived in the smug faith that every bit of needed knowledge was provided by the Galenic commentators; he himself had not believed that, and now he was certain that it was humbug.

On his return to Padua, the great work began in earnest. Calcar drew as Vesalius dissected. Error after error of Galen was exposed, discussed, mapped out, and recorded by the two young men. In all, more than two hundred inaccuracies were identified. Some of the most cherished linchpins of Galenic lore could not be found in real people, among them that jewel in the diadem of medieval medical theory, the *rete mirabile.*

The researches were done with the cooperation of the Paduan authorities, who by then had become accustomed to providing dead criminals to the tireless Belgian professor, even to the extent of postponing executions until he was ready for his next subject. As Calcar drew the final form of the illustrations, Vesalius busied himself with the narrative. His text stressed to the members of his potential audience the importance of verifying his statements by making their own dissections, and he provided instructions for doing just that for each part of the body. Structures must be dissected and redissected in cadaver after cadaver, he taught, to rule out variations between individuals and to confirm evidence. No authority must be allowed to be sacrosanct, including the authority of Vesalius himself, who now declared for all the world to know that Galen had been "deceived by his monkeys." Neither the monkeys, nor the generations of compilers and translators, nor even the old Greek himself was to be permitted to deceive anyone ever again.

Until this period, Vesalius had exhibited considerable respect for the contributions of Galen. His own insatiable delving into the original Greek texts had left him in awe of his illustrious predecessor's methods, and had doubtless given considerable impetus to his own investigative enthusiasm. But by the time he had completed his studies for the *Fabrica,* his contempt for the degradations to which ancient Greek science had been subjected, and for the practices of his contemporaries who styled themselves Galen's disciples, was being openly expressed:

After the ruin spread by the Goths, when all the sciences that had previously flourished and been properly practiced went to the dogs, the more fashionable doctors . . . began to be ashamed of working with their hands, and delegated to slaves the manual attentions they judged needful for their patients. . . . All the preparation of food for the sick they left to nurses; compounding of drugs to apothecaries; surgery to barbers. . . .

This deplorable dismemberment of the art of healing introduced into our schools the detestable procedure now in vogue, that one man should carry out the dissection of the human body, and another give the description of the parts. The lecturers are perched up aloft in a pulpit like jackdaws, and arrogantly prate about things they have never tried, but have committed to memory from the books of others, or placed in written form before their eyes. . . . Thus everything is wrongly taught, days are wasted in absurd questions, and in the confusion less is offered to the onlooker than a butcher in his stall could teach a doctor.

The very frontispiece of the *Fabrica* proclaims its author's new method of teaching. There is no more emphatic statement to be found anywhere in the book than that made by this pictorial masterpiece attributed to Calcar. Every student who saw it must have been struck by its departure from the scene depicted in Ketham's 1491 text. In an article written in 1943 to celebrate the four-hundredth anniversary of the *Fabrica*'s publication, the University of Chicago philosopher Max Fisch called the frontispiece "the manifesto of an educational reform." Here is seen the professor himself, dissecting the open cadaver (actually one of the few women's bodies he was able to obtain) in the presence of a crowd of observers. What we are seeing here is a public demonstration of anatomy. A skeleton is hung close by for orientation, and small animals are ready to be studied. Spectators of every age are present, and it should not escape notice that several of them are members of the clergy. A few tiers above Vesalius stands a young artist, sketching the dissection into a notebook—he is Jan Stephan van Calcar.

A reproduction of that frontispiece hangs in my surgical consulting room. On the wall next to it are two other of Calcar's bursts of virtuosity, his so-called "muscle men." These are drawings of the muscular outer layer of the body. Each of the figures is in motion; each muscle is outlined as though it is functioning. We are seeing the *fabrica,* the workings. As if meant to emphasize the living quality of the anatomy, the backgrounds of the muscle-men drawings are real. When placed alongside each other in proper sequence, they can be shown to provide a continuous scene of the Euganean hills southwest of Padua. We are dealing here with the reality of the human body. Anatomy begins with this book, and so does modern scientific medicine.

If the plates of the *Fabrica* are masterworks of accuracy and craftsmanship, the text was, for its time, a triumph of pedagogy. In spite of his sometimes windy style, Vesalius' generally direct method of addressing the reader in a conversational manner and his excellent organization of the material demonstrate his understanding of the needs of students and serve to overcome a certain tendency toward obscure language. Although the going is tedious compared to the more even flow of today's colloquial textbook prose, the elegance of the *Fabrica*'s rhetoric and the grammatical correctness of the Latin made it a great advance over previous medical books. T. R. Lind, a prominent translator of Vesaliana, has written that "his style is among the best Latin styles written by the Renaissance thinkers." Absent are the glib pronouncements and fuzzy circumlocutions that earlier writers had used to hide their ignorance. (Occasionally Vesalius allowed himself an illustrative anecdote such as the following, in which a "cunning Spaniard," by the piecemeal swallowing of a prostitute's necklace while she was deep in postcoital sleep, proved that the stomach outlet is bigger than had been taught by Galen: "She kept it hung around her neck, even in bed, lest it be stolen. The Spaniard, gazing greedily upon the necklace that would repay him the price of the prostitute's services, employed himself as lustily as possible so that she might fall into a pleasant sleep: thereafter he unclasped the necklace and swallowed the pearls one by one, then the cross and the clasp, lest any trace of his

theft remain. Hence it is clear that the lower orifice of the stomach, even if it is more constricted than the upper, nevertheless is sufficiently ample so that it sometimes transmits even very large objects.")

The *Fabrica* is characterized by a painstaking attention to detailed textual description and by marginal notes that refer to significant characteristics in each of the precisely executed illustrations. There had never been anatomical drawings created with such exactitude, and there had never

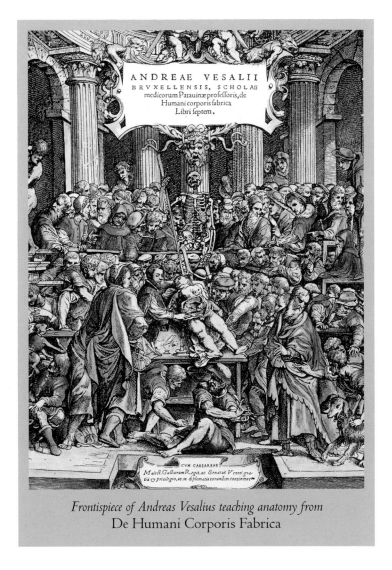

Frontispiece of Andreas Vesalius teaching anatomy from De Humani Corporis Fabrica

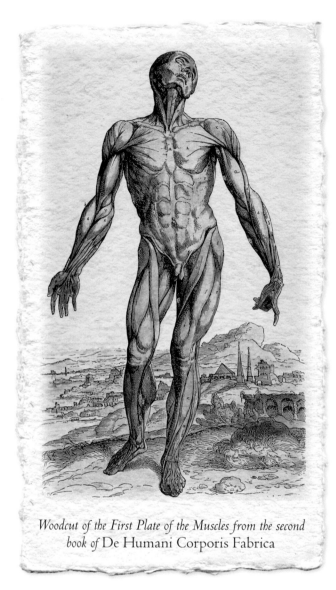

Woodcut of the First Plate of the Muscles from the second book of De Humani Corporis Fabrica

tory of ideas. The fervent pace of his preparations for publication, the compulsive attention he gave to every detail of production, his discriminating choice of artistic and printing collaborators, and his meticulous personal oversight of all facets of the final outcome give ample evidence that he recognized that he was about to bestow a gift of monumental value on the world of medicine. He was aware as well that the cadaveric viscera he was showing his readers were not the only guts that would be exposed in his pages. He was laying out his own innards to the judgment of every critic and every detractor who was willing to riffle through a few pages; at the age of twenty-eight, he was making a very risky bet on his own future.

With all this at stake, Vesalius naturally sought out the most skilled available craftsman to help him in the process of production. Since the greatest of the woodblock cutters were to be found in Venice, it was to one of these that he entrusted his precious illustrations. Although we do not know that man's name, his abilities may be gauged by the quality of the woodcuts and the fact that they remained in relatively good condition well into the twentieth century. Finally, man erased what nature could not—the surviving blocks were destroyed along with the library of the University of Munich, where they were being stored, in an Allied air raid on July 16, 1944.

By August 1542, all of the work for publication had been completed. From Vesalius' experience with the superior printing houses of Basel, he knew that he must go to that city, to the press of Joannes Oporinus. The blocks were carefully wrapped and labeled, scrupulously detailed instructions were written out, and the long, peril-

been a medical book all of whose structural parts were so well integrated with one another. It was the perfect union of words and pictures. Vesalius told his readers that they must do their own dissecting, and he provided instructions for doing so. Paradoxically, the vast erudition and seemingly three-dimensional clarity of his book made it possible to master the subject of anatomy without following his advice.

Andreas Vesalius knew that his *Fabrica* would mark one of the great turning points in the his-

ous journey began, over the Alps on the backs of mules. Vesalius followed soon after, remaining in Basel until he was satisfied with the accuracy and progress of the work. While he was there, he and posterity became the fortunate beneficiaries of an episode of local marital discord. A bigamist, having murdered his first wife in order to simplify his more recent domestic arrangements, was executed by the authorities. As soon as the hangman had retrieved his rope from the swollen neck of the evildoer, the corpse was presented to the visiting anatomist for public dissection followed by reconstruction of the skeleton. Parts of that bony souvenir of connubial disharmony can still be seen today in the anatomical institute of the University of Basel.

Work on the *Fabrica* was completed in June 1543. When it became available for sale in August, with its 663 folio pages, including eleven large plates and almost three hundred other illustrations, it was recognized immediately as an epochal event in the art of bookmaking. Even the severest of critics could not help but admire the workmanship of the publication they now hastened to examine.

The text, as indicated by the title, *De Humani Corporis Fabrica Libri Septem,* was organized into seven books, in the following order: bones; muscles; blood vessels; nerves; abdominal and reproductive organs; organs of the chest; brain. Facing the first page, there appeared a picture of the author dissecting that most intricate of nature's mechanical creations, the human hand. Despite a certain unexplained disproportion of its parts, Vesalius is known to have been very fond of this likeness, which is the only certifiably authentic portrait of him. An introduction dedicated the book to the Holy Roman Emperor Charles V, to whom its author presented a copy.

Wishing to have a "pony" that might be used in the classroom, Vesalius had prepared a summary of his book, which he called the *Epitome.* Published at the same time as the *Fabrica,* it was referred to by its author as a *semita,* or "pathway," to the major work. Although written in Latin, the *Epitome* was produced in a German translation two weeks later, which made even greater the accessibility of this inexpensive minor miracle of condensation, especially to the barber-surgeons. It was dedicated to the emperor's heir apparent, who later became Philip II of Spain, he of the luckless Armada.

The message of the *Fabrica* was heard and, by most, believed; before long its author's prediction began to come true, that physicians would "eagerly communicate to their friends" that a new edifice of medicine was being built. The conservatives, however, refused to retreat. Some of them railed at Vesalius, and a few tried to breathe new life into the moribund old explanation of Galen's errors, that anatomy had changed since his day as the result of the general degradation of the human species after the classical period. Their salvos did not significantly stem the relentless advance of modern thinking, but they wounded one of its messiahs. Most painful to Vesalius were the attacks of his old Paris teacher, Jacobus Sylvius. Sylvius became quite hysterical in his condemnation, perhaps because he saw that in developing new ideas, his former pupil was rejecting to the point of scorn what he had been taught in Paris. After eight years of frenzied outcries, the seventy-three-year-old professor concentrated all his rage into a book with the not very subtle title *A Refutation of the Slanders of a Madman Against the Writings of Hippocrates* and *Galen*, published in 1551. The work was aimed at exposing what its author called "the error-ridden filth" of "that insolent and ignorant slanderer who has treasonably attacked his teachers with violent mendacity." Vesalius, himself certainly no amateur in the uses of invective, was stunned by the fury of Sylvius' rhetoric, which exceeded the bounds of decency even in that age renowned for verbal jugular-slashing. Here are a few choice selections from the book's concluding lines:

> It would have been easier to cleanse the Augean stables than to remove even the worst lies from this hodgepodge made up of thefts and bloated with slanders. . . .
>
> I implore his imperial Majesty to punish severely, as he deserves, this monster born and bred in his own house, this worst example of ignorance, ingratitude, arrogance, and impiety, to suppress him so that he may not poison the rest of Europe with his pestilential breath. He has already infected certain Frenchmen, Germans, and Italians with his deadly exhalation, but only those ignorant of anatomy and the rest of medicine. . . .
>
> Loyal sons of Aesculapius, Frenchmen, Germans, and Italians, I beseech you to come to me as recruits and to assist me in whatever further defense of your teachers may be needed, since I am wearied by my years and my labors. If this hydra rears some new head, destroy it immediately; tear and tread on this Chimera of monstrous size, this crude and confused farrago of filth and sewage, this

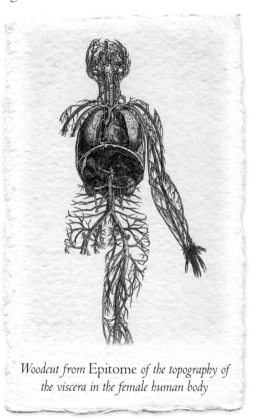

Woodcut from Epitome *of the topography of the viscera in the female human body*

work wholly unworthy of your perusal, and consign it to Vulcan.

Such attacks had varying effects on those who read them. Although some were driven away from the Vesalian teachings, others became more firmly converted, recognizing the desperation of Sylvius and his fellow reactionaries. But Vesalius, who had always chafed under criticism, now began to see evidence that disagreement was turning into intrigue. He was not mistaken. Back in Padua, his former assistant Realdo Colombo, teaching in his absence those very students who had been drawn to the medical school by the magnetic presence of the Belgian, disparaged the message of the *Fabrica* and ridiculed its author. Collegiality, then as now, was a word whose reality often contradicted its dictionary definition.

Though the gathering opposition would prove to be less a storm than a bluster, it was more than Vesalius had patience for. Having presented his shining truth to the world, he held his last public dissection in Padua in December 1543, of a body he described as that of "a beautiful prostitute, taken by the students from a tomb in the Church of San Antonio." Shortly thereafter, he made a dramatic gesture that symbolized his disgust with the odious squabbling in which he was becoming embroiled. He gathered all of his notes and manuscripts into a large pile and put a torch to them. His priceless annotation of Galen, the notes for planned publications in medicine and surgery, and his paraphrase of Rhazes all perished in the flames.

But what seemed on the surface to be the impetuous act of a rejected prophet had a certain deliberateness about it; it was as though he had to be sure that he was destroying the means by which he might be tempted to remain in Padua—he was burning every bridge over which his return was possible from a great decision that he was resolved to make unalterable: to become a clinical doctor caring for the sick. He had already accepted an offer from Charles V to serve as physician at the imperial court; he planned never to return to research.

The literature of Vesaliana is oversupplied with discussions of why its subject left Padua to become a working doctor. He is portrayed by some as having fled in anger, impulsively, spitefully, and in a cutting-off-the-nose-to-spite-the-face frame of mind—"I'll show the bastards, I'll go away and sulk." Zilboorg has a field day with this episode, referring to its "suddenness" and "intensity." Ignoring Vesalius' many known friendships, the public nature of his work, his willingness to travel in support of his doctrines, and his popularity among students, he writes: "Such shut-in persons seldom perform any transition from one mode of living to another, but if they do, they do it impulsively, aggressively, destructively."

The writers, and Zilboorg is only one of many, who explain Vesalius' decision on the basis of spite, frustration, or psychopathology seem to me to be guilty of the sin most commonly denounced at the same time that it is most commonly committed by historians—they attribute the values of their own age and their own minds to situations that are distant in both years and character. No matter what pains historiographers take to avoid that well-marked pitfall against which they warn the rest of us, it is a rare soul who cannot, at some point or another, be found to have been the victim of its subtle seductions.

Fortunately, several Vesalian scholars have maintained enough historical objectivity to recognize that what appeared to be a sudden outburst of reckless impetuousity was actually a logical step in a long-standing life plan. Vesalius had always believed that the primary reason for knowing anatomy was to be a better doctor. He had said as much at the age of twenty-three, in the paraphrase of Rhazes he had written as a thesis while a candidate in medicine. Nicolaus Florenas, to whom that publication was dedicated, was a friend and patron of the young student's, but he was also physician to the emperor, a fact that may have weighed heavily in Vesalius' decision to so honor him. The *Tabulae* was dedicated to the emperor's chief physician, Narcissus Parthenopens, the *Fabrica* to Charles himself, and the *Epitome* to his son Philip—one begins to suspect that the groundwork was being

> *Vesalius had always believed that the primary reason for knowing anatomy was to be a better doctor.*

laid for an eventual position at court, long before the seemingly precipitate actions of the winter of 1543–1544. Vesalius was nothing if not ambitious; it would be surprising if he had not given considerable thought to the deference and security that would be his as the emperor's doctor, especially in view of his family's long history of service at court. Modern society holds its leading scientists in far greater esteem than it does its clinical physicians, but in those dawning years of Renaissance science, a professor's tenure was uncertain and his pay inadequate, and he was the subject of the animus and envy of his colleagues more often than he was of their respect. As for the vast majority of the populace who were without education, what did they know or care of science, or universities, or of professors? But every person in every station of life knew the honor due the emperor's personal physician. In leaving academia to become a doctor to royalty, Vesalius was, quite simply, moving to a better job.

These must have been important considerations, but the historical image of Vesalius should not be weighed down by the heavy burden of pragmatic motivation alone. The practice of medicine was, to him, the most sacred of the arts. It was on his mind constantly—every chapter of the *Fabrica* contains comments on the anatomical changes produced by disease. He viewed the study of anatomy as the proper and direct preparatory pathway to a career devoted to the care of the sick. This was a route that would be traveled by many of the luminaries of later ages of medicine, particularly in the nineteenth century. *Gray's Anatomy*, the most enduring medical textbook ever published, was written in 1858 with the aim of preparing the way for its author's

entry into the rewarding life that was open to the surgeons of the renowned London teaching hospitals. As another eminent researcher-surgeon, Harvey Cushing, wrote:

From the publication of the Fabrica *almost to the present day the intimate pursuit of descriptive and topographical anatomy has constituted the high road for entry into the practice of surgery, and not only have surgically inclined graduates usually sought places as prosectors in dissecting rooms, but in many schools until recent times professorships of anatomy and surgery have often been combined. It bespeaks the enlightened attitude of the Court that Vesalius, who was largely responsible for this trend, should have been appointed, soon after he turned thirty, to serve as the Emperor's physician.*

Thus, the greatest anatomist of his time, or of any time, left his researches behind him and entered the service of the emperor. It did not prove to be the satisfying experience he had expected. The possession of a full purse and expensive clothes that were not permeated with the stench of decaying organs was not compensation enough for the loss of the investigative excitement that had filled his days at Padua. Charles V, moreover, ate too much, drank too much, and never listened to his doctors; he suffered from asthma, gout, and a variety of gastrointestinal disorders caused by his gluttony and intemperance. The scant heed he paid the advice of his physicians left him free to pay attention to any medicine-mixer who happened to be passing through his court. All doctors have a few patients like this; for Vesalius the situation was made particularly difficult not only by his patient's lofty rank but also by the fact that his chief *raison d'être* now lay in keeping this one impossible fellow in some semblance of good health—an objective that, notwithstanding his considerable clinical skill, he was never able to achieve. He did fare better with the several hundred members of the court who were also his patients, but the case of his imperial rule-breaker became an increasing source of frustration for him.

The situation was not mitigated by the presence on the emperor's medical staff of a predominance of Galenists, strongly opposed to the precepts of the *Fabrica* and openly hostile to Vesalius himself. Although the terms of his appointment made him second in rank only to the elderly chief physician, his daily round was conducted in an atmosphere of grumbling discontent. Charles himself treated his young doctor with warmth and kindness despite his disregard of orders, but the general tone of the court was not conducive to relationships of trust. In all, the better job soon proved itself to be a mistake that its holder came to regret bitterly. Even the challenges of the military surgery that came with the emperor's many campaigns did not satisfy the intellectual yearnings of one who was daily finding more evidence that the life of an academic, though more frugal and uncertain, carried rewards that the life of a doctor to the pampered rich did not. Padua, seen dimly across the gaping emptiness left by those burned bridges, looked better and better. There would never again be a time as golden as those former days that he now recalled as "that glorious period of undisturbed labor among the gifted scholars of divine Italy."

Whenever an opportunity arose, Vesalius seized upon it to do some bit of scholarly work.

Should the constant travels of the court bring him to the vicinity of a medical school, he hurried off there to dissect and demonstrate. When the emperor remained in Augsburg for the prolonged period of fourteen months between August 1550 and October 1551, the erstwhile professor revised the text of the first five books of the *Fabrica* for a second edition. The constant campaigns and peripatetic habits of the court left him little other time for such concentrated study, so that it was not until the summer of 1555 that the volume was completed.

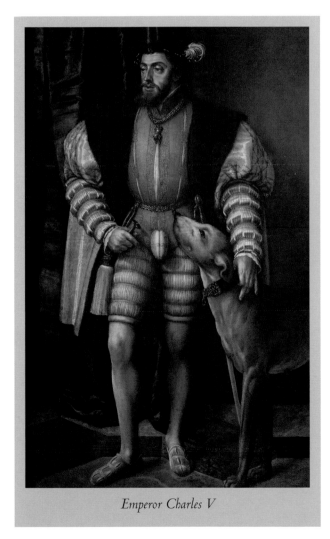

Emperor Charles V

Vesalius had married in 1544, after his anatomical labors were over and his enlistment in the imperial service had assured his ability to support a family. The following year, a daughter had been born to the couple. Whatever may have been his thoughts about leaving the emperor, such a step was thereafter impossible. Not only had he agreed to serve for the duration of Charles' rule, but his domestic needs could never be met on a slim academic salary. Perhaps it was this latter consideration that led him to seek further royal patronage even after his ruler abdicated in 1556.

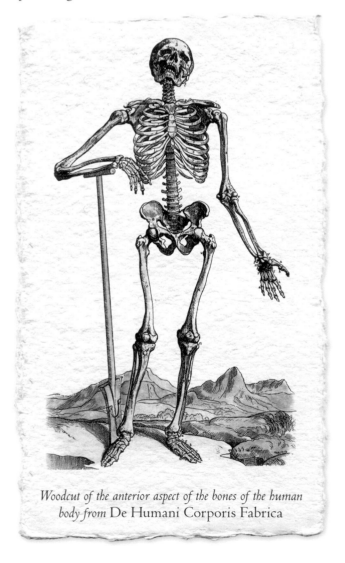

Woodcut of the anterior aspect of the bones of the human body from De Humani Corporis Fabrica

He signed on as physician to the Netherlanders at the court of Philip II, now King of Spain. Before long, he had developed a flourishing practice among the households of foreign embassy officials in Madrid.

The atmosphere in Spain, however, proved to be even more suffocating than that at Charles' court, and when the then Professor of Anatomy at Padua, Gabriele Fallopio, died in 1562, Vesalius petitioned Philip to let him leave Spain so that he might return to Italy. Philip refused. The details of what followed are somewhat hazy, but it is known definitely that shortly thereafter, Vesalius set forth on a pilgrimage to Jerusalem. At least one contemporary observer wrote that the journey was undertaken in gratitude for recovery from a serious illness; several other sources tell a story that seems more apocryphal. By these accounts, Vesalius is said to have unwittingly begun an autopsy on the body of a woman declared dead, but whose heart was found to be still beating faintly when her chest was opened. The horrified dissector had to get out of town for a while.

Whatever the true precipitating event, it is most probable that the real reason Vesalius set out on his pilgrimage was to escape from Spain so that he might return to Padua. He took ship from Venice in April 1564, and it is known that he set sail on the return trip sometime during the early fall. One Pietro Bizzari, writing in 1568, made a statement, considered accurate by historians, that soon after the pilgrim embarked for the Holy Land, "the illustrious Senate called Vesalius to the famous University of Padua, with a very honorable stipend, in place of the learned Fallopio who a little earlier had passed to a better life." Since the newly chosen professor must have known of his appointment prior to the return voyage, it seems certain that he had no intention of returning to the Spanish court.

Here should begin a glorious saga of the prodigal scientist returning to embark on a series of unparalleled successes. Instead, the tale ends in tragedy. The pilgrim ship on which Vesalius was traveling homeward was overtaken by a furious storm that threw it off course and tossed it about on the sea for days. When the food and water began to run out on the inadequately provisioned craft, passengers were thrown overboard one by one as they died or became too weak to justify expenditure of the dwindling supplies. Finally, just when all seemed lost, the storm abated, and the ship was able to make port at the small island of Zante, off the western coast of the Peloponnesus. Vesalius left the craft unaccompanied, and almost immediately fell victim to a serious illness, whose details are not known. Within a few days, according to Bizzari's account, "he miserably closed and terminated the course of his life in a vile and impoverished inn in a solitary place, without any human assistance." A Venetian goldsmith whose ship had stopped at the island chanced to learn that the famous anatomist had fallen ill and died. Bizzari goes on: "With great difficulty he gained permission of the islanders to bury him, and with his own hands prepared the grave and buried the body so that it might not remain as food and nourishment for wild beasts." No one knew who the goldsmith was—the grave he dug on that October morning has never been found.

And so passed the glory of Andreas Vesalius. In five feverish years of inspired research he showed the way for the entry of medicine into the world of modern science, and then spent the rest of his life in frustration and regret. The *enfant terrible* of anatomy never grew up to be the mature investigator who might have shortened the tortuous path to the next necessary stage in the progress of the art of healing—the realization that each symptom of disease is caused by a specific, usually anatomic, change in some structure or tissues of the body. There is evidence in the pages of the *Fabrica* that he might have ventured in this direction had he been able to free himself of his obligations to the emperor. Of Andreas Vesalius, it is proper to utter the saddest words of tongue or pen.

But, no matter what might have been, the *Fabrica* was the embodiment of the spirit of the Renaissance, an accomplishment of such magnitude that its creative energy could only have come from a utopian vision of the future of science. In that future, researchers would use only the evidence of their senses, as the Hippocratics had done; their only inferences would be those that follow logically from the tangible facts before them. And then they would seek out the finest technology of their time, and the fruits of its culture, to produce a record of their observations that would teach the world what they had learned, so that others might add more to the sum of man's knowledge. That was the role of Vesalius in the history of medicine—it is impossible to think of the man without thinking of his book, for both were of the same intellectual essence. Walt Whitman probably never laid eyes on a copy of the *Fabrica*, but he knew about such things:

Camerado, this is no book, Who touches this touches a man.

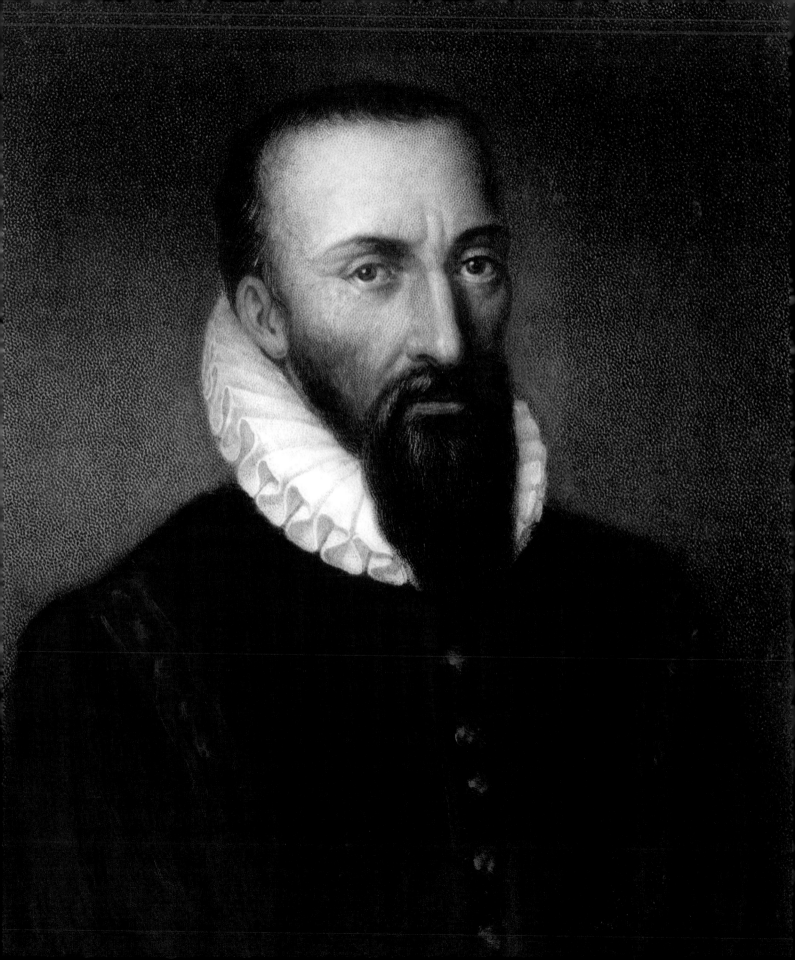

4

THE GENTLE SURGEON

Ambroise Paré

*S*urgery is an exercise in the use of the intellect. Heckling internists, with tongues only barely in cheek, would prefer that surgical specialists be viewed merely as dexterous craftsmen who carry out the routine errands assigned to them by their more cerebrally endowed medical overseers. I attribute this teasing raillery to a kind of good-natured fraternal envy, not so much of our celebrity status, but rather of the visibility of the cures we surgeons achieve and the particular personal gratification we have while doing it. It might seem strange to describe the daily doings of a surgeon as fun, but not many non-physicians can appreciate what a good time we are having, almost always. The fun arises from the challenge, and the major challenge lies not in the doing of wonders with our fingers, but in doing them with our minds.

Even surgery's most dramatic component, the operation, is no more a feat of manual dexterity than is the painting of a beautiful landscape. The operation is the moment during which the mind of the healer makes his or her hands carry out a bidding based on a sensitive wisdom about the ways in which the human body is supposed to work and the ways in which it has failed. It is familiarity with a disease's evolution, from its very beginning to the time of the curative intervention, that enables the operator to comprehend what he sees so that he may choose from among the several paths that can be taken to correct the malfunction in the body of the patient.

Once the diseased recesses have been exposed, there begins a process of deliberation and decision that is virtually instantaneous, by which a plan is formulated that is then carried out in an orderly sequence of successive steps. In the directness of its effect on the life of a fellow human being, an operation may be the most realistic and practical kind of work a man or woman can do; on the other hand, the technical esoterica of its minute details places it certainly among the most abstract. The seemingly automatic exactnesses of cutting and stitching and knot-tying are servants to a process of intellectual synthesis and logic that is one of the highest accomplishments of both the cerebrum and the psyche. Although no one would go so far as to accuse surgeons of excessive modesty, the members of the specialty do have a certain tendency to underestimate the range of their capabilities. When the early-nineteenth-century English surgeon Astley Cooper listed his colleagues' necessary attributes as the "eye of an eagle, heart of a lion, hand of a woman," he diplomatically avoided the resentment of his medical colleagues by omitting what he knew to be his own most important attribute, the mind of a scholar.

And yet, having a scholar's mind will avail naught if the technical skill is absent. If his hands are unequal to the task demanded by his brain, the surgeon is no surgeon; if he cannot do the job with gentleness, he is no healer. The hand that injures tissue cannot cure it; the surgeon who allows himself to be rough cannot expect to see a postoperative recovery that is smooth.

This elementary fact was not always appreciated. There are passing references to it in the writings of Hippocrates and Galen and their disciples, but not until the sixteenth-century teachings of Ambroise Paré became the standard of surgical care did it take hold. Paré led his followers along the irregular path to modern surgery, carrying the message of gentle care that remains to this day his most significant legacy.

Paradoxically, the gentle treatment of tissues was a concept introduced in the midst of the turbulent destruction of a war. War has always benefited the surgeon's art. The immediacy and the complicated nature of military wounds demand an equivalent immediacy of cure. During every major American conflict of the twentieth century, great advances have been made in some particular area of surgical treatment. In World War I, it was surgery of the intestine; in World War II, chest surgery; in the Korean war, vascular surgery; in Vietnam, rapid transport of trauma victims. In every conflict, hospital methods, resuscitation techniques, and surgical skills in general have taken dramatic steps forward. In each case, there has been a spin-off of major improvements in various aspects of internal medicine as well. The silver that lines the heavy gray clouds of war has a luminescence which in the long term may brighten quite as many lives as are blighted by the catastrophe.

Among the reasons that each new war demands yet further improvements in medical care is the fact that it invariably brings with it more efficient methods of destruction. The injuries are more complicated, requiring increasingly sophisticated knowledge of the body in order to treat them. No matter how highly developed becomes the technology that enables us to heal, it seems always to lag one step behind the technology that enables us to maim. In these days of nuclear fission and the threat of world-kaput, it is hard to imagine the terror that gripped medieval Europe following the introduction of gunpowder as a medium of devastation. Probably invented in China around the year 1000, the lethal substance was brought to the West by the Arabs, who seem also to have made the first firearms. Small guns were used in the battles of the early fourteenth century, such as Crécy in 1346, but it was not until the Italian Wars of the sixteenth century that artillery was put to its first major sustained test, as well as its first major confrontation with the healing powers of medical science. In this contest, the long-robed contemplative professors of medicine proved unequal to the challenge. In the end, it was the humble, uneducated barber-surgeon Ambroise Paré who understood what was needed, and provided a solution.

Before describing the circumstances under which that solution was revealed, its discoverer might best be introduced by a quotation from his writings, which illustrates the greatness of the problems he faced and reveals something of the greatness of the man:

From the same wretched shop and magazine of cruelty, come all sorts of mines, countermines, pots of fire, trains, fiery arrows, lances, crossbows, barrels, balls of fire, burning faggots, and all such fiery engines and inventions. Closely stuffed with fuel and matter for fire, and cast by the defenders upon the bodies and tents of the assailants, they easily catch fire by the violence of their motion. They are certainly a most miserable and pernicious kind of invention, by which we often see a thousand unsuspecting men blown up with a mine by the force of gunpowder. At other times, in the very heat of the conflict you may see the stoutest soldiers seized upon with some of these fiery engines, to burn in their harnesses, no waters being sufficiently powerful to restrain and quench the raging and wasting violence of such fire cruelly spreading over the body and bowels. As though it were not sufficient to have arms, iron, and fire for man's destruction, in order to make the stroke more speedy we have furnished them, as it were, with wings, so as to fly more hastily to our own perdition, furnishing scythe-bearing death with wings so more speedily to oppress men, for whose preservation all things contained in the world were created by God. Verily, when I consider all the sorts of warlike engines which the ancients used, they seem to me to be mere childish sports and games in comparison with those I am describing. For these modern inventions are such as easily exceed all the best-appointed and cruel engines which can be mentioned or thought upon, in the shape, cruelty, and appearance of their operations.

For what in the world is thought more horrid or fearful than thunder and lightning? And yet the hurtfulness of thunder is almost nothing to the cruelty of these infernal engines, which can be seen by comparing their effects. Thunder and lightning commonly gives but one blow, or stroke, and that commonly strikes but one man of a multitude; but one great cannon at one shot may spoil and kill a hundred men. Thunder, being a natural thing, falls by chance, one time upon a high oak, another on the top of a mountain, and sometimes on some lofty tower, but seldom on man. But this hellish engine, tempered by the malice and guidance of man, assails man only, and takes him for his only mark, and directs his bullets against him. The thunder, by its noise as a messenger sent before, foretells the storm at hand; but, which is the chief mischief, this infernal engine roars as it strikes, and strikes as it roars, sending at one and the same time the deadly bullet into the breast and the horrible noise into the ear. Wherefore we all of us rightfully curse the author of so pernicious an engine; on the contrary praise those to the skies, who endeavor by words and pious exhortations to dehort kings from their use, or else labour by writing and operation to apply fit medicines to wounds made by these engines.

It was in their perception of what constituted a "fit medicine" that the doctors of the sixteenth century made their greatest error in wound treatment. The error was due to their mistaken belief that gunshot wounds are somehow poisoned by the gunpowder, and must therefore undergo a cleansing with boiling oil. Not only was the underlying theory erroneous, but the treatment was ferociously traumatic. The resultant pain was as intolerable as was the destruction of tissue that accompanied it, and yet the therapeutic iniquity persisted, enforced by the wrong-headed dogma that the "poisoned" wounds must be detoxified.

Ambroise Paré accepted this principle, learned in Paris during his apprenticeship as a barber-surgeon, and he had no reason to doubt its correctness. He was well versed in the proper way to prepare the "oil of elders, scalding hot, in which should be mingled a little treacle." He knew how to soak his packing or bandages in it, and then to apply them directly into missile wounds or onto the large areas of burned skin surface of a struggling, screaming soldier. At the age of twenty-six he had completed four years as a *compagnon chirurgien,* or resident surgeon, at the renowned Paris hospital the Hôtel Dieu. Too poor to pay his entrance fee, he had not been able to undertake the examinations that might qualify him for official admission to the corps of barber-surgeons. Somehow, he managed to obtain an appointment as personal surgeon to Marshal de Montejan, a general of the French king, Francis I.

The army, having successfully defended itself against an invasion of Provence by the Holy Roman Emperor Charles V, pursued the retreating forces into Italy, and thus it was that the young Paré found himself at the siege of Turin, in the year 1537. It was his first campaign, and his first exposure to fresh wounds. There were far more injured soldiers than he had prepared for, and before long he used up all of his boiling oil in cauterizing their burns and plugging their gunshot holes. With the boldness of desperation, and the God-given ingenuity he had been born with, he had the inspiration to design a battlefield clinical experiment: instead of applying "the said oil the hottest that was possible into the wounds," the novice surgeon hit upon the idea of making up a bland, soothing lotion. He was taking a chance and he knew it—if his unorthodox treatment failed, he would certainly lose his position, or worse. He describes what happened:

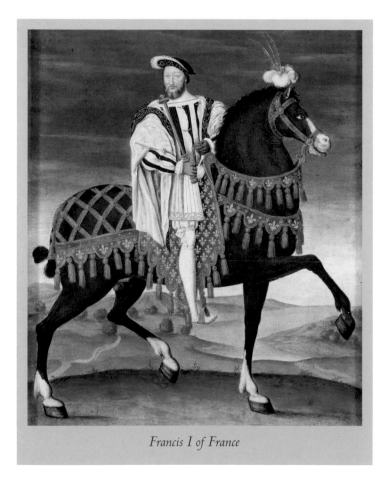

Francis I of France

At last I wanted oil, and was constrained instead thereof, to apply a digestive of yolkes of egges, oil of Roses, and Turpentine. In the night I could not sleepe in quiet, fearing some default in not cauterizing, that I should find those to whom I had not used the burning oil dead impoisoned; which made me rise very early to visit them, where beyond my expectation I found those to whom I had applied my digestive medicine, to feele little paine, and their wounds without inflammation or tumor, having rested reasonable well in the night: the others to whom was used the said boiling oil, I found them feverish, with great pain and swelling about the edges of their wounds. And then I resolved with my selfe never so cruelly to burne poore men wounded with gunshot. . . . See then how I have learned to dresse wounds made with gunshot, not by bookes.

The fledgling surgeon was astonished by the marked contrast between the two groups of soldiers. Those treated with hot oil, whom we may view as the experimental controls, had spent the usual sleepless pain-racked night, while those treated with the gentle emollient were comfortable and without evidence of worsened tissue damage. As Paré viewed the results, his mood changed from apprehension to a kind of awestruck excitement. His conversion from primitive healer to modern was instantaneous and complete.

With this one critical experience early in Paré's career was born the principle of gentleness in the treatment of wounds. The young man was destined to become the greatest surgeon of his time, and for all his scorn of what was to be found in books, he left a series of writings that would stand as the canon of surgery for centuries afterward. Widely translated and widely read, his treatises were the means by which most European surgeons learned the details of their art. They served as the standard reference works, handbooks, manuals,

Before Paré, only Hippocrates had created such a watershed of change for surgery, and after him only John Hunter would create another.

and theoretical surgical texts of the period. Like his contemporary Andreas Vesalius, Paré recognized at an embryonic stage in his own professional development that the teachings of his predecessors held few immutable truths, so that the authentic principles of his craft still awaited discovery, demonstration, and recording. Lacking a formal education, and therefore being ignorant of Latin, Paré did his recording in French. When he was criticized by the lofty professors of the University of Paris for not using the language of learning, he replied that Hippocrates himself had written in his own native tongue.

As the story of Ambroise Paré unfolds, it will become apparent that his influence upon the art of surgery was so vast that it cannot be measured in terms merely of concrete innovations, but rather should be thought of as the triumph of a philosophy. The role of the surgeon and the role of surgery were changed by his life's work—he created a new image of what a surgeon should be, how he should think, and the heritage he should leave to those who come after him. Before Paré, only Hippocrates had created such a watershed of change for surgery, and after him only John Hunter would create another. There have been other historic schools of surgery, and there have been many other surgical innovators, but only three times in the long history of western medicine has surgical philosophy and practice, not to say its horizons and self-image, undergone a virtual transformation from what had been before. And so the names of Hippocrates, Paré, and Hunter deserve to be writ larger than the rest.

As a result of Ambroise Paré's work and his writings, the ignominious role of the barber-surgeons in the hierarchy of healers was elevated to the level where it was no longer possible to ignore their knowledge of disease or their ability to treat it. Their social status rose, their rights and privileges increased, and better men were attracted to the profession. This set the stage for the improvements in ethics and training that resulted in the great clinical advances of the succeeding centuries, as surgeons found themselves in a position to benefit from and contribute to the rapidly increasing store of medical knowledge.

Paré wrote voluminously, and he wrote well. Because he wrote in the plain conversational French of his fellow surgeons, his works were soon translated into plain English, German, Dutch, and other languages which were available to colleagues throughout Europe. The result was not only an expansion of surgical knowledge, but a rapid dissemination of Paré's ethical philosophies and his approach to the evaluation of evidence.

It is here, in his ways of evaluating medical evidence, that Paré's greatness is most manifest and his influence was most long-lasting. He began with a wide-ranging knowledge of the work of his predecessors. He used this as a background against which to measure his own observations, which were gathered up in a vast experience of surgical problems. He approached these observations with an objective eye that allowed enough distance to see his own errors and those of his fellows. And finally, he applied to his great knowledge and his great number of experiences his equally great powers of analysis and reason. The result is apparent to any modern surgeon who reads his writings: his ideas about diagnosis, surgical technique, wound treatment, healing, prosthetics, and prognosis are astonishingly accurate. Thousands of experimental protocols followed in hundreds of laboratories over the past century confirm what Ambroise Paré taught about surgical care four hundred years ago. In the introductory pages of one of his books, he vows to offer precepts that he "will prove by authority, reason and experience." He succeeds so well because he keeps his promise.

Paré's authority came from his extensive knowledge of the work of Hippocrates, Galen, and more recent surgical authors; his reason came from his own gifted intellect; his experience came from war. Two long-term historic conflicts were waged during his lifetime, one coming hard on the heels of the other, so that his career consisted really of a long series of battlefield adventures. These were the Italian Wars of 1495 to 1559 and the so-called Wars of Religion of 1562 to 1598.

It is helpful to have some understanding of the background against which the portrait of Ambroise Paré's long life, from 1510 to 1590, will emerge in the following pages. Specifically, it is important to appreciate that the state of French politics and the state of French surgery provided, respectively, a laboratory plentiful with investigative opportunities and a virtually clean notebook to fill with experiences, experiments, and extrapolations. Paré's life spanned the sixteenth century, which, like our own, will be remembered for both its great achievements and its great cruelties. The cruelties were largely the result of those two series of bloody campaigns, during the first of which the Holy Roman Empire struggled with France decade after decade for the control of Italy, and during the second of which the power of the Catholic kings was directed at the suppression of the Protestant Reformation in France.

The sixty-five years of the Italian Wars were marked by an unrelieved sequence of murderous battles that finally concluded with the victory of the then emperor, Philip II of Spain. The Treaty of Cateau-Cambrésis that formally closed the hostilities did not bring an end to strife and slaughter, however. One of the factors that had forced France's Henry II into peace with Philip was Henry's desire to devote his energies to countering the increasing power of Protestants within his realm. In fact, so much did he wish to draw the Catholic King of Spain to his cause that he gave his daughter Elizabeth in marriage to Philip. This was a political coup, but it resulted in a personal disaster when the French king died of a wound sustained in a tournament which was part of the wedding festivities. The death of his son Francis II after a one-year reign allowed power to fall into the hands of Henry's widow, the Italian-born queen mother Catherine de Médicis, a shrewd, po-

litically astute manipulator whose primary interest was to consolidate the power of her other sons, first Francis III and then his successor, Henry III. Catholic-Protestant animosities were heightened, and on March 1, 1562, an incident in the town of Vassy resulted in a massacre by French troops, and the religious civil war was on.

The most famous event of that conflict began on August 24, 1572, when several hundred Huguenots were butchered in a four-day killing spree that became known as the St. Bartholomew's Day Massacre. But far from breaking the will of the Protestants, the bloodshed only stiffened their resolve. Murders, battles, pestilence, treachery, and politically expedient conversions characterized the whole period, until the godless conflict being waged in the name of God finally ended with the accession to the

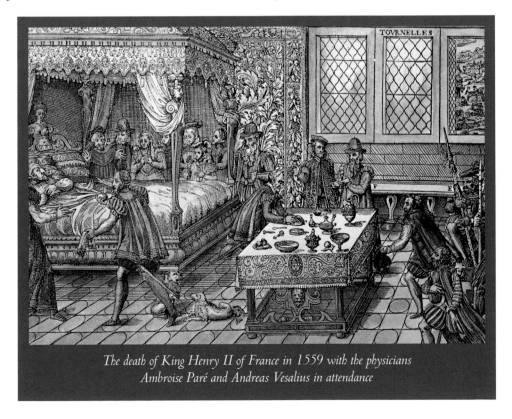

The death of King Henry II of France in 1559 with the physicians Ambroise Paré and Andreas Vesalius in attendance

throne of the former Protestant Henry IV. "Paris is well worth a mass," he is supposed to have said, as he embraced Catholicism with pragmatic fervor in 1593, the first Bourbon king.

To return to a metaphor used earlier: if the battlefields of western Europe were Paré's laboratories, the immature state of French surgery and the lowly position of surgeons provided the vast number of blank pages that his contributions would fill. In fourteenth- and fifteenth-century Paris, the care of the sick had been entrusted to a hierarchy of three groups. The first of these, in both knowledge and socioeconomic level, was the physicians, who were members of the Faculté de Médecine of the University of Paris. Like most of the doctors of Europe, they were trained in Latin and

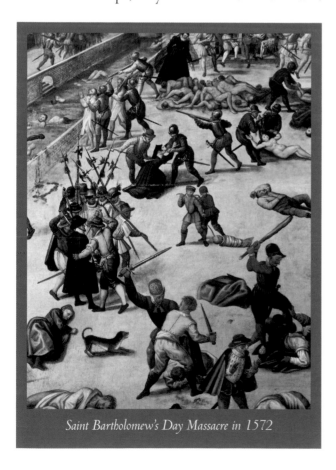

Saint Bartholomew's Day Massacre in 1572

Greek, were considered highly educated, and did their healing with medicines and advice. Their elite position and grand status allowed them not only to look down on the lesser groups but to exercise significant control over all aspects of medical and surgical practice and teaching. Their undisguised contempt was directed particularly at the lowest group in the tripartite hierarchy, the barbers; these were considered little better than those minimally trained near-quacks who roamed Europe as itinerant bonesetters, hernia-cutters, tooth-pullers, and the so-called lithotomists who "cut persons laboring under the stone."

Between physicians and barbers there existed a group that was unique to Paris, and not to be found elsewhere. This was a brotherhood of surgeons, known as the Confraternity of St. Côme, later called the College of St. Côme when their status was somewhat elevated early in the sixteenth century. The members of the organization were characterized by an arrogant and often ridiculous attempt to claim the ritualistic dignity of university professors. But wearing robes (they were called "the surgeons of the long robe"), carrying out quasi-academic ceremonies, and granting degrees do not an academic faculty make. What they did make was a constant state of friction with the real academics in the Faculté de Médecine and the real surgeons, who were the lowly barbers.

For the brothers of St. Côme were not real surgeons. With their pretensions to the status of the scholarly physicians of the University of Paris, they had, over a period of many decades, gradually taken on a certain remoteness from hands-on care. They rarely did operations, preferring to treat surgical problems with medicaments, lordly advice, or the application of the hot cauterizing iron to inflamed or bleeding wounds. Their confraternity existed primarily to protect their own rights, aping the physicians and fighting to preserve what today we would call their turf against the steady encroachments of the barbers. The College of St. Côme was, in the words of Paré's nineteenth-century biographer Joseph Malgaigne, "much less celebrated . . . for services rendered to science than

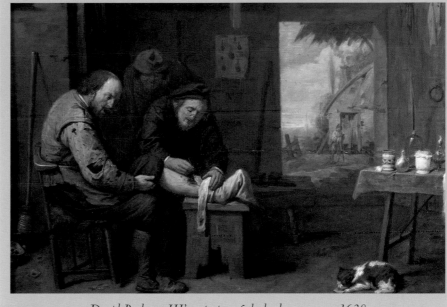

David Ryckaert III's painting of the barber-surgeon, 1638

for the secular fights it maintained against the barbers and against the physicians of Paris."

Another word about the barbers. Throughout Europe, the treatment of minor wounds and sores had been in their hands for centuries. When a physician ordered a bleeding or a scarification, the actual procedure was done by a barber. Gradually, as practical surgical procedures came to be disdained by physicians, they fell more and more into the hands of the barbers, except in Paris, where the brothers of St. Côme attempted to suppress the barbers' activities in their own interests. The outcome of all this is best described by Montaigne: "The barbers tended unceasingly to approach the surgeons [of the College of St. Côme] and to encroach on their domain; the surgeons sought at once to destroy or to submerge the barbers and to approach the physicians; and finally the physicians, occupied at first only with repulsing and submerging the surgeons, later would be

carried along by the force of things to use the barbers as assistants."

The struggles continued for two hundred years, with petitions, lawsuits, decrees, and constant rivalry, not only over turf but over who should teach what to whom, and in what language. Finally, in the first decade of the sixteenth century the Faculté de Médecine made several definitive decisions. First, it formally legitimized the position of the barbers, who were henceforth to be known as the corps of barber-surgeons. The barber-surgeons were to attend lectures in anatomy and surgery given by the Faculté, and would be required to pass not only the master-barber's examination, but another to be given under the university's auspices. Thereafter, they were to be admitted to the College of St. Côme and the brothers of the College were to be admitted as doctors regent to the Faculté de Médecine. Although rivalries continued, the level of chronic enmity lessened. Such

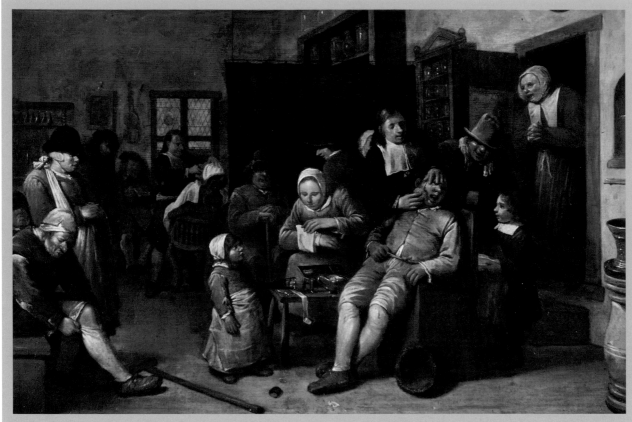

Egbert van Heemskerk III's The Village Barber

was the state of affairs when Ambroise Paré began his surgical career in 1536.

This cabinetmaker's son was born in 1510 in the city of Laval, in what was then the province of Maine, bounded on the north by Normandy and on the west by Brittany. There is much reason to believe that the family was Huguenot, which may have made Paré's position difficult during the Wars of Religion, as will be discussed later. His first teacher was a chaplain, with whom he was sent to board. Later he was apprenticed to a barber-surgeon, and within a short time he obtained the position of *compagnon chirurgien* at the Hôtel Dieu, from which, four years later, he went off to war with Marshal de Montejan to the walls of Turin, where occurred that decisive episode already recounted, of the boiling oil.

When Marshal de Montejan died in 1539 (apparently of liver disease, that traditional French catch-all ailment), his successor urged Paré to stay with the army, in view of his good results and his increasing reputation. However, the young surgeon preferred to return to Paris, where the money he had earned at war enabled him to sit for his qualifying examinations in 1541. He married during that same year and settled near the end of the Pont St. Michel on the left bank of the Seine, where he bought a shop and set up practice as a master barber-surgeon. When his wealth increased in later years, he came to possess a number of buildings in this neighborhood (which is represented by the present-day Place St. Michel) and in Meudon, a few miles southwest of Paris. Interestingly, the curé of Meudon at the time was none other than the masterful François Rabelais. Although it is difficult to believe that Paré and the brilliant physician-priest did not know each other, there is no written record of a relationship.

In 1542, Paré returned to the military, this time as surgeon to M. de Rohan, grand lord of Brittany. It was in the campaign of Perpignan that another of Paré's oft-recounted adventures occurred. The Marshal de Brissac had taken a musket shot near the right shoulder blade, and three or four of "the most expert Chirurgeons of the Army" were unable to locate it. By requesting that the marshal put his body into the position in which it had been when hit, Paré was able to find the ball and remove it. As simple and as logical as that maneuver was, we know of no previous mention of it in any medical treatise, and it was probably an entirely new idea.

By this time, Paré's reputation had grown. When the series of campaigns ended, he returned to Paris to find himself invited to meet with the great physician of the Faculté de Médecine, Jacques Dubois, called Sylvius (the same Sylvius who was first the teacher and friend of Andreas Vesalius and later his most hostile critic). Sylvius urged Paré to write of his experiences with wound treatment, a suggestion that resulted in the publication in 1545 of the thirty-five-year-old surgeon's first book, *The Method of Treating Wounds Made by Arquebuses and Other Firearms, Darts and Such; Also on Combustion Made Especially by Cannon Powder*.

Some of the motivations of any writer can be discerned readily by his readers, some are more difficult to identify, and some remain hidden, even from the author. Among those of Ambroise Paré which are distinct and clear is his wish to guide young surgeons in their practice as they accumulated experience. The following is Wallace B. Hamby's translation of the preface to this first of Paré's books:

TO YOUNG SURGEONS OF GOOD WILL

My friends and brothers in the surgical profession, to comply with your request, I am constrained to write you in this little treatise the method I have followed and found correct for good practicing surgeons, as much in wars (which are frequent) as elsewhere, in the care of wounds made by firearmes and by arrows, darts, and such weapons, also of burns, especially made by cannon powder. Not presuming in my present capacity of being able to teach you (for which more instruction would be necessary) but to satisfy your desire in part, and also to stimulate some higher spirit by writing in this way, so we can all give it greater attention. Now I ask you humbly to take this little book kindly; which if I know you are agreeable, will cause me to do something more, such as my small mind can undertake. For such I pray the Creator, brothers and friends, to happily support our work by his Grace, always increasing our good affections so that something fruitful and useful can come of it, to the support of the infirmity of human life and to the honor of the One in whom are hidden all the treasures of Science, who is the Eternal God.

How well Paré succeeded in his attempt to educate others is shown, first, by the wide circulation this and his later writings enjoyed, as they were translated into other languages to satisfy the needs of surgeons throughout Europe; and second, by the poor condition in which such books are likely to be found, when they occasionally turn up in the collections of bibliophiles today—a natural consequence, as a knowledgeable antiquarian has explained to me, of the heavy use to which these volumes were put for two centuries after their publication. It was not until the great work of John Hunter (1728–1793) that more specifically useful surgical texts were written, especially concerning the treatment of gunshot wounds. The medical historian Fielding H. Garrison wrote, "Up to the time of John Hunter, surgery was entirely in French hands, and Paris was the only place where the subject could be properly studied." That this was true was due largely to the pervasive and continuing influence of Ambroise Paré.

A great deal has been written about Paré's deep piety, his devout Christian faith. Surely the last sentence of his preface to *The Method of Treating Wounds Made by Arquebuses* would seem to confirm this, as would the fact that his clinical case reports are sprinkled with the frequent humble reiteration of "I dressed him, and God healed him." It may seem more than a little mean-spirited to quarrel with such a pious image, but it should be remembered that Paré lived at a time when scholarly writings were often punctuated with paeans to God and to the lordly patrons who supported His work on earth. Religion pervaded every aspect of daily life, and the hand of the Divinity was seen in all things.

There were, moreover, precious few agnostics in the sixteenth century, a time when a confession of atheism was akin to a confession of madness. Those few illustrious scientists who came into conflict with the Church did not admit to rejecting a scintilla of their religious commitment—they simply tried to convince the bishops that new knowledge was not inconsistent with dogma. Galileo Galilei (1564–1642) is the most obvious and most distinguished example.

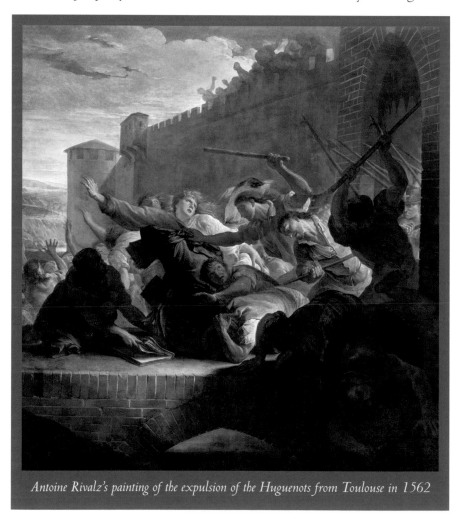

Antoine Rivalz's painting of the expulsion of the Huguenots from Toulouse in 1562

Invoking God constituted a subtle implication that one's noble patron, like oneself, was also a good and religious man. Great compliments were thereby implied to great seigneurs. *The Method of Treating Wounds Made by Arquebuses* was dedicated as follows: "To the very illustrious and very powerful Lord, Monseigneur René, Viscount de Rohan, Prince de Léon, Count of Porhouet, of la Garnache, of Rauais-sur-Mer and of Carantan." It does not take away from our conception of the profound moral goodness of Ambroise Paré, or detract from the evidence of his extraordinary compassion, to be skeptical about his formal faith.

Such skepticism becomes particularly appropriate when we consider his religious affiliation. Almost certainly born a Huguenot, with occasional references in his and other writings to support that probability, he somehow lived through the Catholic persecutions of his coreligionists without losing his life or his position. Many high-ranking Huguenots were murdered during the Massacre of St. Bartholomew, but he was spared, probably at the direct intervention of Charles IX. His second marriage, in 1573, took place in a Catholic church. Moreover, he was surgeon in Catholic armies during the Wars of Religion and seems not to have felt compromised by it. From what we know of his openness and of his honesty it is hard to think that Paré hid his Huguenot origins from his Catholic patrons, or that he compromised his loyalties for the sake of professional advancement. Nor is there any evidence that he converted after St. Bartholomew. It is easier to believe that he wore his official religion lightly. By this I mean that the formalities of religion had no great significance in his life. He certainly did believe in God, and it is clear that he entrusted his patients to divine healing after his own methods had brought them as far as was possible. But his thinking was primarily that of a humanist, dedicated to the travails and glories of this world.

Paré's great-hearted compassion is expressed in every portion of his writings. He hesitates not at all to describe those times when he was frightened for his life or for his reputation. This too has teaching merit for young surgeons. One of the most valuable unspoken dividends of the long years that characterize the surgical training programs of today is that we have all seen our own senior professors when they have been unsure, afraid, or wrong. We have been present when those whom we most respect have committed technical, intellectual, or even moral errors. Those moments have made it possible for us to continue when our own occasional failures strike hard at self-esteem.

So, his personal philosophy was Ambroise Paré's most important heritage: compassion, honesty, gentleness, curiosity, loyalty, and a deep belief that human lives are worth saving. All of these he tried to teach to his peers and to the generations of surgeons who would follow after. The rewards he sought were his own satisfaction and the regard of the colleagues he respected. These he had in good measure, as well as a material success: he was surgeon to four French kings, he became a wealthy man, and he came virtually to rule over French surgery.

But I have leaped ahead of the story, and in the leaping I have given away the punch line. Throughout his writings, Ambroise Paré reiterated again and again his simple credo as a surgeon: "I dressed him, and God healed him." Things are no different today. Whether determined by God or nature, there is a point in the process of healing past which no physician can take a patient. Though modern science is constantly decreasing the distance, the final cure remains largely in the control of as yet unknown factors at which we can only guess. It is the role of the doctor to bring the patient to the farthest reach of contemporary methods of healing. Once there, the conduct of the rest of the journey must be turned over to the uncertain forces of faith or physiology, or perhaps both. No physician should ever be arrogant enough to think otherwise.

About the time of the publication of *The Method of Treating Wounds,* an interval of relative peace began for the people of France. The death of Francis I in 1547 put his son Henry II on the throne. Ambroise Paré, meanwhile, had remained at home, working on anatomical studies and probably practicing surgery. In 1550 he produced his second book, *Brief Collection of the Conduct of Anatomy.* There is a passage in the preface to that volume which is implicit in every scientific contribution that reaches the printer's page, but authors seldom openly assert it. Here is Ambroise Paré to say it for us all:

> *If someone more advanced than we are is displeased by glancing at this book and says that I have not reached the perfection desired or that I have made errors, I affectionately request him to remember that I am not divine, but human, and for the good of the republic to undertake to clear it up better than I, or to content himself with*

> *teaching the aspirants to our profession better. Assuring him that such would not offend me, I shall be the first to thank him and even to praise so worthy an enterprise.*

Following the publication of this book, Paré worked on a second edition of his volume on gunshot wounds; he completed it just in time to respond to the call for mobilization of the army in Champagne, rejoining the forces of the Viscount de Rohan for an invasion of Lorraine in 1552, in which the cities of Metz, Toul, and Verdun were easily taken from Charles V. It was during this series of battles that he saved the life of a common soldier whose wounds were so severe that his comrades had already dug a grave for him—and the ordinary soldiers began to recognize that the compassion of the viscount's surgeon extended to them as well as to the noble captains.

At the siege of Danvilliers, which was part of the Lorraine campaign, a major event occurred in the evolution of Paré's methodology. In the second edition of his book on war wounds he had still recommended the use of the hot iron to stop the bleeding in amputations. Nevertheless, he had begun to give considerable thought to using ligatures to tie the major vessels, as some surgeons were doing in treatment of ordinary wounds; the battles of Danvilliers presented the opportunity to make the trial. When one of the viscount's officers was shot in the leg, Paré tied off the vessels in the amputated stump, and spared him the cauter-

> *Throughout his writings, Ambroise Paré reiterated again and again his simple credo as a surgeon: "I dressed him, and God healed him."*

izing iron. A second great forward step had been taken, which would be communicated throughout Europe by Paré's writings, by his students, and by his increasing fame.

Not only did the fighting in Lorraine provide the opportunity to make an important advance in surgery, it also resulted in an important advance in the innovator's career: his abilities became known to Henry II, who appointed him, although only a barber-surgeon, to be one of his "surgeons-in-ordinarie."

Angered at the loss of the three bishoprics of Toul, Verdun, and Metz, the Emperor Charles V now took personal charge of his army and besieged Metz. The mortality among the wounded soldiers was frighteningly high, and Paré's services were requested. He was virtually smuggled into the surrounded city, to the great relief of the French officers.

Somehow, under the guiding military genius of the Duc de Guise, the French troops withstood the emperor's attacks, and the siege was lifted the day after Christmas, 1552. In his writings Paré chronicled the misery of the subsequent imperial retreat through deep snow with a mixture of sympathy and ridicule, the latter arising out of his anger at the barbarous behavior exhibited by the Spanish soldiers during the siege. Ironically, and as if by way of some grand historical retribution, 250 years later it would be an Emperor

of France who would suffer a disastrous defeat at a besieged enemy city, and see his dreams of victory disappear in an ignominious retreat through snowy, hostile territory. Just as Napoleon's withdrawal from Moscow marked the start of a long decline that led eventually to the loss of his empire, Charles, on that bleak winter day in front of Metz, set out on the dreary road that ended in his abdication and the reign of Philip II.

But the emperor still had a few fights left in him, although not in Lorraine. In 1553, Paré, who had returned home, was once more summoned by the king, this time to Hedin, in Picardy, "where I had much work cut out, so that I had no rest night nor day for dressing the wounded." The battle was fierce; there are few descriptions of premodern warfare that are as vivid and horrifying as that which Paré has left us of the events of those few days. Finally, the French garrison capitulated, only to fall victim to treachery as the Spanish soldiers tortured and slaughtered their prisoners in violation of the surrender terms agreed upon.

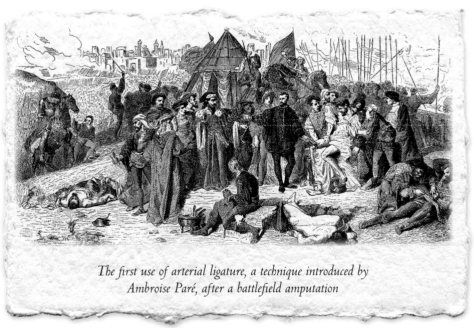

The first use of arterial ligature, a technique introduced by Ambroise Paré, after a battlefield amputation

Fame has its dangers. Fearful of being slain if he could not pay ransom, Paré exchanged clothes with a plain soldier and remained in attendance on one of the wounded French officers. Recognized as a surgeon because of his obvious knowledge, but still not as the renowned surgeon of the king, he managed to gain his release by curing a chronic leg ulcer for a colonel in the enemy army. Once safely away, he reported to King Henry, and then returned again to Paris.

Now forty-four years old, the master barber-surgeon was much sought after by patients and colleagues. The brothers of St. Côme, previously so anxious to subjugate the barbers, knew that having Ambroise Paré on the faculty would add luster to their college. Not only was he an acknowledged leader of European surgery, but he was a friend of the king and had the confidence of much of the nobility. Waiving the requirement for a Latin examination, they admitted him as a master surgeon on December 18, 1554. In 1557, Henry sent him off again following the battle of St. Quintin, at which a severe defeat had been inflicted on the French. In the following year, as the Italian Wars sputtered to an end, he saw action once more, at Dourlan.

All this time the Protestants had been increasing their power. They now had more than two thousand churches in France, and the Huguenot nobility had begun to take over active leadership from the clergy, even making alliances with the German princes and the Queen of England. It was necessary, in Henry's mind, to crush the heresy and to assert his political control. Peace was made with the new Holy Roman Emperor Philip II and cemented, as noted earlier, by Philip's marriage to the Princess Elizabeth, daughter of the French king. Henry's accidental death during the marriage festivities resulted in the one-year reign of Francis II, whose eleven-year-old brother was crowned Charles IX in 1560, leading to the ascendancy already mentioned of Catherine de Médicis. Paré, who had been surgeon to Francis, now was made surgeon to Charles.

Civil war became inevitable as the Court Council, which was predominantly Catholic, sought to suppress the Huguenots. The massacre of the Protestant congregation at Vassy was the spark that ignited the explosive mixture. All of Paré's remaining military experiences took place during the nearly forty years of skirmishes, lootings, and massacres that followed, dignified in history books as the Wars of Religion. It was after the siege of Rouen that he was elevated to the position of premier-surgeon to the king.

The fact that such a position was now held by a barber-surgeon had enormous significance for the future course of French medicine. It signified the realization that the greatest knowledge in treating injuries and certain illnesses no longer lay either with the physicians or with the surgeons of St. Côme. Rather, in the person of their leading authority, the once lowly barber-surgeons were recognized as the well-trained and skillful practitioners they now were.

In 1564, Paré published an interesting volume entitled *Ten Books of Surgery with the Magazine of the Instruments Necessary for It*. Filled with a series of clear illustrations of the instruments used by the author, the treatise has chapter headings ranging from a title as surgical as "On the Extraction of Arrows" to another as overtly in the province of internal medicine as, in the rendering of its English translator, "General Treatment

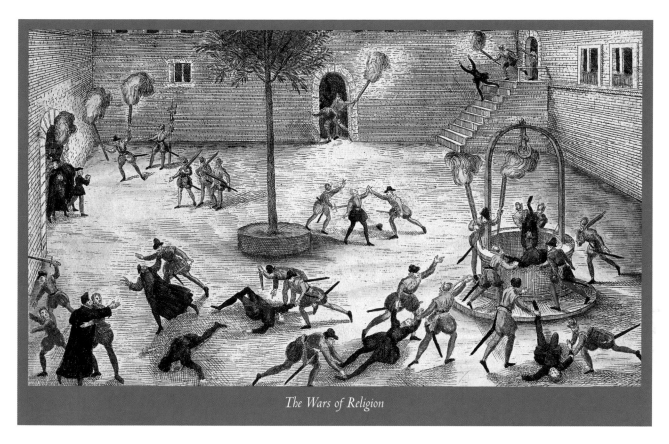

The Wars of Religion

of Hot-Piss," on the treatment of urinary-tract infections.

Although he was periodically called away to one or another campaign, much of Paré's life after this 1564 publication was spent in Paris, in anatomical investigation and writing. When Charles IX died in 1574 his brother, Henry III, not only retained Paré as premier-surgeon, but made Paré *valet de chambre* as well.

Ambroise Paré lived long enough to witness the climax of the Wars of Religion in 1589, as Paris was besieged and Henry III assassinated, thus setting the stage for the accession of the converted Protestant Henry IV. Then, just as peace seemed finally within reach, the illustrious surgeon, who had so narrowly escaped a violent quietus countless times on the battlefield, died at the

age of eighty in the comfort of his own bed on December 20, 1590.

That Ambroise Paré left such an authoritative legacy to later generations of surgeons is due mainly to the soundness of the books he wrote; because he wove into his clinical descriptions a narrative of many of the most significant events of his life, we are privileged to have a great deal of biographical information as well. His two major volumes in particular, the *Complete Works* of 1575 and the *Apologie and Treatise* written a decade later, are rich both in medical learning and personal lore.

Paré was at the height of his power and influence when the first edition of his magnum opus, *The Complete Works of Ambroise Paré, Councilor and Premier Surgeon of the King*, appeared. The response that greeted it provides direct evidence of its author's stature among the surgeons of Europe and his lasting effect upon later medical teaching. Four editions were required by the time of Paré's death fifteen years later, and the demand continued long thereafter, necessitating multiple posthumous ones, ending with the thirteenth in 1685.

The *Complete Works* were translated into English in 1634 by Thomas Johnson, a London apothecary. A short excerpt from the prefatory note addressed by Johnson to his readers sheds further light on the significance of Paré's work to his contemporaries:

I travelled over Germany, and then for four years space I followed the Spanish army in the Low-Countries; whereas I did not only carefully cure the wounded soldier, but also heedfully and curiously observe what way of curing the renowned Italian, Germane, and Spanish Surgeons observed, who together with me were imployed in the Hospitall, for the healing of the wounded and sicke. I observed them all to take no other course than that which is here delivered by Parey. Such as did not understand French, got some pieces of this Worke for large rewards, turned into Latine, or such Languages as they understood, which they kept charily, and made great store of; and they esteemed, admired, and embraced this worke alone, above all other workes of surgery, etc.

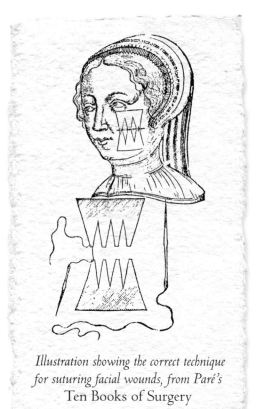

Illustration showing the correct technique for suturing facial wounds, from Paré's Ten Books of Surgery

Paré's most famous work was the *Apologie and Treatise*, which was originally published as part of the fourth edition of the *Complete Works*, although it has usually been printed separately. As pointed out by the English medical historian Sir Geoffrey Keynes (brother of the economic theorist John Maynard Keynes), the *Apologie and Treatise* "contains what amounts to an autobiography covering fifty years of Paré's life from the age of twenty-five to seventy-five." The book was the outgrowth, as we shall see, of a feud.

Modern scientists may disagree with each other in print, but direct insult is considered bad form. Editors censor out comments of questionable taste before they reach the printed page; even the oral discussions at academic meetings tend to be polite these days. That does not mean, of course, that we really harbor no animosity toward our professional rivals, only that we are less overt about expressing it. But there was a time, not long past, when verbal combat was considered an art form, or at least a legitimate means of dialogue. Originally blunt and blunderbussy, it evolved into the kind of thrust-and-parry which went on through much of the nineteenth century, gradually shading by degrees into a finer and subtler form, before finally becoming inaudible and invisible altogether.

But four hundred years ago, such rhetorical altercations were often Olympian in magnitude—as illustrated, for instance, by Sylvius' attack on Vesalius. The one involving Ambroise Paré and the dean of the Faculté de Médecine, Étienne Gourmelen, was another example. The probable origin of the feud lay in Gourmelen's book *Surgical Synopsis*. When it was translated from Latin into French by one of the surgeons of St. Côme in 1571, both author and translator expected the vernacular text to be a great success among their colleagues. However, its popularity was totally eclipsed when Paré brought forth his own next publication, *Five Books of Surgery,* the following year. Alas, poor Gourmelen; neither his Latin text nor its French translation ever required a second edition. He and his supporters craved revenge, and the charges bounced back and forth for a while. The affair reached a head in 1581, when Gourmelen produced three new books on surgery, and used them as a vehicle with which to attack Paré. Unfortunately for him, he made the mistake of concentrating the major ordnance of his offensive against the doctrine that Paré could most easily defend, his use of the ligature in amputations. Attempting to defeat a more powerful enemy by frontal attack on his strongest position has never been a recommended tactic in any war, and it resulted only in the annihilation of Gourmelen by his adversary. Paré responded by writing his *Apologie and Treatise,* in which he not only fought back, but went on to an overwhelming counterattack characterized by his usual "authority, reason and experience," and also by sarcasm and an autobiographical catalogue of his contributions extending over a surgical lifetime. Gourmelen was left figuratively twitching in the dust, with his only reply being a paper best described in Montaigne's words as "feeble in reason and rich in insults." He dared not even sign this libelous attack, which appeared over the name of one of his pupils.

Still, posterity should be grateful to Gourmelen. Otherwise forgotten, his writings did serve a useful purpose: they stimulated the greatest surgeon of the premodern period to write a short, highly literate account of his experiences, his teachings, and his times. That book, Ambroise Paré's last published work, has come down to our generation as one of the gems of surgical literature.

The *Apologie and Treatise* plunges directly into its purpose. As promised, the voice of authority

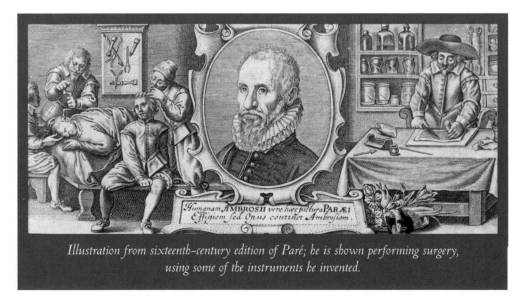

Illustration from sixteenth-century edition of Paré; he is shown performing surgery, using some of the instruments he invented.

is invoked first. It might be asked how it came about that a barber-surgeon whose only language was French should be so familiar with the writings of authors both ancient and recent, virtually all of whom used either Latin or Greek. Although historians point out that translations of many of Paré's sources were becoming available, this cannot be the only answer. We know that he became rich, and we know that he accumulated a large library. It is probable that he paid scholars to translate sections of medical books for him, and he may even have sometimes arranged the Renaissance equivalent of the modern-day reference search. It is otherwise difficult to imagine how he could have been familiar with so many sources. In fact, two hundred authors are listed as bibliographic references in the *Complete Works*.

Having invoked the voice of authority, he turns to reason to support his argument and then provides a series of case histories. So much had Paré's own accomplishments by this time served to elevate his position, as well as the status of the surgical art generally, that he feels free to insult the lofty professor of internal medicine. Not only does he address him as "my little master," but he ridicules a group of operations recommended by Gourmelen in his own surgical text. He compares his adversary to a presumptuous "young lad of Brittany, of plump buttocks" who claims to be able to play the organ when all he can do is to blow on the bellows. Book learning is worth nothing without practice, he chides; "you have not gone from your study or the schools. . . . The labourer doth little profit by talking of the seasons, or discussing of the manner or tilling the earth, or showing what seeds are proper to each soil; all of this is nothing if he does not put his hand to the plough,

and couple the oxen together." He quotes the first-century medical encyclopedist Cornelius Celsus: "Diseases are not to be cured by eloquence, but by remedies well and duly applied." The remainder of the brief volume describes those "remedies well and duly applied," beginning with Paré's first campaign in 1537 and ending with the voyage to Flanders in 1569. By the time of that voyage Ambroise Paré was at the peak of his fame; he was generally considered to be the leading surgeon of Europe. Other than the great contributions of Vesalius himself, there were no books more influential than those written by his pen. His method of dramatic narrative, appearing deceptively simple in construction, was so skillfully handled that there could be found no way to improve upon it. One would have had to look to the writers of the Bible to find such turbulent events recounted in so plain a declarative style, such profound lessons being taught with such economy of language.

Ambroise Paré's method of communicating his message affected the future of surgery as profoundly as the message itself—a situation that has reappeared again and again in the history not only of medicine but of all knowledge. For Paré, the medium was vernacular writing. Before his time, the barber-surgeons did not publish their experiences, nor did they have easy access to the authorities of previous ages, who wrote in Latin. Teaching was by master-barbers, and it was practical, verbal, and visual. Even the lofty surgeons of the College of St. Côme used Latin, as they found it so necessary to imitate the better-educated medical faculty. Occasionally a volume would be translated into a contemporary language, but the chosen works were sometimes undistinguished and the translations often stiff and difficult to follow. Then, along came Ambroise Paré to write in a simple conversational French comprehensible to all. His familiarity with classical writers, his excellent training at the Hôtel Dieu, his vast experience on the battlefield, and his logical method of problem-solving gave him the paradigmatic qualifications to learn, to invent, and to instruct. To these he added an almost artless lucidity of expression that makes him an exemplar of the highest standard in the narrative method of medical teaching. Living as he did in an era when it was commonplace for competing luminaries to attack one another in print, he had the added advantage of being able to anticipate or answer objections from less skillful thinkers. All in all, as the phrase-smiths of our time would say, a good read.

In the books of Ambroise Paré are to be found any number of passages that are of considerable interest to modern readers. Not only do such passages illuminate Paré's thinking, but they sometimes reveal a level of surgical sophistication that may seem surprising for four centuries ago. For example, at the defeat of the French at Hedin in 1553, he was called upon to treat an officer among whose other injuries was a gaping wound through which air was being sucked into the chest. He packed the wound with an oil-soaked sponge "to stay the flow of blood, and to hinder that the outward air did not enter

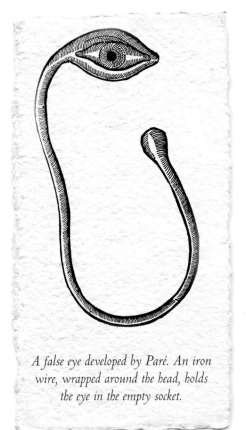

A false eye developed by Paré. An iron wire, wrapped around the head, holds the eye in the empty socket.

into the breast." He placed the sponge in such a way "that egress might be given for the blood that was spilt within the Thorax." From his description it appears that he had created a loosely packed wad that functioned as a one-way valve until he was able to prepare the plasters and bandages that were used to stabilize the patient's flailing chest.

It is clear that observation of many such wounds had convinced him of certain cardinal points of treatment that thoracic surgeons would only begin to appreciate 350 years later: stop the uncontrolled to-and-fro of air, relieve pressure by evacuating blood, and stabilize the chest wall.

Paré was captured during this battle, but he secured his release, as described earlier, by the successful treatment of a chronic ulceration on the leg of one of the emperor's colonels. His description of this event contains a scene reminiscent of present-day bedside rounds made by an attending surgeon for junior house staff, as he demonstrated to the colonel's medical retainers not only the physical findings in the patient's leg, but also the fact that the ulcer was associated with "a great varicose vein which did perpetually feed it." His treatment consisted, as would that of a twentieth-century vascular surgeon, of excising the ulcer, and applying a paste-boot up to the knee. Bed rest was ordered, and the leg gradually healed. The only thing missing from a modern clinical report is the skin graft. And for those who think that before-and-after images began with the elegant cameras of latter-day plastic surgeons, it should be noted that Paré had an equally effective means of demonstrating improvement. He "took a piece of paper, and cut it the largeness of the ulcer, which I gave him, and kept as much myself," to convince his patient of the progress of the cure, should there be any doubt.

Paré's only mention of any form of anesthesia occurs in his chapter on the battles in Flanders. Herein he recommends that opium and henbane be used to help an injured patient sleep. In spite of the scarcity of references to such things, he must have used these drugs frequently, as did virtually all surgeons of the time. Even the most stone-hearted of surgical artisans tried to lessen the agonies of their operations with these agents, or mandrake, or strong spirits. They were also commonly employed to soothe convalescing men, or to ease the way of others toward the grave.

In these electronic 1980s, the armamentarium of slumber-device technology is vast, and includes one enterprising manufacturer's tape recording of gently falling rain to lull even the most thought-tossed mind into the gentle embrace of Morpheus. How would the mahatmas of the U.S. Patent Office react if they were told that Ambroise Paré had thought of it first? "One may cause it to rain artificially by pouring down from some high place into a kettle, so that it makes such a noise that the patient may hear it, and by these means shall sleep be provoked on him." Renaissance or modern, a good idea is a good idea.

There are other rewards in the *Apologie and Treatise*. Some of the phrasing quoted earlier from the author's declamation against the use of gunpowder and firearms is reminiscent of the exhortations of the Biblical prophets raging against the sins of mankind. To wit: "The thunder, by its noise as a messenger sent before, foretells the storm at hand; but, which is the chief mischief, this infernal engine roars as it strikes, and strikes as it roars, sending at one and the same time the deadly bullet into the breast and the horrible noise into the ear."

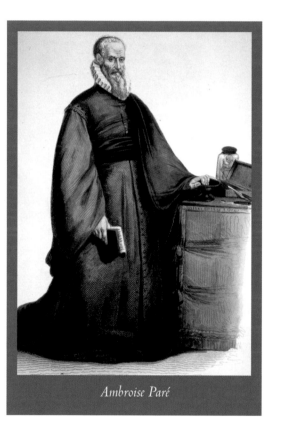

Ambroise Paré

The repeated resonances appear to be a deliberate literary device, aiding the author in his effort to make the chapter "an ornament and grace to this my whole treatise." Likewise, the correspondence of ideas expressed in two successive lines which is so characteristic of Old Testament poetry is detectable in the following passages, which are here again quoted, this time printed in such a way as to emphasize the point, in two distinct verses:

Thunder and lightning commonly gives but one blow, or stroke, and that commonly strikes but one man of a multitude; But one great cannon at one shot may spoil and kill a hundred men.

And:

Wherefore we all of us rightfully curse the author of so pernicious an engine; On the contrary praise those to the skies, who endeavor by words and pious exhortations to dehort kings from their use.

This is expository poetry of a Biblical sort, composed by a Renaissance prophet whose first teacher was a chaplain, and whose first textbook had been translations of the ancient scrolls of Israel.

There has been more than a modicum of jumping back and forth in this chapter, as I have sought to put the life and the contributions of Ambroise Paré into the context from which they arose. I have attempted to describe his humanity in an age of cruelty, his simplicity in an age of arrogance, his objectivity in an age of superstition, his originality in an age of conservatism, his independence in an age of authority, his logical rationality in an age of illogical irrational theories, and his deep moral sense in an age when pragmatic hypocrisy reigned and massacres were perpetrated in the name of sectarian religion.

With his extraordinary powers of observation and his ability to draw universal conclusions from the evidence of his experience, Ambroise Paré begins to approach the great clinical scientists of a later era. But there is a difference, and it is a difference which brings him closer to the ancients than to the moderns. For Ambroise Paré was much less fascinated by the process of disease than he was by the patient, a fellow human being in distress.

This was the old Hippocratic concept, and it was to the objective of restoring the inner equilibrium of the total person that much of Greek therapy was directed. Because this approach led to serious errors in the understanding of the specifics of disease, it gradually came to mean less, as the study of pathologic anatomy came to mean more, near the end of the eighteenth century. As medical investigators focused first on organs, then on cells, then on molecules, it became more and more difficult to see the whole frightened, sick patient who had come for help. To our enchantment by the details of the disease process we owe the great strides that modern medical science has made. But it is to that same driving force that we owe our lessened ability, although we would wish it otherwise, to appreciate the burdens of those who suffer the diseases we treat so well.

So, Paré's motivations were less to understand a pathological process than to relieve the suffering of a wounded or sick patient. This is clear from every description he writes. He looked for methods that worked, and he taught them to everyone who would learn. In this he was more like his predecessors than like his successors. He discarded those ideas of his medical forebears that did not seem to result in effective treatment, and he championed those ideas that he could confirm. He was a giant standing on the shoulders of giants—of Hippocrates, of Galen, and of his near-contemporary Andreas Vesalius. He planted his feet firmly where their teachings supported the weight of his experience, and he avoided the soft places where they could not hold him up. Thus securely braced, he saw further than any surgeon had ever done, and he saw more clearly.

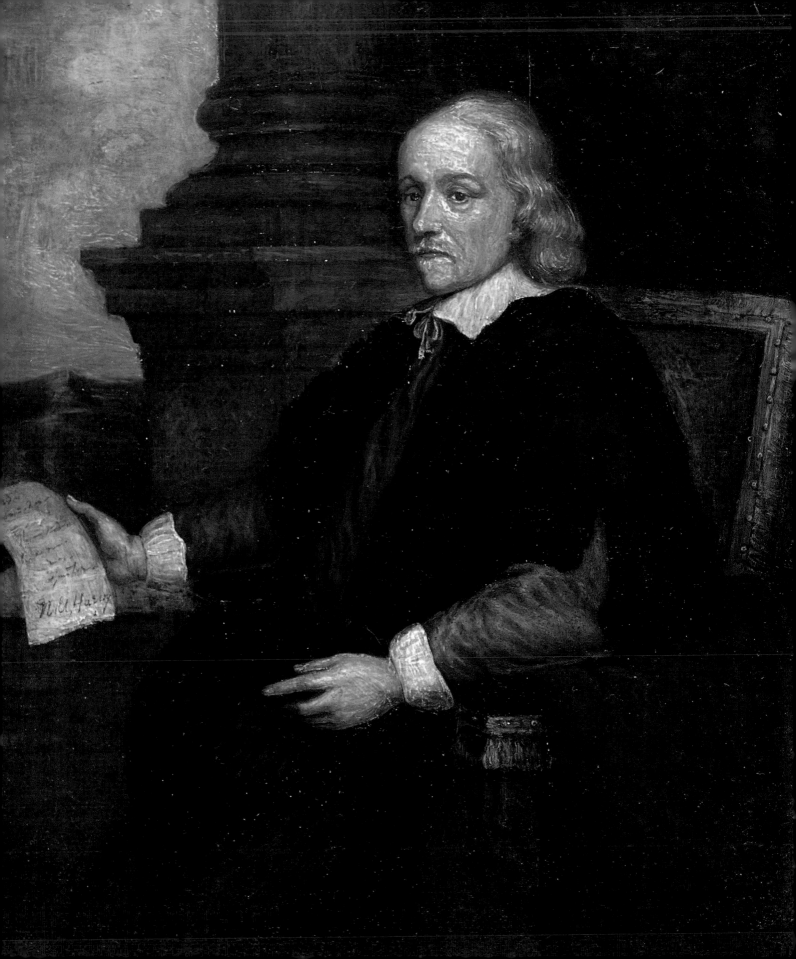

5

"NATURE HERSELF MUST BE OUR ADVISOR"

William Harvey's Discovery of the Circulation of the Blood

Dr. William Harvey was a student of the classics. Fluent in Greek and Latin, schooled in the works of the ancient world's greatest writers, he admitted only a few post-antiquity scholars into his personal pantheon of literary immortals. For the contemporary men of letters whose publications were widely read in seventeenth-century England, he had no use at all. He referred to the era in which he lived as "this age, in which the crowd of writers devoid of taste is as numerous as a swarm of flies on a very hot day, and we are almost stifled by the stench of their thin and trifling productions." He did not hesitate to offer his opinion of that "crowd of writers" in the blunt and earthy terms that so easily slipped off the tongue in those more direct days—he called them a pack of shit-britches.

A listing of the shit-britches whose works were popular at the time would include some familiar names, among them Ben Jonson, Christopher Marlowe, Edmund Spenser, Francis Bacon, and the three Johns: Donne, Dryden, and Milton. The most befouled undergarments of the day must surely have been those worn by that prolific producer William Shakespeare. If the list does not bring much honor to the memory of Dr. Harvey, there are nevertheless not many people who would deny him forgiveness. In the first place, no one has ever demanded of scientists that they be paragons of literary taste. And, more to the point, William Harvey can be forgiven just about anything; criticism of his few quirks is properly drowned in the clamor of humanity's gratitude. For it was he who bestowed the greatest gift ever made by one man to the science and art of medicine—the discovery of the circulation of the blood.

With that single step, Harvey solved the most elusive puzzle that had delayed the progress of medicine, while at the same time introducing, or rather reintroducing, physicians to the concept of experimentation, and making it a principal medium of biological research. With the unique exception of Louis Pasteur, he is the most honored of all of the great contributors to medical knowledge. There are Harvey Societies, Harvey Prizes, and periodic Harvey Commemorations. One of the highest distinctions that can be awarded to a leader of British medicine is to be chosen to deliver the Annual Harveian Oration of the Royal College of Physicians; to be named Harveian Orator is to be recognized for a lifetime of singular accomplishment. In the cold index of worth that serves in the marketplace, the small volume in which Harvey propounded his doctrine in 1628 has become the most valuable medical book ever written, each of the few remaining copies of the first edition having reached a sale price of more than $300,000, and rising fast. By the time you read these words, the book will cost much more.

To appreciate the grandeur of Harvey's achievement, it is necessary to map out the terrain on which it took place. In 1543, Andreas Vesalius had made a revolution in anatomy. The Galenic image of man's body had been overthrown, and the reality of human structure was no longer the subject of inference and conjecture. But the young Belgian had done more than merely replace the ancient errors with facts; in disagreeing with revered authority, he had demonstrated the importance of skepticism, of believing nothing valid unless it could be verified by anyone who took the pains to evaluate evidence. More than anything else, he had created an atmosphere in which anyone who cared and dared to make independent observations was no longer hampered by the inherited erroneous speculations that were the accepted wisdom of the time. It was an intellectual mood that nurtured the curiosity of Galileo, Newton, Boyle,

and a small group of somewhat less brilliant but equally determined men of talent. To that mood we owe the fact that modern science was born in the seventeenth century. Among the foremost of its begetters was William Harvey.

Though no longer able to suppress the emerging truths of anatomical structure, the long-dead hand of Galen still lay cold and heavy on all understanding of bodily function. To the physicians of the early seventeenth century, the liver continued to be the source of all the blood, which was thought to be constantly manufactured in that organ's ample spongy depths from the digested food brought to it from the intestine. Once the food was converted into blood, it was sent out to all parts of the body via the veins, drenching the tissues with dark red fluid which was constantly being replenished as it was consumed by the tissues, as in some ceaseless irrigation system. The right side of the heart was seen merely as a specialized part of the system of veins, functioning to transmit blood to nourish the lungs. Galen further taught that some of the blood that reached the right side of the heart flowed through pores in the septum dividing it from the left. Although Vesalius had not been able to find those pores, that exploder of Galen's anatomy remained so strongly under the influence of his predecessor's abstruse theorizing that he assumed the blood to make its way to the left side by some process similar to sweating. In the left ventricle, it presumably mixed with the pneuma, the spiritual essence which had been inhaled through the lungs. The mixture of blood and this vital substance, warmed by the innate heat, was then driven out into the arteries by the ventricle. There were thus two separate sorts of blood, the darker venous kind, which supplied nourishment, and the bright-red arterial kind, which brought life itself by means of the pneuma and the innate heat. Galen had no idea of the circulation to and from the lungs, believing that the blood flowed into those structures merely to nourish them. The lung's imagined function was to inhale the pneuma into the body and to transport it to the left ventricle. That there was not a shred of evidence to support any of this theoretical formulation seemed to bother no one. It was true because the immortal Galen said it was true, and it had been accepted without question for nearly a millennium and a half.

(Several writers had actually understood the true nature of the passage of blood between the heart and lungs, the so-called lesser circulation. However, their explanations never reached the light of general awareness. One of them, the Spanish physician Michael Servetus, produced a generally correct description which was written into a tractate, the *Christianismi Restitutio,* considered heretical by the church, as were other of his publications. In Calvinism's capital, Geneva, with the connivance of Calvin himself, Servetus was put to the stake in 1553, and his writings on the lesser circulation were consigned to the pyre along with the book of his life.)

The man who was destined to advance medical knowledge far enough to put it out of the reach of both Galenic authority and religious stricture was born on April 1, 1578, in Folkestone, on the Kentish coast of England. William Harvey was the first of "a week of sons" and two daughters of Joan and Thomas Harvey, the latter a self-made man of business and international trade. As young William grew up, his father's enterprises prospered, so that the boy never wanted for comfort or the good uses to which money can be put. He was the only one of Thomas' sons who was not attracted to the world of commerce. Five of them became foreign traders of the type known in the City of London as Turkey merchants, so called because they were engaged in trade with the East. They saw to it that their talented eldest brother had ample means to pursue his medical interests. Eliab Harvey, who eventually became the wealthiest of the clan, went so far as to manage William's financial affairs for him, so that throughout his life he had no need to think about such worldly matters as might distract less well-attended men.

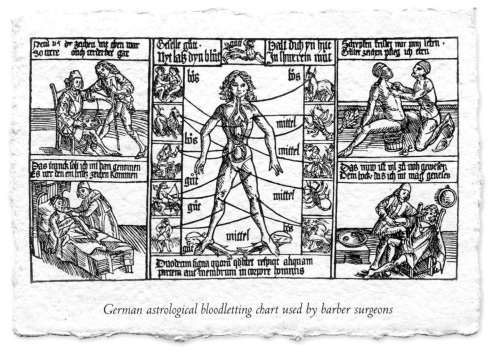

German astrological bloodletting chart used by barber surgeons

Young William began his formal education at the age of ten, being sent to Canterbury to enroll at the King's School, whose statutes demanded of its students that "whatever they are doing, in earnest or in play, they shall never use any language but Latin or Greek." Thus, like his predecessor at Galen-smashing, Andreas Vesalius, William Harvey learned early in life to be at ease with the rhythms and nuances of the languages of antiquity. When he was sixteen, he enrolled at Gonville and Caius College of Cambridge, whose latter name derived from the Dr. John Caius who had for a time shared lodgings with Vesalius at Padua. As might be expected, Caius College attracted students who were interested in the study of medicine, as it continues to do today. When Harvey was in attendance, the bodies of two executed criminals were dissected each year for the purpose of instruction in anatomy, so that by the time he received his B.A. degree in 1597, he had had considerable exposure to the difficulties inherent in the interpretation of observed anatomical structures.

It was only natural that the embryonic physician should next matriculate at Padua. For the reasons given in Chapter 3, that university provided the most open atmosphere in Europe in which to study any of the classical four disciplines of law, theology, medicine, and philosophy. So safe an academic haven was it for Protestants and Jews that when Pius IV, Pope from 1559 to 1565, tried by papal bull to prevent non-Catholics from obtaining degrees, Venice replied by turning over the degree-granting power to the Palatine counts, thus taking it away from the Pope. Padua had the added advantage of being a university organized around its students; indeed, the young men controlled much of the governance of the school,

including the employing of the faculty. The students from various countries were organized into groups called "Nations," each of which elected a representative councillor, and the councillors, together with the rectors, constituted the executive body of the university.

But the primary attraction of Padua was its galaxy of faculty stars, past and contemporary. Its greatest adornment in the eyes of William Harvey was Giralomo Fabrizio, called Fabricius of Aquapendente, the successor of the equally talented Gabriele Fallopio, for whom are named the delicate tubes through which each generation's eggs must pass on their way to reproductive assignation. The fact that Galileo Galilei was Professor of Mathematics at the university seems not to have been a factor or an influence. It was Fabricius who became Harvey's most adored teacher, his studies of the chick embryo and the formation of the fetus determining in large part the direction which some of the English physician's later research would take. Perhaps of most specific effect on the eventual discovery of the circulation was Fabricius' description of the valves in the veins. Late in his life, Harvey would tell Robert Boyle that it was his realization of the one-way function of the valves directing blood back to the heart that led him to his great contribution, an insight that grew out of the anatomical findings of his mentor and friend Fabricius.

Harvey thrived in the academic and social freedom of Padua. He was elected Councillor for the English Nation, a distinction which entitled him to have his coat of arms, or stemma, painted in a prominent place in the Great Hall of the university. Two of Harvey's self-designed stemmata can be seen to this day on the curved ceiling of the lower loggia as one leaves the location of the old anatomical theater. The Master and Fellows of Caius College had them restored soon after their rediscovery in 1893. They are identical to the coat of arms which appears on William Harvey's doctoral diploma from Padua, dated April 25, 1602.

The diploma itself is an ornate thing, enumerating its owner's qualifications and privileges in the hyperbolic terms that were the style of the day. It goes on to provide a graphic description of the graduation ceremony:

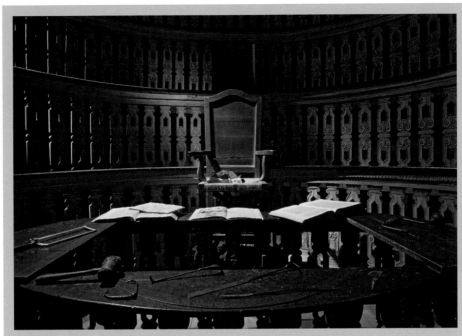

In this amphiteater at Padua, demonstrations in anatomy were made as early as 1500.

> *Johannes Thomas Minadous did then solemnly decorate and adorn the same noble William Harvey (who in a most perspicuous oration asked for and accepted them) with the accustomed Insignia and ornaments belonging to a Doctor: For he delivered to him certain books of Philosophy and of Medicine, first closed and then, a little while after, open; he put a golden ring on his finger, he placed on his head the cap of a Doctor, as an emblem of the Crown of Virtue, and bestowed on him the Kiss of Peace with the Magistral Benediction.*

The diploma was granted by Sigismund de Capilisti, Count Palatine, a nonecclesiastical appointee of the Venetian Senate. It was in the count's palace that the ceremony took place.

Harvey took his ring, his cap, and the lingering traces of Minadous' scholastic smooch and headed back home to England. He applied for, and was granted, membership in the College of Physicians, and he soon began to take an active role in its affairs. In the same year, 1604, he married Elizabeth, daughter of Dr. Lancelot Browne, formerly a physician to the Virgin Queen and now performing the same office for King James I. Ironically, Elizabeth Browne had a brother named Galen.

Very little is known about the marriage, except that it was childless, that Mrs. Harvey owned a pet parrot, and that she predeceased her husband by more than a decade. Indeed, not a great deal is known about William either, if we are seeking clues to his personal life or his character. We must rely on a few traces that are to be found in contemporary writings, and these are sketchy at best. The most detailed source is a relatively brief biographical essay written by John Aubrey, who became a friend of Harvey's in 1651, when he was twenty-five and the famed physician was seventy-three. The essay was included in the volume later published as *Aubrey's Brief Lives*, which also contains material concerning Shakespeare, Milton, and Hobbes. Aubrey's biography of Harvey is a hodgepodge of unorganized observations, judgments, and just enough hearsay to cast doubt on the historical value of some of its details. Because he knew Harvey well only in the great doctor's later years, he depended on secondhand information for many of the statements he made about his subject's character and his reputation as a physician during his professional career. A certain wryness, moreover, seems to have crept into the old man's personality in his last years, as witness his comments on literature. Sir Geoffrey Keynes, author of the definitive study of William Harvey's work, says of Aubrey that he was "curious, credulous, and unmethodical. It is admitted that he was often inaccurate, but he was never untruthful, a distinction of great importance in estimating the value of reportage such as he provides." In a letter to Anthony Wood, the seventeenth-century Oxford historian, Aubrey commented on his own attitude toward the writing of biography:

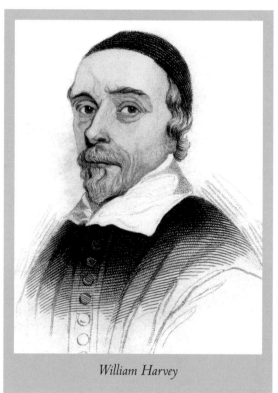
William Harvey

I here lay down to you the Trueth, and as neer as I can and that religiously as a Poenitent to his Confessor, nothing but the trueth; the naked plain trueth, which is here exposed so bare that the very pudenda are not covered, and affords many passages that would raise a Blushe in a young Virgin's cheeks. So that after your perusal, I must desire you to make a castration and to sowe on some Figge-leaves—i.e., to be my Index Expurgatorious.

For better or for worse, Aubrey is virtually all we have to go on, so it is his description on which we must rely. Of Harvey's appearance, he tells us, "He was not tall, but of the lowest stature, round faced, olivaster like wainscott in complexion, little eie, round, very black, full of spirit; his hair was black as a Raven, but quite white twenty yeares before he died." The reliability of these details, at least, is supported by portraits of Harvey made when he was in his middle years.

Unlike Galen, Paré, and Vesalius, William Harvey did not wax autobiographical in his writings. We therefore have no way of analyzing his own words or using his self-descriptions to fill out the many gaps in the vague general image of his personality that has been left to us. Aubrey would give us to believe that he had in him an irascible streak that was easily roused: "He was, as all the rest of the Brothers, very Cholerique; & in his younge days wore a dagger . . . but this Dr. would be apt to draw out his dagger upon every slight occasion." That this meant he was so easy to anger as to reach for his blade at minimal provocation is less likely than the more satisfactory interpretation that he was simply fidgety, with a superabundance of energy. We have a brief note in a letter by Harvey's friend Lord Arundel that supports this contention, in which the nobleman refers to him as "the little perpetual movement called Dr. Harvey." Had the frequent unsheathing of his dagger meant anything more provocative than a bit of nervous hyperactivity, we can be sure that he would not have survived whole into his eightieth year. Aubrey further tells us, "He was hot-headed, and his thoughts working would many times keepe him from sleepinge; he told me that then his way was to rise out of his Bed and walke about his Chamber in his Shirt till he was pretty coole, i.e., till he began to have a horror [a chill], and then returns to bed and sleeps very comfortably."

What emerges, then, is the image of an olive-complected, dark-eyed man of quite slight stature, filled with nervous energy of the high-output kind. But though his physical movements may have been fitful, his brain was filled with purpose, and there was nothing aimless or twitchy about the way that gifted cerebral organ functioned.

Year after year, decade after decade, century after century, Harveian Orators have found themselves stymied for original ways to describe the great man of whom they must speak. The magnitude of the problem has been discussed by many of them, but has never been better stated

that it was in 1929 by Sir Wilmot Herringham. His comments on the matter are to be found not in his actual address, but in a series of letters he wrote to his American friend Harvey Cushing during the months of preparation. The Yale Medical Historical Library contains a collection of the Orations dating from 1661 to 1975, most of which were originally the property of Cushing. While reading through them I found several handwritten notes tucked into the slim volume of Sir Wilmot's speech, one of which begins with the following plaintive gnashing of literary teeth:

Dear Cushing:
Jan. 13, 1929
 You are quite right. This beastly little man is making me work night and day. The little brute wrote practically no letters, or rather there are hardly any preserved—and there is nothing to go upon but casual remarks in other documents. Even these are extraordinarily sparse. Etc.

By the time Herringham came to deliver what he called in this letter "the Oration, which may the devil damn," in October, he had cooled down enough so that he expressed all of his investigative frustration in the opening sentence, whose calm words provide for us a fine example of the understatement for which his nation is so justly celebrated: "Harvey seems to have had an unusual capacity for slipping through the world unnoticed."

Now, all of the foregoing should be looked upon as an explanation of just why it is that the remainder of this essay deals almost not at all with the man Harvey who did scientific work, but rather with the scientific work itself, and its significance to medical progress.

Shortly after being elected a full Fellow of the College of Physicians in 1607, Harvey was named

Assistant Physician to St. Bartholomew's Hospital, a distinction that added significantly to the growth of his private medical practice. Throughout his life he would remain what we call in the twentieth century a clinician-researcher, a doctor who is both an investigator and a healer of the sick. Actually, his practice was from the beginning a flourishing one, at least if one uses his attractiveness to high-bred patients as a criterion; in time he became physician to James I and later to Charles I, as well as to many members of the aristocracy, among them the Lord Chancellor, Sir Francis Bacon.

There is a touch of irony here. It is to Bacon that historians give credit for being the first elucidator of the method of inductive reasoning, and therefore of what we are pleased to call the "scientific method" (of which more later). It is to Harvey, though, that the credit is given for being the first physician actually to apply the Baconian approach. Bacon himself never used his own formulation, and there is no evidence that Harvey, who did use it, was influenced by Bacon at all. In fact, the two seem to have had very little regard for each other as scientific thinkers. Harvey said of his distinguished patient that he "writes philosophy [the word "philosophy" was often used synonymously with "science"] like a Lord Chancellor; I have cured him of it."

During these early years of practice, Harvey found time to carry out investigations in anatomy and in physiology, the ways in which the various parts of the body function, and he rapidly became known not only as a very capable physician, but also as one who was already well on his way to becoming a productive researcher, if we may use that term for the relatively primitive studies that could be done by medical men of that period. In 1615, he was appointed, although still considered a very junior physician, to the major post of Lumleian Lecturer of the College of Physicians. This lecture series had been founded by John, Lord Lumley, in 1582 for the purpose of instruction in anatomy and surgery. By its terms, a leading Fellow of the College was appointed to give two public lectures each week in a six-year cycle, the appointment being for life. Harvey served until 1656, when he voluntarily gave up the office at the age of seventy.

William Harvey gave his first Lumleian Lecture on the morning of Tuesday, April 16, 1616, exactly one week before the death in Stratford-on-Avon of William Shakespeare. His lecture notes were for two centuries thought to be lost; they were rediscovered in the British Museum in 1876. Since then, those manuscripts have been subjected to such meticulous scrutiny that it is possible to say with certainty that Harvey began to consider the great themes of his magnum opus on the circulation long before its eventual publication in 1628. What follows is a general outline of his thesis and the way

> *Throughout his life he would remain what we call in the twentieth century a clinician-researcher, a doctor who is both an investigator and a healer of the sick.*

in which it developed, as gleaned from the lecture notes and the book itself, *Exercitatio Anatomica de Motu Cordis et Sanquinis in Animalibus*, (in English, *Anatomical Studies on the Motion of the Heart and Blood in Animals*), or, in historian's shorthand, *De Motu Cordis*.

Excellent studies by several scholars in recent decades point to the probability that Harvey's discovery of the circulation took place in two quite separate stages, apparently as much as ten years apart. In this view, presented in its most articulate form by Jerome Bylebyl of the Johns Hopkins Institute of the History of Medicine, Harvey originally set out to solve the ages-old mysteries of the heartbeat and the pulse, and the relationship between the two. Having accomplished this, which he is thought to have done by the time he gave his first Lumleian Lecture in 1616, he wrote a treatise on the subject. Because the first half of *De Motu Cordis* stands as a coherent whole in which the physiology of the heart and arteries is analyzed and explained (without any reference to the circulation), it is thought that this section of the book is the original treatise. The remaining chapters, on the other hand, which introduced the concept that the blood travels through the body in a never-ending circular cycle, were written later. So it seems that in *De Motu Cordis* we have two separate pieces of research done at two separate periods of their author's life, and later joined together by him to form a complete description of the way in which the heart drives the blood around its circuit through the arteries out to the tissues and back again via the veins. In Bylebyl's words:

Thus it would appear that De Motu Cordis, *like the work which it reports, evolved in two distinct stages.*

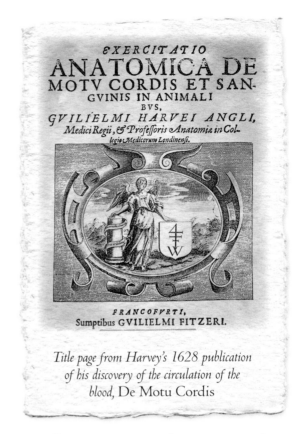

Title page from Harvey's 1628 publication of his discovery of the circulation of the blood, De Motu Cordis

Originally, Harvey seems to have written a self-contained treatise on the heartbeat and arterial pulse. Subsequently he changed his plans and decided to include the circulation as well. He then inserted chapters eight through sixteen into the earlier work, prefixed . . . a new introduction to the expanded treatise, and thereby transformed an important work into one of the greatest scientific masterpieces of all time.

The heartbeat and its relationship to the pulse had puzzled scholars since the days of Aristotle. Part squeeze, part squirm, each cardiac pulsation throbs and thrusts with such eye-wink quickness that physicians despaired of ever finding the secret of its mechanism or the sequence in which the stages of each major movement occur. In the words with which William Harvey begins the first chapter of *De Motu Cordis*, "When

I first tried animal experimentation for the purpose of discovering the motions and functions of the heart by actual inspection and not by other people's books, I found it so truly difficult that I almost believed with Fracastorius [Giralamo Fracastoro, a sixteenth-century Venetian polymath] that the motion of the heart was to be understood by God alone."

But Harvey persisted. Determined to decipher the meaning of what must at first have seemed to him to be a series of poorly coordinated twitches, "coming and going like a flash of lightning," he made observation after observation on a host of vivisected animals, before finally settling on creatures of the cold-blooded sort, particularly snakes, because of the slow beating of their hearts. He took advantage also of the opportunity presented "if one carefully observes the [dog and pig] heart as it moves more slowly when about to die. The movements then become slower and weaker and the pauses longer, so that it is easy to see what the motion really is and how made." Having myself spent many hundreds of hours in laboratories of surgery and physiology in the overseeing of dog hearts giving up their grasp on life, I can vouch for Harvey's veracity when he describes the pauses between beats and the almost languid motion of a mammal's last few cardiac pulsations before fibrillation or arrest.

By repeated experiments, Harvey proved to his own satisfaction that the heart contracts forcibly during the phase of its action called systole, so as to drive its contained blood out into the major arteries. As the heart contracts, it thrusts itself forward so that its apex strikes the chest wall, simultaneously with an expansile dilating of the arteries. Thus the pulse is synchronous with the

heart's contraction and is caused by it. This constantly reproducible finding disproved the old theory that an artery undergoes pulsatile dilatation on its own, as a result of independent active expansion of its wall. The Greeks, it will be recalled, had believed the pulse to be due to rhythmic expansion of the pneuma contained within the arteries. Harvey proved that it is produced by the heartbeat.

Further experimental observations showed that the atria (the upper reservoir chambers of the heart) contract just prior to the ventricles (the two powerful pumping chambers). Harvey demonstrated what a few earlier writers had only guessed at: once the blood leaves the ventricles, the great cardiac valves prevent its return into the heart, so that the flow of blood in the arteries is always outward to the periphery.

By the year 1616, Harvey had arrived at the major argument of his original treatise, the first half of *De Motu Cordis:* while the heart is relaxing between beats it is passively filled by blood flowing in from the periphery of the body by way of the two great veins entering its right side (the venae cavae) and by the great veins entering its left side returning blood from the lungs (the pulmonary veins). As the atria fill and overflow into the ventricles, they begin to contract, so that, as Harvey put it, they "arouse the somnolent heart." The atrial contraction is followed immediately by a similar contraction of the ventricular chambers, forcing the blood out of the right ventricle and into the main artery to the lungs (the pulmonary artery) and simultaneously out of the left ventricle into the main artery to the periphery (the aorta). This means that the only active coordinated movement of the heart is the contraction of the atria spreading to the ventricle, which expels blood centrifugally out into the major vessels to produce the pulse wave, the effect of which is that "all the arteries of the body respond as my breath blown into a glove."

The circuit within the chest had been established—the blood enters the heart from the venae cavae, is driven through the lungs by the right ventricle, returns to the left side, and is then pumped out by the left ventricle into the aorta and thence to the rest of the body. This is the thesis that grew out of the experiments described in the early chapters of *De Motu Cordis:* a complete understanding of the motion of the heart and major vessels, and an explanation of the movement of blood through the lungs. So far, all conclusions had been based upon observations made during experiments in which the cardiac and vascular structures were exposed to Harvey's scrutiny. It should not escape notice that all of the observations had thus far been qualitative—no measurements had been used. Above all, not a word had yet been said about the general circulation to the body.

It is in the second half of *De Motu Cordis* that Harvey grappled with a question to which his predecessors had never thought to turn their attention, since its answer was believed to be known—

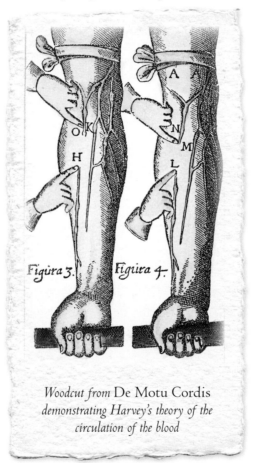

Woodcut from De Motu Cordis *demonstrating Harvey's theory of the circulation of the blood*

the actual pathway followed by the blood en route to the tissues. In mapping the correct pathway, he was aided by something new and something old. The something new was his introduction into medical research of the use of measurement. All historians would agree with the statement made by Chauncey Leake in a footnote to his 1913 translation of *De Motu Cordis:* "The introduction of quantitative evidence into physiological problems was Harvey's great philosophical contribution, and he apparently realized it, for he uses it again and again with telling effect."

Harvey's "quantitative evidence" was, by today's exacting standards, crude. But in the long history of science, no single set of measurements has ever been made to greater effect. He estimated the fluid capacity of the human ventricle to be approximately two to three ounces. Given a normal cardiac rate of seventy-two beats per minute, over the course of one hour the heart must expel 2 × 72 × 60 or 8,640 ounces—that is, 540 pounds—of blood into the aorta. (Crude or not, Harvey's estimate agrees quite well with the results of cardiac output studies done today, using the finest artistry available to our space-age cardiologists.) But this is more than three times the weight of the average man, clearly disproving the Galenic doctrine that the blood is constantly being made anew in the liver from ingested food, and sent out to drench the tissues. Since such a vast amount of blood is discharged into the aorta, and since its source had already, in the first treatise, been shown to be the venae cavae, the obvious question is, from where does the venae cavae blood come? Its only possible source is the veins. The next logical step was to prove that blood in the veins travels only in a centripetal direction toward the venae cavae and the heart.

This is where the something old comes in. Harvey's teacher, Fabricius, had described the valves in the veins, but he had no idea of their purpose. Based on the Galenic doctrine that blood traveled centrifugally from the liver to nourish the tissues, he presumed that they functioned to slow the flow, in order not to inundate the periphery of the body. By the simple experiment of running a finger outward along a filled superficial vein, you can demonstrate on your own arm that the vessel fills from its more distant portion to its more central. Even the valves can be identified this way, as they bulge out, preventing backward flow. Several illustrations in *De Motu Cordis* show how this little auto-experiment can be done by any armchair physiologist.

Now, in Chapter VIII Harvey wrote:

On these and other such matters I pondered often and deeply. For a long time I turned over in my mind such questions as, how much blood is transmitted, and how short a time does its passage take. Not deeming it possible for the digested food mass to furnish such an abundance of blood . . . unless it somehow got back to the veins from the arteries and returned to the right ventricle of the heart, I began to think there was a sort of motion as in a circle.

Once the explanation had been considered, there was no denying its truth. Harvey summarized his theory of the circulation of the blood in Chapter XIV. The entire chapter is only one paragraph long, but what a thunderous paragraph it is:

It has been shown by reason and experiment that blood by the beat of the ventricles flows through the lungs and heart and is pumped to the whole body. There it passes through pores in the flesh into the veins through which it returns from the periphery everywhere to the center, from the smaller veins into the larger ones, finally coming to the vena cavae and right atrium. This occurs in such an amount, with such an outflow through the arteries, and such a reflux through the veins, that it cannot be supplied by the food consumed. It is also much more than is needed for nutrition. It must therefore be concluded that the blood in the animal body moves around in a circle continuously, and that the action or function of the heart is to accomplish this by pumping. This is the only reason for the motion and beat of the heart.

The last sentence deserves particular attention. No more pneuma, no more innate heat, and no more Galenic hocus-pocus. As Harvey wrote elsewhere, the concept of pneuma or vital spirit is "the common subterfuge of ignorance." The heart, once its function has been demystified, is found to be a straightforward mechanical device whose only purpose is to pump the blood continuously around its circuit. Harvey's theory is one that would have delighted the strictest of the Hippocratic physicians: it can be verified by simple observation and simple experiments. But for the first time in medical research, measurement had played a role as well.

There remained only one fly in the unguent of Harvey's new physiology—he could not explain the exact pathway by which the blood passed from the smallest arteries in the periphery into the smallest veins, so that it might start its journey back to the heart. He therefore hypothesized the existence (and thereby predicted the discovery) of what he called "pores," doubtless expecting that some future scientist would find them. His expectation was fulfilled. In the very year in which *De Motu Cordis* was published, the man was born who would, in 1660, demonstrate with a microscope the existence of capillaries, those filamentous miles of conduit through which blood streams on its way from the arterial to the venous side of the circulation. Five years later, that same skilled investigator, Marcello Malpighi of Bologna, proved the presence of red corpuscles, the little disks in which oxygen rides as though in high-speed railway cars to bring breath to the cells of the body.

Harvey mentioned another kind of pores in his dissertation, those that according to Galen allowed blood to pass from right ventricle to left so that it might mix with the vital spirit. These were the pores that Vesalius could not find, and over whose absence he sweated enough to compromise his usual principles in a weak-kneed disclaimer. Harvey was more forthright: "Damn it, no such pores exist, nor can they be demonstrated," he proclaims in the introduction to his book.

All of "the common subterfuge of ignorance" concerning the motion of the heart and the blood had been laid to rest. First with Andreas Vesalius and now with William Harvey, the medical world was beginning to awaken from the long sleep induced by the opiate of Galenism. Along with the rest of science and of culture, medicine stirred it-self during the course of that glorious seventeenth century and shook off the shackles of ignorance, of authority, and of the ancients. In 1664 one of the earliest of the scientist-philosophers, Henry Power, captured the essence of his era when he wrote of it:

This is the Age wherein all men's souls are in a kind of fermentation, and the spirit of wisdom and learning begins to mount and free itself from those drossy and earthy impediments wherewith it hath been so long clogged, and from the insipid phlegm and Caput Mortuum of useless notions, in which it has endured so violent and long a fixation. This is the Age wherein (methinks) Philosophy comes in with a

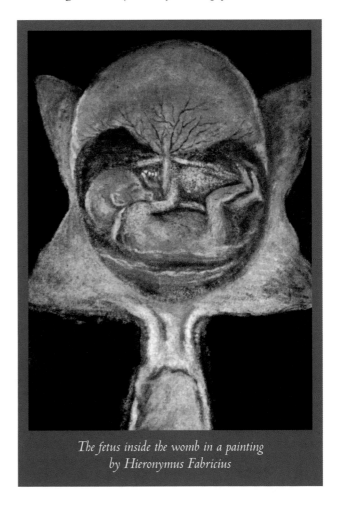

The fetus inside the womb in a painting by Hieronymus Fabricius

Spring-tide; and the peripateticks may as well hope to stop the current of the tide, or (with Xerxes) to fetter the ocean, as hinder the overflowing of free Philosophy: methinks, I see how all the old rubbish must be thrown away, and the rotten buildings be overthrown, and carried away with so powerful an inundation. These are the days that must lay a new foundation of a more magnificent Philosophy, never to be overthrown, that will empirically and sensibly canvass the phenomena of nature, deducing the causes of things from such originals in nature, as we observe are producible by Art and the infallible demonstration of mechanics. And certainly this is the way, and no other, to build a true and permanent Philosophy.

The seventeenth was the century of emergence. A profusion of genius appeared, in a quantity seen by no previous era in the history of western civilization, to bring the sciences and the humanities alike out of the long night. Harvey is almost lost in the throng of names whose mere listing will suffice to enumerate the great things that were accomplished in those hundred years. Only the best known are here mentioned, alphabetically for want of a more imaginative way; I tremble to think whom I may have left out: Bacon, Bernini, Bernouilli, Boyle, Brahe, Caravaggio, Cervantes, Corneille, Dekker, Descartes, Donne, Dryden, El Greco, Galileo Galilei, Halley, Hals, Hobbes, Hooke, Inigo Jones, Jonson, Kepler, La Fontaine, Leibnitz, Locke, Malpighi, Milton, Molière, Monteverdi, Newton, Pascal, Pepys, Racine, Rembrandt van Rijn, Rubens, Scarlatti, Shakespeare, Spinoza, van Leeuwenhoek, Velázquez, Vermeer, and Wren.

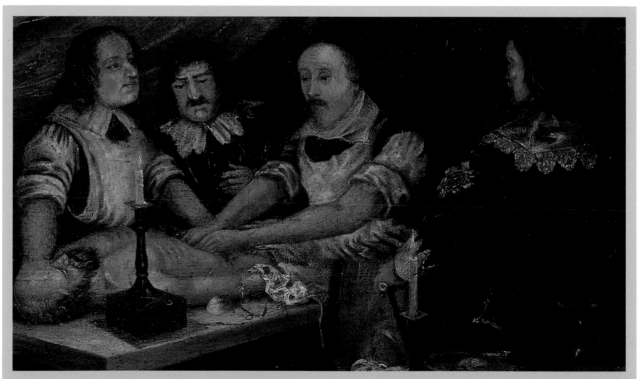

William Harvey dissecting the body of Thomas Parr, a man who supposedly lived for 152 years

These men inherited a darkened world and illuminated it. Their predecessors believed that everything was known that needed to be known. For them, the wisdom of the ancients was unassailable and their books as holy as scripture. But these builders of the seventeenth century were new men. They were the philosophers, and scientists, and writers, and musicians, and artists whose "souls are in a kind of fermentation." The scientific thinkers among them sought the truth that only experience and experiment could teach them, through the evidence of their senses. The ultimate test of that truth was that it could be demonstrated and confirmed by anyone who had the desire to learn—it had to be convincing to the most skeptical. Every one of those contributors to "the days that must lay a new foundation of a more magnificent Philosophy" knew the ground rules. William Harvey expressed them in a letter to the President and Fellows of the College of Physicians, which he used as a preface to his great book. Here are a few of the things he said:

I was greatly afraid lest I might be charged with presumption did I lay my work before the public at home, or send it beyond seas for impression, unless I had first proposed its subject to you, had confirmed its conclusions by ocular demonstrations in your presence, had replied to your doubts and objections, and secured the assent and support of our distinguished President. . . . For true philosophers, who are only eager for truth and knowledge, never regard themselves as already so thoroughly informed, but that they welcome further information from whomsoever and from whencesoever it may come; nor are they so narrow-minded as to imagine any of the arts or sciences transmitted to us by the ancients, in such a state of forwardness or completeness, that nothing is left for the ingenuity and industry of others;

very many, on the contrary, maintain that all we know is still infinitely less than all that still remains unknown; nor do philosophers pin their faith to others' precepts in such wise that they lose their liberty, and cease to give credence to the conclusions of their proper senses. Neither do they swear such fealty to their mistress Antiquity, that they openly, and in sight of all deny and desert their friend Truth. . . . I profess both to learn and to teach anatomy, not from books but from dissections; not from the positions of philosophers but from the fabric of nature. . . . I avow myself the partisan of truth alone; and I can indeed say that I have used all my endeavors, bestowed all my pains on an attempt to produce something that should be agreeable to the good, profitable to the learned, and useful to letters.

Farewell, most worthy Doctors,
And think kindly of your Anatomist,
William Harvey

De Motu Cordis is a small book of seventy-two pages, in quarto size of 5½ by 7½ inches. Viewed as an example of the printer's art, it is an undistinguished little product. When held in the hand, it seems of such minimal distinction as to be hardly worth notice. Some years ago, while visiting the medical library of a great American university, I was told a short sad story that speaks eloquent volumes about the humble appearance of the book. In the late 1940s the school's curator of medical history had discovered on the shelf of a London dealer an unrecognized one of the fifty-five copies of the modest little monograph still in existence. He paid the fifty-odd cents demanded for it by the unsuspecting merchant, and triumphantly bore his treasure home with him, where it became the jewel of his university's collection. Thirty years later, when its market value had soared to $125,000, it disappeared from the library while the collection was being moved into a new building; during the course of the move, it had been placed in a plain brown paper bag so as to conceal its true value. Because its rediscovery has never been reported by any of the small fraternity to whom such a treasure would probably be brought if stolen, it is presumed to have been thoughtlessly thrown into a heap of trash by a mover who took a quick glance at the apparently worthless contents of the bag.

As with the *Fabrica*, and all others of those revolutionary books of science, the publication of *De Motu Cordis* was greeted with approval by some and angry dissent by others. William Harvey was not a man who enjoyed acrimony or controversy. He did design some new experiments to strengthen a few of his arguments, and he even went so far as to reply to several of his critics, but beyond this he saved his restless energies for other things. In the Harveian Oration of 1662, Sir Charles Scarburgh, Harvey's devoted friend and personal physician, quoted him as saying:

It is of no great importance that I for my own gratification, should molest for a second time the republic of letters. I will not be the author or sponsor of any new controversial doctrine. Let my thoughts perish if they are worthless, my experiments if they are erroneous, or if I have not properly understood them. I am satisfied with my industry. It is not in my nature to upset the established order. If I am wrong (for after all I am but a man), let what I have written turn sour with neglect, but if I am right sometime at least the human race will not disdain the truth.

What is more notable than the controversy over Harvey's book is the fact that the new theory had little effect on the medical practice of the time, even in the hands of those who believed in it, including its author himself. This was because the long-accepted concept of to-and-fro motion of the blood had been used to explain the great majority of symptoms seen in daily clinical work, and it seemed to do so quite satisfactorily. It was believed that blood was capable of rapid changes in concentration and location in response to various sorts of stimuli. Thus emetics, poisons, foods, temperature changes, and local in-

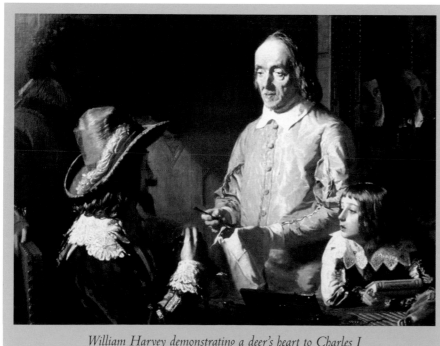

William Harvey demonstrating a deer's heart to Charles I

jury might cause blood to rush to or from a particular part of the body. Its increased presence might then be manifested in the form of redness, swelling, fever, bounding pulse, distended veins, or similar such identifiable signs; its relative absence might result in pallor, numbness, fainting, coldness, or weak pulse. Blood was thought to be capable of rapid movement inward to become concentrated in the center of the body or outward to the extremities. Because of this ability to expand, contract, or concentrate its volume in any area, an armamentarium had grown up of local or general treatment to stimulate the appropriate transport in such a way as to overcome the symptom-producing stimulus. This was done by bleeding, cupping, massage, and the application of tourniquets, all of which seemingly changed the volume of blood in a given location. The doctors of the time thought their treatment system worked. Even Harvey himself was unwilling to abandon the therapeutic methods which his experience told him were effective simply because he had disproved the theory on which they were based. Harvey's theory had to await more studies and better practical understanding of disease before it could become useful to physicians. More than a century went by before this began to happen.

Although the publication of *De Motu Cordis* had little effect on the way Harvey treated his patients, it did influence the course of his practice. Aubrey reports:

I have heard him say that after his Books of the Circulation of the Blood came out, that he fell mightily in his Practize and that 'twas beleeved by the vulgar that he was crack-brained. . . . With much ado at last, in about 20 or 30 yeares time, it was received in all the Univer-

sities in the world, &, as Mr. Hobbes sayes in his book de Corpore, he is the only man, perhaps, that ever lived to see his owne Doctrine established in his life-time.

Whatever decrease in his practice resulted from the publication of his book, Harvey seems after this point to have devoted more and more time to his relationship with King Charles, and less to his more ordinary patients. In addition, both before and after *De Motu Cordis*, he pursued ongoing researches in an area in which he had first become involved during his student days in Padua, the development of the embryo. Because there are references to generation, as it was called, in *De Motu Cordis*, it is very likely that Harvey had by 1628 already done considerable work on the problem and may even have begun to write a book. Over the years, he accumulated a wealth of observations, made with his naked eye and the use of a simple lens. Because the compound microscope was then on the verge of magnifying the visibility of the entire world of biological research, his conclusions proved to be of no lasting value, in spite of their general accuracy. The book he published in 1651, *De Generatione Animalium (The Generation of Animals)*, is nevertheless of continuing interest because it sheds light on those methods of gathering evidence which had resulted in the discovery of the circulation. Particularly in the introduction to the treatise, its author describes the ways in which he sought out truth. From these and other writings, there emerges a palpable reconstruction of a thinking pattern that in all branches of knowledge characterized the differences between the thinkers of the seventeenth century and (almost) all who had gone before. We are dealing here with the origins of the scientific method.

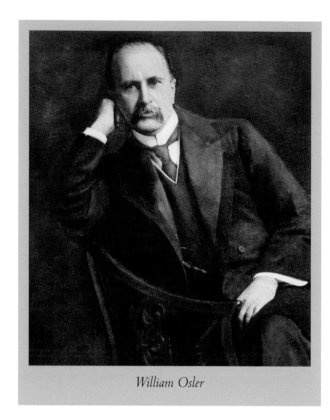

William Osler

If a single particular may be said to differentiate this developing science of the period from the thought patterns that preceded it, then it is this: the philosophers of the seventeenth century were more interested in answering questions that begin with the word *how* than in trying to figure out the *why*. Harvey himself put it quite clearly when he wrote, "I own that I am of the opinion that our first duty is to enquire whether the thing be or not, before asking wherefore it is." In other words, the objective of the scientist must not be to look for the causes of a thing, but only to find out the observable facts. Teleology is an ideology, not a science. When one declaims of primary causes and reasons why, objectivity is lost and every observation is made to fit into a scheme in which all is preordained. The Hippocratic physicians had known better than to look for causes—the

strength of their system lay in its dictum of seeking predictable mosaics in the evidence obtained through the use of their senses. When Galen ignored that most basic of their teachings, it was at his own peril. He interpreted what his senses showed him by using what his heart told him. He filled in the empty spaces in his already biased knowledge with speculation based on his concept of how things would be if constructed by a Creator of infinite wisdom. And so, to use Alexander Pope's term, he misunderstood "Whatever is" because he had predetermined what "is Right."

William Harvey played by a different set of rules. He understood that it is not in the scientist's realm to learn *why*, but only to learn *how*. What is observable and measurable is the stuff of science; that which could only be the subject of mystical speculation was to be banished. In learning *how*, he became the first physician to use the scientific method, a method characterized both poetically and very accurately by the English physiologist Sir George Pickering in his Harveian Oration of 1964 as "disciplined curiosity."

Harvey's point of departure from his predecessors is a point indeed, an abrupt, sudden leavetaking from which there could be no return. Though it had been delayed a millennium and a half by the pervading miasma of Galenism, the leap forward now took place. Sir William Osler, the greatest of medical teachers and the greatest of medical humanists, told his audience at the College of Physicians in 1906 that

here for the first time a great physiological problem was approached from the experimental side by a man with a modern scientific mind, who could weigh evidence and not go beyond it, and who had the sense to let the conclu-

sions emerge naturally but firmly from the observations. To the age of the hearer, in which men had heard, and heard only, had succeeded the age of the eye, in which men had seen and had been content only to see. But at last came the age of the hand—the thinking, devising, planning hand; the hand as an instrument of the mind, now reintroduced into the world in a modest little monograph of seventy-two pages, from which we may date the beginning of experimental medicine.

The word "reintroduced" has a particular historical significance. By choosing it, Osler was reminding his listeners that Galen had taught physicians how to do experiments, but they had forgotten. Because the methods he had shown them uncovered truths that he put into a system of speculation by which he meant to explain everything, no one thought it was necessary to explore further. In this sense, the Galenists were themselves the most flagrant violators of one of the major precepts of their progenitor, the precept embodied in his injunction that one "should put his trust not in books on anatomy but in his own eyes," and "alone by himself industriously practice exercises in dissection." Andreas Vesalius and William Harvey, applauded as the Galen-busters, were actually the first real disciples of the master of experiment whose teachings had become bastardized by centuries of misinterpretation. Galen is not alone among the prophets to have been dealt this particular form of undeserved fate.

Harvey reintroduced experimental physiology, but this time it came to the world free of the encumbrances of speculation and teleology, in a form in which it would remain so that, henceforth, scientists might "weigh evidence, and not

go beyond it." It is evidence, after all, that the scientific method is all about. Classically, the researcher sees evidence, analyzes it, recognizes a pattern, and comes up with a hypothesis to explain it. He then tests the hypothesis with carefully designed reproducible experiments. And what is an experiment? It is nothing more than a planned occurrence that allows the researcher to make observations under controlled conditions. It may be looked upon simply as an enlargement of

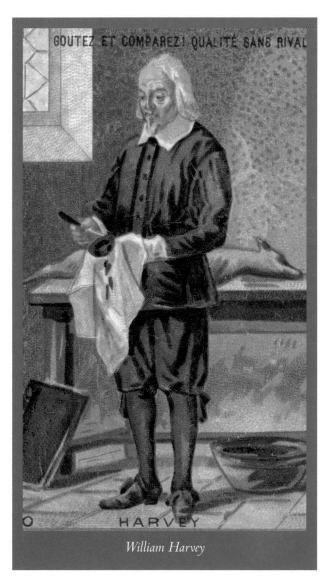

William Harvey

his experience, unhindered and unblurred by extraneous influences that might mar his ability to assess objectively what he observes.

Having made appropriate experiments whose results support his hypothesis, the researcher presents it to the world in the form of what is called a theory. The real scientist, that idealized form rarely encountered in these pragmatic days of academic competition, will always remember that no one knows what truth is, or what constitutes irrefutable proof. So he will never go beyond calling his conclusions by the name of theory—a word which in its etymology implies that it is only a credible way of looking at something. Even when supported by every "proof" of which modern research technology is capable, it remains, in the words of William S. Gilbert's song, "in spite of all temptations to belong to other nations," a theory, and it is greatly to the credit of a dispassionate science that no further special plea is made for it. No matter the certainty, no matter the conviction with which he may proclaim it to the world, no researcher dares to claim anything of his conclusion but that it is a useful way of looking at a thing, of explaining *how*, a way that has achieved credibility by the results of his experiments. Only an ideologue knows the truth; the scientist knows only a theory.

De Generatione Animalium appeared when its author was seventy-three years old. From what is known of the details of its publication, it represents studies and writing done many years earlier. It is probable that Harvey did very little original work during the last two decades of his life. He had given up his London residence in 1648, and gone to live with his brothers Eliab in Roehampton and Daniel in Lambeth, probably also

retiring from the active practice of medicine at the same time. In July of 1651 he donated funds to the College of Physicians so that a building might be erected to house a library, a museum, and a meeting room. The Fellows reciprocated by commissioning a statue of their illustrious benefactor. Some time after this, Harvey was offered the presidency of the College of Physicians, which he declined because he was in poor health. Besides the gradually increasing infirmities of old age, he was victimized by gout, which he treated by immersing his feet in cold water when the pain became intolerable. The vigorous, fiery little researcher had become a frail old man hunched over a leaky wooden tub, wiggling his agonized toes in the icy water to keep up the flow of the circulation he had described to the world four decades earlier.

From time to time, colleagues would write to him, and some of them would try to arouse his "disciplined curiosity" to study some new problem in physiology, but he always declined. To one such correspondent in 1655 he wrote: "My now too long a tale of years causes me to repress from sheer weariness any desire to pursue new subtleties, and after long labors my mind is too fond of peace and quiet for me to let myself become too deeply involved in an arduous discussion of recent discoveries."

The last years were lived out quietly. Harvey enjoyed the company of friends, who saw in him none of the airs and pretense with which aged greats sometimes puff themselves up. Aubrey writes: "Ah! my old friend Dr. Harvey—I knew him right well—he made me sit by him 2 or 3 hours together discussing. Why! had he been stiffe, proud, starcht & retired, as other formal

Doctors are, he had known no more than they." Aubrey appears not to have been the only young person in close proximity to the old widower, as he relates it: "I remember he kept a pretty young wench to wayte on him, which I guess he made use of for warmth-sake as King David did." Age has its privileges, but they probably helped Harvey not a whit more than they did the sweet singer of Israel: *And the damsel was very fair, and cherished the king and ministered to him; but the king knew her not.*

The reigning monarch of medical research wanted only to end his years peacefully. On April 24, 1657, he wrote to a colleague, "I am not only ripe in years, but also—let me admit—a little weary. It seems to me indeed that I am entitled to ask for an honourable discharge." His wish was soon granted. Two months later, on June 30, he suffered a stroke, and died within a few hours. Among his pallbearers was his young friend John Aubrey.

In his preface to *De Generatione Animalium*, William Harvey spelled out the precepts by which the new scientists of the seventeenth century studied the phenomena of nature. Though indebted to Greek thought, they recognized the incompleteness of the knowledge to which it had left them heir. Of equal importance, they acknowledged the fallibility of even the most revered of the ancient authorities and the books they inspired. "Nature herself must be our advisor" was their credo. Not content merely to cast off the old restraints, they created a new attitude toward science, nowhere better expressed than in Harvey's preface: science

is awash with serendipity; science is hard work when done properly, but in the hard work there is joy and in the discovery there is abundant reward; science functions by inductive reasoning—the discovery of general principles from the evidence of individual facts, a process described by Harvey in almost heroic phrases: "We confer with our own eyes, and make our ascent from lesser things to higher."

As Aubrey noted, William Harvey did see his doctrine established in his own lifetime, at least in the sense that his doctrine was the circulation of the blood. Though medical use of the principles of the circulation was still a long way off, the significance of his discovery was not lost on many literate people. In his old age he was applauded and lauded, and rendered the ultimate homage of being called an "immortal." But the greater part of his teaching, the part exemplified by his description of science, had to wait at least another hundred years to be understood and accepted by any but that select vanguard of clear thinkers of the seventeenth century—each of whom seems to have come upon it independently of the others, as is so often true of truth. Any one of them might have written the words here abstracted from the preface to *De Generatione Animalium*:

> *Nature herself must be our advisor; the path she chalks must be our walk. For as long as we confer with our own eyes, and make our ascent from lesser things to higher, we shall be at length received into her closet-secrets.*

> *"We confer with our own eyes, and make our ascent from lesser things to higher."*

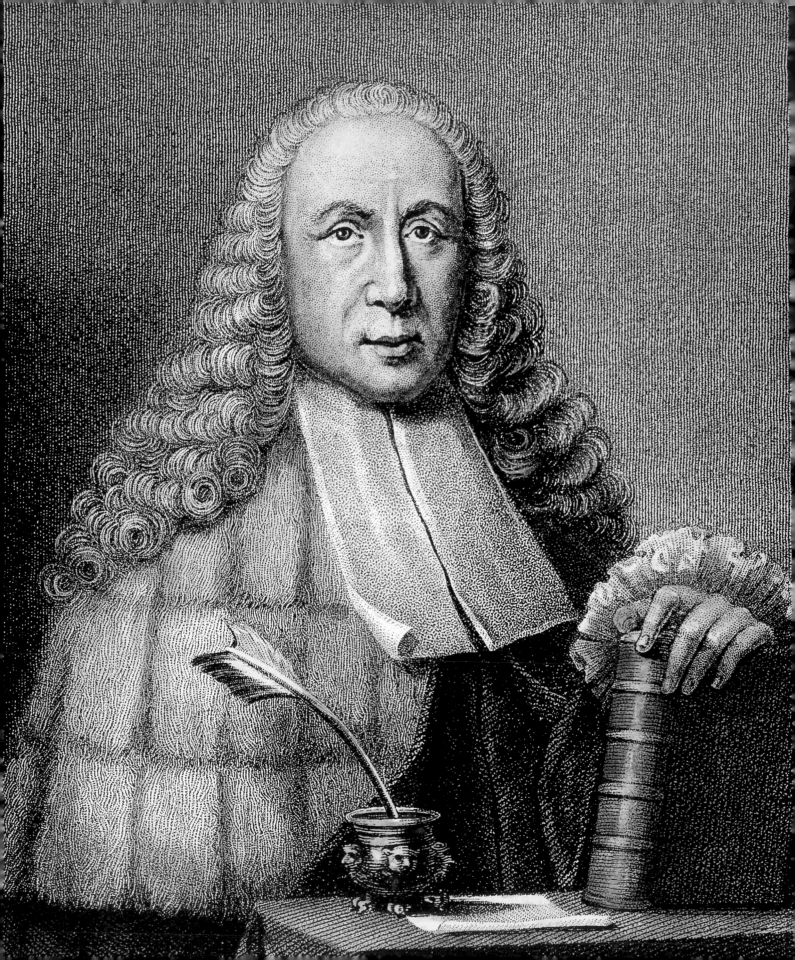

6

THE NEW MEDICINE

The Anatomical Concept of Giovanni Morgagni

A clinical case history of the early eighteenth century:

An old man of seventy-four years of age, of a slender build, and fond of his wine, had for the past month begun to walk in such a manner as to bear his weight chiefly on his left leg. Although his servants had noticed the limp, he himself had said nothing about it, nor had he complained of any discomfort. After twenty-two days of this lameness, he was seized with a generalized pain in his belly. He medicated himself with powder of theriaca, a popular standby for such symptoms since the days of antiquity. The pain left him. About noon twelve days later, he began to have a severe oppressive ache in the right lower quadrant of his abdomen, which he described as being "like the gnawing of dogs." The painful area was swollen, and a hard mass could be felt when deep pressure was applied with the hand of the physician he now consulted. The doctor noted that the pulse was rapid, a strange, sunken look had made its appearance in the sockets of the eyes, and the tongue was dry. The patient passed a poor night.

The following morning, the pulse was large and bounding. The pain and the mass had now extended themselves out as far as the middle of the lower abdomen, and soon reached the left side. The physician ordered that the old man be bled seven ounces. When this was done, it was observed that the resultant clot had a thick yellow sickly-looking crust on its surface. The patient had become nauseated, but had not vomited. The second night was extremely bad.

The next day, the pulse was weak, and the old man was belching up a bitter acid fluid from his stomach. His speech was slurred, and he slipped into and out of delirium. By the following morning he was having frequent convulsions lasting as long as a quarter of an hour at a time. His pulse was so weak that it could be obliterated by a light touch of his physician's fingertips. Foul liquid was being vomited up; it smelled like feces. Respiration became very labored. That evening, with his mind inexplicably having cleared itself of delirium, the old man gasped once, convulsed, and died.

At the autopsy which was done the next morning, the most striking findings were, as expected,

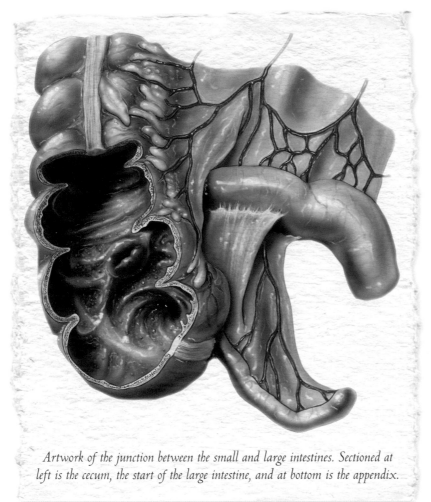

Artwork of the junction between the small and large intestines. Sectioned at left is the cecum, the start of the large intestine, and at bottom is the appendix.

tion crept into the contiguous intestine, and other circumstances that I have described, there is no chance to explain." Nor would there be a chance to explain for more than another century and a half, since the underlying cause of the patient's symptoms was a disease that was as yet unrecognized on that day in 1705 in the city of Bologna, where the autopsy took place. The old man died, as you may by now have guessed, of a ruptured appendix.

The disease had nothing to do with humors, innate heat, the patient's environment, or the season of the year. It was a specific pathological process involving a specific area in the body. The symptoms presented by the patient had been the result, not of a holistic generalized imbalance, but of a highly localized badness whose seat was

in the right lower quadrant of the abdominal cavity. The beginning of the large intestine, called the base of the cecum, was a mass of gangrene where it lay upon the muscles leading toward the leg. A foul-smelling abscess penetrated into those muscles so deeply that it could not be separated from them without cutting into it, whereupon a large collection of pus and serum burst forth.

The seat of the symptoms had thus been identified, but there was no way to discover the original cause from which the evolving process had originated. In the words of the physician who did the autopsy, "But in what manner the inflamma-

in the cecum. The case history you have just read was one of the first in a series of seven hundred that its dissector would collect over the course of the subsequent half-century. Those cases, organized in the form of seventy letters, affirmed the vision of the ancient Cnidians—the key to the origin of every disease is to be found in some local disturbance of an individual organ. To seek out that local disturbance was to be the First Commandment of the new medicine.

On that morning in 1705, the young dissector had just started on his pilgrimage up the steadily rising mount of cadavers from which he would one day descend to bring the medical world its long-awaited keys to the kingdom of scientific clinical thinking. Thereafter there was a new bible of healing, whose canon would never be closed to the discoveries of observation and experiment. When that by then aged anatomist finally published his findings in 1761, his book joined the *Fabrica* and *De Motu Cordis* as the third cornerstone of the pyramid in which the old medicine could be embalmed and buried forever.

At the time he did the autopsy, the dissector was a twenty-three-year-old assistant to the University of Bologna's Professor of Anatomy, Antonio Valsalva. His name was Giovanni Battista Morgagni, and he was destined to change the way in which physicians viewed the essential nature of disease. Something that may be said of William Harvey and Andreas Vesalius may also be said of Morgagni: it was as though he had been placed on earth to carry out a mission for which the medical world had been preparing itself, and which needed only the appearance of a single unifying intellect to achieve. The mission was the bringing of a message. The message itself was a simple one: it is useless to seek the causes of disease among the foggy vapors of the four humors or any variations of such theories. Diseases are not general imbalances of an entire patient, but rather are quite specific derangements of particular structures within the body. Each disease, to state it another way, has a seat in some organ that has gone wrong. It is the job of the physician to identify that seat.

Later writers gave a name to Giovanni Morgagni's message. They called it the anatomical concept of disease, and it became the foundation stone of all subsequent medical thought.

Symptoms are, in its author's words, "the cry of the suffering organs." We now know that not only organs, but tissues, cells, and even subcellular structures and molecules may be seats of disease. But no matter how detailed and submolecular may become our knowledge of the process of sickness, the principle elucidated by Morgagni two hundred years ago will remain at the core of our seeking. *Ubi est morbus?*—Where is the disease? That is the question that must be answered by every doctor for every patient. Only then can treatment begin.

There is no physician trained in the twentieth century who would, in his wildest imaginings, question the obvious statement that distinct anatomical or biochemical changes in organs, tissues, and cells underlie all disease processes. The real burden of medical research in modern times has been to identify the primary etiological factors that cause such changes to occur. Thus, investigators in microbiology, genetics, immunology, psychology, public health, cell biology, and a score of other subspecialties work to elucidate the most basic instigating influences on pathological occurrences.

It is difficult for most of us to imagine a time when the great majority of physicians saw little relationship between a patient's symptoms on the one hand and the accompanying pathological derangements on the other—when they did not attempt to identify the suffering organ by the sound of its cry. To modern clinicians, the first function of a history-taking and a physical examination is to enable a reconstruction of the series of anatomical and physiological events that have led to the presenting findings, and thereby to make an accurate diagnosis, which can then be substantiated with studies of body fluids and tissues, and by various imaging techniques.

Of course, it was not always so. In fact, it is a little disquieting to realize just how recently it was not so at all. The establishment of the independence of the United States as a sovereign nation in 1776 is a convenient date to remember as the approximate time at which the thinking of many physicians began to be affected by the perception that symptoms of disease are due to some sick thing that has happened to an organ. The theories invoking humors and spirit, or those of even more mystical etiologies, generally held sway until that time. Obscurities and uncertainties were hidden behind quasi-scientific terminology. The vestiges of Hippocratic and Galenic formulations still existed; mixed with theoretical concepts of vital life principles gone awry, miasmas, and moral badness, they were used to account for much of the disease of the day by most physicians, inadequately trained as they were. Even Andreas Vesalius and William Harvey, in spite of their scientific approach to research, turned to the old ways in the actual diagnosis and treatment of their patients. The direct evidence of organ pathology that they saw in the dissecting room radically altered their understanding of anatomy and physiology; in pragmatic day-to-day clinical practice, however, they never freed themselves from the suffocating grip of Galenic inertia.

> "*To admire and follow not antiquity, not novelty, not tradition, but only the truth, wherever it might be.*"

But there were nests of attentive observers in some of the European universities, particularly Padua, where centuries of tradition had given inspiration to a succession of scientific contributors, including Vesalius and Harvey, whose medical thinking was based on careful observation and personal experiment meticulously recorded. In the credo of Giovanni Morgagni can be heard the echo of the philosophy of his two distinguished predecessors: "To admire and follow not antiquity, not novelty, not tradition, but only the truth, wherever it might be."

What Giovanni Morgagni accomplished in his pursuit of the truth was the creation of another of those literary monuments that have marked the most significant turning points in the development of medical science. Like most of the other titles of works that represent critical course changes, his book's title is a summary of its message: *The Seats and Causes of Disease Investigated by Anatomy*, or in Latin, *De Sedibus et Causis Morborum per Anatomen Indagatis*. He was telling his fellow physicians that it is not in speculative pronouncements of invisible fluxes that disease is to be understood, but in the dissection of the cadaver itself—anatomy is the key to diagnosis, and the physician's five senses are the key, as was first taught by the Hippocratics, to truth. Obviously, it was not a message never heard before, but after Morgagni it could no longer be ignored. By the time the young dissector of Bologna was ready to present his thesis to the world, he had become the sage old Professor of Padua, a man admired to the point of reverence not only for his scientific achievements but for his nobility of character as well. In the intervening six decades, he was never afflicted with any of the hotheaded ambitious striving of Vesalius, nor did he have the impetuous nervous energy of Harvey. On the contrary, he was a serene Gibraltar of emotional substance, as gentle in his personal manner as he was reliable in his habits. His stature as a man was not exceeded by his stature as the most respected anatomist of his day.

Morgagni's worthiness of character was of the sort that William Osler must have been extolling in his memorable 1901 address at the Boston Medical Library, "Books and Men." Osler, the most distinguished of American professors of medicine, was also one of the foremost historians of science at the turn of the twentieth century. In that oft-quoted Boston oration, he said of those persons of the past whose works we must cherish and whose lives we must emulate, "They would remind us continually that in the records of no other profession is there to be found so large a number of men who have combined intellectual pre-eminence with nobility of character." Although such a hunk of grandiloquent hyperbole only proves that even the great Osler could indulge himself in a little exaggeration from time to time, there are nevertheless a few figures in medical history for whom it rings true. Foremost among them is Giovanni Morgagni. Iconoclasts have never wasted their time in vain attempts to soil his unassailable image, nor have historians ever turned up a datum of his life that does not add a few candlepower to the golden glow in which he is remembered.

Among Morgagni's virtues was patience. He delayed publication until he had proved his case to the point where it was invulnerable. When his book finally appeared in 1761, he was seventy-nine years old. This seems to be the world's record for medical research, a field notorious for the beardlessness of many of its major contributors. The aforementioned Osler, by the way, spoke in another famous oration of the comparative uselessness of men above forty years of age and the *absolute* uselessness of those beyond sixty. He went so far as to muse over the advantages to the world of providing such superannuated sages with what he called "a peaceful departure by chloroform." I would sooner have wished Osler to chloroform himself, or even the wizened Copernicus, before delaying the progress of clinical science by putting the lethal bottle to the nostrils of such as Morgagni.

There being no Osler and no green-gas anesthetic poisons in the eighteenth century, it was given to Giovanni Battista Morgagni and to the world which reaped the benefits of his great contribution that he should have a long, productive, and secure life. His years were characterized by regularity of habits and consistency of devotion to his scientific work, to his large family, and to the religious principles that guided both his search for truth and the stability of his spirit. As one reads the descriptions of his personality that have come down to us, the image that emerges is that of a serene scholar, much admired by his students of many nationalities and by his friends, among whom were included several of the most powerful figures of the day, such as Pope Benedict XIV and the Holy Roman Emperor Joseph II. He enjoyed warm professional relationships with some of the great medical thinkers of his time, including Hermann Boerhaave of Leyden, Albrecht von Haller of Berne, Johann Meckel of Göttingen, and Richard Mead of London, a group whose spectrum of interests reflected Morgagni's own, ranging from education to research to the care of the sick.

Morgagni was born on February 25, 1682, in the little northern Italian town of Forli, some thirty-five miles southeast of Bologna. At the age of sixteen he went to the latter city to study medicine and philosophy, soon coming under the patronage of Antonio Maria Valsalva, the great anatomist who had been a pupil of Malpighi. Upon receiving his degree with distinction in 1701, the nineteen-year-old Morgagni became Valsalva's assistant for six years. Following more than a year of postgraduate study between 1707 and 1709, he returned to his hometown of Forli to be a practicing physician. Here his tall, robustly handsome appearance, his engaging personality, and his great abilities soon made him a successful practitioner and a much-sought-after consultant, in spite of his youth. He married Paola Verzeri at this time, the daughter of a noble family of the town. Together they raised twelve daughters and three sons, eight of the girls becoming nuns and one of the boys entering the priesthood.

In 1711, Morgagni was invited to Padua, to assume the post of junior Professor of Theoretical Medicine. So effective was he in this position that he was named only four years later to become the successor to Vesalius, Fallopius, Fabricius, and Spigelius as Professor of Anatomy, the oldest and most esteemed chair at the university. He was thirty-three years old. Within a very few years he had established himself as the outstanding anatomist of Europe, and thereafter scholars came from all over the known world to visit and to study with him. He was elected to many foreign scientific organizations, most prominent being the Royal Society of London, the Royal Academy of Science at Paris, the Royal Academy of Berlin, and the Imperial Academy of St. Petersburg.

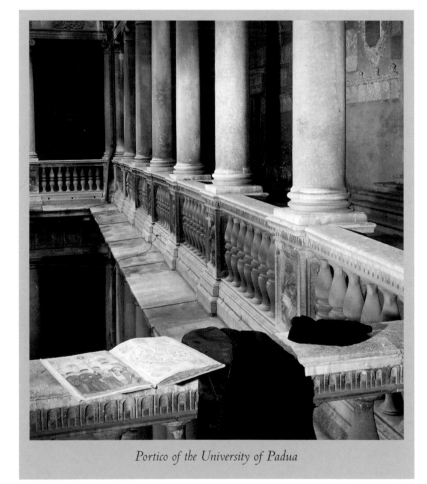

Portico of the University of Padua

Although Morgagni was primarily an anatomist, his ultimate accomplishment arose out of his own sense that he was first and foremost a physician, one whose responsibility it is to care for the sick. Anatomy was his best tool in the effort to understand disease, and it was thus his means of becoming a better doctor. He did indeed practice medicine throughout his long career, and was sought out as a consultant by colleagues from most of the countries of Europe. Many of his consultations, or *Consulti*, were made in the form of letters, since the patients were at such a distance. A hundred of his reports, which he gave to his pupil Michele Girardi shortly before his death in 1771, have been edited, and translated into English by Saul Jarcho. In Jarcho's words, "While we are warranted in believing that he regarded anatomical study as a means and not an end, it proved to be one of the most important sources of his clinical strength." In an evaluation of the ways in which the consultations reveal Morgagni as a healer of the sick, Jarcho writes, "In a few cases the *Consulti* actually enable the reader to see the behavior of a great physician at the bedside. In all cases the *Consulti* should be valued for their depiction, within well-defined limits, of Eighteenth Century academic medicine at its very best."

So the Morgagni who should take form in our historical memory was less a scientist than a doctor at the bedside. In his self-image and in the motivations that led him to study his patients as carefully as he did, healing was the final objective. His deep interest in clinical medicine and his ongoing experiments in physiology led him to seek reasonable and observable explanations for the phenomena of disease, with the aim of classifying and explaining each disease process as a distinct entity.

Using the approach they learned from *De Sedibus*, Morgagni's successors formulated the basic principles that lie at the core of all modern clinical medicine. In 1894, Rudolf Virchow, in whose brilliant hands the field of pathological anatomy reached its grandest fulfillment, pointed out that medicine did not attain its true importance until *De Sedibus* had appeared. Speaking of Morgagni's influence on the leading centers of medical teaching and research in the nineteenth century, he said, "The full consequences of what he worked out were harvested in London and in Paris, in Vienna and in Berlin. And thus we can say that, beginning with Morgagni and resulting from his work, the dogmatism of the old schools was completely shattered, and that with him the new medicine begins." The medical researchers of the nineteenth century steered their courses by the guideposts that had been planted in Padua by the painstaking observations and methods of the Professor of Anatomy.

It is impossible to overestimate the magnitude of Morgagni's accomplishment. In 1874, a century after *De Sedibus* was published, W. T. Gairdner, the president of the Glasgow Pathological and Clinical Society, told his audience of leaders of Scottish medicine:

All the more eminent moderns, and even the men of our own time, although they work with new means and appliances, amid a flood of new light from physiology and histological [microscopic] anatomy, and amid a science of organic chemistry . . . are all of them successors and legitimate heirs of Morgagni's labours and method. . . . For it is this method and this spirit that make the essential distinction of the modern-minded physician or surgeon and that separate him . . . from the man whom

Molière has depicted for us in outrageous caricature. . . . . I claim not only the professed and exclusive morbid anatomists, but also, and still more, almost all the greatest physicians and surgeons of our own and the last century, as the legitimate successors of Morgagni and the inheritors of his method of working. . . . That diagnosis has been rendered exact, and statistical conclusions possible, are results which we owe simply to a rigid application by many and varied minds, of principles derived in great part from the work of Morgagni.

Gairdner spoke of Morgagni's method, which, in the long term, was more significant even than the observations which arose from it. His was the method of science: observation, hypothesis, experiment, recording of data, and cautious inference based upon repeated, reproducible studies. The specific pillars that supported it in his work were fourfold—clinical, pathological, experimental, and literary. Each of his seven hundred case reports details a clear clinical history followed by a report of the pathology found at autopsy. Relevant experiments are done where indicated, and a search is described of the extant literature on the subjects of investigation. This is the model for a form of teaching exercise that physicians of a later era came to call the clinicopathological conference, or CPC. Every week, in teaching hospitals throughout the world and in the pages of the *New England Journal of Medicine*, a CPC is presented, in which a physician attempts to make a diagnosis from a clinical case history, after which his conclusion is confirmed or denied by the pathologist's report of the autopsy, operation, or biopsy. After two and a half centuries, the CPC is still one of the most useful methods of teaching medicine. It was one of Giovanni Morgagni's gifts to the ages.

Morgagni was not the first, of course, to relate disease manifestations to derangements of specific structures. Even Galen, whose works were the most persistently inhibiting factor in the advance of scientific medicine, had suggested such a correlation. In his book *On the Affected Parts*, the Greek physician wrote, "There are very few essential symptoms of disease which do not point to the affected part. In fact, the alterations of function point directly to the affected part." It was one of the great Galenic paradoxes that statements like these were forgotten, and only their author's humoral theories were remembered and taught.

Even had Galen's enunciation of the anatomical concept of disease been remembered, the strong Greek and then Moslem injunctions against dissecting the human body would have prevented any elucidation of Galen's lost precept. Not until his writings were a thousand years old do we begin to find occasional descriptions of autopsies, and even a few which were done with the purpose of ascertaining the cause of death. The helpful role played by the Catholic Church when it began to allow dissections in the thirteenth century affected the study not only of normal anatomy but of disease as well. For example, Pope Clement VI did not merely permit but actually ordered autopsies to be done on the bodies of the victims of a plague epidemic that occurred in Sienna in 1348.

As more physicians began to dissect to learn anatomy, there were increasingly frequent descriptions of pathological findings as well, but always interpreted within the context of the theory of the four humors. Andreas Vesalius was convinced of the importance of studying pathological organs, and wrote of his intention to publish a book that dealt with the subject. Although he accumulated a goodly number of such investigations, his records were apparently lost, and the publication never saw the light of day.

Scattered throughout the writings of William Harvey too are references to his own studies in pathological anatomy, which he viewed as an essential follow-up to the examination of patients he had treated during life. This represents a very modern attitude, gradually beginning to take root among the leading physicians of that remarkable seventeenth century. In a letter to the French physician Jean Riolan, Harvey wrote:

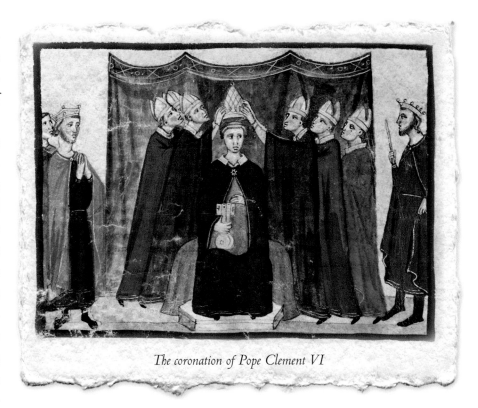

The coronation of Pope Clement VI

I intend putting to press my Medical Anatomy, or Anatomy in its Application to Medicine . . . that I may relate from the many dissections I have made of the bodies of persons diseased how and in what way the internal organs were changed in their situation, size, structure, shape, consistency and other sensible qualities from their natural forms and appearances such as they are usually described by anatomists . . . I venture to say that the examination of a single body of one who has died of consumption or some other disease of long-standing, is of more service to medicine than the dissection of ten men who have been hanged.

Harvey's promised publication suffered the same fate as did that of Vesalius—it never appeared.

Even before Harvey, Francis Bacon, the greatest of the seventeenth-century philosophers of science, had urged, in his 1605 *Advancement of Learning,* that autopsies be done when patients die, because "in the differences of the internal parts are often found the immediate causes of many diseases." (This observation was consistent with the core of Bacon's well-articulated principle that in order to know a thing we must understand its causes and its antecedents.) And the very same Dr. Nicholas Tulp whose anatomy lesson was the theme of one of Rembrandt's most honored paintings was the author in 1641 of *Observationes Medicae,* which contained not only autopsy reports, but drawings of pathological specimens as well.

In spite of this slowly rising tide of clinicopathological correlations, however, the causes of disease were still thought to be based upon humoral imbalances, even by the more farseeing physicians. Thus, a 1661 autopsy report on a patient who was found to have succumbed to perforated ulcers of the lower small intestine ascribes the findings to "an overflow of sharp and corrupted biliary humors." The dissector was not a small-town country doctor—he was the eminent Danish anatomist Thomas Bartholin, one of the leading researchers of the century.

Ultimately, Harvey's discovery of the circulation began to affect the interpretation of postmortem findings. By demonstrating the way in which the heart and vessels actually do their work, his book stimulated at least some physicians to seek anatomical evidence that might explain why function had gone awry badly enough to cause death. The landmark example of this is the case of the Swiss physician Johann Jakob Wepfer, who had become convinced of the importance of autopsies in the study of patients whom he had treated during life. In his declining years Wepfer suffered from slow irregular pulse, chest pain, swelling and coldness of the legs, and shortness of breath worsened by lying flat, all now known to be symptoms of chronic congestive heart failure. Shortly before his death at the age of seventy-five in 1695, he requested that his son-in-law Johann

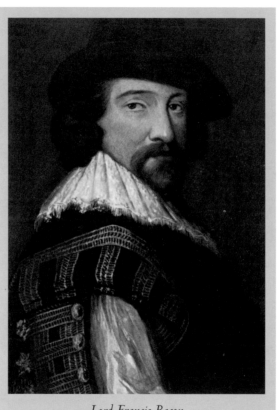

Lord Francis Bacon

Conrad Brunner examine his cadaver. Brunner published a detailed report of the case history and autopsy, whose findings included fluid in the chest and abdomen, enlargement of the heart, and hardening of the aorta and the other major arteries. A drawing of the blood vessels that was included with the case report is the world's first illustration of arteriosclerosis, hardening of the arteries. In an impressive correlation of the clinical with the pathological findings, Brunner attributed his father-in-law's death to failure of the circulation and slowing, or stasis, of the bloodflow. Brunner's publication leaves no doubt that he is to be included with the moderns; he declares, "Those who adhered to the beliefs of the ancient writers would have attributed death to the loss of vital heat. But exactly in our case the error of such a concept is evident; it is blood, indeed, which is responsible for the body's natural heat. If deprived of circulation, the external parts become cold, and this was the symptom of which Wepfer complained so frequently."

The edifice of humoral theory was beginning to show its first few lines of stress, but it was far from being ready to crumble. Up to this point, postmortem correlations between symptoms and their organs of origin had been the work of only a few investigators. Several others of equal stature, however, including England's leading physician, Thomas Sydenham, had rejected them as useless. The grounds for disagreement with the dissectors were outlined by Sydenham's friend the renowned John Locke, who was also a physician: "Though we cut into the inside, we see but the outside of things and make but new superfices to stare at . . . Nature performs all her operations in the body by parts so minute and insensible that I think nobody will ever hope or pretend even by the assistance of glasses or other inventions to come to a sight of them." That he made such a statement should not detract from Locke's stature as a philosopher; it simply means that he was a poor prophet.

Until that time, autopsies had not been particularly well planned, nor had clinicopathological correlations been deliberate and systematized. Most evidence was casually obtained and anecdotally described. There was as yet no good reason for the scoffers not to heap scorn on those who were loosening their allegiance to the traditional time-honored theories. The first major attempt to present an organized argument in favor of the congruence of premortem symptoms with postmortem findings was published in 1679 by Theophilus Bonetus of Geneva, with the title *Sepulchretum Sive Anatomica Practica*. The English translation of the book's complete title indicates its thesis: *Repository of anatomy practised on corpses deceased of disease, which reports the histories and observations of all alterations of the human body and reveals the hidden causes. Indeed, it [anatomy] deserves to be called the foundation of real pathology and of proper treatment of disease, even the inspiration of old and recent medicine.* Unfortunately, Bonetus was not equal to the prodigious task he had set for himself. It would require the sound scholarly precision of Giovanni Morgagni to bring it to a fruition worthy of its majestic title.

What Bonetus did was to assemble from the available literature almost three thousand cases in which clinical histories had been correlated with autopsy reports and commentary. That so many examples existed is a testament to the attention that was increasingly being paid to postmortem studies, albeit haphazardly. Even more revealing is the fact that there were 470 authors whose writings Bonetus was able to quote in the seventeen hundred pages of his text. But there were serious problems with the *Sepulchretum*, to which more were added when an enlarged second edition, compiled by Mangetus, appeared in 1700. These defects, which made the work virtually useless to scholars, included misquotations, misinterpretations, and inaccurate observations. Moreover, the book lacked a proper index, making retrieval of information laborious when it was possible at all. In a later century, René Laennec would dismiss the entire text as an "undigested and incoherent compilation."

The young Morgagni, nevertheless, pored over the *Sepulchretum*. It became clear to him that because the concept upon which it was based epitomized a fundamental truth, the medical world required a revision of the work that would be both accurate and usable. Rewriting the massive tome would have seemed wildly impossible to any but an impetuous youth not yet sufficiently impressed with the onerous demands of the academic medical life. Morgagni later wrote of his decision to begin the job:

I remember, likewise, that as young men are generally presumptuous enough to entertain thoughts of the most

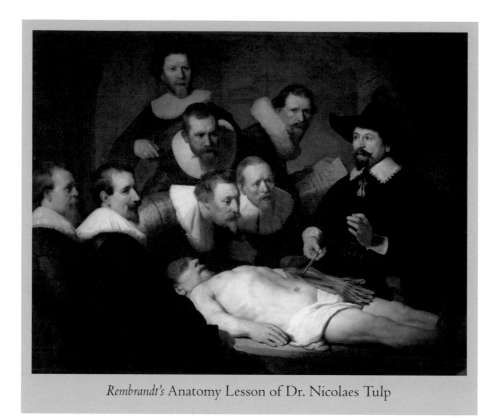

Rembrandt's Anatomy Lesson of Dr. Nicolaes Tulp

who had chosen to call themselves the Academia Inquietorum—Academy of the Restless. As implied by their organization's name, these were young men who were impatient with the theorizing of their predecessors, and whose loyalty to the medicine of the ancients had been superseded by their curiosity to unearth the hidden truths of nature. It was that society which became the Academy of Sciences of Bologna, in 1714; thus Morgagni was probably about twenty or twenty-one years old when he began to collect the material which would eventually grow up to be *De Sedibus.*

difficult and laborious undertakings, I did not even then despair, but if I should have sufficient leisure in future time, I should not only be able to supply the deficiencies that I have pointed out in the Sepulchretum, *and others besides these, but also that I should be able to reform the indexes; and I even thought of a plan whereby this might be done, and communicated my plan to that respectable society, which is now called the Academy of Sciences.*

The wording of this last sentence provides a clue to the period in which Morgagni first took up his labors. Upon graduation from medical school in 1701 at the age of nineteen, he had been invited to substitute for his teacher Valsalva, who was at that time in Parma. His popularity soon brought him the presidency of a society of scientifically minded students and recent graduates

While Morgagni may have set out merely to revise the *Sepulchretum,* what came of his original plan was an entirely new work, based on careful clinical descriptions most of which involved patients dissected by himself or by Valsalva. His observations were sound, and were uncluttered by those insignificant details that less skilled physicians could not distinguish from the salient points in the evolution of a disease process. His interpretations were rational, he used occasional physiological experiments to support certain of his conclusions, and all of his writing rested on a well-researched historical background. To this enormous undertaking he brought his considerable talents as a practicing physician, his towering preeminence as an anatomist, his resourcefulness as an experimental physiologist, and his infinite patience with detail. Morgagni's scholarly ability to integrate and synthesize information, as well as his determination, enabled him to complete a task that medical science was, at that moment in its development, waiting for. Without that step, whether contemporary physicians perceived their situation or not, progress in diagnostic and therapeutic methodology could proceed no further.

De Sedibus et Causis Morborum per Anatomen Indagatis is organized in the form of seventy letters written to a young man whom Morgagni had met during the intermediate stages of his work. This young man, described by the author as being "much given to the study of the sciences, and particularly to that of medicine," asked Morgagni to write to him after the manner of the *Sepulchretum*, describing the cases and observations he had been collecting. Apparently the then fifty-nine-year-old professor began, in 1741, to send one after another of his meticulous analyses to his anonymous (or perhaps fictional) friend, until five books had been completed, entitled by category: (1) Diseases of the Head, (2) Diseases of the Thorax, (3) Diseases of the Belly, (4) Surgical and Universal Disorders, and (5) Supplement, to which is appended the series of indexes for easy reference.

Each of the five books is dedicated to a leading foreign physician, two in Germany and one each in France, England, and Russia. The seventy letters provide case-history materials correlated with autopsy findings, including the appropriate references to other authors and historical background, the discussion sometimes being expanded with descriptions of those experiments carried out by the author in order to elucidate the disease process. An objective of *De Sedibus* was to provide guidelines by which the practicing physician might trace each symptom to its origin within his patient's distressed body.

The style is gentle and conversational. The reader feels as though he is listening to a master teacher revealing to him the experiences and insights of a lifetime, as each case analysis gradually unfolds itself. Historical background is given, the evolution of contemporary thinking is reviewed, authorities are quoted, their opinions are discussed, and the logical development of the professor's conclusions, step by step, becomes clear. Commentators on the original Latin text have been struck by the literary quality of the case histories, so carefully written that it is possible to reconstruct every symptom as it must have felt to the patient and appeared to his medical attendants.

Morgagni allows his reader to be an observer of each step of the autopsy and to accompany him to his library of references. All of this is done in a form addressed in the first person to the individual reader, who is treated not like a novitiate, but like an esteemed colleague, as are the anonymous young man and the various foreign professors to whom the salutations are inscribed. Thus the young man becomes the medium through whom each reader is given private instruction.

So *De Sedibus* was indeed far more than its author had originally intended. A text which started out as a revision of the *Sepulchretum* had grown into a vast literary museum of clinical medicine, arranged in such an orderly way that every exhibit and every case could be found without effort and indexed to further facilitate reference. One of the indexes enables the reader to find pathological data by referring to clinical symptoms and diseases, while another does the opposite—reference to a postmortem finding identifies the page on which may be found the clinical symptom it caused prior to the patient's death. A third index lists the subject of each letter as in a table of contents, and a final index is appropriately titled "Names and Passages Most Worthy of Notice." The indexes thus serve as a catalogue to Morgagni's museum of medicine, whereby every subject is made instantly available. The function of the indexes is described by the author:

So that if any physician observe a singular or any other symptom in a patient and desire to know what internal injury is wont to correspond to that symptom, or if any anatomist find any particular morbid appearance in the dissection of a body and should wish to know what symptom has preceded an injury of this kind in other bodies; the physician, by inspecting the first of the indices, the anatomist, by inspecting the second, will immediately find the observation which contains both (if both have been observed by us).

With the publication of *De Sedibus*, the first distinct sounds of the humoral theory's death knell were heard. An entirely new basis had been presented upon which to understand the nature of

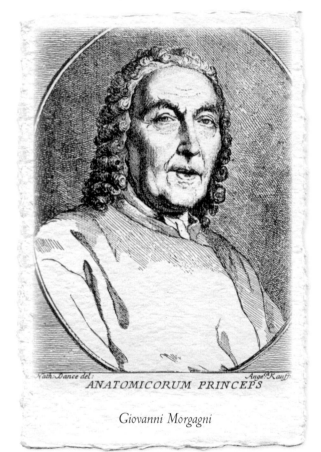

ANATOMICORUM PRINCEPS

Giovanni Morgagni

disease. Henceforth, the human body was to be viewed as composed of a group of coordinated physical-mechanical structures working in faultless harmony. These are the organs and the groups of organs which we call systems. The cause of disease would be seen, therefore, as a failure in some part of the machinery. The purpose of postmortem dissection is to identify the seat of the breakdown, and to study the ways in which the sick organ produced the symptoms of which the patient complained prior to his death.

To his credit, Morgagni did not speculate about the underlying stimuli which initiate the process of breakdown. This more basic step could not be taken until such disciplines as bacteriology and biochemistry were developed in the nineteenth century. His intent was to discover the seats of disease and, at least in part, to explain those outward manifestations of inner-organ derangements which we call signs and symptoms. As a result of his work, it was made clear to the generation that succeeded him that his "Index the Second" was more than a mere alphabetical list of patient complaints matched with pathology—it was a paradigm for the way in which sickness can be diagnosed back to its seat, its deranged organ.

Just as one can look up a symptom in that index and find its hidden origin within the body, it is the physician's duty to identify all clues that are discoverable by questioning and examining his patient, in order that they may direct him to the internal pathology that is being sought in the process of diagnostic evaluation.

The Hippocratic physicians had developed a sophisticated type of physical examination to help them to determine the nature of the humoral imbalance in their patients, and to prognosticate. Now, twenty-two hundred years later, the long-forgotten art of physical evaluation was about to be revived and improved, as a new generation of medical investigators built on Morgagni's teachings to identify the keys to diagnosis. It was during this period that there was perfected the physical examination as we know it today, with its four cardinal principles of inspection, percussion, palpation, and auscultation—looking, tapping, feeling, and listening with the stethoscope. More will be said in later chapters about the development of presentday techniques of diagnostic evaluation, but it is sufficient for now to point out that its purpose lies in Morgagni's thesis: to identify the suffering organ, one must learn to interpret its cries. Every X-ray and scan, every blood, urine, or tissue sample, every microbiologic or chemical analysis, has as its function to trace the disease process to its site of origin, and to determine how the pathological process evolved into the state at which the patient presents himself to his doctor.

Morgagni thus becomes more than the father of pathological anatomy, which is what the historians call him—he is the founder of modern medical diagnosis. With him another step is taken in the rise of scientific medicine; with him

the anatomic concept took such strong root that even a century after his death, it would still be, in the words uttered by Rudolf Virchow in 1894, "the concept of the future." As Virchow so correctly put it, "This future marks the beginning of its chronology from the days of Morgagni. I Iis be the honor!"

Though the honor is Morgagni's, the spirit of his work is that of the age in which he lived, an era which has been given a titular designation that deserves to be capitalized, uppercased, underlined, italicized, or in any other way vociferated enough to stress its distinctiveness from any other. It was the period during which the modern world gestated and was brought forth. It was the Age of Enlightenment.

Ignorance, tradition, dogma, and a lack of curiosity had characterized what came before the seventeenth century and its Enlightenment offspring in the eighteenth. This newborn infant, the modern world, would be skeptical of every iota of accepted wisdom that had been handed down to it. In medicine, most of the accepted wisdom was erroneous. That it had endured for so many centuries is attributable to the ways in which human beings had been accustomed to explaining the phenomena of nature. Through the ages, the human mind has been endlessly fascinated by the making of theories. Unfortunately, we have been prone, even in recent times, to do this whether or not we have enough information to justify drawing conclusions. Put in terms of today's pop-speak, we have too often proceeded without a sufficient data base. We choose a few easily available observations, assume a posture which we subjectively call objective, and before long we have brought forth a comfortable gener-

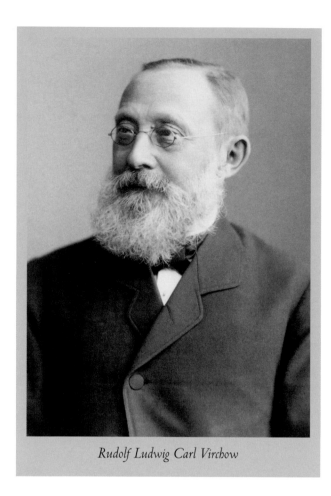

Rudolf Ludwig Carl Virchow

eral tendency to intellectual chicanery and self-deception. And as our species has lived longer in an atmosphere of increased learning, more of its members have become aware of that certain intellectual laziness, of that great human propensity to explain without first exploring, of looking at things without really making observations about them. Many of us now recognize that in searching for systems of thought that may explain the universe and our fellow man, our history has been one of succumbing to speculation.

As long as fanciful all-embracing systems of ideas could be used to shroud what was unexplainable and smother what was unpalatable, there was a certain fragile order to things. But since the Enlightenment, educated men and women have been shown just how perilous it is to ignore the flimsiness of the fabric from which the dogma-shroud is woven. It is at our own peril that we deny that it is only by the cleansing force of truth that we can construe a reality that is consistent with our highest good and our organism's biological needs.

The systems of speculative thought that have failed us in the history of medicine were wildly supernatural, quasi-rationalistic, or weirdly based on mechanistic principles that were meant to imitate stricter disciplines, such as mathematics or physics. When physicians began to realize that aims must be more modest, science began. When the power of simple, reproducible data, of unbiased observations, of proof, and of inductive reasoning was demonstrated, then the philosophers of disease became more like scientists. At that point, medicine's modern era was ready to begin.

Because all of us carry large pieces of the old inherited baggage, we can understand why it took

alization to explain how we have arrived at some point from wherever it is we think we started. One of the rules of this kind of philosophizing is that the theory which results from it is usually such a nonthreatening one that it fails to challenge the worldview to which our culture, our experiences, and our genes have predisposed us. This is a poor enough approach to understanding abstract phenomena like love or politics, and it is absolutely no way to learn about nature.

Nevertheless, there have always been a few people in every generation who allowed themselves to see realistically and reason rationally, regardless of the effect on their basic assumptions. Somehow, such as these have been immune to the genso long for science, and particularly medical science, to make its entrance. When it finally arrived, it did so because the world had prepared itself, in the words of Immanuel Kant, for "man's emergence from his nonage." The Germans gave a name to the philosophical movement that developed when we began to think and to reason in the new ways—they called it the *Aufklärung.* The English, who seem to have started the whole thing in the first place, translated that perfect word into "Enlightenment," and that is what we have called it to this day.

It was the spirit of the Age of Enlightenment that pervaded the atmosphere in which European and American philosophers worked during most of the eighteenth century. The thinkers of that intellectual epoch were characterized by a willingness, actually more like a crusading zeal, to question every given that had been bequeathed to them. In politics, in religion, in literature, and in art, new forms were developed and a new skepticism made its appearance. In such a time, is it any wonder that natural science (or natural philosophy, as it was then called) should come to the forefront of men's thoughts? Even a devout Italian Catholic with as committed a Christian name as Giovanni Battista could hardly have avoided inhaling the exhilarating air of its fresh incoming breezes. Though the Enlightenment agnostics and Deists had no effect on Morgagni's religious faith, he was as intoxicated with the new spirit as any clear-thinking person could be. He crystallized the evolving objectivity of medicine's scientists, and he gave form to a logical system that would result in a veritable outburst of progress in the generation that followed him.

The keen accuracy of observation found in Morgagni's conversational monographs (for that is really what his letters are) makes them in many ways as fascinating today as they must have been to readers two centuries ago. Unlike the "57-year-old white female gravida 3 para 2 right-handed computer programmer" of today's CPCs, the patients in *De Sedibus* are such as "a butcher, who had been disorder'd in his senses for fourteen months, from the effects, as was said, of a love-potion, [who] at length died, in the beginning of the year 1719, by the violence, as was suppos'd of the very cold season, from which he took no care to secure himself." At postmortem, the brain of the butcher was found to be the site of a kind of hardening or sclerosis that is consistent with one of the forms of cerebral degeneration that are today recognized.

We read in *De Sedibus* of a type of patient who is instantly recognizable from the very first sentence of the case history: "N. Ferrarini, a priest of Verona, who had formerly been suppos'd consumptive at Venice, and had been treated for one-sided headache ten years before at Padua, having now completed his forty-third year, the hair of his head was grey, and his face was sometimes too red; his habit of body was slender, yet not lean; and though he seem'd sprightly and joyful, he was very anxious with dissembled cares, and was very prone to anger." It is not surprising to read that Father Ferrarini died suddenly one day, and was found at autopsy to have been the victim of a brain hemorrhage, no doubt due to bursting one of his cerebral blood vessels as a result of hypertension.

Some of Morgagni's descriptions create vivid scenes of the circumstances surrounding the onset of an illness, and reconstruct them so well that every intern of today could recapitulate them in his sleep, from his own experience with such time-transcendent problems: "A certain man, who was a native of Genoa, blind of one eye, and liv'd by begging, being drunk, and quarrelling with other drunken beggars, receiv'd two blows by their sticks; one on his hand, which was slight, and another violent one at the left temple; so that blood came out of the left ear. Yet soon after, the quarrel being made up, he sat down at the fire with them in the same place; and again fill'd himself with a great quantity of wine, by way of pledge of friendship being renewed; and not long after, on the very same night, he died."

Our modern-day intern, on hearing this case history, would correctly predict that postmortem dissection should reveal that the boozing beggar had died because his cerebral cortex was compressed by a blood clot that lay between the skull and the membranous envelope that surrounds the brain, what is today called an epidural hematoma. On rounds the next morning after discussing such a presentation, the intern would very likely refer to it by a term of which young doctors are inordinately fond—he would call it "a classical case," by which he would mean that even someone as old as his

most senior attending physician had probably seen a few exactly like it during his own internship in those long-ago pioneer days of medicine. To clinch the diagnosis the intern would need one of the newest bits of medical gadgetry, and to cure the disease he would use one of the oldest—a CT scanner and a drill, respectively.

Morgagni could not make diagnoses as we know them today, since very few of the conditions he so accurately described had yet been classified or given names. His exploration of a disease process is restricted to describing the postmortem findings and attempting a recapitulation of the way in which they clarified the premortem symp-

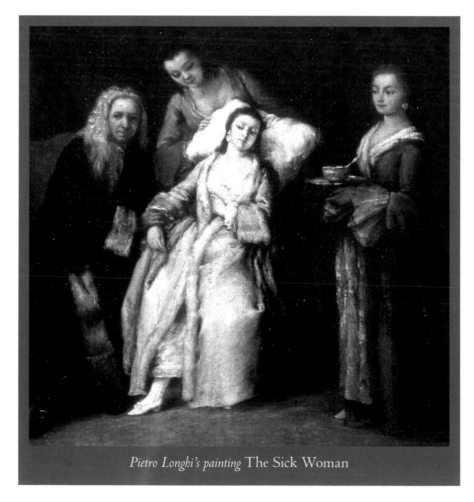

Pietro Longhi's painting The Sick Woman

toms. His method of analysis is so clear that not only all-knowing interns but even their older colleagues can supply many of the diagnoses from the information provided in the pages of his great work. Browsing through *De Sedibus* has warmed my soul on many a cold New England evening.

One of the major motivations that leads men and women to study history must surely be the feeling of sanctified security that comes with musing over the memories and artifacts of bygone times. The historian's trade is a safe one—he is the Monday-morning quarterback of every game that civilization has ever played. He has knowledge that was unavailable to those who were participants in the harsh realities he ponders, and he has the leisure to contemplate it. Snugly harbored in his archives and stacks from the swirl of contemporary events taking place outside his sanctum, he tells the rest of us that he studies yesterday in order to illuminate today. Yesterday, as it turns out, is a comfortable place to be.

When I feel overwhelmed by the pressures of keeping up with the rat-tat-tat of today's rapid-fire breakthroughs (they are always breakthroughs, in the same cliché-ridden way that surgeons are always brilliant) in such high-tech areas as tumor immunology and surgical techniques, I flip the latest medical journal up to the top of a ceiling-scraper pile of its fellows, and I turn to something a few hundred years old. Safe, sound, smart, and cozy, I can slip instantaneously into a medical world that sits still and lets me examine it. With the smug advantage of a century or two of science, I discover things the old docs never suspected might be under their very diagnostic noses. The warmth generated by my own self-satisfied pleasure permits me to forget, at least for a moment,

how ignorant it makes me feel to scan the titles of the articles in this month's *American Journal of Physiology*, or sometimes even (may God forgive me for admitting it) the *Annals of Surgery*.

Morgagni is my favorite antidote. When I turn to the past to escape the present, he is always there with a beautifully detailed case history that presents just enough of a challenge to let me strut my stuff like some kind of diagnostic Walter Mitty. In his twenty-four hundred pages I have found cases, among them the first ever described, of diseases that are recognizable as every one of the following: lobar pneumonia, aneurysm, coarctation, and syphilis of the aorta as well as incompetence and stenosis of its valves, Stokes-Adams heart block, pulmonary stenosis, tetralogy of Fallot, mitral stenosis and regurgitation, endocarditis, tuberculosis of the lungs, femoral artery embolus, nephritis, syphilis of the brain, stomach and bowel cancer, intestinal polyps, ulcerative colitis, Crohn's disease, recto-vesicle fistula, Richter's hernia, cirrhosis of the liver, pancreatitis, and enlargement of the prostate. There remains plenty of undiscovered treasure to be dug up on future winter evenings.

Morgagni described the hardened obstructed coronary arteries that accompany the pain of angina pectoris, and he was also the first to show that stroke is caused not by a lesion in the substance of the brain, but by pathological changes in its feeding blood vessels. Each of these descriptions was a giant leap forward in the understanding of disease. The patients, sometimes by name and always by occupation, figuratively step forth from the pages of text, bringing to mind that awe-inspiring statement that is to be found engraved on the walls of so many modern hospital autopsy rooms: *Hic est locus ubi mors gaudet succurso vitae*— This is the place where death rejoices to come to the aid of life.

There are other sparkling nuggets in *De Sedibus,* some of which I hesitate (but only for a moment) to mention because they border sometimes on the ribald and sometimes on the lurid. The worthy Morgagni is not a man to be accused of trying deliberately to arouse his readers' prurient interest, but he does it nevertheless, willy-nilly. He recounts the tale of a young woman of easy virtue whose final moments were spent in such a lusty transport of venereal delight that she tore her aorta's lining up its middle and died, presumably at the height of a particularly strenuous sexual contortion. Autopsy revealed the cause of the lethal event to be what we today call a dissecting aortic aneurysm with hemopericardium. Here is Morgagni's dispassionate description of a clinical history which may represent the first report of a rare hereditary condition that would become known as Marfan's syndrome, after a Frenchman of that name wrote a case review in 1896:

> A strumpet of eight and twenty years of age, of a lean habit, having complain'd for some months, and par-ticularly for the last fifteen days, of a certain lassitude, and a loathing of food, and almost of every thing, for this reason made less use of other aliments, and more of unmix'd wine; to the use of which she had been always too much addicted. A certain debauchee having gone into the house to her, and after a little time having come out, with a confus'd and disturb'd countenance, and she not having appear'd for two or three hours after, the neighbours, who had observ'd these things, entering in, found her not only dead but cold; lying in bed with such a posture of body, that it could not be doubted what business she had been about when she died, especially as the semen virile was seen to have flow'd down from the organs of generation.

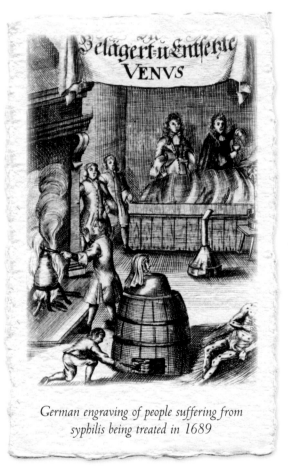

German engraving of people suffering from syphilis being treated in 1689

Sometimes a case history presented by Morgagni is so horrifying that it stretches the imagination of his readers. In the year 1704 a man was admitted to Bologna's Hospital of Incurables with an aneurysm, a bulging weakened section of his aorta due in his case to syphilis, about to burst through the skin of his chest:

> It began to exude blood in one place; so that the man himself was very near having broken through the skin (this being reduc'd to the utmost thinness in that part, and he being quite ignorant of the danger which was at

hand) when he began to pull off the bandages, for the sake of showing his disorder. But this circumstance being observ'd, he was prevented going on, and order'd to keep himself still, and to think seriously and piously of his departure from this mortal life, which was very near at hand, and inevitable. And this really happen'd on the day following, from the vast profusion of blood that had been foretold, though not so soon expected by the patient. Nevertheless, he had the presence of mind, immediately as he felt the blood gushing forth, not only to commend himself to God, but to take up with his own hands a basin that lay at his bed-side; and, as if he had been receiving the blood of another person, put it beneath the gaping tumour, while the attendants immediately ran to him as fast as possible, in whose arms he soon after expired.

In death, this unfortunate fellow presented a sacrificial offering to medical science. Like the old man with appendicitis, the prostitute with Marfan's syndrome, and the seven hundred others whose organs were described by Morgagni, his case history became one of those studied by physicians throughout Europe and America, so that they might emulate the methods of Padua. Those five professors to whom Morgagni had sent copies of De Sedibus recognized its value immediately, as did many of the members of the learned societies to which its author belonged. Within three years of its publication, demand for the book required the printing of a second and then a third edition. When Morgagni was visited by the Philadelphia physician John Morgan in 1764, the American wrote in his diary that De Sedibus was "in ye highest Estimation throughout all Europe, and all ye Copies of the last [third] Edition allready bought up." In that same year, Samuel Bard, a founder of what is now the Columbia University College of Physicians and Surgeons, wrote to his father from Edinburgh that De Sedibus was a book "from which the learned here seem to have great expectations."

The great expectations were fulfilled. From the pages of De Sedibus, physicians learned that the symptoms of their patients point the way to the internal seats of disease. After Morgagni, it would no longer suffice merely to listen to a patient relate his history, to look him over, feel his pulse, and stare at his urine. New kinds of cries would henceforth be sought from the suffering organs, cries that were more subtle, cries that took a great deal of listening in order to hear. More careful histories were taken by the physicians who learned their lessons from De Sedibus, and probing questions were increasingly asked, in an attempt to turn up information not volunteered. That most sensitive of the physician's arts, the art of physical examination, traces its real origins not to the irretrievably lost skills of the Hippocratics, but to

> *That most sensitive of the physician's arts, the art of physical examination, traces its real origins not to the irretrievably lost skills of the Hippocratics, but to the techniques developed in the century following Morgagni.*

the techniques developed in the century following Morgagni. Palpation became more thorough and more dependent on a three-dimensional knowledge of anatomy; percussion, the tapping out of differences in tissue density, was described by the German physician Leopold Auenbrugger in 1761, not fully appreciated, and then had to be rediscovered much later by Morgagni's French disciple Jean-Nicolas Corvisart. The most cherished moment in the growth of physical diagnosis finally occurred in 1816 when René Laennec invented the stethoscope, which spurred physicians on to yet greater discoveries of examination methods.

As impressive as was his reputation before 1761, Morgagni became looked upon thereafter as the leading sage of medical science. In his journal, James Boswell relates an amusing story of Samuel Johnson suggesting to him that he write to Padua to request that the professor dissect a scorpion in order to settle a biological debate which the two of them were having. Boswell, on his grand tour of the continent, called on Morgagni, whom he describes in his memorandum for June 27, 1765, as a "fine decent old man" who felt that he had devoted too many of his eighty-three years to study: "I have passed my life amidst books and cadavers." Boswell's biographer Frederick Pottle tells us that the purpose of the young Scotsman's visit was "partly to meet a very famous man, partly to get professional advice" about the ever-recurrent gonorrhea that plagued him after so many of his frequent amatory dalliances. Morgagni told him to live soberly, take little exercise, and stop syringing himself, none of which pieces of advice Boswell seems to have heeded. The professor's approach to medicine and life is exemplified

by one of the statements he made to his British visitor: "A physician takes his cue from Nature, who does things step by step, never by leaps and bounds." Leaping and bounding being Boswell's usual style, he was doomed to a long and intimate association with his dripping affliction.

A year before Boswell's consultation, Morgagni had been visited by the previously mentioned Dr. John Morgan, one of the original faculty of the College of Philadelphia, the institution that was to become America's first medical school. In his journal entry for July 24, 1764, Morgan recorded his impression of the old anatomist: "Went to pay my Respects to the celebrated Morgagni to whom I had letters from Dr. Serrati of Bologna. He received me with the greatest Politeness imagineable, and shew'd me abundant Civilities with a very good grace. He is now 82 y'rs of age, yet reads without spectacles and is as alert as a Man of 50." Morgan tells of a poignant moment that took place as his host was showing him the paintings of his predecessors that were on display in Padua's anatomy museum. Among them hung two crayon portraits of beautiful young women. Upon being asked who they were, Morgagni replied that these were his youngest daughters. His eight girls had gone off in pairs to four different convents. The two last had chosen a strict order of Franciscans in which they were required to go always barefoot and veiled. "Before they were shut up thus for Life, ye celebrat'd female Paintress Rosalba as a Friend of Morgagni drew these Portraits and made him a present of them before he knew she had any intention to draw them. As the others are of Orders less strict and may be seen without Veils, there was less occasion for their Portraits." And so, among the impedimenta and souvenirs of a lifetime spent "amidst books and cadavers" hung the portraits of the two much-loved young daughters, Margherita and Luigia Domenica Rosa, as they looked to their adoring father when he gazed on their faces for the last time.

The steadfast and tender union of Giovanni Morgagni and his devoted wife, Paola, came to an end with her death on September 2, 1770. The aged widower did not tarry long on this earth after the departure of his mate. He whose work had so clarified the pathological basis of stroke now succumbed to one himself, just as had his teacher Valsalva and his teacher's teacher Malpighi. He died in the house in which he had brought up his family, at 3003 Via S. Massimo, where a memorial plaque may still be seen bearing the simple sentence "Giamb. Morgagni, after founding pathological anatomy, died here on Dec. 6, 1771."

Eight years before his death, the city fathers of Morgagni's native Forli had placed in their municipal hall a marble medallion bearing an effigy of their most renowned native son. In typical small-town fashion, the medallion's inscription overreached the extreme boundary of its subject's proper station in the history of mankind: "Giovanni Battista Morgagni—nobleman of Forli. In the year 1763 the townspeople of Forli erected a marble statue because he distinguished himself for his country and all the people of the world with his discoveries and excellent books. As learned men sincerely believe, Morgagni is the foremost in the history of the human race."

We have been left no record of the unpretentious Morgagni's reaction when he first read the inscription. Most likely, he smiled indulgently in benevolent recognition of the town's need to honor itself by so honoring him. Too considerate to offend the mayor by disclaiming the medallion's bombastic exaggeration, he probably thanked the committee, shook hands all around, got back in his carriage, and returned to Padua to dissect.

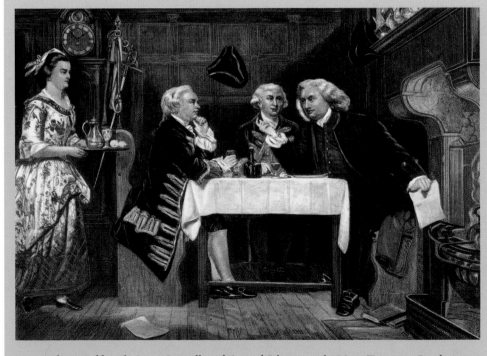

Oliver Goldsmith, James Boswell, and Samuel Johnson at the Mitre Tavern in London

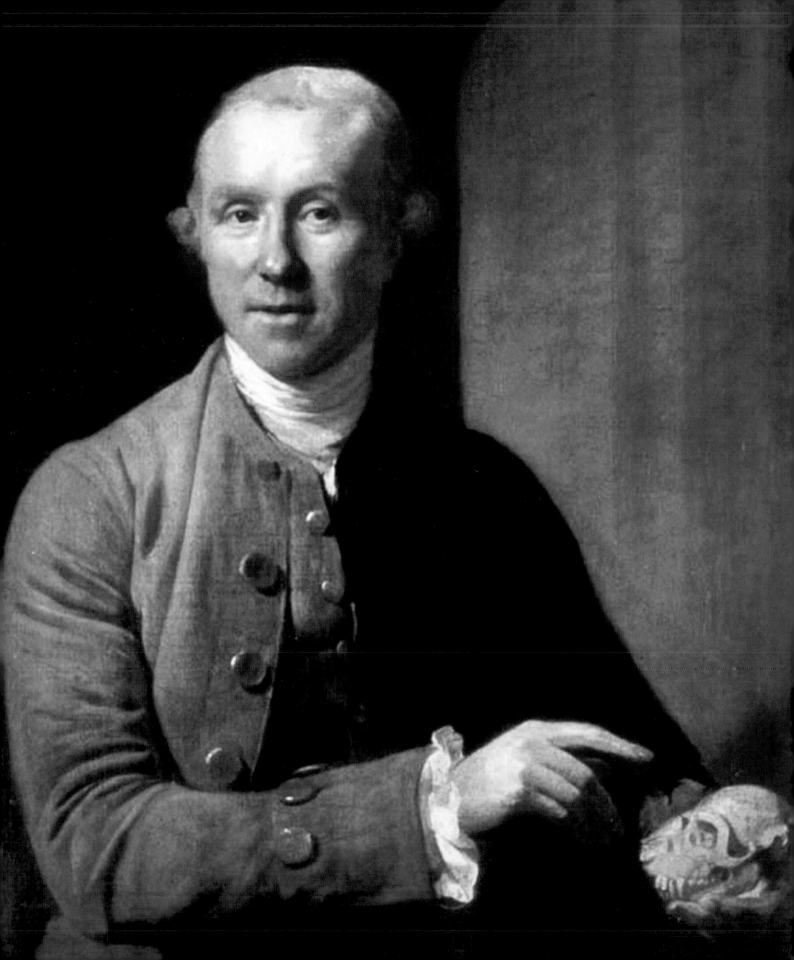

7

"WHY THE LEAVES CHANGED COLOR IN THE AUTUMN"

Surgery, Science, and John Hunter

No natural phenomenon can be adequately studied in itself alone, but to be understood must be considered as it stands connected with all nature.
—Sir Francis Bacon

Francis Bacon proclaims a basic tenet in the gospel of science. The essential unity that joins all natural phenomena ordains an interweaving of the work of every scientist of every discipline of every period in history with the work of every other. It forges a familial bond between all who have felt the tickling excitement of prying into Nature's elusive concealments, whether their sights are turned up at a star or down at a molecule. There is not a man or woman who has ever wrenched or seduced so much as a single new bit of information from Mother Nature's treasury who would fail to appreciate the vivid image created by Bacon's contemporary William Harvey: "to be received into her closet-secrets" conveys a sense not only of the lusciousness of victorious discovery, but of a sharing of company also, with all scientific curiosity-seekers since the forebears of Aristotle, and with Nature herself.

During most of the years when Giovanni Morgagni was restricting his gaze to a deliberately narrow focus in order to peer into Mother Nature's closet, another of her snooping sons was exploring her affairs by doing exactly the opposite. John Hunter took the entire realm of life and living to be his rightful investigative domain. He considered his purview to be all things that have to do with animal structure and function from the moment of conception to that instant when the vital flame is extinguished. He was eager to know everything—how the animal body works when it is working well, why it breaks down, and how it fights off the forces that lurk ever-present to destroy it.

Neither the quality nor the scope of Hunter's restless wonderment is describable in terms that apply to other men and women. To invoke the concept of genius is the only way in which any sense can be made out of his life and his accomplishments. Otherwise, we would have to believe in such vaguenesses as prescience, luck, or divine inspiration. The intellectual and social constraints that bind the rest of us do not frame fences around such people. There is no point for them on the bell-shaped curve of human abilities. To the John Hunters, formal schooling is superfluous and the normative methods of acquiring knowledge are a hindrance. We should not attempt to judge them as fellow human beings, nor should we try to puzzle out the sources of their creativity. It is enough that we can benefit from their time upon this earth.

John Hunter was the creative artist of medical science, a savant of unorthodoxy who created his own standards and made his own way, pointing out the new pathways to a retinue of talented disciples who transformed the image not only of the craft of surgeons, but of the entire profession of medicine as well. He wondered about everything that lives, and his wonder made him attentive to nature with a scrutiny so perceptive that he saw things no one else had ever imagined.

Hunter's great strength was the same as that which sustained the efforts of Vesalius, of Harvey, and of Morgagni. All of them, ignoring the pap of their predecessors, relied exclusively upon their own abilities to recognize what was significant, to describe it, and to correlate a large group of accurately made studies. All were gifted with the extraordinary faculty of distinguishing what is important from what is not. But although he

covered thousands of pages with his writings, Hunter never brought forth a *De Sedibus* or a *De Motu Cordis*, and certainly not a *Fabrica*. There was no single Hunterian magnum opus, but rather a lifetime of steady discovery of basic mechanisms of health and disease. Some of his steps were small, and some were as large as though made with twenty-league boots, so that the intellectual distance covered in the scientific journey of his career was immense. His masterpiece was not a book, but himself—a man who believed with a fervent certainty that by curiosity and hard work he could answer every question.

The greatest bounties of Hunter's vision were given to his fellow surgeons. After him, there was a new consciousness of the role that they could play in the elucidation of the processes of disease. But even more important than this was his introduction to his surgical colleagues of the concept that theirs was no longer to be considered merely an empirical craft but should thereafter employ the methods of the scientist. Had this greatest of all medical naturalists left no other heritage but this one, he would have deserved every encomium that has been heaped upon him by generations of his successors. As Fielding Garrison has written, "Hunter found surgery a mechanical art and left it an experimental science."

Expanding the scientific horizons of his fellows, Hunter's example brought them into a new arena of societal prestige, which only a few of them had previously enjoyed. One of his colleagues remarked, "He alone made us gentlemen." The ascending spiral of professional stature that had begun its slow upward winding with Ambroise Paré now started a rapid acceleration—increased prestige attracted better-educated and more highly motivated people whose achievements added to the status of the profession, and so on, and so on, and so on. Within a century after Hunter's death, it could be said with confidence that many of the greatest advances in the science of medicine had been made by surgeons, by then the most honor-laden of healers.

Hunter demonstrated that surgery is a profession worthy of the best minds. There is no doubt that his work influenced many to become surgeons who might otherwise have turned to internal medicine or gone into some other field entirely. In studies of the evolving rise of any profession, there are two quietly understated background stimuli that are consistently found to exert a powerful driving force: the improving intellectual status of entering members of the group and the development of professional societies. The fact that there was such a man as John Hunter served as a magnet that drew brighter and more enterprising workers to surgery and to medicine in general, and brought greater recognition to their organizations.

Hunter's students—and in a sense every surgeon trained around the turn of the nineteenth century was his student—made a catalyst of his memory. He was the instigator for a host of discoveries that brought added luster to his name and a solid base of support to his methods. As things turned out, it was his favorite disciple who became the one most famous, the young man to whom he once wrote, "I think your solution is just; but why think? Why not try the experiment?" His advice to that young surgeon, Edward Jenner, inculcated an attitude toward research that years later led to Jenner's discovery of vaccination for smallpox.

What the Royal College of Physicians did to honor their own First Scientist, William Harvey, the Royal College of Surgeons did for Hunter: each year on his birthday, February 14, an eminent speaker is chosen to deliver the laudatory Hunterian Oration. At the banquet for the 1963 Oration, the speaker, Sir Stanford Cade, found himself sitting near two foreign diplomats who

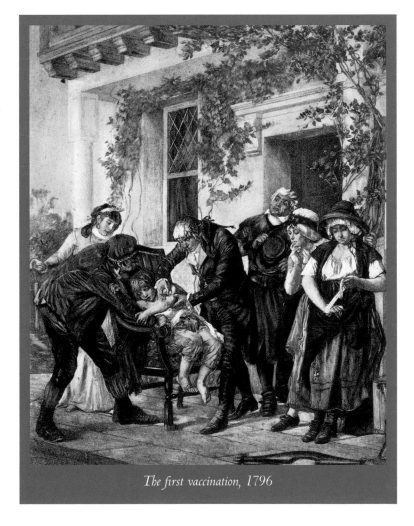

The first vaccination, 1796

sought information about the great surgeon. To the Italian ambassador he said, "Hunter is our Leonardo da Vinci," and to the French ambassador he explained, "He is to us what Ambroise Paré is to France." These are interesting comparisons, for they refer not only to men whose lives transcended the times in which they lived, but men who were largely self-taught, to the extent that they were often misunderstood by the contemporary conventional authorities. Equally appropriate was the comment of the nineteenth-century Edinburgh anatomist Robert Knox, who said of Hunter, "He not only was not formed by his age, but in direct antagonism to it. . . . He overcame all, and left in his museum a monument like the Cena of Leonardo, to tell posterity, five hundred years hence, that great men are not formed by the times they live in, but the times by them."

> *The earliest manifestation of Hunter's resistance to the standards of his day was his attitude toward school—he never let it interfere with his education.*

The earliest manifestation of Hunter's resistance to the standards of his day was his attitude toward school—he never let it interfere with his education. While other boys were becoming entrapped in the constricting mazes of Latin, Greek, and mathematics, young John was finding his freedom among the ecological miracles that he could daily discover in the Lanarkshire Scottish countryside where he was born in 1728. Not one iota of his childhood curiosity was ever dampened by any necessity of forcing his unique intellectual powers into the tight patterns that pedagogues

demand. He was fascinated from early boyhood to the end of his days by the wonder of biological forms, and by the various ways in which nature has succeeded in creating them and preserving them. There seems never to have been a time before which he did not recognize that the answers to his questions could not be found in books.

Others misunderstood. Hunter has been described by most authors as having wasted his youth until the age of twenty. Hunterian Orations and biographies are studded with such statements as the following, which was written by his first and otherwise most worshipful disciple, his brother-in-law, Sir Everard Home: "He was sent to the grammar-school, but not having a turn for languages, nor being sufficiently under control, he neglected his studies, and spent the greatest part of his time in country amusements."

Comments such as Home's set the tone for most of the future assessments of Hunter's youth. His most prominent late-nineteenth-century biographer, Stephen Paget, wrote of him in 1897:

We find no tales of early enterprise, no childish love of nature, no signs of future mental power. . . . It seems strange that a mind so remarkable as John Hunter's, so robust and self-willed as it proved, should not have shown or felt its power till, as if by chance, it was brought to scientific work. He had not lived in darkness or among dull people; his father was a shrewd and sensible man; his mother well educated; his two brothers were persons of remarkable mental power. With these, his mind had had opportunities of exercise and culture, but he had neglected them as to him useless. He had lived among the same wonders of the organic world, the same truths and utilities in nature as moved him, in his later years, to restless study; yet he seems to have given no heed to them. No desire of knowledge was stirred in him till he was under the influence of scientific minds. . . . His mind had no motive power till it was set to its right work, and in right working found happiness.

Home, Paget, and the others mistook their man. John Hunter offered up his entire life to indulging his God-given fascination with nature; so much was he in thrall to it that he seemed to others to have spent his youthful years skipping idly after moonbeams and rainbows. The self-education of surgery's first scientist was conducted in a school without walls, by wordless teachers who used no books and followed no syllabus. His youth was one prolonged, even perpetual, field trip.

Perhaps it was the cloistered rigidity of their own schooling that prevented so many of those who have studied John Hunter's life from comprehending the real meaning of his seeming lack of interest. Had they truly understood the significance of his lifelong romance with nature they might not have overlooked the evidence of his own words, written many years later: "When I was a boy, I wanted to know all about the clouds and the grasses, and why the leaves changed colour in the autumn; I watched the ants, bees, birds, tadpoles, and the caddis-worms; I pestered people with questions about what nobody knew or cared anything about." His niece, Agnes Baillie, said of his boyhood, "He would do nothing but what he liked, and neither liked to be taught reading nor writing nor any kind of learning, but rambling amongst the woods, trees, etc., looking after bird's nests, comparing their eggs—number, size, marks, and other peculiarities."

This was no ordinary Lowland rustic. This was a young man with the insatiable curiosity of a scientist and the wisdom to perceive that nature's secrets can only be learned by the methods of observation and analysis. One's powers of observation can be improved by the constant practice that teaches what to look for and points the way to understanding what is seen. Learning to categorize observations is the key to analyzing them. This was the self-education of John Hunter: to observe keenly enough to appreciate what was really being seen, to categorize observations well enough to analyze them, and then to seek some general principles. He was teaching himself the method of inductive reasoning, but its purpose would eventually be to use those general principles to derive clues to individual biologic observations. Thus his approach was, in the ultimate sense, deductive—reasoning from a major principle to explain specific phenomena. Without planning it or knowing what was happening, John Hunter spent his youth training himself to think like a scientist. And all the time, he thought he was only trying to satisfy his curiosity.

It had been Robert II, the first Stuart King of Scotland and the son of Robert the Bruce, who had given the Hunter family its Lanarkshire estate in the fourteenth century. Even in the best of times, life was hard for small landowners in the counties around Glasgow, and the two decades preceding John Hunter's birth had been particularly bleak. A series of bad-weather years had de-

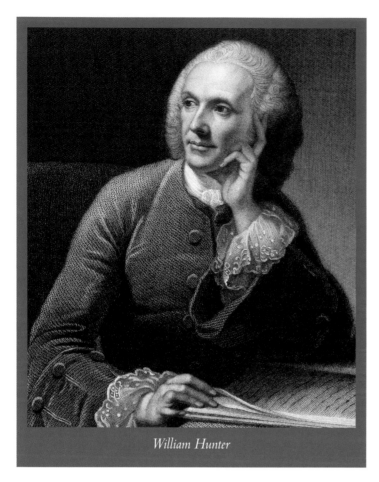

William Hunter

and its leading practitioner of obstetrics. He was bookish, he was fastidious, and he had the well-deserved reputation of being as adept in the lecture hall as he was in the dissecting room. His patients included some of the most fashionable and influential members of society, among whom he moved with an easy air of belonging.

Offering a decided contrast to the elegant, gentlemanly physician William Hunter was his stubby, brash, sartorially heedless fire hydrant of a brother. Where William was inclined to be courtly, John was gruff. The niceties of civil behavior that one learns in a drawing room are of no use in animal barns and fields—there were those of William's genteel friends who thought his brother's too forthright manner more suited to the stable than the salon, and they were right. Lack of an occupation drove him to his brother's door in 1748. He arrived in London an outspoken, high-spirited youth whose good intentions were often frustrated by his insensitivity to the feelings of the ordinary mortals around him. He had the type of personality that is called feisty by those who admire it enough to indulge its sharpnesses, and deplorable by everyone else. It required a tolerant patience to pick through the Scottish burrs to the underlying warmth and good nature of the man.

When to a disposition like John Hunter's is added an all-pervasive sense of honesty and an outspoken contempt for humbug, the possessor of such a constellation of qualities is virtually certain to spend much of his energies immersed in conflict. Quickness to anger, contentiousness, and a quarrelsome combativeness were part of the

pressed the harvests and the spirits of the countrymen so that even a "small Scots laird" might have trouble feeding his family, especially if he had ten offspring, as did John's father. By the time this last of his children was born, the senior Hunter had seen a little prosperity return, but only to be accompanied by his own ill health. When he died in 1741 at the age of seventy-eight, the responsibility for the family fell to his twenty-three-year-old son William, who, having completed his training as a physician, was then practicing in London. By the time young John reached the age of twenty, seven years later, William had prospered in the imperial capital, and was well on his way to becoming England's foremost teacher of anatomy

constitutional makeup of both Hunters, but the pragmatic William had at least trained himself in the elements of self-control; John never did learn to give a damn. The outspoken rough-edged elements of his personality remained unchanged until the day of his death.

When John first arrived in London to seek his vocation, William, not knowing quite what to do with the bumptious boy, put him in nominal charge of the dissecting room of his anatomy school. In a very short time, John began to realize that there among his brother's specimens he had found the ideal focus for his curiosity about nature. But before settling down completely to hard work, he had to get a little of the country-boy wildness out of his system. Newly arrived in the big city with a pocketful of wild oats, he proceeded to sow them all over the fleshpots and public houses of London. Drewry Ottley, in his 1835 biography of Hunter, described how at first "he mixed much in the society of young men of his own standing, and joined in that sort of dissipation which men of his age, and freed from restraint, are but too apt to indulge in. Nor was he always very nice in the choice of his associates, but sometimes sought entertainment in the coarse, broad humour to be found amid the lower ranks of society."

William's chagrin at his brother's dissolute habits soon changed to admiration, as the younger man quickly demonstrated his talent at dissection. That he had great manual skill was no surprise to Dr. Hunter, but his ability to marshal a newfound sense of discipline was an unexpected source of gratification. The wild oats were sown in a shorter time than anticipated; within less than a year the aspiring healer had begun to study surgery under the famous William Cheselden at the Chelsea Hos-

pital. Soon afterward, his brother appointed him demonstrator in his school. When Cheselden died in 1751, John became a pupil at St. Bartholomew's Hospital, where Percival Pott had succeeded to the role of England's leading surgeon.

Hunter dissected and taught in his brother's school whenever he could free himself from his clinical obligations on the wards. Finally he had to make a decision—in order to qualify as a surgeon at St. Bartholomew's, he would have to apprentice himself for five years, which would necessitate abandoning his cherished dissecting. There was no such rigidly demanding training at St. George's Hospital, so it was there that he chose to take his apprenticeship in 1754. The following year, he decided to give formal education one real chance. In July 1755 he enrolled, probably at William's instigation, at Oxford. Not surprisingly, that venerable university could no more make a conventional scholar of him than had the Kilbride Latin School. In his own words: "They wanted to make an old woman of me; or that I should stuff Latin and Greek at the University; but these schemes I cracked like so many vermin as they came before me." He left Oxford before the year ended.

Despite the failure of his plan to reform his free-spirited brother's academic disinclination, William's pride in his performance continued to grow, and he did everything he could to advance John's career. He was destined to remain disappointed, however, in his sibling's performance as a lecturer to anatomy students. Untutored in the niceties of grammar and elocution, and never having been impressed with the importance of verbal communication of ideas, John Hunter did not take naturally to the lectern. This oratorical deficiency was to plague him, and his students, for the rest of his life; in later years, we are told by Home, he "never gave the first lecture of his course without taking thirty drops of laudanum to take off the effects of his uneasiness." He rarely looked up from his lecture book. The worst of his sins may have been what students perceived as inconsistency, since he would on occasion contradict statements he had made in a previous lecture, not because his mind was wandering but because more study had caused him to change his views. The new theoretical concepts he was presenting required a kind of elucidation that he was quite incapable of providing; students who expected to be spoon-fed found his lectures indigestible. His classes never drew more than thirty students, whereas the superior lecturing abilities of his pupils John Abernethy and Astley Cooper, teaching much the same material they had learned from Hunter, would later attract hundreds at a time.

That John Hunter became one of the great teachers of surgery thus occurred in spite of, rather than because of, his method of teaching. It was his example and his knowledge that attracted those who were later to become outstanding members of the next medical generation, in Europe and the United States. It was the Hunterian excitement that captivated them and the Hunterian philosophy of objectivity that made adoring disciples of them. They became the messengers who translated what seemed like obscurities into comprehensible language and thus converted scores of surgeons to a scientific and experimental approach to healing.

In 1756, Hunter was appointed house surgeon to St. George's Hospital, a post similar to an internship, which he held for five months. His du-

ties included the day-to-day care of the patients of the various senior surgeons, the treatment of most of the fracture cases, and some minor operative procedures. Except for this brief period, he spent all of his nonteaching time between 1756 and 1759 in the study of anatomy, both human and comparative. This was the period of Hunter's life during which he evolved the pattern of investigation which was to remain with him for the next four decades. Since many parts of the human body are too complex for their structure and function to be easily understood, Hunter decided to start with simpler animals, and began laying the foundation of his collection of lower forms. He did everything in his power to get his hands on rare animals, even going so far as to make an arrangement with the keeper of the wild beasts in the Tower of London so that he might get their corpses when they died. He made similar bargains with circus owners and anyone else who had access to unusual creatures.

The constant miasma of the dissecting room took its toll on the young anatomist, however, and for reasons of health (or possibly because he needed the refreshment of a change from his brother's oversight), in the autumn of 1760 he enlisted in the army as a surgeon. England was at that time embroiled in the Seven Years War, a conflict which, in the words of the historian Samuel Eliot Morison, "should really have been called the First World War; hostilities were waged over as large a portion of the globe as in 1914–1918." As in so many of the wars in which the United Kingdom has been involved, the British began by losing one battle after another, but somehow managed to turn the tide and emerge victorious, gaining ascendancy over North

America and India, and once more asserting their supremacy over the seas.

John Hunter was given his commission on October 30, 1760, two months after the French surrendered in North America at the end of the portion of the hostilities called the French and Indian War. Between then and the final sputtering of the conflict to a close with the Treaty of Paris in February 1763, his time was largely taken up with the care of soldiers sick with the fevers, agues, and dysenteries that have plagued armies since the beginnings of organized battle. But he did gain one unexpected dividend from his military service—his first exposure to marine biology. He had never studied seabirds before, nor had he had any contact with the fauna to be found along the shore, such as sea urchins, anemones, squid, crabs, and eels, and contemplating their myriad forms, he began to consider the possibility that animals might be classifiable in some sort of phylogenetic series. It may not be too much to claim for Hunter that his studies anticipated Darwin's. Had he lived longer, he might have left behind a system of classification that would have made a theory of evolution a virtual inevitability.

Although Hunter's sentiments concerning his military-hospital colleagues are probably best conveyed by his reference to them as "a damned disagreeable set," he did form one solid friendship, with the surgeon to General John Burgoyne's regiment of light cavalry, Robert Home. Home's daughter Anne became Mrs. John Hunter in 1771, and her brother is the Everard to whom reference was made a few pages back.

Whatever had been the scattered quality of Hunter's training up to this point, he was a surgeon when he returned from the army. It was time to go into practice. During this period, surgery was not a calling noted for the material well-being it afforded its practitioners; it was said, in the words of a contemporary, "not to provide its members bread until they have no teeth to eat." But while the new surgical practice did not prosper, Hunter's army half-pay and the small income he derived from teaching anatomy allowed him to

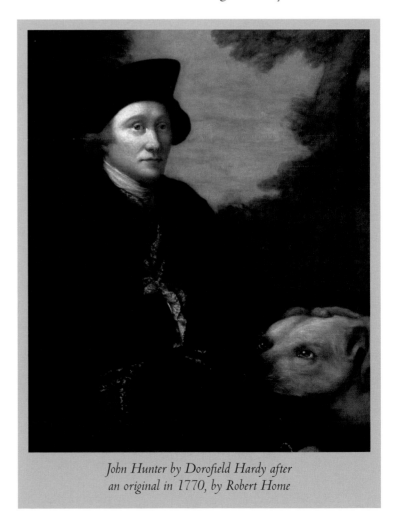

John Hunter by Dorofield Hardy after an original in 1770, by Robert Home

survive the difficult early days. In 1765, he bought a plot of land in Earl's Court, at that time two miles out in the country, in order to build a house and a small menagerie. He was ready to begin in earnest his studies in comparative anatomy—studies that were, in truth, the proper study of mankind.

At the time John Hunter began his practice, all surgical treatment was based on the isolated experiences of individual practitioners. There was neither in surgery nor in medicine any understanding of the general principles of disease, or even of the way in which the body functions when it is healthy. Although surgery was a practical art and medicine a theoretical one, they were both filled with sources of error. The one used pragmatic methods introduced by its leading figures, while the other still depended for its philosophy on the residues of Galenic traditions. Except insofar as Morgagni's new *De Sedibus* demonstrated those of the manifestations of disease that were visible to dissectors, no one had any idea of the ways in which the disordered processes of sickness are related to the natural processes of health, nor how things go awry to cause specific syndromes. Least of all was there any appreciation of nature's methods of cure.

John Hunter clearly perceived what was lacking. He set himself the task of furnishing a solid foundation for the understanding of human physiology, both normal and deranged. He believed, and rightly, that in order to "know" man-

kind, the entire animal series must be understood. It was to this task that he now dedicated himself. Drewry Ottley summarizes the master plan as it stood on that day in 1765 when his subject took up the work: "It was no less an undertaking, then, than the study of the phenomena of life, in health and disease, throughout the whole range of organized beings, in which Hunter proposed to engage; an undertaking which required a genius like his to plan, and from the difficulties of executing which, any mind less energetic, less industrious, and less devoted to science than his own would have shrunk."

As before, Hunter let it be known that he was on the lookout for animals, and he got them. Sir John Bland-Sutton, in his Hunterian Oration of 1923, describes the atmosphere at the Earl's Court ménage-cum-menagerie:

Leopards and jackals lived in the den, buffaloes, stallions, sheep, goats, and rams occupied the stables. A mulberry tree furnished leaves for the silkworms, and St. John's wort supplied pollen for bees. There was a pond for the ducks and geese which laid eggs for the table and for embryological studies. He made observation hives for the bees, discovered that their wax is a secretion, and left some excellent notes of the relation of vegetables to animal fat.

Actually, the wilder animals lived in outbuildings, and the leopards were usually tied up in some way, but the general picture of a research farm is perfectly accurate. This is where so many of the

> *He believed, and rightly, that in order to "know" mankind, the entire animal series must be understood.*

great experimental studies were done. It was also the home to which he brought the lovely young Anne as his bride, in 1771. It is hard to imagine what attracted the sensitive, dignified, good-looking daughter of Robert Home to the blunt-spoken, short (five feet two inches, by all accounts), round-faced animal dissector with whom she honeymooned among that host of winged, scaled, and furry chaperons at Earl's Court. But the marriage brought them both happiness. They seemed to have great admiration for each other's talents and abilities. Anne Hunter brought out in the abrupt and quick-tempered John a softness and a gentle consideration that could be elicited by few others. She was well educated in literature and music, and had many friends who shared her interests; her writing talents were such that some of her poems were set to music by Joseph Haydn. She was one of those ladies to whom the term "bluestocking" was applied in those days, when educated women were beginning to discuss literature and eschew the incessant card-playing in which most people of their class indulged.

Three years before his wedding, John Hunter had taken over the lease of his brother's house in Jermyn Street. After their rural honeymoon at Earl's Court, the couple took up residence in the town house, which served also as the place of Hunter's private practice. Later, in 1783, they left Jermyn Street and moved to Leicester Square, continuing to use the Earl's Court main house as a country home.

The Hunters had four children, all born during the first four years of their marriage, and they eventually built up a household which would be considered huge by any standards, even those of the time. William Clift, who became John's amanuensis near the end of his life, listed all of its almost fifty members by name, including those who did domestic work and those who were involved in the animal and experimental undertakings. The costs of the household, the expenses associated with the Earl's Court laboratory and research, and John Hunter's propensity for spending all available funds on his scientific collections kept him captive his whole life to the need for ready cash. There was never enough.

Much of his money went for the purchase of specimens for the museum which he established in the Leicester Square house. By the time of his death in 1793, he had become the world's leading authority on comparative anatomy, and the one to whom naturalists would bring any rare specimen that fell into their hands. He dissected everything, and he kept samples of everything. His collection came to contain nearly fourteen thousand specimens, described in ten volumes of his written manuscripts and notes. Overall, he would spend some £70,000 on his museum—a monumental sum then, and a virtually incalculable one in today's terms. Though his practice in its greatest years yielded him an annual income of £6,000, every spare penny of it went into his research and museum. The other property he left at his death was barely sufficient to pay his debts.

But all this was only in its beginning phases in 1765. The great experiments were just getting under way, and one of them was an experiment on the researcher himself. In February 1766, Hunter broke his left Achilles' tendon, the heel cord of the leg. It has been presumed that this happened while the ebullient surgeon was dancing, but since the event took place at four in the morning, by his own account, "while jumping and lighting upon my toes without allowing my heels to come to the ground," he may have been engaging in the eighteenth-century equivalent of jumping-jacks to relieve the tedium of writing up an experiment. In any case, what followed is characteristic of Hunter's ability to take advantage of every opportunity to make observations that came his way. In addition to recording the way in which his ruptured sinew healed itself, he turned his attention to a study of torn Achilles' tendons in general, cutting the structure in a series of dogs, through a tiny needle hole in the skin. The dogs were killed at different intervals, and Hunter was thereby enabled to demonstrate for the first time that tendons heal just as do bones, by means of a strong scarlike substance that the body produces to cement the ends together in a firm union.

In 1767, Hunter was elected a fellow of the Royal Society; the honor seems to have come to him primarily on the basis of future promise rather than any solid accomplishment, since it would be five years before he published a complete paper in the Society's *Transactions.* His brother William, ten years his senior and ten years longer in London, was not elected until a few months later.

As John Hunter became better known, the demands for his surgical and consulting skills grew rapidly. His working day needed more hours. He would begin his dissections before six in the morning, and continue until he took some breakfast at nine. He would then see patients in his home until noontime, when he began a round of house and hospital calls, which included any operations that might be necessary. The main meal of the day comes at four, after which he took a nap for about an hour. He spent the evening delivering or preparing lectures, or dictating the results of his research to an amanuensis. At midnight, when the family went to bed, the butler brought in a fresh lamp so that his master might continue his labors for a few more hours. The image brings to mind the words of the English essayist William Hazlitt: "Men of genius do not excel in any profession because they labour in it, but they labour in it, because they excel."

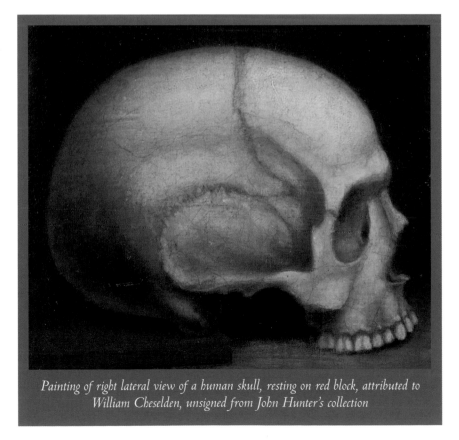

Painting of right lateral view of a human skull, resting on red block, attributed to William Cheselden, unsigned from John Hunter's collection

In the same year that Hunter was elected to the Royal Society, he carried out what was to become one of the most famous self-experiments in the whole history of science: he inoculated himself with venereal disease in an attempt to show that syphilis and gonorrhea are two separate manifestations of the same "morbid poison" (although a few scholars question whether Hunter was indeed the anonymous subject to whom he refers in his writings, it is otherwise generally agreed that this was an auto-experiment). This is a story that has been told, and mistold, so many times that those who know very little else about Hunter remember him as the selfless fellow who gave himself a case of both clap and syphilis in the name of science, and spent the next three years analyzing his drips and sores.

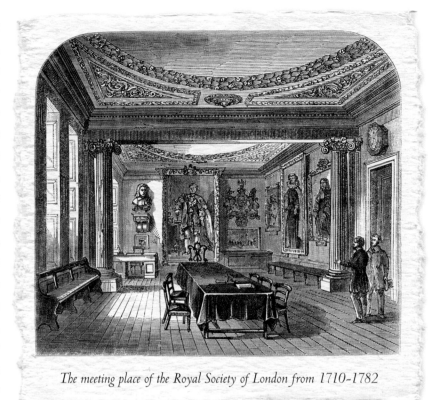

The meeting place of the Royal Society of London from 1710-1782

The sequence of events is described in a book published by Hunter in 1786, entitled *A Treatise on Venereal Disease.* In May 1767 he dipped a lancet in gonorrheal pus and then inoculated himself by puncturing the foreskin and head of his penis. The symptoms of gonorrhea developed rapidly, followed by those of syphilis. The areas that were involved early in the course of the disease were treated by cauterization, a local chemical burning. The later symptoms were medicined with mercury applied locally, in the style of the time. These were often effective treatments. In fact, mercury worked so well that in its various forms it remained a mainstay of syphilis treatment even after Paul Ehrlich's introduction of the "magic bullet" of Salvarsan in 1910. Until the large-scale use of penicillin near the middle of the present century, every medical student contemplating licentious assignation had to take into consideration the well-known maxim that a night with Venus might lead to a year with Mercury.

Because Hunter contracted both gonorrhea and syphilis as a result of his auto-experiment, he was strengthened in his conviction that the two diseases were really one, presenting in different ways in different tissues of the body. The source of his error is to be found in the source of his pus—he had unknowingly infected himself from a subject who harbored both diseases. Although its major conclusion was wrong, Hunter's experiment proved to be a scientific success. Over the course of the three years of his recurring symp-

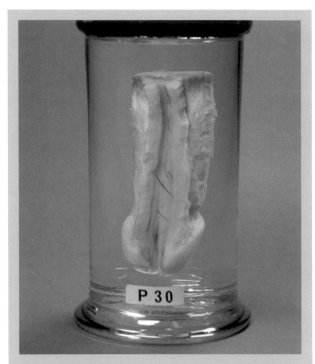

Ventral part of penis with gonorrhoea at time of death. This specimen is listed in Hunter's earliest catalogue and was probably prepared in 1753. In his Treatise on Venereal Disease, *John Hunter described procuring the bodies of two felons executed at Tyburn in 1753 whom he knew to be suffering with 'severe gonorrhoeas'.*

toms, he made a series of remarkably accurate observations that resulted in the first thorough description of the clinical course of venereal disease. For decades afterward, his publication stood as an oft-emulated example of the proper way to study the evolution of a pathological process in a human subject. Granted, no one knew that Hunter himself was the experimentee, but it became clear to his legions of readers (the book required a second edition and numerous translations during its author's lifetime) that the correct method of researching a chronic disease was to make repeated observations on the same patient from the instant of infection until the resolution of the process.

Syphilis is in many ways a model disease for study. Because it has the potentiality of involving every tissue of the body, it presents an opportunity to observe the ways in which individual organs respond to infection. Most particularly, it provides a paradigm of the way in which the process of inflammation both harms the disease victim and is the mechanism of his cure.

Inflammation is the process by which the body responds to injury. When a living tissue is damaged, whether by chemicals, trauma, or the effects of microbes, it protects itself by a series of local reactions at the site of insult. In general, the sequence is initiated by the injury itself, which starts up certain changes in the microscopic vessels in the area, resulting in the outpouring of plasma proteins, corpuscles, and other elements of the blood, either because they leak through the vessel walls or because the capillaries, arteries, and veins are actually torn open by the injuring agent. In these blood constituents, which are collectively called the inflammatory exudate, can be found all of the elements that are needed for the process of healing.

The task of the inflammatory exudate is to destroy the offending agent, to limit its spread, and to neutralize its effects. If this counterattack is successful, the invader's destructiveness rapidly ends, and the process of inflammation goes on to its next phase, which is to repair the injured tissue. Should the body, on the other hand, not be able to adequately combat its enemy at this initial encounter, the affected area enlarges and the inflammation intensifies to the extent of producing an overt disease. The disease may remain relatively localized, as in the case of an ulcer or a burn, for example, or it may become generalized by spreading through adjacent tissues or the bloodstream, as in many infectious syndromes.

It is perfectly clear to anyone who has ever had even the most minor injury or disease that the inflammation itself causes its own symptoms, which become part of the symptomatology of the disease. The classical evidence of the presence of inflammation is the quartet which has been recognized since Hippocrates: rubor, calor, dolor, and tumor—redness, heat, pain, and swelling. Thus the very symptoms which we find so distressing when we are sick may be the evidence that our bodies are fighting off the noxious forces. On the other hand, they may be evidence of something else entirely: sometimes the whole system goes awry; in such cases, the inflammation gets out of hand and itself becomes part of the enemy's attack. Uncontrolled inflammation added to an overwhelming injury is a common cause of death in lethal sickness. Many of the most dangerous of the diseases flesh is heir to are those that kill by the inflammatory reaction they produce in their host. Among them are those two lingering ravages of mankind, tuberculosis and syphilis.

Until the work of John Hunter, no one had ever undertaken a serious study of inflammation. It was to be the enduring triumph of Hunter's life that not only did he produce a body of work that elucidated some of its most basic principles, but his example stimulated the generations following him to recognize its fundamental importance to an understanding of disease. The studies of an entire career went into his *A Treatise on the Blood, Inflammation, and Gunshot Wounds,* completed just before his death and published posthumously. In this book can be recognized the same scrupulous attention to detail that characterized every piece of research that he had ever done. His observations on the evolution of syphilis may be viewed as a prelude to his observations of the role of inflammation in all diseases.

Although the *Treatise* is about injury and repair, its author used the term "inflammation" to mean primarily that part of the process by which diseased parts are healed—it was the example of his Achilles' tendon expanded to a universality. Since a surgical operation consists essentially of a planned, controlled injury which depends for its success on a predictable healing pattern, the fundamental nature of such research is apparent. The *Treatise* became, as had Hunter's investigations of syphilis, the basis of ongoing studies throughout the entire nineteenth century. To the present day, all over all the world, the most sophisticated methods of modern technology are being used to continue the investigation of inflammation that was begun by John Hunter more than two hundred years ago.

The two treatises, on venereal disease and inflammation, became prototypes of clinicopathological description and of research in physiology, respectively. It was through such publications that John Hunter brought the previously mechanical art of surgery into the field of scientific medicine. Henceforth, surgeons would be concerned with the same kinds of problems in human functioning as were their internist brethren. No longer was operative technique the only interest of the surgical specialists. For the first time, they turned their attention to the ways in which the body responds to all forms of sickness. They became physiologists and pathologists, and thus truly worthy of full membership in the ranks of the healers.

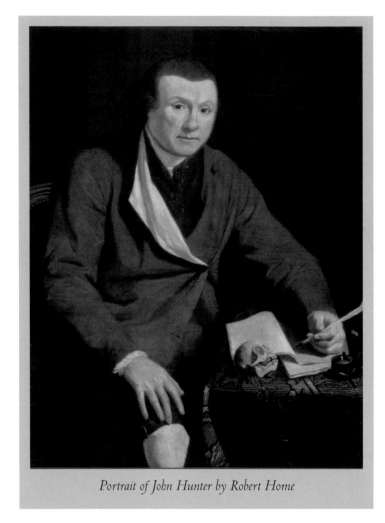
Portrait of John Hunter by Robert Home

of action to restore them to that state wherein a natural mode of action alone is necessary: from such a view of the subject, therefore, inflammation in itself is not to be considered as a disease, but as a salutory operation, consequent either to some violence or some disease. But this same operation can and does vary; it is often carried much further even in sound parts, than to acomplish union, producing a very different effect, and forming a very different species of discharge from the former; instead of uniting and confining the parts, rather separating and exposing them, which process is called suppuration, and varies with circumstances. However, even this in sound parts leads to a cure, although in another or secondary way; and in disease, where it can alter the diseased mode of action, it likewise leads to a cure; but where it cannot accomplish that salutory purpose, as in the cancer, scrofula, venereal disease, etc. it does mischief.*

Hunter's abilities as a descriptive scientist had to rise above the obscurity and opacity of his prose. He never did learn to express himself much more clearly on the printed page than at the lectern. His innovative approach to punctuation didn't help—it was called execrable by the nineteenth-century Philadelphia surgeon Samuel Gross. Here is the unschooled John Hunter explaining that inflammation is beneficial to the body but can sometimes become part of the problem:

Inflammation is to be considered only as a disturbed state of parts, which requires a new but salutory mode

It is the experimental studies described in the *Treatise on the Blood, Inflammation, and Gunshot Wounds*, not the language of their description, that explains such praises as the tribute of Fielding Garrison. Once penetrated, the book reveals itself as exemplary of its author's inductive and deductive reasoning: the experiments that he carried out and the observations that he made allowed him to induce the general physiological principles of inflammation, from which he then reasoned deductively back to the elucidation of specific diseases, such as osteomyelitis, peritonitis, phlebitis, and trauma.

Hunter had never read Francis Bacon and seems not to have known of his work—he had apparently come upon the principle of inductive reasoning by himself—yet he introduced Baconian logic to surgery, and by doing so, introduced surgery to the logic of science. Hidden away in one of his essays, "Observations on Digestion," is a statement that demonstrates the stout ties which bind great truths and great truth-seekers in all generations to each other. Compare the following words of Hunter with those of Bacon which were quoted at the outset of this chapter. Allowing amply for the former's punctuation and prolixity, we find him saying exactly what his predecessor did, if not with the same elegance:

> *It should be remembered that nothing in nature stands alone; but that every art and science has a relation to some other art or science, and that it requires a knowledge of these others, as far as this connection takes place, to enable us to become perfect in that which engages our particular attention.*

Several of John Hunter's experiments have become part of the legend and lore of medicine. Among them are his studies of transplantation of tissues, of which he said, "The most extraordinary of all circumstances respecting union is by removing a part of one body, and afterwards uniting it to some other part of another. . . . The possibility of this species of union shows how strong the uniting power must be. By it the spurs of the young cock can be made to grow in his comb, or on that of another cock; and its testicles, after having been removed, may be made to unite to the inside of any cavity of an animal. Teeth, after having been drawn and inserted into the sockets of another person, unite to the new socket, which is called transplanting." The result of one of Hunter's experiments, in which he transplanted a human tooth

into the center of a cock's comb, can be seen today in the Hunterian Museum of the Royal College of Surgeons in Lincoln's Inn Fields, London.

Another of the classic experiments was the one in which was demonstrated the principle of collateral circulation. When a major artery is obstructed, small vessels will develop from a point above the obstruction to carry the blood to a point beyond it, so that the tissues supplied by the artery continue to get some nourishment, albeit less than might have been carried were the main pathway not obliterated. These smaller channels are called collateral vessels, and they have saved many an organ or limb from gangrene when a large artery has become plugged by arteriosclerosis. John Hunter was the first to

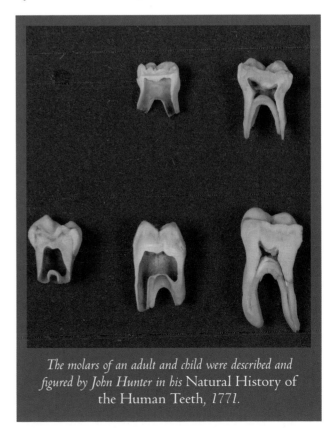

The molars of an adult and child were described and figured by John Hunter in his Natural History of the Human Teeth, 1771.

demonstrate their presence experimentally, in the following way.

He asked that a young stag be caught for him in London's Richmond Park. While several keepers held it still, he obliterated the major blood vessel in one side of its neck, the carotid artery, by tying a tight thread around it. As expected, the pulse in the velvet of the buck's antler disappeared immediately, and the antler became cold. Within a few days, the appendage was noted to have stopped its normal growth, whereas its opposite number remained warm and healthy. But before two weeks had passed, warmth had returned to the affected antler and it was growing once more. Upon sacrificing the animal and injecting colored fluid into its carotid artery, Hunter found that the circulation had been restored through collateral vessels; he then used this finding to devise an operation by means of which he was able to save the legs, and probably the lives, of several patients with aneurysm, or a weakened bulge in the wall of an artery.

It is of considerable interest these days, when so much progress is being made in the various forms of laboratory-induced pregnancy, to note that the very first successful human artificial insemination was done by John Hunter. In 1776, he was consulted by a man with hypospadias, a congenital deformity of the penis which made it impossible for him to impregnate his wife. Using a warmed syringe, Hunter injected the husband's masturbated semen into the cervix of the wife's uterus. The outcome, if the use of this word is permissible in such a context, was a successful fertilization. Thus the world's first modern democracy and its first artificially conceived baby were created in the same year.

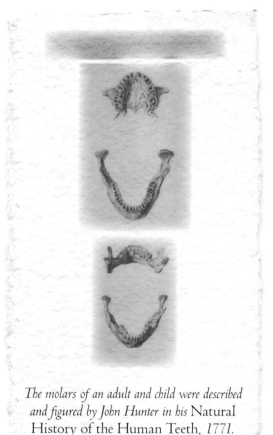

The molars of an adult and child were described and figured by John Hunter in his Natural History of the Human Teeth, 1771.

John Hunter seems to have accomplished the same sort of upgrading for dentistry as he did for surgery, writing two books on the teeth which required many editions and translations. At the time they were published, dentists were as low in prestige as itinerant bonesetters, those often unskilled craftsmen who knew a few tricks. Extraction methods were clumsy, and the remainder of dental work consisted of creating false teeth of bone, ivory, or wood, and primitive attempts to fill decayed cavities. Most practitioners were little more than quacks, trained, if at all, by other quacks. The mere fact that a surgeon of such stature as John Hunter would turn his attention to problems of the mouth had an impact, to choose the appropriate word for it. The structure and development of the jaws, their muscles, and their movement were particularly well outlined in his books, and the permanent teeth and their calcification described. The anatomic classification which is in use today derives from his work. Whenever your dentist mentions a cuspid, bicuspid, molar, or incisor, he is using terminology introduced by Hunter. He treated, among other topics, inflammations of the gums and bone, pyorrhea, tic douloureux, and salivary-duct stone, and he was the first to point out the necessity for removing plaque before it causes irritation, receding gums, and disease of the socket.

Sometimes Hunter's investigations of nature led him into situations of high adventure or low comedy. An example that demonstrates both is an episode that took place at his Earl's Court menagerie. One evening, hearing the sound of uncontrolled frightened barking, he rushed out into the yard from which the loud yelps were coming, finding several of his best dogs in a state of abject terror. Two of the captive leopards, having broken their chains, had the canines cornered and were emitting those low-pitched snarling growls that come just before the lethal leap. Impulsive as ever, Hunter dashed between the cats and their prey, seized the nape of a leopard's neck in each hand, and dragged the snarling beasts back to their cage. Immediately upon snapping shut the lock, he realized what he had done, and promptly fell to the ground in a dead faint.

On other occasions, it must be admitted, the scientist's relentless pursuit of research material led him into situations of intrigue or even thoughtless deceit. The tale of the Irish Giant, Charles Byrne (a.k.a. O'Brien), has been twice told even by storytellers who have forgotten the names of the protagonists or the background against which they played out their conspiratorial roles. The saga of Byrne is one of body-snatching. More than that, it is a saga that epitomizes the heedless way in which, until quite recently, some of the best medical scientists have gone about the business of studying the machinery of the human body.

There are two versions of the story. The first is the better-known one, originally told in Drewry Ottley's 1835 *Life of John Hunter.* The second is not as familiar, but nevertheless is probably more authentic, since it is the narrative of John Clift, Hunter's amanuensis during the last years of his life. What follows is based on Clift's account.

Charles Byrne was born in 1761 of quite ordinary-sized parents in the small village of Littlebridge near the border between the counties of Tyrone and Derry in the north of Ireland. By his late teens he had reached the height of eight feet two inches. These days, such gangling young men buy themselves an athletic supporter and a pair of sneakers and head off to Madison Square Garden. But professional basketball not having been invented, the long-legged lad undertook to exhibit himself at fairs, theaters, and anywhere else that curious country folk might willingly be separated from a few coins. Recognizing the pecuniary advantages that might accrue from a larger and better-heeled audience, an enterprising fellow in the neighboring village of Coagh, one Joe Vance, took it upon himself to become Byrne's agent. Finding a star-quality *nom de théâtre* for his client did not tax the inventiveness of the small-town hustler—the sobriquet of Irish Giant was the obvious choice, and London was the obvious destination for two country boys setting out on the road to show-biz fortune. The impresario and his would-be star arrived in the big city on April 11, 1782, and two weeks later placed this advertisement in a London newspaper:

Irish Giant. To be seen this, and every day this week, in his large elegant room, at the cane shop, next door to late Cox's Museum, Spring Gardens. Mr. Byrne, the surprising Irish Giant, who is allowed to be the tallest man in the world; only 21 years of age. His stay will not be long in London, as he proposes shortly to visit the Continent. . . . Hours of admittance every day, Sundays excepted, from 11 till three; and from 5 till 8, at half-a-crown each person.

At first, things went well. But the shiny coin of the realm soon showed its other side—too much of it too quickly was the ruin of our provincial Mutt and Jeff. Byrne took to drink just about the time that the novelty of his size began to lose its hold on his audiences. The crowds of spectators grew smaller, his advance-man Vance left him for greener pasture-boys, and he was victimized by thugs who found him easy to rob during his frequent

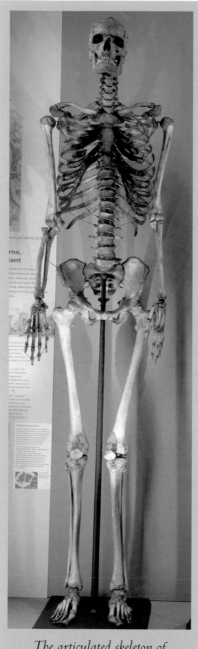

The articulated skeleton of Charles Byrne (1761–1783), known as the "Irish Giant." Although contemporary newspapers claimed Byrne to be over 8 feet tall he was actually about 7' 7".

booze-sodden episodes of coma. His country-bred lungs, accustomed to the invigorating freshness of Irish air, could not tolerate the oxygen-poor smogginess of London's humid filth. When he awoke in the muddy gutter one morning coughing blood, he knew that he had fallen prey to the scourge of the city—tuberculosis.

By June of 1783, Byrne lay dying. John Hunter, who had been watching his decline from afar, yearned to have his skeleton and sent his man, Howison, to keep close surveillance over all of the Irish Giant's movements, in the hope of laying hands on his body immediately after death. Howison was like his master—he pursued his quarry without subtlety or secrecy. Byrne soon learned that his cadaver was to be anatomized by the great surgeon, and the thought of it kept him in a constant state of terror. He had hoarded a residue of his dwindled little savings, which he now paid to some Irish friends, that they might carry his remains far out into the North Sea and sink them in an oversized lead coffin.

Hunter was able to learn the name of the undertaker

whom Byrne had chosen to prepare his body for its aquatic burial, and he set about attempting to bribe him to turn it over for dissection as soon as it made its appearance in his parlor. Never has a scientist borne a more suitable surname. The hunter and the mortician met in an alehouse, where they proceeded to haggle. Unfortunately for the zealous collector's pocketbook, he was well known for his willingness to pay high prices for a valuable biological trophy, be it derived from man or beast. His first offer of fifty pounds was refused. Each time he raised his bid, the mortician scurried out to discuss the new price with a hastily summoned brain trust of his cronies who had assembled in the alleyway. Sensing the eagerness that Hunter could not hide, they drove the price higher and higher. Finally, agreement was reached on a figure of five hundred pounds, which the perpetually cash-short surgeon had to go out and borrow.

When Byrne died a few days later, confident that his earthly remains would soon be safely consigned to Neptune, the well-bribed undertaker volunteered to accompany the corpse to its marine mausoleum. Clift has left a colorful description of the atmosphere in which the cortege wended its funereal way northward from London on that day in early June, to the small quayside from which the departed was to depart: "The road was long, the weather hot, the coffin heavy, the bearers and escort Irish. They kept up a walking wake as they went along, stopping to liquor up at convenient distances as hostelries occurred."

Finally, coming to an inn whose door was too narrow for the coffin, the undertaker suggested that the bulky box be locked up in an adjacent barn. For safety's sake, the key was given to the leader of the bodyguards, and the entire troupe of besotted mourners retired to the comforts of the tavern. Byrne's hired protectors could not have known that this whole scenario had been worked out beforehand by the undertaker, who had accomplices and tools hidden behind a pile of straw in the barn. In less time than it takes a gang of modern young hoods to strip a parked car in New York, the coffin lid was unscrewed, the body removed and hidden under the straw, and its weight replaced by paving stones. After suitable refreshment, the funeral party returned, unlocked the barn door, and resumed their staggering journey to the sea. As soon as they were out of sight the corpse of Charles Byrne was suitably packed and stowed on a springboard wagon for the return trip to London.

In the dead of that night, the Irish Giant's fugitive hearse drew up alongside a fashionable private carriage. Peering impatiently through the partially drawn curtains was the grand orchestrator of the entire cloak-and-dagger scheme. In a few moments, Byrne had been transferred, and Hunter, with his huge and now quite stiff passenger propped up in the seat next to him, was clattering his way home to Earl's Court. Fearing discovery, he immediately cut up the corpse, separated its flesh by boiling it in a vat specially built for such purposes, and prepared the skeleton. In later years, the unusual brown discoloration of the bones would be remarked upon by many a visitor, unaware that the tinting had been caused by rapid boiling in a pot.

The story of the Irish Giant is usually told (and I have told it this way) as one of those amusing if somewhat gruesome anecdotes that footnote the pages of medical history. Much of the amusement, in fact, arises from the very gruesomeness of the details, the terror of the victim, and its stark contrast with the sang-froid of the doctor-hero dispassionately going about his investigative work. Modern physicians and laymen alike see it as a Halloween prank of suspense, coffins, and skeletons, too far removed from their ordinary experience to be threatening to the desired humanitarian image of doctors or the ordinary person's sense of his safety from such maraudings. Looking at it in any other way would force both physicians and laity to remember the distasteful truth that until relatively recent times, many a researcher used his role as a scientist to elevate himself not only above the law of the land, but also above the more fundamental moral law that governs the relationships between human beings. The more single-minded a medical investigator was, the more zealous in his pursuit of Nature's secrets, the more likely he was to violate, deliberately or not, the rights of Her creatures.

His freedom from self-doubt and the shackles of society's rules made him, in the eyes of many, the ideal medical scientist.

To the ardent investigator who is the hero of this chapter, the Irish Giant was not a person, but just another of those samples of "research material" to whose pursuit he devoted all his energies. To his disciples of the next generation, who would narrate and record the Byrne story, Hunter's quest justified his means. If those means were a bit reprehensible, so be it. He was, after all, the great John Hunter, and his methods were more to be envied than criticized. His freedom from self-doubt and the shackles of society's rules made him, in the eyes of many, the ideal medical scientist.

The attitudes exemplified in the story of Charles Byrne would vex physicians and laity alike for the next century after Hunter's death. The attitude of lay people was one of fear and indignation; the attitude of the medical profession was one of ambivalence. On the one hand, there seemed no other way to gather certain kinds of scientific information than to bypass the ordinary pathways that society allowed; on the other, it took a degree of hard-hearted arrogance, or at least a dulling of moral sensibility, to use unsuspecting patients as if they were experimental animals, or their dead bodies as if they were anatomical preparations.

As the nineteenth century progressed, however, compunctions became more common, the protests of the people became louder, and solutions to the dilemma began to be found. When Sir Astley Cooper, one of Hunter's foremost disciples, appeared before an investigating committee of Parliament in 1828, and told its members that there was not one of them whose corpse he could not obtain from grave-robbers within a day of death, it was clearly time to act. In Britain and elsewhere, anatomy laws were drafted providing means by which cadavers might be donated by survivors or by civil authorities. The atmosphere of cooperation between the profession and the people gradually improved as each group became more sensitive to the other's concerns, and to the concerns they shared in their mutual goal of improving the health of succeeding generations. Although there were instances of abuse by medical researchers (particularly against minorities and the poor) until well into our century, the more flagrant examples became ever fewer. Behavior was eventually codified into statements of ethics reflecting the concern of scientists with the welfare and the rights of those they studied. It is a source of considerable pride to the medical profession that the physician members of today's Human Investigation Committees are the staunchest protectors of the same rights and dignities of patients that their forebears of a century ago felt so free to violate in the name of science.

All through the long period of productive research, John Hunter's private practice grew. Beginning in 1775, the first year in which he earned more than a thousand pounds, it reached a level that allowed him greater freedom to purchase whatever specimens and technical help he needed. His practice became even larger after he was named Surgeon Extraordinary to the King in 1776. Upon the death of Percival Pott in 1788, Hunter was acknowledged by all as the first surgeon of Great Britain. He was named Surgeon-General of the Army and Inspector-General of Regimental Hospitals, both of which added to his income, but demanded time and effort.

In spite of his success in practice, Hunter never enjoyed the more routine aspects of patient care. He would not hesitate to travel anywhere to see an interesting case or help out with a difficult problem in clinical management, but he chafed under the necessity of taking care of everyday problems. Heedless of amenities, he often made his irritation known to those many wealthy Londoners who came to him with minor complaints. He considered his huge daily practice to be the source of support for his research endeavors, and he made no attempt to act otherwise. On one occasion, he said to his pupil William Lynn, as he was going off to make a house call, "Well, Lynn, I must go and earn this damned guinea, or I shall be sure to want it tomorrow." And yet he would sometimes refuse a fee when he felt his patient was too poor or judged that he had not been helped by the treatment.

Hunter believed, as do all good surgeons, that the healer's greatest skill is his judgment, especially the judgment that restricts surgical operations to situations in which more conservative measures are to no avail. In that era before either antisepsis or anesthesia, such a philosophy was not only prudent but mandatory, although many disagreed. He once compared the practitioner who resorted to surgery unnecessarily to "an armed savage who attempts to get that by force which a civilized man would get by a stratagem."

When he moved his family to 28 Leicester Square in 1783, Hunter's income from practice had reached five thousand pounds a year and was going up. He had enough money to convert his house in such a way that it could provide him all the living and working space he needed. It took two years and six thousand pounds to complete it, but he considered the money well spent, even though it meant that his income would henceforth never exceed his expenditures. The sumptuous main house adjoined the museum, a room fifty-two by twenty-eight feet, having a gallery all around, with a skylight for a roof. Beyond the museum, a glass door twelve feet high opened into the Great Salon or Converzatione Room, a beautifully decorated chamber one hundred by fifty feet, hung with valuable paintings. Another door separated this room from a semicircular lecture theater whose walls were lined all around with shelves holding the specimens that Hunter used to illustrate his lectures. Next to the lecture hall was a drawing room which could be used for meetings. Behind all of this was a courtyard, part of which was glasscovered. Upon crossing the courtyard, one entered the back of another house in the adjoining Castle Street, also owned by Hunter, and used as a home for his house-pupils and for

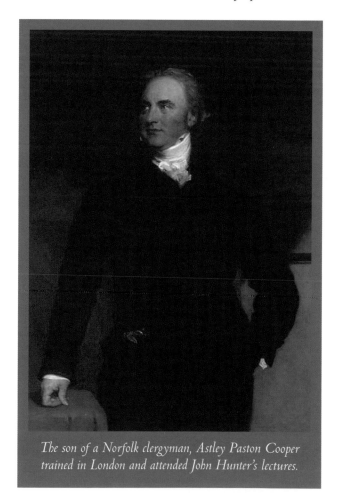

The son of a Norfolk clergyman, Astley Paston Cooper trained in London and attended John Hunter's lectures.

offices, including the place from which he published his own monographs and books. In all, the grounds made up a large estate, on the equivalent of three building lots.

Although a dreadful lecturer, Hunter was a teacher without peer to his private pupils. To be with him daily, to see him solve difficult clinical problems, to help him with his experiments, and to observe his mind at its sublime work—there could be no better way to learn the art and science of medicine. Each pupil paid a fee of five hundred guineas, and was bound to his teacher for a period of five years. Those privileged to live in his family as house-pupils were the most fortunate of the lot. They were the ones who came to understand him best, who knew that he spoke as an oracle of the coming science. They learned to interpret the words and the rhythms of his wisdom, and they learned that his speech had the sound of truth.

Leicester Square was not unaccustomed to famous men. Isaac Newton had lived in a house that fronted on it in St. Martin's Street, and William Hogarth had come with his new bride to set up a household in 1733. When John and Anne Hunter bought their property, they were well aware that Joshua Reynolds would be their neighbor at number 47, where he had made his home since 1760. Living on the opposite side of the square, the Hunters were bound to become friendly with Sir Joshua and his sister, especially in view of Anne's interest in the arts.

Colleagues, and no doubt Reynolds himself, frequently urged Hunter to sit for his neighbor, but were always refused. Finally, at the insistence of another friend, the engraver William Sharp, he agreed to go through the disagreeable procedure. Impatient, fidgety, and regretting every moment of the lost time, he was a predictably poor subject. It took a great deal of travail and grumbling, but at last the portrait seemed to be nearing a barely satisfactory state of completion. And then one afternoon, just as Reynolds had given up on the possibility of producing a truly fine portrait, a remarkable thing happened. For a few minutes, Hunter seemed to forget where he was, and fell into a state of reverie, as though communing with the sources of his genius, listening to "whisperings from the Infinite." Without disturbing the stillness of that enchanted instant, Reynolds turned his almost-finished portrait upside down and made a new sketch of his subject's transported face between the legs of the old. He started his painting all over again. What he laid down over the previous picture was considered a masterpiece when it was exhibited the following year at the Royal Academy of the Arts.

In the portrait, Hunter is surrounded by the souvenirs of his life. Among them are a preparation of the injected blood vessels of the lungs, an opened folio volume of his manuscript on what he called the "graded series" of comparative anatomy, and the lower limbs of Charles Byrne's discolored skeleton. Each year on the occasion of the Hunterian Oration, the portrait is hung facing the assembled audience, above the Orator. Lost in thought among his most prized mementos, John Hunter speaks more eloquently to his fellow surgeons at these assemblies than ever did any invited professor.

In 1785, when he was fifty-seven years old, Hunter began to experience episodes of chest pain. At first occurring only during strenuous exertion, they began after a time to grip him on much less drastic provocation. As always, he made

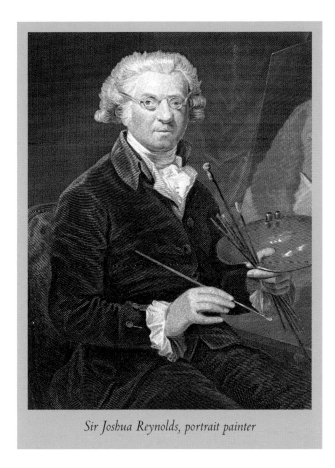

Sir Joshua Reynolds, portrait painter

good use of his infirmity, rushing to a mirror on more than one occasion of seizure in order to see on his own face the expressions of pain and fright that accompany an attack of angina pectoris. Gradually, he learned to avoid the rapid activity and stair-climbing that brought on his spasms, but he had no control over his turbulent thoughts, nor could he acquire at this stage in his life a serene disposition. For every one of his students and close friends who adored him for his essential goodness, there were five men who despised every cell in his pugnacious body. For every person whom he had helped through life with acts of genuine kindness, there were a dozen others he had insulted. He had all his years been contemptuous of mediocre men, and his greatest rages of

learn the prophylactic value of walking away from a confrontation. By his sixty-fifth birthday, angina had become an old adversary, to whom John Hunter knew he must lose the last battle. "My life," he said, "is in the hands of any rascal who chooses to annoy and tease me."

The final collision took place in the boardroom of St. George's Hospital on October 16, 1793. Hunter was hotly involved in a debate occasioned by his support of two young Scotsmen who had applied for admission as surgical students. When a statement he made was contradicted by one of his opponents in the discussion, he rushed out of the room in a fury, his mortally wounded heart shrieking its last painful warning. He collapsed lifeless into the arms of a physician who chanced to be standing near the door. The healing principle had departed from John Hunter's body.

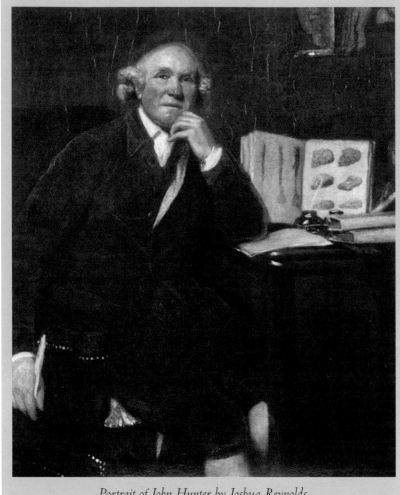

Portrait of John Hunter by Joshua Reynolds.
Notice the Irish Giant's skeleton hanging in the background.

combativeness erupted when those mediocrities took positions antagonistic to his own. It was not so much a question of being unable to suffer fools gladly—he couldn't suffer them at all.

Unfortunately, now Hunter's Celtic emotions poured forth from a heart that was but poorly nourished by hardened coronary arteries. In moments of stress, its blood-starved muscle cried out a warning that was always forgotten the next time he allowed his anger to get the better of him. He was aware that he lived in peril, but he refused to

Thus died the most illustrious of surgeons. It is fitting that his grateful countrymen, after a lapse of sixty-six years, would transfer his body to an honored spot in Westminster Abbey from its near-forgotten first resting place in the crypt of St. Martin-in-the-Fields church near Trafalgar Square. It is fitting also that one of the earliest proponents of Darwin's theory of evolution, Charles Lyell, should lie at his head, and Ben Jonson, another kind of poet, at his feet. There in the north nave of the abbey may be seen the brass plaque that reminds the living world of what it owes to John Hunter:

The Royal College of Surgeons of England has placed this tablet on the grave of Hunter to record admiration of his genius, as a gifted interpreter of the Divine power and wisdom at work in the laws of organic life, and its grateful veneration for his services to mankind as the founder of scientific surgery.

None of the written biographies or Hunterian Orations has ever done justice to the towering mountain of information, anecdotes, data, and hints that form the historical heritage of John Hunter. Even the major books that have been published tend to emphasize certain directions that his spirit took, at the expense of the several others. Perhaps in some future time the appropriately intuitive and voracious reader and thinker will appear who can focus the proper talents on the work. He or she will have to be gifted with a narrative style that is equal to the task of weaving a literary tapestry manycolored and multifibered enough to show the whole panorama of the man. That writer will have to be a surgeon, a naturalist, a psychoanalyst, a historian, a philosopher, a physiologist, an embryologist, a dentist, a social critic, and a very sensitive soul.

No other surgeon has ever had the commanding effect on his art, on his science, and on the quality of the contributions of those who followed him that John Hunter did. And yet he was, in truth, less a surgeon than he was a naturalist. One of his biographers, William Qvist, has written of him, "John Hunter worshipped Nature with profound humility. He was not just a disciple of Natural History—he was its High Priest." More than that, he was its small boy, never losing his gift of looking at life through the wondering eyes of childhood, wanting "to know all about the clouds and the grasses, and why the leaves changed colour in the autumn."

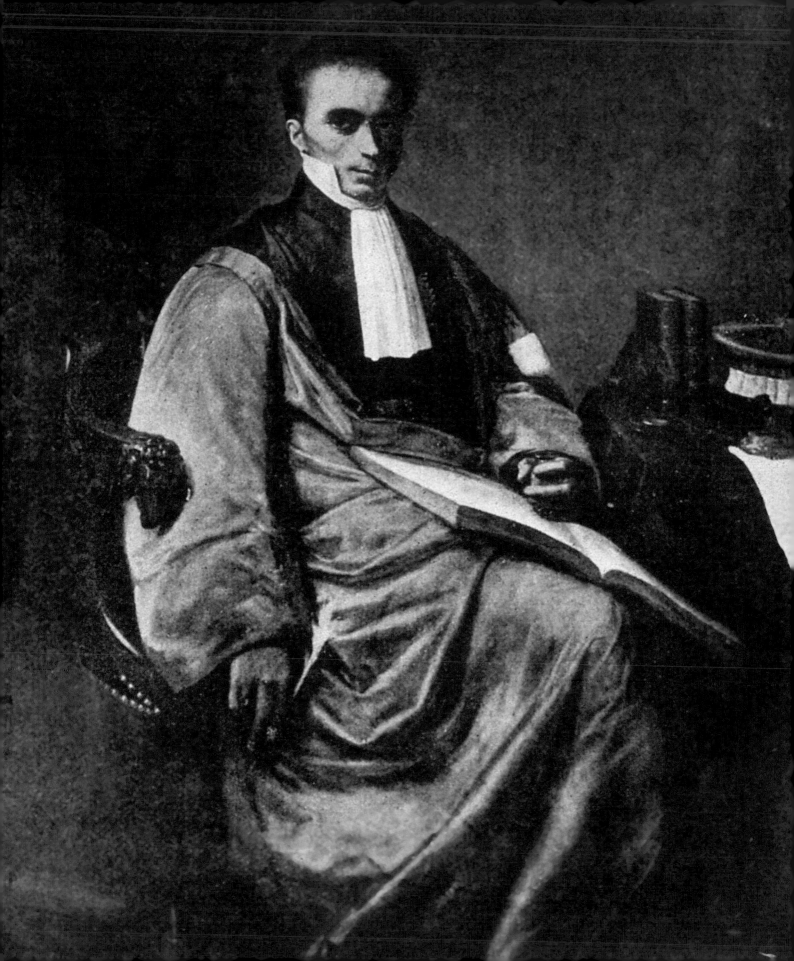

8

"WITHOUT DIAGNOSIS, THERE IS NO RATIONAL TREATMENT"

René Laennec, Inventor of the Stethoscope

Die Frucht der Heilung wächst am Baume der Erkentniss. Ohne Diagnostic keine vernünftige Therapie. Erst untersuchen, dann urtheilen, dann helfen.
The fruit of healing grows on the tree of understanding. Without diagnosis, there is no rational treatment. Examination comes first, then judgment, and then one can give help.
—Carl Gerhardt, Würzburg, 1873

Tomorrow is Alumni Day at my medical school. Because I remained in New Haven after my class dispersed itself to internships in other parts of the country, I like to think that I serve the university as a changeless memento of the good old days—everybody's good old salad days. Actually, it is not I who am changeless, but rather my image of each year's returning old grads. In the effervescence that results from the bubbling up of bright memories, every alumnus and alumna seems forever young, as though some gentle fixative had preserved all of them just as they were at the palmy conclusion of those four years

of professional ripening. What I see when I greet an old classmate is what I saw on graduation day in 1955, and what we talk about in the first minutes of our conversation is what we were talking about then. That initial instant of recognition at every reunion is golden. It re-creates youth and reconstitutes the optimistic verve with which we first set out to conquer, quite literally, the ills of mankind.

Before we old classmates let the conversation shift to matters of present-day concerns, there is likely to be, as in all such enthusiasms, some jocular talk of "Do you remember the time when . . . ?" And even if not spoken, even if we don't get around to articulating it during the course of the weekend, there is the flood of quite specific remembrances that is evoked by each newly arrived face. Ours was a small class—only seventy-six men and four women traveled those eventful four years together—and we shared a lot. We were in company constantly for the first two years and never farther than a few corridors away from each other during the final two. We all bought our first stethoscopes on the same afternoon.

Now, that was one glorious day. The ceremony of the buying of the stethoscopes, immediately dubbed "hearing-irons" by a classmate from Oklahoma, marked the second of four well-spaced rites of passage that sequentially brought us the full inheritance of Hippocrates. The first had been the timorous moments of introduction to the cadaver, the very instant of initiation into the priesthood of medicine. Then toward the end of the sophomore year was bestowed the right to ownership of the sacred stethoscopic badge of office, acquired in exchange for seven or eight dollars at the local medical bookstore, called the White Shop and presided over by a tutelary tradesman named Meyerowitz. Six months later, with hesitation scarcely less tremulous than the well-remembered anxiety of our first contact with corpse dissection, we were permitted to examine a live patient. And finally, there came step number four: when courses were completed, exams passed, and no balance remained on the bursar's bill, we became real doctors, or at least we were so certified by a school which, having been at the business for almost 150 years, was considered by the state licensing authorities to know what it was doing.

Of all of the four stations on our way, none marked a transition more significant than the buying of the stethoscope. By the wearing of that insignia, we became instantly recognizable as doctors. In those days, nurses might be granted its momentary use in order to take a blood pressure, but no one else dared presume to touch the venerated instrument or to carry it necklaced around the collar. It was at once a medal for achievement, an insignia of rank, and a symbol denoting power; all of us, including the women, thought of it as the doctor's phallus. As third-year medical students, we quickly learned to comport our stethoscoped selves with that casual air that conveys both insouciance and wisdom. I know of no more telling commentary on the present egalitarian status of all segments of what are today euphemistically called the health-care professions than the fact that the stethoscope is no more the sole property of the physician than is the white coat. The legatees of the long-dead Meyerowitz have never been busier.

Whatever its function as a symbol of rank, the stethoscope was an amazingly efficient instrument in the days when I first learned to use it, and it remains so today in spite of MRI, CT, and all other alphabetized and acronymic modernities. Although it is nothing more than a device to conduct sounds to the ear, its invention in 1816 opened up an entire new range of diagnostic possibilities to physicians, and much medical thought for more than a subsequent century was devoted to describing the various ways in which it could be used to detect subtle clues to disease. Riding lightly in the coat pocket of the physician, it was a readily available companion in diagnosis and an invaluable aid in teaching students the elements of pathological processes. This chapter is about its invention and its inventor.

The Hippocratic Corpus contains the first mention that there is a usefulness in listening to the sounds that emanate from within the recesses of the body. In *De Morbis* is written: "You shall know by this that the chest contains water and no pus, if in applying the ear during a certain time on the side you perceive a noise like that of boiling vinegar." The sloshing of air and fluid in the thorax, called succussion splash, is another sound recorded by one of the Hippocratic authors, as is the "creaking like new leather" that is heard when a bit of injured lung rubs against the inside of the chest wall. In the seventeenth century, both Robert Hooke and William Harvey described the sound of the beating heart. It was Hooke, in fact, who predicted the diagnostic riches that would in later centuries be found by studying the noises produced in man's internal machinery. In an astonishing bit of prescience, he went so far as to suggest that it might prove possible to augment the ear's ability to appreciate the individual sounds and the differences between them:

Who knows, I say, that it may be possible to discover the Motions of the Internal Parts of Bodies, whether Animal, Vegetable, or Mineral, by the sound they make, that one may discover the Works perform'd in the several Offices and Shops of a Man's Body, and thereby discover what Instrument or Engine is out of order. . . . And somewhat more of Incouragement I have also from Experience, that I have been able to hear very plainly the beating of a Man's Heart, and 'tis common to hear the Motion of Wind to and fro in the Guts, and other small Vessels, the stopping of the Lungs is easily discover'd by the Wheesing, the Stopping of the Head, by the humming and whistling

Noises, the slipping to and fro of the Joynts in many cases, by crackling, and the like. . . . To me these Motions and the other seem only to differ secundum magis & minus, and so to their becoming sensible they require either that their Motions be increased, or that the Organ be made more nice and powerful to sensate and distinguish them (to try the contrivance about an Artificial Tympanum) as they are, for the doing of both of which I think it not impossible but that in many cases there may be Helps found.

The modern process of examining patients attained its present form because of Giovanni Morgagni. His work led ineluctably to the era in which the art of physical examination was developed. In his *De Sedibus*, Morgagni described some seven hundred cases in which the symptoms of illness could be traced after death to their organs of origin. As strange as it may seem to us two hundred years later, his findings were a revelation which many contemporary physicians greeted with astonishment, accustomed as they were to blaming disease on such vaguenesses as ill winds, lax morals, miasmas, and a much-maligned Deity. That brief period of wonderment was succeeded by a long era during which the main interest of medical investigators was to find means of identifying the organ abnormalities while the sick patient still lived. This is, of course, the purpose of the modern physical examination—the looking, and tapping, and listening, and feeling that elicit the evidence of disease and localize it to its organ of origin. In the evolution of that art, there is no greater contribution than the invention of the physician's first and most useful diagnostic instrument, the stethoscope, a product of the uniquely French approach to Morgagni's work.

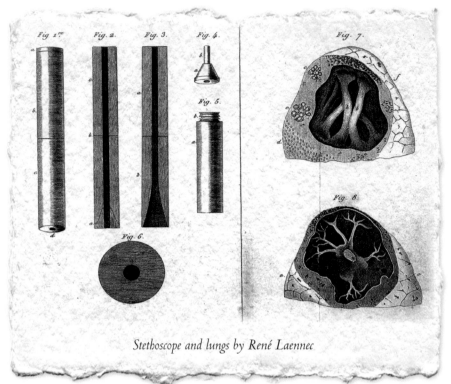

Stethoscope and lungs by René Laennec

empty keg, he might begin by percussing at the bottom and then gradually moving the tapping higher. As soon as the air-filled upper portion of the keg is reached, the flat sound is replaced by a deep hollow tone. It is not surprising that percussion was invented by an inn-keeper's son, the Austrian physician Leopold Auenbrugger.

Although the story may well be apocryphal, the young Auenbrugger is said to have made his discovery while tapping out the contents of his father's beer barrels. What is known for certain is that he did his research on the technique after he had grown up to be Physician-in-Chief to the Hospital of the Holy Trinity in Vienna. Having recognized the potentialities of percussion, he spent seven years studying the method on his patients and confirming his results at autopsy. In addition, he conducted experiments on cadavers to test his hypotheses.

Auenbrugger was a skilled musician. He understood such things as resonance, pitch, and tonal quality. He made good use of his knowledge during his studies of percussion, but, being a modest and good-natured fellow, did not delude himself into thinking that others would necessarily value or even understand his contribution. Here follow a few sentences from the preface to the book in which he described his discovery:

I have not been unconscious of the dangers I must encounter; since it has always been the fate of those who

But before narrating the story of the stethoscope, there is an equally interesting and much shorter tale to be told about the origins of another method of physical diagnosis which preceded it by almost half a century—the technique of percussion. Most patients who have had their chests thumped by the family doctor have probably wondered just what sort of information can be obtained from that mysterious procedure. The physician places the flat of his palm on one's trunk and delivers a few smart taps on his outstretched middle finger with its fellow of the other hand. The resulting sound, if listened to carefully, is heard to be either dull or resonant, depending upon whether the underlying area of chest or abdomen contains a solid or a hollow structure. The note may be as resounding as a drum or as flat as a block of wood. If one wished to determine how much beer, for example, is left in a partially

have illustrated or improved the arts and sciences by their discoveries, to be beset by envy, malice, hatred, detraction and calumny. . . . What I have written I have proved again and again, by the testimony of my own senses, and amid laborious and tedious exertions;—still guarding, on all occasions, against the seductive influence of self-love.

The preface concludes with a sentence that should serve as an inviolable rule for all scientific writing: "I have not been ambitious of ornament in my mode or style of writing, being contented if I shall be understood."

Auenbrugger would probably have welcomed a little envy, malice, hatred, detraction, or calumny, because such responses would have signified that someone was paying attention to his work. As it was, the scientific community of Europe responded with neglect or aloofness. Not being one to push himself into the public eye, Auenbrugger did not do more to advance his ideas than to publish a second edition of his book two years later. In fact, by the time of that second edition he had resigned his hospital post and begun to enjoy, at the age of forty, the *gemütlich* life of a successful Viennese practitioner who was a favorite of the empress, a lover of the opera, and the adoring husband of a beautiful wife.

Percussion was doubtless a useful technique, but it arrived on the medical scene too early. The work of Morgagni had not yet become well known, and so the search for methods of physical examination had not begun. Auenbrugger announced his discovery at a time when observations of the pulse and breathing were the only known methods for evaluating the chest. His book was written on the very brink of the time when Morgagni's work would make the search for physical signs such a valuable part of diagnosis. It vanished into obscurity, to be saved half a century later by a French physician who rediscovered it in 1808, one year before Auenbrugger's death. That physician, Jean-Nicolas Corvisart, translated the German text into French and popularized its message, demonstrating the many ways in which percussion could be used. So lost had Auenbrugger's great contribution become that it would have been a simple matter for Corvisart to claim it as his own, but he refused, stating later of his predecessor, "It is he and the beautiful invention which rightly belongs to him that I wish to recall to life."

Of all of the countries of Europe, France was the most prepared to savor the freshness of those new breezes of medical discovery. It was, after all, the land of revolution. Among the results of 1789 were the closing down of the old medical colleges and the beginnings of a new spirit of inquiry, using the criteria of close observation and unbiased interpretation. In this atmosphere, French physicians of the early nineteenth century, inspired particularly by the example of Corvisart and a few others, turned their attention to the seeking out of correlations between the symptoms of the sick and their findings at postmortem. Corvisart was not only a gifted doctor, he was his own pathologist. He was the true founder of the French school, in which each patient became part of a wide-ranging three-part study: first, to identify the ways in which certain groups of symptoms consistently occur together to produce some specific disease which can be classified into a general category of sicknesses; then to find the anatomical changes that are responsible for the symptoms;

finally, to add to the description of each disease a list of those findings that a physician can recognize by a careful physical examination. Thus did Corvisart became the *accoucheur* at the birth of modern clinical medicine.

It is not surprising that foreign visitors to the French hospitals in those days wrote home to their colleagues that the entire Parisian school was "sensualist." In medical terms that particular word implied high praise. It implied that the physicians of Paris had abandoned conjecture and in its place seized upon the visible, palpable, audible, and even tastable and sniffable realities that were available to their five senses. Hypothesis and guesswork no longer held pride of place in the diagnostic armamentarium, which thus became much more a useful set of tools than a bag of tricks. Corvisart, the personification of the new objective approach, referred to his great book, *Essay on the Diseases and Organic Lesions of the Heart and Great Vessels,* as "a work of pure practice founded on observation and experience." On the wall of his lecture room was printed the admonition "Never do something important following pure hypothesis or simple opinion."

Like a few other renowned medical personages, Vesalius among them, Corvisart succumbed to the blandishments and dazzle of the court; he became

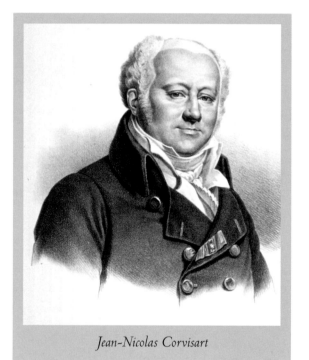

Jean-Nicolas Corvisart

Napoleon's physician in 1804, and his retirement from medicine was complete after the emperor's final defeat in 1815. But before he allowed himself to be drowned in courtsmanship and the flatteries of the First Consul, his far-reaching influence on French medicine had attracted a group of distinguished pupils, of whom none brought greater honor to his fellow physicians and to France than did the sickly young Breton who was destined to be remembered as the inventor of the stethoscope, René-Théophile-Hyacinthe Laennec.

The life of René Laennec (1781–1826) spanned first those Dickensian best of times and worst of times, and then the Napoleonic and post-Napoleonic periods. These were tumultuous years for France. She was a land both cursed and blessed, and the same might be said of the life of her son Laennec, the tubercular genius who became the greatest physician of the early nineteenth century.

So far west on the peninsula of Brittany that it lies due south of the English city of Plymouth is Quimper, a charming country town nestled among heather and forest-covered hills. The seat of the bishop of Rennes, it has a beautiful cathedral not far from which may be seen a statue erected by the physicians of France in Laennec's honor. He was born there on February 17, 1781, to Mme. Michelle Laennec, who died, probably of tuberculosis, when the boy was six years old. His father, Théophile, was throughout his life a vain, somewhat eccentric fellow who fancied himself a poet, but who derived his precarious living from minor political posts. Finding himself a widower, with René, his younger brother Michaud, and the one-year-old Marie-Anne on his hands, he set about unburdening himself of his onerous parental obligations. He sent the little girl to be brought up by his aunt, and he shipped the two boys off first to live with an uncle who was a parish priest, and after one year to the nearby city of Nantes, to the custody of their other uncle, Dr. Guillaume Laennec.

Guillaume was no ordinary local doctor. He had begun his medical studies in Paris, moved on to one of the German universities, and obtained his degree from the ancient school at Montpellier. Drawn by the magnet of John Hunter's teachings, he next moved to London and attempted to enroll as a surgical pupil at St. George's Hospital. When his application was refused, he returned to Quimper in 1775, and finally settled in Nantes, where his talents were so highly regarded that within two years he had been appointed rector of the faculty.

It was therefore into the home of one of the most distinguished citizens of Nantes that the two motherless boys were welcomed in 1788, to be brought up with their three-year-old cousin Christophe. Christophe would one day become a famous lawyer, and Michaud, when he died at the age of twenty-seven, was also well on his way to great success in that profession. That all three boys did so well in their careers was due in no small measure to the example of Guillaume,

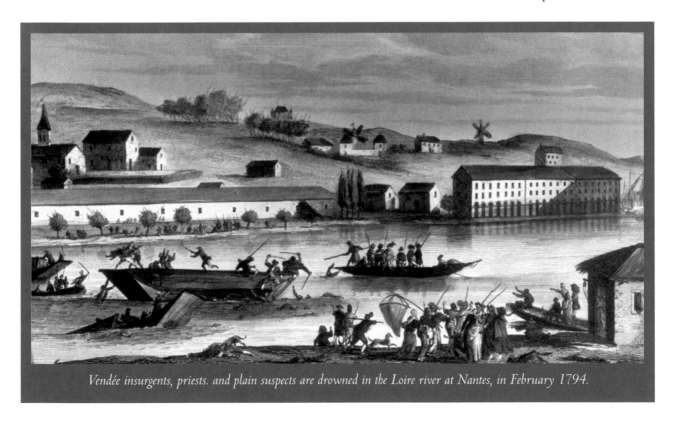

Vendée insurgents, priests. and plain suspects are drowned in the Loire river at Nantes, in February 1794.

a man of high intelligence and scholarly attainment, who set proper academic standards for the three talented boys of whose upbringing he so enthusiastically took charge.

In the movements of revolution and counterrevolution that began in 1789, the Laennecs were not much affected until the so-called Wars of the Vendée broke out in the west, including Brittany, in February 1793. They started as a revolt by the peasants in protest against military conscription and taxation; their spread resulted in harsh reprisals by the Republican government. The Vendée, as the uprisings were also called, was, in fact, only the premonitory out-break of a much larger movement that was beginning all over the country. Dissatisfaction with the decrees of the National Convention, anger over the January 1793 execution of Louis XVI, and a deteriorating military situation led to movements of counterrevolution, with some proroyalist elements, throughout France. The result was that the infamous Committee of Public Safety was appointed by the National Convention, and the Reign of Terror began. Between the summers of 1793 and 1794 more than forty thousand "enemies of the revolution" were put to death. Finally, in July 1794, moderates overthrew the leadership of the radical Robespierrists and began to undo their work; in October 1795, a new government was instituted, with a conservative constitution and a five-man Executive Directorate.

The excesses of the Terror were at their worst in Paris, but Nantes also was particularly hard hit, with three thousand citizens being executed. A guillotine was set up in the Place de Bouffay, on which the windows of the Laennecs looked out. But the guillotine was not fast enough to satisfy the zealous patriots of Nantes, who found that they could kill people more efficiently by mass drownings in the river, a quasi-judicial form of execution which became known as the Noyade de Loire, with a particularly degraded variant, *le mariage républicain,* in which naked men were tied to naked women and thrown in pairs into the water. A somewhat more merciful type of mass execution was the herding of people together so that they could be mowed down by chain shot.

Though the boys were kept to the back of the house as much as possible, René saw approximately fifty heads roll into the

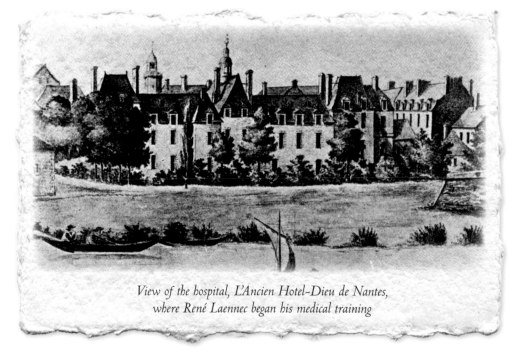

View of the hospital, L'Ancien Hotel-Dieu de Nantes, where René Laennec began his medical training

guillotine's basket. He very likely heard about the shootings and drownings, and may well have been surreptitiously present at some of them. He spent one period of six weeks in constant fear for his uncle, who had been thrown into prison as a suspected nonsympathizer with the local "government."

Even during the worst of the killing, however, certain ordinary activities continued to proceed with a modicum of normality, and among them was education. The three Laennec boys went on uninterruptedly with their schooling, absorbing all they could under the constraints of the Terror, and winning academic prizes for their efforts.

Although he briefly considered a career in engineering, the influence of his scholarly uncle and his own fascination with nature led René to decide on the less prestigious profession of medicine. In the month of Vendémiaire (September) in the Revolutionary year III (1795), at the age of fourteen, he enrolled at the University of Nantes to begin his professional studies.

René's emotionally distant father having married a well-provided widow and been appointed a judge in the bargain, there was a little money to support his educational venture, though never very much; his correspondence of the next few years is peppered with pecuniary requests to Théophile. He continued to depend on his uncle Guillaume for spiritual fathering, and for his daily subsistence.

It was during René's studies at the hospitals associated with the University of Nantes that the first indications appeared of his physical frailty. Smaller than most boys his age, and bearing what was thought to be a hereditary predisposition to tuberculosis, he was watched over carefully (and watched overcarefully) by his devoted uncle. When Guillaume's own twenty-month-old child died, as, he wrote in a letter to Théophile, "an unconscious victim of Revolutionary conditions," he became even more vigilant of his aesthenic nephew's health than previously. In that same letter of May 1796, he expressed the hope that René's life achievements might console him for the loss of his own child.

It was clear that Guillaume nurtured the fond hope that his nephew would one day succeed him in his practice. But it was not enough that the boy become his professional heir, he had to be every bit as proficient at his work as was the rector himself. René was constantly exhorted to be diligent in his studies that he might be fit to bear the responsibilities that would eventually be his. "Our calling," Guillaume told the boy, "is like a set of chains that one must carry at all hours of the day and night."

Théophile, on the other hand, wished mightily that René would choose to become a businessman or a lawyer, both occupations higher on the social scale than medicine. The boy, however, decided to continue with his medical studies—a decision probably due more to his uncle than to any certainty that he was doing the right thing—and proceeded to throw himself into the work with the spirited eagerness that would characterize his professional labors for the rest of his life. Not content to restrict his learning to the simple knowledge that passed for clinical training in those days, he studied chemistry and physics, which he felt were necessary in order to properly understand the functioning of the human body. Even this was not enough. He squeezed sufficient money out of his tight-fisted father to allow him to take courses in Latin and Greek as well as art and dancing. And he learned to play the flute, an instrument that was to provide him with many hours of amusement and inspiration during the difficulties of the years ahead.

Before long, he had set his candle aflame at both ends; the wax in the middle began to show the first signs that it was susceptible to meltdown. In the spring of 1798 he developed a prolonged fever, exhaustion, and some difficulty with breathing. He was treated with laxatives, as called for by contemporary medical dicta when the body was thought to need purging of some undesirable flux. He recovered after many weeks, probably in spite of his treatment and certainly not because of it.

> *Before long, he had set his candle aflame at both ends; the wax in the middle began to show the first signs that it was susceptible to meltdown.*

Young Laennec's illness left him physically weakened, but determined to pursue his career. Over the next two years, during small outbursts of civil war, he and Uncle Guillaume negotiated with Théophile in hopes of gaining his commitment to support René's medical studies in Paris. Meantime, the youth marked time by repeating his hospital work over and over, while holding some minor posts that gave him experience in treating the wounded. Finally, on November 10, 1799, the life histories of both France and René Laennec took a dramatic turn toward stability. On that day, in the city of Nantes, bells were set to pealing, celebratory cannons were fired, and the townspeople shouted grateful hurrahs to the skies—Napoleon Bonaparte had been named First Consul of the Republic.

The optimism of the moment seems to have lightened even the parsimony of Théophile Laennec. Having sent Michaud to Paris to train as a lawyer, he could no longer resist the importunings of the aspiring young physician and his uncle. In April 1801, with six hundred of his father's francs in his pocket, René Laennec set out on foot for Paris. He walked the two hundred miles of the journey in ten days, arriving weary but elated at the end of the month. As soon as he had settled himself with his brother Michaud in a room in the Latin Quarter, he enrolled as a medical student at one of the great hospitals of Paris, the Charité. The choice was not difficult to make—at the Charité was the clinic of France's foremost teacher, Jean-Nicolas Corvisart.

Had he planned it, young Laennec could not have begun his professional training at a more fortuitous time. Thanks to the philosophies of the Revolution, the entire French system of education was undergoing a complete revision, with science and medicine being major beneficiaries of the reforms. The basis of the new medical pedagogy was the hospital itself, with the method of instruction being clinical in the sense that it used the hospitalized patient, alive and dead, as its primary teaching example. Paris provided the ideal situation for this kind of instruction. In the last decades of the eighteenth century and the first few of the nineteenth, the city became a haven for large numbers of young people either uprooted or seeking their fortunes in the metropolis. The force that moved them to their nation's capital was the tide of revolution—first the French and then the industrial. The increased population, the straitened circumstances in which so many of the migrants lived, and their dislocation from the nurturing care of their families created a chronic state of crisis that kept the wards of the city's forty-eight hospitals filled (the in-patient census was reported as 20,341 in 1788), and strained the capacities of the autopsy rooms. The endless human tragedy unfolding on the streets of Paris was the grim fodder that nourished the rapid growth of French medicine.

During all of this period, reorganization was taking place. After 1790, all hospitals belonged to the state. They were centrally directed after 1801 under a general council. The Faculté de Médecine of Paris, which had controlled teaching since the Middle Ages, was dissolved in 1790, leaving the training of doctors, as the philosophy of the new Republic demanded, to the realm of individual enterprise. Whatever may be the merits of such a system in other areas of endeavor, it has never done anything for medical education except create chaos. Soon after, the country was at war, the need for physicians became even more urgent than it already was, and something had to be done. The something was the founding of three new medical schools, or écoles de santé, in Paris, Montpellier, and Strasbourg.

Faculty remuneration at the écoles de santé was legislated in a manner that made it a forerunner of what we today call the geographic full-time system. So that the professors should not be dependent upon direct fees from those whom they taught, they were paid a reasonable salary, though not enough for much luxury; accordingly, they were also allowed an unrestricted private practice, a privilege which seems not to have been much abused.

As might be imagined, the prestige, the income, and the sheer excitement of a professorship in one of the new schools made those positions desirable to the leading members of the profession. True again to its revolutionary principles, the National Convention established a system of public competitions, called *concours*, to fill the Chairs and the equal number of adjunct professorships they had created. In addition, each institution had a dean, a librarian, and a curator of the anatomical collection. As has often been true at the birth of great schools of medicine, a goodly proportion of the outstanding members of the faculty were under the age of forty. Corvisart, forty-six years old when René Laennec enrolled as his pupil, was the sage of the Charité.

Since the hospitalized patient and his corpse at autopsy were the focus of instruction, the entering student was on the wards and in the dissecting rooms from the very first day of training. He was taught by the guiding precept "Read little, see much, do much" *(Peu lire, beaucoup voir, beaucoup faire)*. In the early nineteenth century, this was an apt approach; most of what was then in clinical books was theoretical claptrap, not worth the value of the candle by which it was read.

The Charité, located on the Rue des St. Pères, had been founded in 1607 by the Brothers of

Charity of the religious order of St. Jean de Dieu at the instigation of Marie de Médicis, a woman not otherwise well known for good works. Two hundred years later, there was no hospital in the world where a student could be better trained in diseases of the heart and lungs, and probably everything else as well. In a book entitled *The Hospitals and Surgeons of Paris,* the visiting American physician F. Campbell Stewart listed the following as the most frequent diagnoses in the French hospitals during the early part of the century: phthisis, pneumonia, typhoid, cancer, eruptive fever (especially smallpox), puerperal fever, heart disease, and disease of the urinary tract.

The progressive, almost futuristic, medical studies that were being done in the hospital belied the antiquated edifice in which they were carried out. Because virtually no progress had been made in caring for the sick since the Brothers first came from Italy, there had been no need, and now there was no money, to modernize the physical plant. It consisted of a confused jumble of buildings of irregular size and style separated by several courtyards and gardens where convalescing patients were permitted to exercise. Having been built on a small hill, the facility did boast a good run-off system for water, and even a covered drain, which was unusual for hospitals of that day. Also unusual was the fact that the wards were spacious and airy, allowing for a distance of three feet between beds in the men's wards and fully six feet in the women's. Of patients who entered the Charité, five out of six could expect to leave it alive. This statistic, excellent for the early nineteenth century, was thought by one English medical visitor of the time to be attributable to "the large and well-aired wards, and the custom of placing only one patient in a bed."

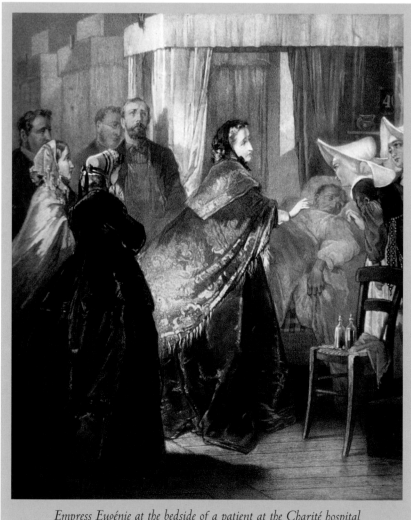

Empress Eugénie at the bedside of a patient at the Charité hospital

The one-bed one-patient policy was a new one. Until the establishment of the Republic it had not been uncommon for four, five, or even six very sick people of both sexes to be clumped together between the same sheets. This meant, of course, that in time of pestilence a newly arrived patient stood a good chance of awakening at some bleak pre-dawn hour tightly packed in among stiffening corpses. It was a variety of horror that may have been the odd necrophile's idea of heaven, but was a preview of hell to everyone else.

By the time of young Laennec's arrival at the Charité, then, an air of cautious optimism had replaced the terror which had permeated hospitals only two decades earlier. Although the therapies available to physicians remained as speculative as ever, the dreaded sick-pens had become oases of respite and attention. The almost three hundred beds of the Charité were filled with men and women hopeful that the gentle attentiveness of the Sisters of St. Vincent de Paul might nurture them back to health. Eight thousand of the afflicted sought the sensitive ministrations of the nuns each year.

There was even some chance now that the physicians might help. In the spirit of Morgagni and Corvisart, every patient was subjected to a new kind of scrutiny, and professors and students alike were ever on the alert for original findings that would lead to diagnosis. Rounds were made at least once daily by the senior professors followed by a retinue of students and by physicians coming in increasing numbers from America and many countries of Europe. The ward had become the laboratory where the young diagnostic medicine was developing that almost a century later

would lead to the beginnings of successful methods of therapy.

Almost as though he divined that he would soon be running a race against his own premature death, René Laennec dashed frenetically into his medical studies. If there was a lecture or an autopsy going on, he was there; if Corvisart was making rounds on the wards, he was there; if there were special courses to be taken, he was there. Wherever there was knowledge to be soaked up, his presence was a certainty. He took classes in anatomy, physiology, chemistry, pharmacy, materia medica (what is now called pharmacology), botany, legal medicine, and medical history. Withal he worked at improving his Greek by attending the École Centrale in moments stolen from his regular classes—he wanted to be able to read the Hippocratic Corpus in the original. Also, he resumed taking lessons on the flute, although one wonders how he found a free breath to blow with.

In physical stature, Laennec can best be described as tiny—five feet three inches tall, with just enough flesh over his bones to keep them from poking through his pale skin. He looked like a wisp and he functioned like a whirlwind; in the words of one of his biographers, "He was but a breath of air, and he thought himself a Hercules." He proudly traced his blue eyes and chestnut hair, as did so many of his fellow Bretons, to remote Celtic ancestors. If his coloring and the diminutive structure of his frame were not enough to give him a distinctive appearance, a prominent forehead and high cheekbones made his face, once seen, not easily forgotten. He was a most unusual sort of man, and he looked it.

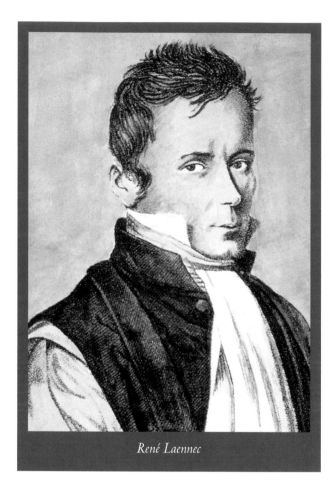

René Laennec

There were two great honors by which a medical student might distinguish himself in Paris. One was to be invited by his instructors to become a member of the Société d'Instruction Médicale, an organization in which students met to criticize each other's clinical and autopsy work; the other was to pass a competitive examination to enter the École Pratique, created for a special group of pupils who did three years of chemistry, dissections, and operative surgery. Laennec achieved both distinctions.

Early in 1802 he published his first scientific paper, a study of the narrowing of one of the heart valves probably caused by rheumatic fever, and called mitral stenosis. Several months later he published on venereal disease, and later that same year on peritonitis. This latter work, done when its author was a twenty-one-year-old student, was an epochal contribution. The lining membranes of the body had only recently been recognized as having an important role in disease. The discovery had been made at the Charité, by a much-admired young teacher and friend of Laennec's, Marie-François-Xavier Bichat. Bichat died in July 1802 at the age of thirty, of tuberculous meningitis, but his work had stimulated Laennec to an appreciation of the significance of the lining of the abdominal cavity, called the peritoneum, and that of the chest, called the pleura, as well as the linings of joints and the coverings of internal organs. The initial result was the paper on peritonitis, in which was first outlined the vital differentiation of diseases of the abdominal organs from those of the tissues that cover them and line the cavity in which they reside. In writing of the various forms of peritonitis, Laennec was the first researcher to describe adhesions, false membranes, and the outpouring of intraabdominal fluid caused by inflammation.

The work of Bichat and Laennec, preliminary as it was, had a significance far beyond its immediate usefulness. It marked the entering of a new phase in the understanding of the processes of disease—a new layer, in a manner of speaking. Morgagni had localized the seats of disease to organs; Bichat introduced the anatomical concept that organs and organ systems are made up of sheets of protoplasm called tissues; now Bichat and Laennec together showed that the concept of disease should include not only organs but also the tissues of which they are composed. Later in the nineteenth century, the development of the principles of medical microscopy would provide the illumination and the enlarged vision, literally and figuratively, to enable the Berlin pathologist Rudolf Virchow to demonstrate that it is in the individual cells themselves, of which tissues and organs are made, that the basis of disease must be sought. (The shift was one not only of focus, but of geography as well, as ascendancy in medical science passed sequentially from Italy, to France, to the German-speaking countries, and finally to the United States.)

Beyond his work on peritonitis, the labors of Laennec while a medical student resulted in a series of important studies in normal and pathological anatomy. It was during this time that he described the fibrous envelopes in which many of the abdominal organs are contained. In his researches on the scarred livers of alcoholics, he took note of a characteristic dull-brown color they acquire. From his use of the Greek word *kirrhos*, or tawny, to describe this color has come our eponymic disease Laennec's cirrhosis. Ask any modern physician the significance of the name of Laennec and he will be sure to mention cirrhosis, but not the stethoscope, so little is it remembered today that the greater discovery is also his.

It had been René's intention to complete just enough medical study to enable him to return to Brittany to join his uncle Guillaume in practice. But the scientific itch was beginning to make itself felt. Not only was he becoming fascinated with his researches into pathology, but he was achieving the honor of a recognition that was difficult for a young man from the provinces to resist. First Bichat and then Guillaume, realizing that in directing his nephew to the study of medicine he had laid the groundwork for a career too important to be confined to Nantes, urged him to stay in Paris. Théophile wrote to René of his uncle, "He is Pygmalion in ecstasy before his handiwork."

Young Laennec was successful not only as a researcher, but also in his primary obligation, which was to be a good student. When the government, in 1803, donated awards to the students of all the special schools in Paris, he entered the competition, winning first prize in medicine and the sole prize in surgery. The two awards carried a monetary sum of six hundred francs, which ameliorated somewhat the difficult financial circumstances in which he had been living. Nevertheless, he had to borrow some additional money from his father in order to be decently enough clothed to appear at the prize ceremony held at the Louvre.

Whether it was the relentlessly hard work, the penury, or a general constitutional disability, at this time Laennec began to suffer occasionally from a shortness of breath which he called asthma, but which, in reality, was probably the insidious progression of a smoldering tuberculosis. He ignored his own lungs, however, and concentrated more than ever on studying the lungs of others. He took on new duties. In November 1803, he began to teach a private class in pathological

> Théophile wrote to René of his uncle, "He is Pygmalion in ecstasy before his handiwork."

anatomy, in which much of the course material consisted of information from research done by himself and one of his colleagues, Gaspard-Laurent Bayle. It was in the presentations to his classes that he defined the notion of the central pathological finding in tuberculosis, the tubercle.

The word "tubercle" originates from the Latin *tuberculum*, a small bump or lump. The disease gets its name because such tiny seedlike lumps are produced by the body's attempt to protect itself, by the process of inflammation, from the invasion of the organism that causes the disease, *Mycobacterium tuberculosis*. The white blood cells that are poured into the area of microbial invasion attempt to destroy the bacteria, and are in turn ingested by larger cells. These larger cells then change shape and quality, and become crowded together to form a clump, which is the tubercle. Microscopic at first, tubercles gradually attain a size large enough to be seen with the naked eye. Laennec, because he disdained the primitive microscopes of the time, made all of his observations with either the unaided eye or a small magnifying lens. What he saw was therefore visible to any physician who was willing to take the trouble to look for it. The looking was made particularly easy by the tendency of the enlarging tubercles to coalesce into quite a substantial size, after which it was not uncommon for the center of the tubercle to undergo a cheesy degeneration, resulting in the production of the well-known cavities so often seen in late stages of the disease.

Although the existence of visible tubercles had been known for more than a hundred years, they had been thought to involve only the lungs. Laennec showed that the lesions could be found in any organ of the body, and even the bones. As a result of his work, the old Hippocratic diagnosis of phthisis was gradually abandoned and replaced by the anatomically accurate tuberculosis. The change is in itself a statement of the progress of medical science. The terminology that arose from the work of Corvisart, Bayle, and Laennec is a reflection of the fact that disease was henceforth to be looked upon as the result of anatomical-pathological causes. In abandoning "phthisis," the Greek word for wasting or decay, the medical world was beginning to abandon also the Greek way of classifying diseases by the only method they knew, in terms of their major symptoms as narrated and exhibited by the living patient. The use of the term "tuberculosis" was an acknowledgment that disease nomenclature, like diagnosis, must be based on pathological changes in tissues and organs.

Even the greatest of researchers, if a medical student, must pass a final rigorous testing in order to qualify for a doctorate. The titles of the courses in which Laennec took his qualifying examinations in the late winter and spring of 1804 give some indication of the curriculum of the best medical schools of the time: anatomy, physiology, internal pathology and nosology (which formalized the wedding of classification to organ derangements), materia medica and pharmacy, hygiene and forensic medicine, and finally internal medicine.

After he had successfully completed his examinations, Laennec moved to a new apartment on the site of the present Boulevard St. Germain. Perhaps his private pathology course had provided enough income to allow him to rent these more presentable lodgings, but it is more likely that he was counting on soon being able to earn a respect-

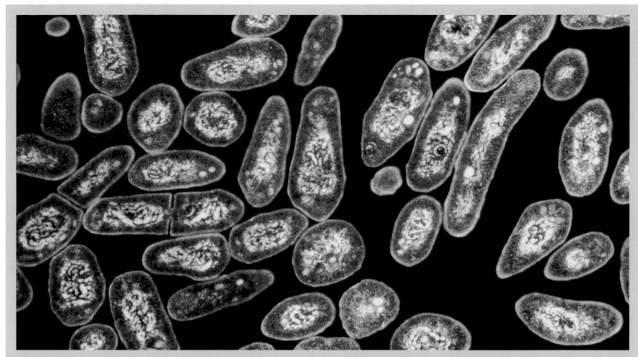

Color-enhanced transmission electron micrograph of Mycobacterium tuberculosis

able income from practice. Michaud had left Paris to take a job as attaché to the prefect of the Oise, and been replaced as a roommate by Uncle Guillaume's eldest son, Christophe.

Laennec now began work on his doctoral thesis, which dealt with the Hippocratic doctrines as they relate to practical medicine. On June 11, 1804, the dissertation was successfully defended before a jury of three professors, one of whom was Corvisart. Théophile, ever on the alert for an opportunity, encouraged his son to dedicate the work to some influential government minister. René never considered the suggestion for so much as a moment—the dedication is to his beloved Pygmalion, Uncle Guillaume.

The young graduate had achieved the highest levels of success that were possible for a French medical student. He was now elected to the Socié-té de l'École de Médecine, the organization that had in prerevolutionary days been the Royal Society of Medicine. Not only was he paid a fee for attendance at the society's meetings, but his membership made him an official contributor to the prestigious *Journal of Medicine, Surgery, and Pharmacy*. Although he had published a number of articles in the journal during his recent student days, the regular appearance of his writings was now to bring him even greater recognition.

Somehow, during all of his other activities, Laennec found the time to develop his burgeoning interest in the culture of his Breton forebears. A sort of Breton revival was under way in Paris, and Laennec was in its forefront. He obtained from his father a Breton grammar, a dictionary, and some books, and began studying the language with a sense of devotion, as though he were

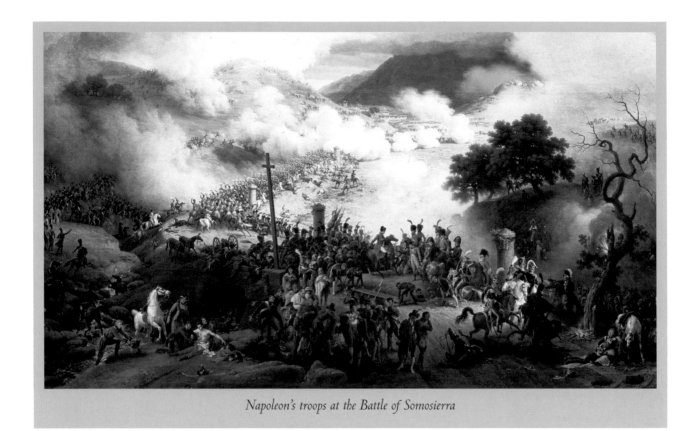

Napoleon's troops at the Battle of Somosierra

consecrated to its survival. In less than a year he was able to demonstrate his new skill in the letters he wrote home, and he sought out other opportunities to speak and to write among the many wounded Breton boys in the hospitals of Paris, who were only too grateful to converse in the Celtic dialect with the young physician whose attentions seemed all the more caring because they were articulated in the mother tongue.

It was also during this period that Laennec turned to his Catholic faith. His childhood had not been a religious one, and his father's ties to the church were flimsy. René changed all of that, evidently finding in his strong bonds both to religion and to the Breton culture a sense of community that sustained him in the dislocated life he led in Paris. His distinctly royalist political lean-

ings may have been a less obvious manifestation of his need for sources of authority and approval.

At last, it was time for the newly qualified physician to properly start up his practice. He had already distinguished himself as an excellent physician, a skillful surgeon, and a teacher whose rounds and lectures attracted ever larger numbers of students. He was a regular contributor to, and he now became an editor of, a major medical journal. He had written almost a thousand pages of a proposed work, albeit one he never published, on pathological anatomy. Not only had he described peritonitis but it is correct to say that he had discovered it. He had been the first to point out that abdominal organs are covered by fibrous capsules, the first to show the existence of the pigmented tumors we call melanomas. And he had used the evidence of over two hundred autopsies to prove that the tubercle is the basic lesion, what is called the pathognomonic finding, of tuberculosis. Through his work, the ancient disease of phthisis was finally understood to be simply tuberculosis of the lungs, one organ's response to a disease that has the capability of striking any part of the body.

The young man who had accomplished all of this was of an age at which modern medical students are just being introduced to their first living patients. His future seemed secure, and yet no hospital appointment presented itself. He poured all of his burning energies into his rapidly enlarging private practice, and he waited. Various teaching posts came up as one senior physician after another passed from the scene, but Laennec was never successful in being appointed or being invited to compete in a *concours*, perhaps because in practice the egalitarian basis of the system was sometimes honored only in the breach; Laennec had no powerful sponsors. He did his writing and continued to record his observations of disease, but almost all of his time was devoted to the care of his patients. In 1810 his brother Michaud died of tuberculosis, as had his mother, but when episodes of chest pains began to complicate his own breathing problems, he called them angina pectoris, and continued stubbornly to diagnose his frequent shortness of breath as asthma.

In the early months of 1814, the declining fortunes of Napoleon's troops filled the hospitals of Paris with the wounded. They brought with them the age-old pestilence of defeated armies, typhus. Because Laennec was by then a prominent practicing physician, albeit one without a teaching post, he petitioned the authorities to let him treat the

soldiers from Brittany in a single hospital. Given special wards at the Salpêtrière facility, he enlisted three young Breton doctors to help him, and set out to provide what he thought his countrymen needed more than materia medica and pharmacy. In the conclusion of a letter to his cousin Christophe he described the treatment that was most effective: "I have to return to the wards, to talk to those patients in greatest need of consolation. For that is the best medicine I can count on in the care of my Bretons."

For most of the first half of the year, Laennec spent hours each day, sometimes whole days at a time, walking the wards of the Salpêtrière, bringing a touch of home and a touch of Christian grace to the soldiers under his care. A deacon sent

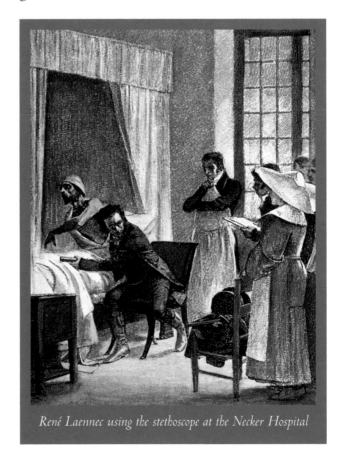

René Laennec using the stethoscope at the Necker Hospital

by the bishop of Rennes gave the last sacrament to those who could not speak French, and a local priest who volunteered to help was given an exhortation translated by Laennec into Breton, by which he might console those whose fitful passage into eternity he was trying to ease.

When the last soldier finally left the Salpêtrière in June 1814, Laennec returned to his practice full-time. His fatigue and respiratory problems had weakened him physically, but he forged ahead with his clinical work during the next two years as though he were in perfect health. The academic career that had seemed so certain appeared now to be beyond his grasp. In 1816, at thirty-five years of age, ten years out of the university, he began to make plans to go home to Brittany. And then, in one ironic stroke of good fortune, the course of his life, and with it the course of medical history, was changed. He was named Physician to the Hospital Necker.

The irony of the appointment lay in the fact that Europe's most brilliant medical researcher got his long-sought-for job not because of his unparalleled abilities or his promise for the future, but strictly on the basis of personal connections. It happened that a friend of Laennec's, one Becquey, became under-secretary of state to the home secretary; he had it within his power to determine which of twenty candidates would take over the newly available post at the Necker. He encouraged his friend Laennec to apply.

At first Laennec resisted. Situated on the edge of Paris far from the university quarter, with only a hundred beds and no tradition, the Necker was not considered a major institution, or even a good one. But whether out of desperation or an unwillingness to offend Becquey, or perhaps, as one his-torian has suggested, because the hospital had a fine garden in which he might exercise, Laennec at last decided to take advantage of the opportunity. He was officially appointed on September 4, 1816.

History did not have long to wait. Within a very short time, the most important medical event of the early nineteenth century took place during his routine daily ward rounds. H. B. Granville, one of the British students who was present at the momentous occasion, gives the date as September 13. The episode is best narrated in Laennec's own words, as they appear in the book he wrote three years later:

In 1816, I was consulted by a young woman labouring under general symptoms of diseased heart, and in whose case percussion and the application of the hand were of little avail on account of the great degree of fatness. The other method just mentioned [the application of the ear to the front of the chest] being rendered inadmissible by the age and sex of the patient, I happened to recollect a simple and well-known fact in acoustics, and fancied, at the same time, that it might be turned to some use on the present occasion. The fact I allude to is the augmented impression of sound when conveyed through certain solid bodies,—as when we hear the scratch of a pin at one end of a piece of wood, on applying our ear to the other. Immediately, on this suggestion, I rolled a quire of paper into a sort of cylinder and applied one end of it to the region of the heart and the other to my ear, and was not a little surprised and pleased, to find that I could thereby perceive the action of the heart in a manner much more clear and distinct than I had ever been able to do by the immediate application of the ear. From this moment I imagined that the circumstance might furnish means for enabling us to ascertain the character, not only of the *action of the heart, but of every species of sound produced by the motion of all the thoracic viscera. With this conviction, I forthwith commenced at the Hospital Necker a series of observations, which has continued to the present time. The result has been, that I have been enabled to discover a set of new signs of diseases of the chest, for the most part certain, simple, and prominent, and calculated, perhaps, to render the diagnosis of the diseases of the lungs, heart and pleura, as decided and circumstantial, as the indications furnished to the surgeon by the introduction of the finger or sound, in the complaints wherein these are used.*

Seemingly in the wink of an eye, the world of clinical medicine had undergone another of its great transformations—through the medium of a rolled-up sheaf of paper. What Laennec had invented was not merely an instrument by which the sounds of the body could be transmitted to the listener's ear—it was an instrument that would teach physicians the difference between evidence that is objective and evidence that can be influenced by the patient or the bias of the examiner. Until the introduction of the stethoscope, diagnosis depended almost completely upon the patient's narrative description of his symptoms, unreliable though it might be. Although the principles of the newly understood pathological anatomy were beginning to make doctors aware that they must seek more trustworthy clues to organ derangements, lit-

tle progress had yet been made in that direction. True, there was more careful laying on of hands to feel deeply lying structures, and certainly more careful looking for visibly obvious findings, but there remained yet a gaping inconsistency between what could be predicted from these beginning attempts at physical examination and what would later be found at autopsy. One had still mainly to trust in the patient's recitation of his history and, to a lesser extent, his appearance.

The history was taken at face value, since most diagnosticians of the day had no reason to deny, for example, that pain was pain or weakness was weakness. It was so if the patient thought it was so. They had not yet come to appreciate that a person's description of his illness is affected by a score of factors, some of which are beyond his conscious control and some of which are not. It was well known that the details of the narration might differ depending on whom they were being related to, but the significance of that phenomenon was minimized—what the afflicted person

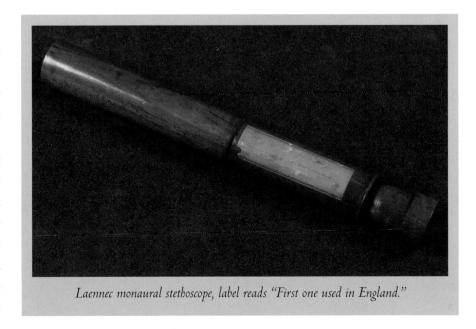

Laennec monaural stethoscope, label reads "First one used in England."

told the most senior examiner was accepted as the true story. The possibility that it might not be remembered or told accurately was considered only in the most obvious cases, or where deliberate intent to defraud was suspected. Some wise physicians, Laennec among them, remained determined that a more exact method must be sought, free of the influence of imprecise information.

And then the stethoscope was invented. Here was a tool that provided audible clues almost as dependable as those which were visible at autopsy; here was a tool that demonstrated to physicians that it is possible to learn things about the workings of the body that are exactly, reproducibly the same regardless of who does the examining; and therefore, here was a tool that taught the healer that he could separate the objective evidences of his own five senses from the subjective responses of a sick person, and that he could do it while the person was still living. This was surely the Hippocratic method of observation brought forward into modern times.

From the date of Laennec's discovery the criterion of objective diagnostic findings has been the hallmark of clinical examination. The quest for examination techniques and for specific visible, audible, or palpable physical evidence was one of the major stimuli to bedside medical investigation throughout much of the nineteenth century. Percussion, which had remained largely neglected even after Corvisart's unearthing of Auenbrugger's contribution, became of great interest, as examiners sought to determine what was solid and what was gas- or fluid-filled, so that they might better evaluate the diseased internal organs which they could not see. Palpation became bolder and deeper, even as it be-

came at the same time more gentle and more surface-oriented. This seeming paradox resulted from an increased familiarity with the pathological changes wrought by illness, so that examiners needed on the one hand to try to feel deeply for the shapes and forms of organs, and on the other—often quite literally on the other—to appreciate vibrations, internal bumpings and grindings, and subtle changes in texture.

The paradigm for it all was the auditory evidence heard through the stethoscope. The instrument's length placed the physician at an objective distance from his patient. He might even close his eyes if he wished, so that he could concentrate more of his receptive abilities on the sounds transmitted to his ear from the invisible recesses of each body cavity. Anyone who has ever leaned back in a soft armchair with the headset of a Walkman snuggled up against his ears must surely appreciate what it is like to become lost in a world of sound, where every note brings its own distinctive message.

The new instrument became the equipment for the playing of a new game. That game was deadly serious in the hands of its inventor, as he tirelessly followed patient after patient from the ward to the autopsy table, correlating what he heard with what he later saw. He learned that a constricted bronchial passage causes one kind of sound when air moves through it, and a dilated one quite another. The large cavities hollowed out of the lungs by the ravages of tuberculosis were found to make a sound all their own, and still another resulted from areas that were solidified by pneumonia. It made little difference what the patients told Laennec when they recited the symptoms of their clinical histories—he listened without skepticism only to what he was told by his stethoscope, and he was rarely misled.

He gave names to the different kinds of messages that the lungs transmitted to him. He called them râles, bruits, fremitus, egophony, pectoriloquy, bronchophony, and the like. Each one, distinct from its fellows, carried its own warning about the process that had produced it. Interpreting the information that came to him was not difficult. In many cases he had merely to wait a few weeks to see with his own eyes, in the autopsy room, the abnormality that had produced the sound. The next time he heard that noise in the chest of a living patient he could predict what mischief lay beneath the open end of his stethoscope. In this way, he identified not only the physical changes that were taking place in the auscultated heart and lungs, but also the diseases that caused them. Thus he was the first physician to be able to differentiate between the diseases called bronchiectasis, pneumothorax, hemorrhagic pleurisy, emphysema, lung abscess, and pulmonary infarct.

These were enormous strides. By the use of a single new instrument which was simplicity itself, a large lumped-up group of amorphous chest diseases had been separated one from the other, defined, described, and given criteria to aid in their diagnosis. When a patient coughed up a bit of blood, a physician skilled with the stethoscope could now determine in moments whether he was most likely to be dealing, for example, with pneumonia, a tuberculous cavity, or a clot in the lung. Diagnosis was affected, classification was affected, and the ability to prognosticate, so highly valued by the Hippocratics and every physician since, was markedly improved. Laennec had introduced the modern era of scientific diagnois.

Though it seemed to have taken place in a moment, though Laennec himself described it so, the invention of the stethoscope was not instantaneous. As a scholar, Laennec was certainly well acquainted with the boiling-vinegar statement of Hippocrates, though he later wrote that he had not considered it to be a valid observation and had quite forgotten about it. He probably also forgot that his own countryman Ambroise Paré had pointed out, "If there is matter or other humour in the thorax, we can hear a noise like that of a half-filled gurgling bottle." But even if such statements were consciously out of his mind, he could not have helped but be aware, from his own clinical experiences and the writings of others, that some chest noises, particularly those of certain ailments of the heart, are audible without any special effort being made to listen for them. His teacher, Corvisart, had dismissed the usefulness of such findings in a brief comment in his book on cardiac disease, but Laennec's friend Bayle took them more seriously, often applying his ear to a patient's chest, and claiming to learn a good deal from the practice. Bayle, who died of tuberculosis in 1816, had worked closely with Laennec on the tubercle research. We know that Laennec had tried his method of listening on occasion, but was reluctant to employ it more widely, not only because it was awkward and embarrassing, but because the skins of the patients at the Charité and Necker were not very likely to be as well washed as his own ear. However, in view of Laennec's great respect for Bayle's abilities, it is not unlikely that he had been for some time considering how he might develop a method of listening that would be less tasteless and less tactile. He can be imagined contemplating the problem on

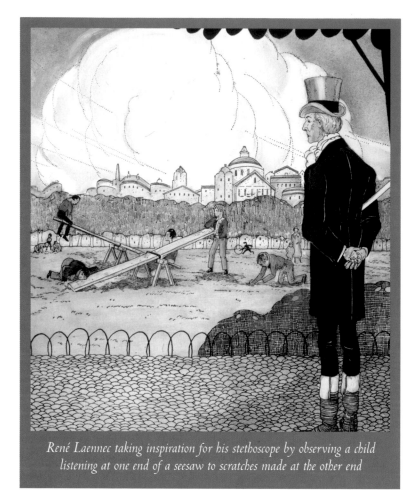

René Laennec taking inspiration for his stethoscope by observing a child listening at one end of a seesaw to scratches made at the other end

a chum scratching with a pin at its opposite extremity. Immediately on seeing this, the delighted doctor realized that his problem was solved. He hailed a passing cabriolet, rushed back to the Necker, rolled up a notebook as tightly as he could, and applied it snugly beneath the left breast of a buxom, intimidatingly pretty wench whose diagnosis had been eluding him. The case was immediately clarified and the stethoscope was invented. The story has the appeal of pure theater, in addition to the fact that it does fit some of the details of Laennec's own, possibly expurgated, description. I like to think it is the way things really happened.

The invention of the stethoscope may also have been in part the product of another of Laennec's array of skills. It must not be forgotten that he was a musician. Accustomed to thinking in terms of sound, and uniquely qualified to appreciate the slightest nuances in auditory stimuli, he seems to have been placed on earth by Aesculapius himself, with the specific mission to develop the art of auscultation. Even his chosen instrument, the flute, must have played its part—what he created was a wind instrument blowing the sad tunes that emanated from the chests of his stricken patients. He had taught his fellow physicians how to listen to the mournful music of disease and death, how to hear the cry of the suffering organs. From that time forward, the search was on: by every means available to them, medical researchers would begin to seek disease clues

more than one humid August morning in 1816, while standing before a shaving mirror scraping the wispy whiskers off his pale, drawn face.

There is a charming little story which it is customary to tell to medical students about the invention of the stethoscope, and it may even be true. According to this tale, Laennec was wandering alone one day, puzzling over the problem, when he chanced to find himself in the courtyard of the Louvre, where some boys were playing a game he knew well from his own childhood days in Brittany. One lad would put his ear to the end of a long piece of wood so that he could hear coded sounds being transmitted by

that were independent of any conscious or unconscious influence of patient or physician.

The first fruit was the development of the principles of physical examination; later in the century it would become possible to study the chemical changes that sickness wreaks on body fluids and tissues; and finally in 1895 came the method that added the definitive power of unbiased sight, the X-rays of Wilhelm Konrad Roentgen. It was Laennec's invention of the stethoscope that demonstrated to physicians not only that it was possible to be truly scientific in diagnosis, but that a technology must be pursued to permit the fulfillment of that promise.

Having been invented, the new instrument needed a name. Uncle Guillaume suggested "thoraciscope," but that seemed too cumbersome and restrictive. After considering several other possibilities, Laennec finally settled on "stethoscope," from the Greek *stethos* or chest, and *skopos* or observer. He himself usually called it simply *le Cylindre*, while to others it became known as a baton, a solometer, a pectoriloquy, or a *cornet médicale*. Whatever one called it, carrying the thing around was an awkward proposition. Laennec made his own instruments, and built them so that they came apart into two segments. These could be tucked into a coat pocket or carried inside a large top hat, clipped in place to prevent them from tumbling out.

The French remained loyal to the cylindrical form of *le baton* through most of the nineteenth century, but British and other European physicians designed stethoscopes that were somewhat flexible and less awkward to use than the short straight tube. In 1829, Nicholas Comins of London suggested that both ears might be used in auscultation. Eventually, in 1855, Dr. George Philip Camman of New York devised such a binaural stethoscope, having an ebony chestplate and two separate ivory-tipped hearing pieces that fit into the examiner's ears. The tubes were constructed of spiral wire covered by gum elastic and cloth. This was the prototype from which the instrument of today has evolved.

On August 15, 1819, the medical-book dealers of France put up for sale a two-volume work in which Laennec presented to the world the results of the studies he had done with his new instrument. The publication was entitled *De l'Auscultation Médiate, ou Traité du Diagnostic des Poumons et du Coeur, Fondé Principalement sur ce Nouveau Moyen d'Exploration* ("On Mediate Auscultation, or A Treatise on the Diagnosis of Diseases of the Lungs and Heart Based Principally on the New Method of Investigation"). *De l'Auscultation Médiate*, as the publication was called, had been preceded by a series of lectures in which its author described the stethoscope and its uses. The first had been given before the French Academy of Sciences in February 1818, and four more were presented in the spring of that year before the Faculté de Médecine.

"Auscultation" was a term coined by Laennec himself, taken from the Latin *auscultare*, meaning not merely to listen, but to listen carefully. It was the perfect choice of words. "Mediate" implied that the auscultation was not direct, as it would be if the word "immediate" were applicable—it was mediated by the tube. And so a new book, a new instrument, a new terminology, a new nosology, and a new philosophy of diagnosis had been introduced in two volumes of print which could be bought for thirteen francs. For three francs more, the publisher threw in a stethoscope, very likely fashioned by the author himself on his own home lathe.

As might be expected, the book and the stethoscope received mixed reviews. To some, the instrument was too short, to others too long, and to still a third group of critics it was a silly affectation. There were those who thought its only function was to impress patients, and others who feared that patients would be put off by it. One group of doctors claimed that only a few of the sounds described by Laennec could be heard, while another group heard so much that they could not differentiate one noise from another.

The complainers had a point. As time went on, Laennec and his admiring followers had begun to describe all sorts of wondrous sounds and diagnoses they claimed to be able to make by auscultation. Variations in pitch and tone so fine that they could be appreciated only by the most astute-

ly musical mind, or perhaps imagined by it, were soon being termed characteristic findings of this or that disease. Major diagnostic decisions were made and nosological categories were created on the basis of a sigh that fluttered some one professor's eardrum and no one else's. To Laennec's credit, very little of the acoustic hype can be attributed to him directly, but it did nevertheless detract from the rapidity with which his writings were accepted. It would, in fact, take more than twenty years before a completely realistic evaluation of the various auscultatory signs would be made, and then it would be by a Viennese physician, Josef Skoda.

Most well-educated physicians, however, were too wise to let the mere existence of some exaggerations blind them to the value of auscultation. To those who were disappointed that they did not hear everything they thought they were supposed to, P. A. Piorry, in the *Dictionnaire des Sciences Médicales* for 1820, responded: "If this method had only a quarter of the utility attributed to it by its inventor, it would still be one of the most precious discoveries of medicine." In that one sentence, he enunciated the basic truth about the stethoscope, then and now.

In June 1820, Lejumeau de Kergaradec set out to write a series of articles review-

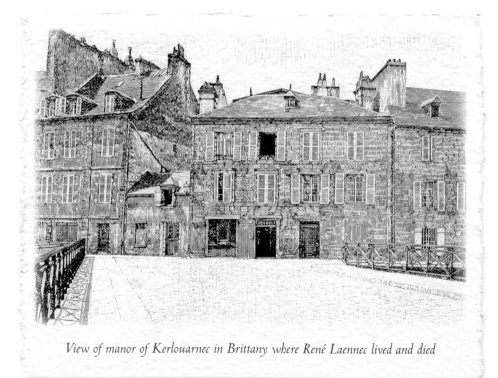

View of manor of Kerlouarnec in Brittany where René Laennec lived and died

ing Laennec's book. Although he had intended to devote the final essay in the series to responding to the stethoscope's detractors, the level of acceptance rose so rapidly that he found it unnecessary to do so. In his fifth and last article, written in August 1821, he stated that the progress in the use and usefulness of the instrument had by then made it superfluous for him to defend it.

Laennec's book was translated into English in 1821, and into German in 1822. Publicized by reviews appearing in American, Dutch, Italian, Russian, Spanish, Polish, and Scandinavian medical journals, as well as by the proselytizing of Laennec's pupils, his teachings became well known and were eventually accepted all over the Western world. The state of affairs is perhaps best summed up by a reviewer for the *Glasgow Medical Journal,* who was able to write, by 1828, "In 1821, the new mode of examination began to attract attention, in this city. Though at first suspected, ridiculed, and sometimes abused as a piece of pompous quackery, it has gradually gained ground in the estimation of medical men. . . . Those who formerly scoffed, would now be ashamed to acknowledge the ignorance in which they then glorified." Of Laennec's place in history, the reviewer had no doubts: "None will dare to deny that he has produced the most complete treatise on diseases of the chest, which exists in any language."

The writing of *De l'Auscultation Médiate* had been an exhausting undertaking for its sickly author. Added to the relentless burden of his practice, the urgent imperative to complete the manuscript encumbered his narrow shoulders with an insupportable weight that could not be borne without stumbling. During the last three weeks of feverish writing, he refused all new patients and turned over his regular practice to a colleague. He did not appear at the Necker during the final frenetic seven days. After writing the last line of his book, on August 6, 1818, he collapsed.

Though he might have wished to think it was nervous exhaustion that had done him in, Laennec was unable to ignore the increasing evidence of his old "asthma" that plagued him during the final few months of his labors. For the first time, he began to admit the possibility that he might be a victim of the affliction that had claimed the lives of so many of his colleagues as well as his mother and brother. Nevertheless, he who knew more about its symptoms and pathology than any other living man continued to deny, at least to others, that he might be suffering from tuberculosis. He preferred to diagnose himself as a case of *taedium vitae,* the contemporary equivalent of today's nervous breakdown.

Unable to resume either practice or hospital work, Laennec took a long holiday in his beloved Brittany. He had inherited from his father's family an old country house called Kerlouarnec, or "place of the foxes" in the native Breton dialect. It was to this small estate that he now repaired to recover from his labors and his breathlessness. Within a few months, his chest was better, his spirits were less depressed, and he felt ready to return to work. After paying visits first to his father and then to Uncle Guillaume, he returned to Paris in November.

To his colleagues, he looked not much better than on the day he had left. He remained thin to the point of gauntness, and seemed often on the verge of fainting. Moreover, what he returned to was not much less enervating than what he had left three months before. The practice was as busy as ever, and the teaching load had, if anything, grown heavier. Although he no longer had to contend with the frenzied throes of writing, he was now required to be the editor and reviser of his manuscript. Somehow, he managed to see it through the press, but not without a recurrence of his breathing problems and general state of depression.

Finally, there could be no further delay—he must give up his career or his life. About a month before the publication of his book, he wrote to Guillaume:

> I expect to say farewell to Paris at the end of August, at the very latest. Many people in my place would be in despair . . . but I am no longer capable, without endangering my life, of the degree of intense mental concentration required for the preparation of a lesson, and my nerves would force me to call it off or else do it badly in twenty cases out of forty. . . . Never could I undertake such a task if I could not do it honorably. I much prefer to go and vegetate, and do as much good as I can at Kerlouarnec. After all, so long as I can make ends meet, I shall be happy there.

He resigned his hospital post, and gave his pathological specimens and some of his books to the library. After selling the rest, he disposed of his household goods and, on October 8, 1819, left Paris in the black cabriolet in which he had so often gone to visit the sick.

For two years, Laennec lived the life of a gentleman farmer while he attempted to restore his health. During the days when he was not supervising some detail at Kerlouarnec, he would take quiet walks in the woods with his dogs or cover long distances on leisurely horseback rides. He played doctor to his tenant farmers and anyone else who needed his services, which gave him the opportunity to demonstrate to the local physicians the stethoscopes he created ever more skillfully on his lathe. He spent countless hours perfecting his Breton speech. Every Sunday, rosary in hand, he would join in the solemn procession of bareheaded fishermen and peasants making their way to the local village church. He became, in all ways, a country squire of Brittany.

In spite of the unhurried pace of life, Laennec's strength came back only slowly. When his cousin Christophe wrote to him in January 1821 that he might be offered a chair by the Faculté de Médecine, he did not take the bait. Uncle Guillaume, who did not realize how far advanced his nephew's illness had become, wrote to tell him that he was behaving like a psychopath for not pursuing the opportunity. One line from the younger man's reply described how exhausting he still found a day's work to be: "I am like Ajax," he wrote. "I can only fight valiantly during the day."

Gradually, however, he began to plan his return. He made the final determined decision at the end of the summer of 1821. Early in October, traveling in short stages and accompanied by his physician nephew Mériadec Laennec, he set out for Paris. Shortly after he arrived, on November 15, he resumed his practice and once again took up his clinical lectures. Although he no longer visited the sick at their homes, he had enough consultation work and wealthy patients so that his income soon became substantial again.

Once more, influence and connections resulted in the most worthy of France's physicians being appointed to a major post under unworthy circumstances. By a royal decree of Louis XVIII, the *concours* had been abolished in February 1816, so that professors were thereafter appointed by the government. On July 31, 1822, Laennec's fellow Breton, the minister Corbières, saw to it that he was appointed professor and royal lecturer at the Collège de France. As the next school year was about to begin, there were some minor student outbreaks to protest the fact that the king had appointed his own almoner to head the university. The government seized on the opportunity to blame the riots on the professors, whose liberal leanings they had long wished to suppress. A royal decree of November 21, 1822, abolished the faculty in an obvious ploy to turn out the men who were obnoxious to the ministers and replace them with others whose political and religious views were more agreeable. Laennec, who did have the properly orthodox religious sentiments and was well known to be a royalist, was one of the few who profited by the upheavals. He was made a member of a small committee appointed to reorganize the faculty, the result of which was that he became the sole professor of medicine in the Collège de France. Other honors followed soon after. In January 1823, he was elected a full member of the Academy of Medicine, and in August 1824 he was made a knight of the Legion of Honor.

The Charité was the appropriate hospital for the Professor of Medicine at the Collège de France. Laennec now moved his clinical work back to where he had spent his student days, in the old buildings on the Rue des St. Pères. Then

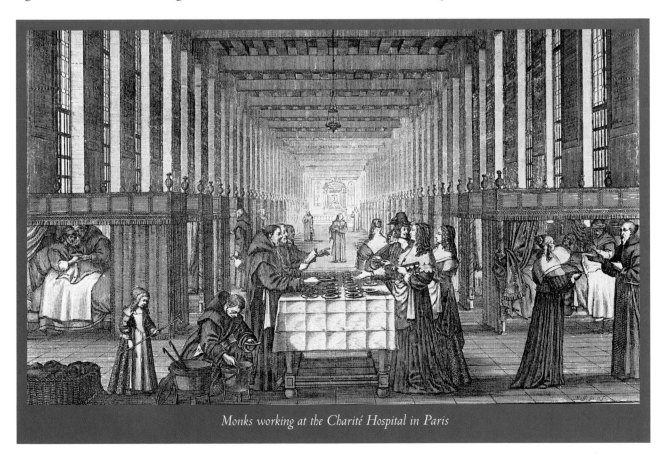

Monks working at the Charité Hospital in Paris

began the truly great days of his reputation as a teacher. He taught others as he had taught himself, by correlating the symptoms and physical examination of his patients with the findings at autopsy. Pathology, in our time a separate specialty of its own, was then an extension of clinical medicine. For teaching and research purposes, it was its most useful part. Lured even more by Laennec's clinical skills than by reading translations of his book, foreign students by the hundreds flocked to the five wards of the hospital which were under his direction. Paris became, even more than before, the world's main stage for the study of medicine, and at the very center of it stood René Laennec.

Except that he began later than the usual six-in-the-morning starting time, Laennec conducted his teaching clinics much as did the other leading physicians and surgeons of Paris. He made his ward rounds at ten, followed by a cortège of junior physicians, students, and foreign visitors. The entire session, excepting only the interrogation of patients, was conducted in Latin, for the benefit of the foreigners who might not speak French. Laennec would stop at the bed of each new patient, take his history, and then demonstrate the proper way to carry out the appropriate parts of the physical examination. Several of the students, French and foreign alike, were then permitted to examine the patient and discuss their findings with the professor. Af-

The doctors of the past had not understood that an entire organism can be made sick less because of general imbalances than because of very specific derangements of organs.

ter rounds were completed, the entire group retired to an amphitheater where Laennec gave a lecture on the cases that had just been seen.

After the lecture, there followed the most important part of the clinic, the performance of autopsies of patients who had died some time after the students had seen them on rounds. It was this "summing up" of the case that gave the Parisian method of instruction its singular quality. Impressed by it and stimulated by it, foreign students returned home and set up similar systems in their own countries. Particularly in London, Dublin, and Vienna, the hospitals and their autopsy rooms became the arena for the transmission of medical knowledge, as a kind of scientific cross-pollination took place. Historians have referred to this method of teaching as "hospital medicine," a process that resulted in the transfer of the site of instruction from university lecture halls to the bedsides of the institutionalized sick.

This was the period of history as well when the central point of medical research shifted from the patient to his disease. The doctors of the past had not understood that an entire organism can be made sick less because of general imbalances than because of very specific derangements of organs. First Morgagni and now the physicians of the Paris school sent out the ringing message that no progress would ever be made in the treatment of people unless specificity took the place of generalities, unless the particular source of every symptom could be found, and unless the diagnostic vision of the healers was permitted to narrow itself to a much smaller and therefore more brilliantly illuminated focus. The Cnidian philosophy had to be allowed to overcome the Coan.

What is implied here is not that the Cnidian emphasis on specificity will prove, in the long run, to be the correct one. When we some future day know much more about such things than we do now, it may well be that our view of disease causation will eventually shift back to something closer to that of Hippocrates, or another model entirely. There is already a strong body of medical evidence suggesting that there are multiple causes for any disease process; those that are genetic, immunologic, environmental, psychological, hormonal, and so forth perhaps all act together to produce a particular outcome that may be different for each person, depending upon his underlying constitutional factors, which in turn are also genetic, immunologic, and all the rest. In other words, we may be approaching in the twenty-first century a new era of Hippocratism, based on science. However, none of this should be taken to diminish the importance, considering where things stood at the beginning of the nineteenth century, of Laennec and the others seeking out direct one-to-one relationships between symptoms and identifiable physical changes in organs. Only when this viewpoint came into ascendancy could disease mechanisms begin to be studied in the way that has led to the enormous expansion of knowledge that is enabling medical science to take the next step, for which it may now be ready.

The philosophy that organ pathology is the root cause of all disease was not taken up without some hesitation, largely on humanitarian grounds. There are numerous statements in the extant letters of foreign visitors that comment adversely on the French tendency to think of patients as little more than material for learning and teaching. So far abstracted did the Parisian clinicians sometimes seem from the sick people they treated that they appeared often to be dealing with pathology divorced from its human context. It is a charge that the medical profession has since grown accustomed to hearing. The accusation is not a product of late-twentieth-century scientific technology, as many would believe, but rather an outgrowth of the anatomical concept of viewing disease. Without it, scientific medicine would almost certainly never have achieved anything beyond humors and hope—it would not even be scientific medicine. But the price paid in humanity and goodness has been high, much higher than the profession has until recently realized.

Pierre Louis, a great clinician of the next Parisian generation after Laennec, began one of his books with a quotation from Jean-Jacques Rousseau which may, at least in part, explain the approach of science, and explain why it was so necessary that there be an emotional distance between a physician and his patient: "I know that the truth is in the things, and not in my mind which judges them. The less I put of my own into these judgments, the surer I am to approach the truth." This was a declaration of objectivity—in diagnosis, a clinician's mind must be closed to anything but the reproducible evidence of his five senses. In this view, anything that interferes with scientific detachment interferes with the search for truth. The bias that is introduced by emotions and personal feelings, as useful as it may be in total patient care, too often stands in the way of exact diagnosis of pathological processes and exact modalities of treatment. That was the credo of the French clinician-researchers of the early nineteenth century and has remained the credo for the scientific aspects of their profession. Of course, there is more to healing than science alone, and every physician knows that. But it is precisely in the Cnidian reduction of disease into terms of its effect on tissues and organs that the Hippocratic hope may best see its fulfillment—to treat fellow human beings who happen to be sick, rather than to treat sicknesses that happen to occur in human beings.

Of all of the groups of students who accepted only reluctantly the seemingly cool detachment of their Parisian professors, the Americans, with their greater feeling for equality, for the human dignity even of the poor, were the most outspoken. But even they recognized the value of concentrating people with pathology in hospitals in such a way that great use could be made not only of their sheer volume but of the orderly way in which disease was subjected to scrutiny. In the twenty years after Laennec's invention of the stethoscope, many an American who had the means to do so traveled to Paris as soon as he had received his medical diploma. (This was made easier by the introduction in 1817 of regular transatlantic packet ship sailings from New York, which meant that travelers to Europe needed no longer to wait weeks or months until

a captain decided that he had a full enough hold or a fair enough wind.) One of the medical visitors to the Charité was Oliver Wendell Holmes, who described the advantages of the French system in a letter he wrote home in June 1835:

If I was asked—why do you prefer that intelligent young man who has been studying faithfully in Paris to this venerable practitioner who has lived more than twice as long—I should say, because the young man has experience. He has seen more cases perhaps of any given disease—he has seen them grouped so as to throw more light upon each other—he has been taught to bestow upon them far more painful investigations—he has been instructed daily by men who know no master and teach no doctrine but nature and her laws, pointed out at the bedside for those to own who see them, and for the meanest student to doubt, to dispute if they cannot be seen—he has examined the dead body oftener and more thoroughly in the course of a year than the vast majority of our practitioners have in any ten years of their lives. True experience is the product of opportunity multiplied by years.

When they returned to the United States, Holmes and his fellow voyagers found nothing to compare with the pedagogical advantages of the French system, and realized, moreover, that the American temperament would not permit such a detached scientific climate to develop. For one thing, the stronger emphasis on classlessness in American society (French professions of *égalité* notwithstanding) demanded a greater sensitivity to hospitalized patients as more than mere "teaching material" in the hands of the professors. For another, Holmes and the others recognized the powerful anti-intellectual strain that existed in the populist young country, where, at the time, Jacksonian democracy was in its ascendancy. Throughout the nineteenth century and for the first few decades of the twentieth, American medical schools lagged as far behind in teaching as did American physicians in scientific research. The "hospital system" would not exist in this country until the founding of The Johns Hopkins University Medical School in 1893, a few years after the establishment of the university's own hospital. Even after that, it took more than thirty years for its principles to take root throughout the United States. As late as World War I, it was only the exceptional American school whose students had any meaningful access to hospitalized patients. The story of the development of a system in which medical schools forged alliances with major hospitals is the

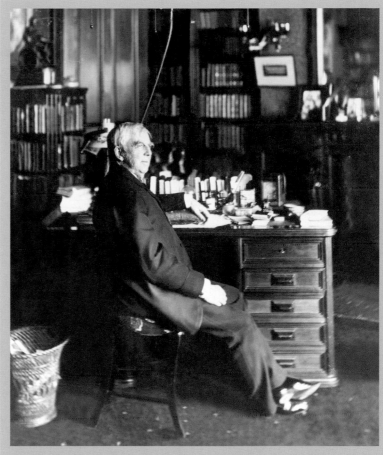

Oliver W. Holmes, photographed in the study of his home in Boston

story of the transformation of American medical education into its present status as the world's best.

The excellence of Laennec as a teacher and diagnostician does not mean that he had much more to offer his patients, once diagnosed, than had his hero Hippocrates twenty-three hundred years earlier. His surgical colleagues, it is true, had made some progress in their ability to deal with a goodly number of externally obvious maladies, and had even developed improved instruments and operations. The physicians, on the other hand, were still attempting to alter the dis-

ordered humoral balance of their patients. They continued to purge, puke, and blister as they always had, although they had created somewhat more sophisticated rationalizations for doing so. This kind of treatment, called empirical because physicians based its usefulness on their own personal experience, sometimes had what would later be found to be, albeit fortuitously, a sound physiological effect; bleeding for the fluid-filled lungs of heart failure is one such example. Because a therapy was seen to be effective on many occasions, it might then be recommended for ailments that seemed to be related to those in which it succeeded, but which were, in fact, quite different. Extending this kind of thinking out in all directions resulted in many therapeutic methods that made very little scientific sense, especially when they were based on Hippocratic theories of disease causation. Fouquier, for example, who was one of Laennec's successors at the Charité, treated fevers with a sedative and severe diarrhea by applying leeches to the anus.

As Professor of Medicine at the Collége de France, Laennec delivered a course of lectures in addition to his teaching rounds at the Charité. His private practice, meanwhile, had grown larger with his increasing fame. In addition to all of this, it soon became time to bring forth a second edition of *De l'Auscultation Médiate*. When it is considered that he also continued to publish papers in the medical journals, it can be appreciated that after his 1822 professorial appointment he found himself working harder than ever—at a time when his chronically deteriorated health must have limited his energies so much that it is a wonder he could work at all.

In October of 1822, Laennec invited the widowed Jacqueline Argou to move into the apartment he shared with his nephew Mériadec, in order that she might oversee the household and thus relieve him of a few of his day-to-day burdens. She was a distant cousin and a devout Catholic, which meant, as he wrote in a letter to Christophe, that "with that and her forty-two or forty-three years, no one could possibly raise any objections." Besides, who would ever be so ungracious as to suggest that the mind of the wizened, tubercular, middle-aged professor could harbor temptations thought to be reserved for healthier flesh?

Apparently, lots of people were that ungracious and worse. Within two years, the Laennec domestic arrangements had become the subject of a great deal of small-minded gossip in Paris medical and social circles. That Mme. Argou was known to be the very substance of virtue and piety, and quite homely to boot, was beside the point. What mattered was a chance to poke malicious fun at the great professor and his pious relative. Finally, on December 16, 1824, Mme. Argou was promoted from widow to wife, probably more to silence the scandal-mongers than out of motives of beatific romance. But she and her new spouse did better than that—in the spring of 1825, Jacqueline Laennec, barely more than a bride, became pregnant. Her husband was resuscitated by his enthusiasm at the thought that he would finally become a father, and he began to make plans that indicate he expected to live to see his child grow up. Sadly, the pregnancy was lost a few months later during a severe illness of uncertain nature that the mother contracted.

By April 1826, when the second edition of the great book went to press, the loss of his wife's pregnancy with its accompanying loss also of optimism, the unremitting hard work, and the relentless advance of his breathing problems had brought the final exhaustion on Laennec. No longer could he deny the lethal reality of his tuberculosis. The chest pain and the fever were beginning to worsen rapidly. He was coughing up thick putrid material from the decaying tissue of his lungs. Mériadec, using the stethoscope, heard for the first time the dread sounds that indicated a tuberculous cavity in the upper portion of his uncle's left chest. On April 20, Laennec drew up his will.

The time had come to go home to his beloved Brittany. Perhaps some strength might be regained there, but regardless of the outcome, Laennec had decided never again to return to Paris. On May 30, cadaverically emaciated and ghostly pale, he made his excruciating way down the stairs of his house in Paris for the last time. Clothed in his customary suit of black, leaning his scant and trembling weight on his wife's arm, he had about him the air of a man descending step by step into his own tomb.

The journey home was a torment. Finally, after ten agonizing, rain-filled days, the hills around Kerlouarnec came into view. The rain had mercifully stopped and the sun was shining in all the splendor of an early June morning as Laennec stepped down from his carriage to be greeted by a throng of local farmers and the peasants from his estate. He had come home, but too late.

The six brief weeks that remained to the dying man were a period of farewell. From time to time he would be taken around the countryside in a small cart pushed by a neighbor. He made many visits to the local chapel of St. Croix, and had his prayers briefly answered by a short period of improvement during which he could walk about his property with the friends and the cousins who came to make what they knew would be their last goodbyes. During the second week of August, the fever returned, and brought with it a state of delirium.

In midafternoon on August 13, Laennec awoke for one last lucid moment. He looked over at his wife sitting watchfully alongside him, raised himself with great effort to an upright position, and slowly removed the rings from his fingers and placed them on the bedside table. "I am doing this," he was barely able to utter, "because otherwise someone would soon have to render me this service. I wish to spare them the painful task." Those were his last words. Two hours later, René Laennec, the foremost physician of the world, the inventor of medicine's first diagnostic instrument, had become yet one more victim of the white death of tuberculosis, the very scourge whose true nature he had exposed.

After Laennec's funeral in the local cemetery, the family gathered to hear the reading of his will. In his last days at Kerlouarnec he had added a codicil bequeathing to Mériadec all of his medical books and papers. He also wrote, "I give him my watch, my ring, and above all my stethoscope, which is the best part of my legacy."

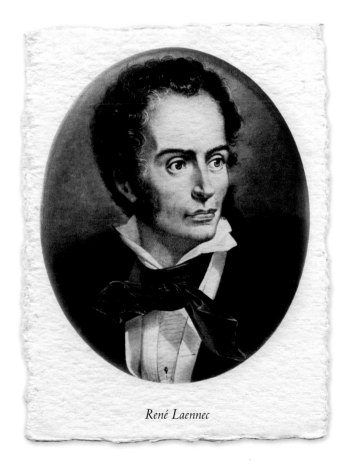

René Laennec

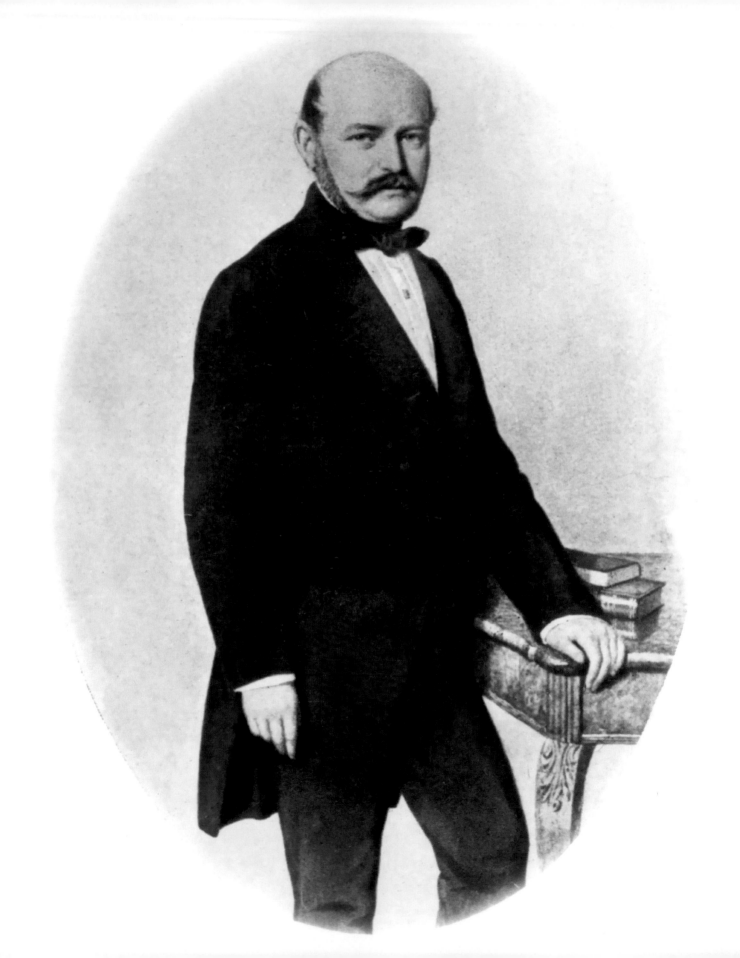

9

THE GERM THEORY BEFORE GERMS

The Enigma of Ignac Semmelweis

Genius was priceless, beneficent, divine, but also was, at its hours,
capricious, sinister, cruel; and natures ridden by it, accordingly,
were alternately very enviable, and very helpless.
—Henry James, *Roderick Hudson*

The many biographers of Ignac Semmelweis have created a mythology that compares the events of his life to those of a Greek tragedy. The biographers, however, would have us believe that it is a tragedy after the manner of Aeschylus, a tragedy in which the hero is destroyed by malevolent gods—by forces beyond his control. Although there is no question that this genius who discovered a method of preventing the lethal disease of childbed fever did live out a tragedy, the facts of his life indicate that it was a tragedy more reminiscent of Sophocles than of Aeschylus. The basic elements of the Sophoclean drama are there: a hero, a truth, a mission, and finally a flight of passionate arrogance resulting in downfall. This was not Aeschylus writing; the fate of a Sophoclean hero is governed not by the actions of the gods but by a fundamental fault in his own nature. The drama of Ignac Semmelweis arose from the classic flaw—having discovered his own truth and his own mission, he created and was inexorably drawn to his own tragic fate. Genius can, as Henry James tells us, be cruel, and those possessed of it, or by it, can be utterly helpless.

The helplessness of Ignac Semmelweis was consequent to the tight grip in which he was held by his self-destroying psyche. He was brought to his tragic fate by his own faulty nature, and not, as popular historians have told us for generations, by the overwhelming gods of a backward medical establishment.

In one sense, however, Semmelweis was ill-used by his stars—his genius led him to a discovery for which the world was not yet prepared. He violated the most basic of the principles that underlie the hunting-rules of those who would track down Nature's secrets: an idea must never be presented before its time. When a seemingly revolutionary leap occurs in science, it proves, almost always, to be but a particularly long step by a particularly bold researcher, in a process for which the stage has been set by the work of others who came before. When the cultural milieu is just right, when the technological tools have been invented, and when enough restless minds have begun to chafe under the status quo, some one spunky spirit comes forward to deliver the enlightening goods. Though only a small number of the restless may at first appreciate the magnitude of the idea that thus makes its appearance, acceptance is in fact inevitable, because the new concept has arisen from such a logical process of discovery. Even when the savants of science do not yet know what to do with some particular bold bound forward, at least a few will always appear who appreciate that it is a valid idea, and therefore must be cherished until the day that its usefulness will become apparent. This latter situation applied in the case of William Harvey's discovery of the circulation, and to a lesser extent in the case of the anatomy of Vesalius and that of the surgical research of John Hunter. For such lucky investigators as Morgagni and Laennec, the response to the new concept was prompt and avid. The number was large of those who were wise enough to value their work, and there was an immediate practical application for it, as well.

Ignac Semmelweis was not so fortunate. He presented a disease concept that was based on the spread of bacterial contamination, but he did it nine years before Louis Pasteur's demonstration that bacteria are the cause of putrefaction. He identified the means by which a lethal infection, childbed fever, can be spread from one patient to another by the very doctors who are trying to cure it, but his forward leap was accomplished almost twenty years before an even greater jump by Joseph Lister, who would prove, in 1867, that wound infections, since they are caused by bacteria, can be transmitted by the hands of doctors.

Nevertheless, Semmelweis should not be viewed as a luckless victim of untimely destiny. His discovery, as will soon become apparent, did arise from the work of predecessors, and did come into being in a milieu that might have allowed its fragile seed to germinate, in spite of its premature planting. That this did not occur is less the result of Semmelweis having awakened, like Leonardo, "too early in the darkness" than of his own obstinate refusal to see that medical science, though not quite prepared, was at the very edge of a readiness that should have brought him the recognition he sought, and saved the many lives that were tragically lost because of his obdurate posture.

Ignac Semmelweis failed, in the final analysis, not only because he was too early, but also because he was too stubborn. So fixed did he become in his self-righteousness that he never did the experiments that might have helped his cause, nor was he able to convince any of the then increasing number of skilled laboratory researchers that his ideas were worth investigating. His should have been the prepared mind that first took up Pasteur's discovery and made it a basic foundation stone of medicine. Instead, it was the patient, selfless Lister who took the colossal step that led to the germ theory of disease.

The life story of Ignac Semmelweis thus becomes one of the cautionary tales of medical sci-

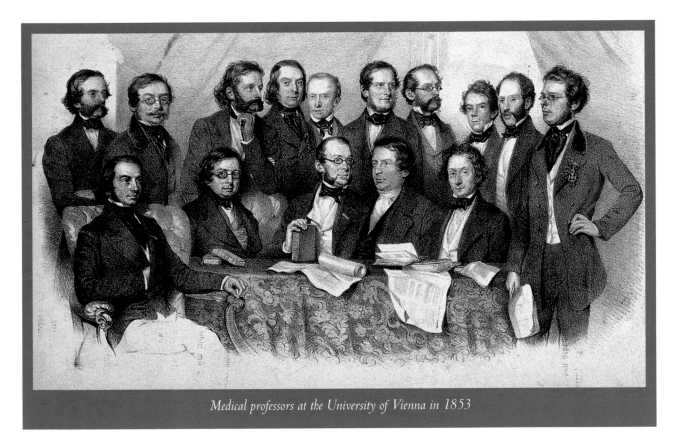

Medical professors at the University of Vienna in 1853

ence. In the procession of successes presented in this book, it is fitting that we should pause to look at a failure. The blind alleys of medical research have been many, and more would-be heroes have fallen by the wayside than have lasted the course. In the "exposition of human ineptitudes" of which Fielding Garrison wrote, the saga of Semmelweis is one of particular poignancy, because its protagonist's ineptitude was not one of talent, but of character. Having for a brief moment done everything right, albeit just a bit before its time, he then spent the rest of his career doing everything wrong. His book, instead of marking one of those great turning points in the history of medical science, marks only the unhappy spot at which a tangent took off, to be forgotten for the rest of the nineteenth century.

At the Vienna Medical School the year 1847 was a time of extreme conservatism, both in national politics and in medicine. Hungary and Austria were both parts of the great Hapsburg Empire, but whereas Vienna was the shining capital, Hungary was a subordinate province dominated by the ascendant Germanic culture. Prince Metternich, the empire's first minister, followed a policy of repression and cruelty in which the diverse national groups of the empire were played off against one another. It was the eve of the unsuccessful revolutions of 1848, which brought about no real improvement in the political arena but which did open the way for increased freedom in matters academic.

The University of Vienna, and most particularly its medical school, became a hotbed of revolutionary activity. The uprisings of 1848 were strongly supported by the younger faculty members, largely because the university was under the stifling control of government ministries. Some of the major positions at the school were held by professors who were old in years and who owed their power to close connections with those very same bureaucrats. They became arrayed against the younger faculty, whose liberal policies and new ideas they opposed, both in research and in concepts of disease causation. Into this setting—the new versus the old, the intellectually liberal versus the conservative, the true scientific understanding of disease versus the fuzzy theoretics of the old medicine—the Semmelweis theory figuratively exploded. Because the theory was the result of methods of observation and analysis that the Young Turks stood for, and because it was a natural outgrowth of the teachings of their three great leaders, it became a battleground along which clear lines could be drawn.

Major battles of the eighteenth and nineteenth centuries not infrequently began at sunrise. There is some poetic truth in saying that what Ignac Semmelweis was, years later, to call "the rising of

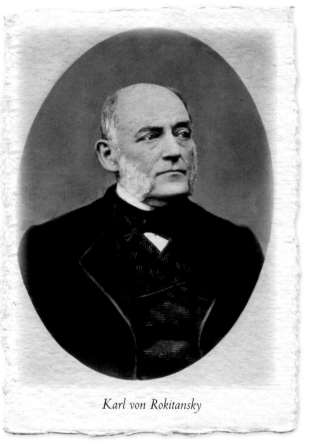

Karl von Rokitansky

the puerperal sun over Vienna" was to signal the call to arms for this major battle in the history of the Vienna Medical School.

Because of the happy coincidence that three brilliant and visionary young men came together, the school entered on the most glorious period in its history. The first, and the greatest, was Karl von Rokitansky, Professor of Pathologic Anatomy, who contended that clinical symptoms are the outward manifestations of pathological changes in organs and tissues. Given breath by Morgagni, and then nurtured through its infancy by the Paris school, the still-young concept was not yet universally accepted when Rokitansky was appointed to his chair in 1844. In his view, it was the role of the dissector not only to identify the organ derangement, but to see it as one evolutionary phase, one instant, in an ongoing dynamic process of disease. Inspired by the French, and by the physiological researches of John Hunter, he sought to describe the way in which a disease process evolves to the point at which it is encountered by the attending physician in the clinic or at the autopsy table. It was no longer enough that the cry could be traced to its suffering organ; one must trace that organ's disordered state directly back to its beginnings, so that the process of disease could be reconstructed and understood.

Rokitansky wanted to know not only the way in which the anatomical change evolved, but also the accompanying change in function, the pathologic physiology. This kind of close observation of the ongoing development of diseases required that its researchers be specialists in such work. With Rokitansky, the study of pathology became a field of medicine all its own. In Vienna, the clinical physician did not do his own postmortem dissections—he came to the autopsy room to see what the pathologist could show him, as do the clinicians of today. The Pathological Institute at the University of Vienna was like a concert hall of medicine, in which the artists of one branch of healing performed what might be called an organ recital for the artists of another. Rokitansky gave approximately eighteen hundred such performances each year, some thirty thousand during his lifetime. The body of every patient who died at the two-thousand-bed Vienna General Hospital was delivered to his department. Before his career was ended he had brought considerable order and system to the classification of disease; Rudolf Virchow called Rokitansky "the Linnaeus of pathological anatomy." He was also at the forefront of a historic process by which the leadership of western medicine was being transferred to the German-speaking schools and hospitals of central Europe, where it would remain until well into the next century.

The pathologist Edwin Klebs, a major contributor to the bacterial theory of disease causation (and, incidentally, the father of one of the founders of my library), wrote of Rokitansky that he "taught us to think anatomically at the bedside and to weave at the autopsy table the individual phases of the morbid process into the pattern of the clinical progress." It was from this master teacher that Ignac Semmelweis learned the wisdom of close observation, learned to differentiate what was significant from what was trivial, and learned how to bring his observations together into a unitary diagnosis in which the clinical findings were correlated with the pathological.

The second member of the triumvirate was Josef Skoda, the leading clinician of the Vienna Medical School. He is best known for his studies on percussion and auscultation in which, like Rokitansky, he accurately correlated the clinical

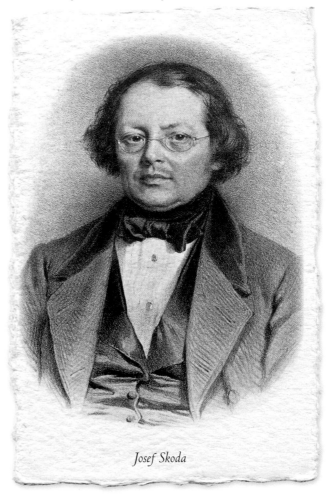

Josef Skoda

findings to the pathological changes that caused them. His approach was somewhat different from that of Laennec and his followers, concentrating more on the physical properties of the structures being auscultated than on their biological characteristics. This made for a system that was less prone to exaggerations than was the French, and was therefore more readily learned by novices. Rokitansky was kindly and generous, but Skoda tended to be cold and rigid and to care not at all for warm personal friendships. What he did care about was clinical science, and to Josef Skoda clinical science meant diagnosis, not therapy. He had not much use for the generally ineffectual treatments of the time, which he dismissed with the brusque truth that *"das ist ja alles eins"*—they are really all the same. He was, however, a proponent of prevention; he believed that the proper approach to disease should be prophylactic, to stop it before it could begin its ravages. To this end he devoted considerable effort to the study of the epidemic diseases such as typhoid and cholera. His was the clinical personality that would enthuse over a theory like that of Semmelweis.

Although he was an advocate of hygiene and public health measures, it was in the area of one-on-one diagnosis that Skoda achieved his lasting fame. Working together with Rokitansky in the autopsy room and applying his findings to patients on the ward, he developed a method of clinical reasoning that caught the imagination of young Semmelweis. Skoda and Rokitansky both recognized that the puerperal-fever discovery was a logical outcome of their own teachings in the new methods of scientific logic. Erna Lesky, in her encyclopedic study of the Vienna Medical School, states that these two rising giants were not only

the supporters of Semmelweis but the "intellectual fathers of his discovery."

The youngest of the three medical leaders was Ferdinand von Hebra. Only two years older than Ignac Semmelweis, Hebra was also a pupil of Rokitansky and Skoda, and applied their principles to the diagnosis and classification of skin diseases. Having been assigned by Skoda to study certain forms of dermatitis, he founded a new school of dermatology based on pathological anatomy. Hebra and Semmelweis became close friends. Because of their closeness, and because of his belief in its validity, the sensitive, kindly Hebra was the first to describe in print the puerperal-fever theory of his reticent friend. In Hebra's mind, the discovery was worth ranking beside Edward Jenner's introduction of smallpox vaccination.

Heroes often seem to come from the ranks of the social or intellectual aristocracy on the one hand, or the poverty-hardened peasant or working class on the other. Our tragedy has an unusual hero; his father was a grocer, a member of the traditionally nonheroic bourgeoisie.

In fact, Ignac Semmelweis was unusual in several respects. For one thing, this Hungarian national hero had a very non-Hungarian name. In their scrupulously researched 1968 biography, Gyorgy Gortvay and Imre Zoltán, by studying parish registers, traced the Semmelweis family back to the small village of Marczfalva in 1570. Very likely descended from a Frankish tribe, this family, like most of the trading population of Buda and Pest, spoke a German dialect called Buda Swabian. Ignac Philip, known as Naci by his relatives, did not properly learn the Hungarian language until secondary school. When, therefore, he enrolled in the University of Vienna in 1837 his German was an awkward dialect, and his Hungarian was freshly mastered in secondary school. Neither in Hungarian nor in the polished Viennese German of his colleagues was he comfortable. At Vienna he entered law school and then transferred to medicine after one year; it was the first of the direction changes that were to occur again and again in his life. Some of the changes were imposed upon him, but others were self-chosen. In the faculty register of the Vienna Medical School, Semmelweis, just prior to his graduation in 1844, stated his intention to return to his home country. For reasons that are not clear, among which may have been the death of his mother one week before he was to receive his degree, he soon determined to remain in Vienna.

If the imagination of the newly graduated doctor was captured by the studies of Rokitansky, it was set on fire by the work being done in forensic pathology by a Rokitansky disciple, Jacob Kolletschka, whom Semmelweis idolized. When he applied for a post as Kolletschka's assistant, however, he was not accepted, for reasons that are unclear. The disappointment must have been great. But Semmelweis also had other interests, and soon thereafter applied to be Skoda's assistant only to be rejected once more; Skoda had promised the job to someone else.

In July 1844 he decided to study obstetrics, and was at the same time given permission by Karl von Rokitansky to dissect female cadavers. Shortly thereafter he became assistant to Johann

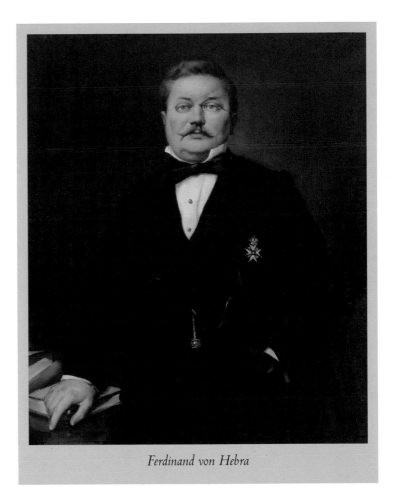

Ferdinand von Hebra

Klein, Professor of Obstetrics, his appointment to extend until 1847. The fact that Klein was among the staunchest of the old guard and a good friend of the politicians in the ministry did not seem to diminish the enthusiasm that Semmelweis brought to his undertaking.

As the young obstetrician did more and more autopsies on the bodies of women who had died of childbed fever, or puerperal fever as it is more commonly called, he began to develop a theory of its pathophysiology—that is, the way in which it evolved. There were at that time a number of different explanations that had been put forward by various authorities in an attempt to understand why so many women died of the dread process in their immediate postdelivery days. In some hospitals, at certain times of the year, the figure had been reported as high as 25 percent of all mothers. Most physicians considered it to be a specific disease entity, like smallpox, for example. The most widely accepted theory of its transmission was that it came and went in epidemics, also like smallpox. There were those who thought it was caused by a miasma, one of those noxious atmospheres invoked since the Greeks to explain disease causation. The theory of Ignac Semmelweis was to change all of this. The series of astute clinical observations and the incisive clarity and logic of the reasoning that led him to develop that theory are revealed in his first publication, which did not appear until eleven years later:

Observation I: At the Vienna General Hospital, the Allgemeines Krankenhaus of the University of Vienna, there existed side by side two obstetrical divisions, exactly the same in every way, each delivering approximately thirty-five hundred babies each year. There was only one difference between them: in Division I, all deliveries were by obstetricians and students, and in Division II, all were by midwives. In Division I, an average of six hundred to eight hundred mothers died each year from childbed fever; in Division II the figure was sixty deaths—one-tenth as many.

These figures had not been easy to ascertain. It was common practice to transfer women who contracted puerperal fever to the general hospital wards to die, and they were therefore not included in the obstetrical mortality rates. This resulted in a skewed picture of the true magnitude of the difference between the two divisions, which Semmelweis was able to elucidate only by careful searching.

Observation 2: While childbed fever raged violently within the hospital, no such epidemic existed outside in the city of Vienna. Mothers delivered at home had a very low mortality, and mothers self-delivered, even in alleyways and streets, had essentially no mortality.

Observation 3: Yearly statistics showed that mortality was in no way related predictably to weather or seasonal variations.

Observation 4: The greater the injury to the cervix and the uterus during delivery, the greater the likelihood a mother would develop childbed fever.

Observation 5: Closing down the ward would always stop the mortality for a time after it was reopened.

From such observations, it became clear to Semmelweis that neither epidemic nor miasma could be the cause. The explanation was to be found in some unexplained factor that existed in Division I and not in Division II.

As Semmelweis pondered the data, looking for that factor, a great tragedy occurred at the Vienna Medical School. Kolletschka, the much-admired teacher of forensic pathology, sustained an accidental laceration during an autopsy and died quickly of an overwhelming wound infection. Semmelweis, who had lost his father only nine months before, was distraught. What came next is best described in words he would write fourteen years later:

Totally shattered, I brooded over the case with intense emotion, until suddenly a thought crossed my mind; at once it became clear to me that childbed fever and the death of

Professor Kolletschka were one and the same because they both consist pathologically of the same anatomic changes. If, therefore, in the case of Professor Kolletschka . . . septic changes . . . arose from the inoculation of cadaver particles, then puerperal fever must originate from the same source. . . . The fact of the matter was that the transmitting source of the cadaver particles was to be found in the hands of the students and attending physicians.

At the Allgemeines Krankenhaus every student and every teacher dissected several cadavers each day, according to a hard-and-fast Rokitansky-inspired rule of the curriculum. Washing was perfunctory. Semmelweis had found his explanation—the transmission of what he called "invisible cadaver particles, recognizable only by their odor" was the cause of puerperal fever.

To Semmelweis, then, puerperal fever was not a specific disease like smallpox; it consisted of a group of pathological changes in organs and tissues transmitted by the purulent material carried on the hands of medical personnel. Unlike smallpox, which could be caused only by another case of smallpox, the pathological changes of puerperal fever could result from contact with any source of pus, be it a sick mother, a putrid cadaver, a lanced boil, or an infection-soaked sheet; moreover, only putrid animal matter (bacteria-laden pus), from whatever source produced the pathology.

At the time, America's Oliver Wendell Holmes, as well as several English physicians, had been describing the problem as a specific contagious disease that might be airborne or otherwise carried without the necessary presence of what Semmelweis called "putrid organic matter." Indeed, Holmes (whose work Semmelweis did not know) had, in 1843, come quite close to identifying the cause, even speculating about what he called a "virus." But only Semmelweis really understood that three factors were required: the source of putrid material, a means of physically transporting it from that source to make intimate contact with the victim, and an injured surface, such as the denuded lining of a postpartum uterus or a lacerated finger. In Semmelweis' own words, "Childbed fever is a transmissible, but not a contagious disease." To return to the very useful smallpox analogy, only smallpox can produce another case of smallpox, and that is what is meant by contagion. An abscessed tooth or an infected uterine cancer cannot cause smallpox. But the pus from them can cause childbed fever.

Using his authority as Klein's assistant, Semmelweis instituted the simple measure of washing the hands in a chlorine solution until the skin was slippery and the cadaver smell was gone. In 1848, the first full year of this prophylaxis, Division I had a puerperal death rate of 1.2 percent and Division II of 1.3 percent, completely comparable and unprecedented. In April 1847, the last month without handwashings, the percentage of postpartum mothers who had died (quite literally) at the hands of their doctors had been 18.3 percent. The cause and prevention of puerperal fever was thus established. The doctrine was simple, logical, and consistent with every observation made by Semmelweis. It was the perfect outcome of the investigational techniques he had learned from Rokitansky and the reasoning methods he had been taught by Skoda. The experiential approach to bedside medicine, introduced by the Hippocratics and given new life by the French, was the triumphant authority behind the entire thesis.

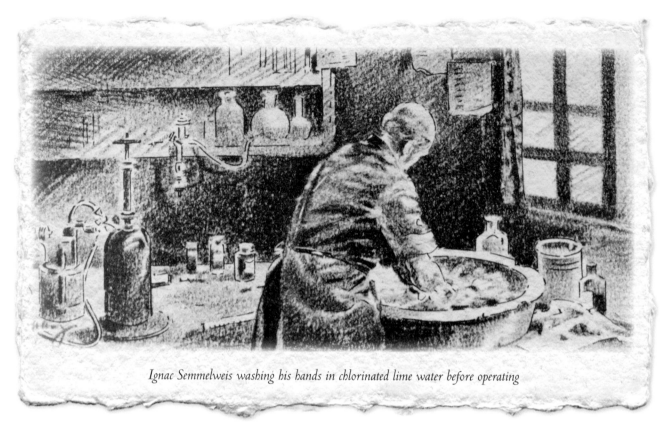

Ignac Semmelweis washing his hands in chlorinated lime water before operating

No longer could the deliberately myopic Krankenhaus obstetricians remain inattentive to the difference in mortality rates between the two divisions, or obscure a great part of it from themselves by transferring patients out to the general hospital wards to die. An explanation had been found, but it brought with it an excruciating accusation and a demand that the old methods give way to new. For many a conscience-stricken obstetrician, already burdened by years of tormented helplessness in the face of puerperal mortality, it would be an appeal to self-condemnation that was too heartbreaking to bear.

As the embodiment of the philosophy of the young professors at the Vienna Medical School, however, the theory of Semmelweis was a standard around which they could rally in their struggle to overthrow the older faculty and the government ministers who supported them. The illustrious Vienna surgeon Theodor Billroth, writing thirty years after these events, pointed out that the term "academic freedom," which we use so frequently these days, first came into popular use in 1848. Billroth wrote of the older conservative Austrian faculty as

> *a generation that had been reared in an intellectual straitjacket with dark spectacles before their eyes and cotton wool in their ears. The young people turned somersaults in the grass, and the old men, whose bodies had been hindered in their natural development by the lifelong burden of state supervision, felt their world tumbling about their ears, and believed that the end of things was at hand.*

What Billroth was describing, of course, was the transition by which the new medicine based on pathologic anatomy was pushing its way into a dominant position. The older men resisted change, and none of them resisted it more than Johann Klein, Semmelweis' chief of obstetrics.

It must have been difficult for the aging Klein to contemplate his own role in the carnage. Accepting the Semmelweis doctrine would have forced him not only to acknowledge the validity of his opponents' logical method of objective reasoning, but also to admit his unknowing complicity, as a teacher of obstetricians, in the death of thousands of young women. That the hand-washing proposal should arise from a series of astute clinical observations made by an argumentative protégé of the very movement he was trying to suppress—this must have been a painful blow, too painful to submit to. He preferred to remain stubbornly steadfast in his conviction that childbed fever was an insoluble problem, to persist forever as the inevitable fate of a great many hospitalized mothers.

The time came for publication. Semmelweis, however, did not write. Instead, in December 1847, Hebra told the world of his friend's discovery, in a local Viennese medical journal. Rokitansky made a strong supporting statement. In April 1848, Hebra published again in the same journal, though like the first article, this one was really an editorial and contained very little detail.

Skoda also spoke out publicly in favor of the Semmelweis theory on several occasions, including one address to the Academy of Sciences, the most important scientific organization in Austria. Not only did he speak, he published his remarks as well.

The mythologists of Ignac Semmelweis' life write of a lonely and misunderstood figure, fighting almost universal opposition before being overwhelmed by sheer weight of numbers and influence, and consequently destroyed. The truth is otherwise. The emerging leaders, who within a few years became victorious at Vienna, were all with Semmelweis. In a portrait made in 1853 of the Collegium of the Medical Faculty, nine of the fifteen professors in the picture are among those who gave active support to the Semmelweis doctrine by speaking, by writing, or by using it in practice. Rokitansky's power and influence were such that he had been elected rector of the Uni-

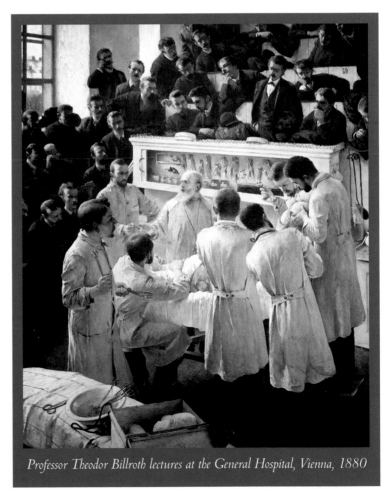

Professor Theodor Billroth lectures at the General Hospital, Vienna, 1880

versity of Vienna in the previous year. Of those pictured, only Anton von Rosas, a close friend of Johann Klein, still remained to represent the opposition. (The other five men pictured took no stand.)

With three separate statements having appeared in the literature, a number of outstanding obstetricians from other European universities were reading of the theory, and some were disagreeing. Ignac Semmelweis himself, however, did nothing to support his own doctrine in a public forum, despite the urging of his powerful friends. Historians have assumed, and no doubt correctly, that his literary ungainliness in the German language held him back. But another factor, corollary to the first, may have been more significant. It is probable that Semmelweis thought of himself as an outsider, the awkward son of a grocer, who spoke a clumsy dialect of German in a university community which, in spite of its generally cosmopolitan character, was basically hostile to certain kinds of foreigners. The otherwise humane attributes of the surgeon Theodor Billroth, for example, obscured a deeply ingrained intolerance for certain minority subgroupings; in a tasteless diatribe written thirty years after the events of which we speak, he referred to those Hungarians whom he called "pure Magyar" as being the acceptable ones. The non-Magyar Hungarians evidently stood only one step above the Hungarian Jews, who, in the authoritative words of the biased Billroth, "have the worst reputation among the Viennese students themselves." Poor Semmelweis was a Hungarian with a Germanic name. It is not stretching the limits of possibility that he may have felt himself suspected, in some quarters, of being Jewish. That his friend Hebra was a Jew

(and a Moravian to boot) and nevertheless accepted in Vienna as an honored colleague apparently made no impression on Semmelweis, who for his part seems almost to have courted rejection.

Yet another factor in the fragility of Semmelweis' self-esteem may have been the position of obstetrics in the academic hierarchy of mid-nineteenth-century Europe. Although there were chairs of obstetrics at all of the major universities, the subject remained an elective course for most students. The great majority of deliveries outside of hospitals were carried out by midwives. It should not be forgotten that Semmelweis himself became an obstetrician only after being turned down for other jobs he preferred, first in pathology and then in medicine.

In studying the details of Ignac Semmelweis' behavior in the several years following his discovery, it is difficult to escape the conclusion that he was living out a self-fulfilling prophecy. He seems to have seen himself as a maladroit, graceless outlander, who came from the wrong place, the wrong social class, spoke the wrong dialect, and had been rejected for the right university jobs; in short, always the outsider clanging and banging on the gates of an academic Pantheon in which he felt unworthy to dwell. The reality of his genius, of his immense discovery, of his powerful friends, of the truly mongrel nature of the Viennese intelligentsia, never overcame his greater sense of unworthiness. That self-concept lived side by side with its seeming opposite—conceit, a rage, and finally a towering hurricane of grandiosity that would eventually sweep him to his destruction.

In the midst of the emerging publicity about his theory, Semmelweis' term as assistant in obstetrics came to an end, on March 20, 1849. Klein, backed by his ministry friends, refused to renew it, in spite of the urgings of Rokitansky, Skoda, and Hebra. Not only had Semmelweis become forcefully obnoxious in the promotion of his beliefs, but he was not averse to letting those who questioned him know that they must think of themselves as murderers if they did not wash their hands with chlorinated solution before examining a patient in labor. He was a hellfire-spewing evangelist and an afflicter of conscience all at once, the kind of righteous goad that no one wants to be near. More than one obstetrician who might otherwise have been favorably disposed to giving his technique a fair trial was put off by the abrasive manner in which he attempted to make them dip and drink at his antiseptic trough of truth.

Klein resisted all appeals, and time passed. Pressed finally into some action by the continued coaxing of the brilliant triumvirate, the now jobless Semmelweis, three full years after identifying the cause of childbed fever, finally consented to speak about it before a forum of his colleagues, the Medical Society of Vienna, on May 15, 1850. Sponsored by his three friends, he had been elected to the society in July 1849, four months after his dismissal by Klein. Perhaps by this time he felt safe because Rokitansky was now the organization's president, but for whatever reason, he is reported to have handled himself so well that at the end of the ensuing debate, which continued into the June and July meetings, the rector stated that Dr. Semmelweis had won a resounding victory for his thesis.

At this point, the Semmelweis theory of puerperal fever stood on the verge of acceptance, in spite of its author's sometimes counterproductive ways of promoting it. It had the support of the emerging leaders of Vienna medicine, and the open debate and resultant clinical and laboratory trials could only ensure its success. But at this very instant, Semmelweis made two serious and self-destructive errors. First, he did not publish his presentation and debate before the Medical Society of Vienna; because he did not submit them in writing, his lectures and comments were published only as abstracts recorded in the minutes, as contrasted with the comments of his opponent in the debate, Eduard Lumpe, which were printed in full. (Lumpe's argument consisted of the old thesis that the large seasonal variations in the incidence of puerperal fever proved that the so-called "cadaver infection" could not be the cause. Since Semmelweis had not yet published, and the writings of his friends were sketchy, Lumpe did not believe that the seasonal character of the disease was more apparent than real.) Second, when Semmelweis was offered a minor clinical appointment that somewhat restricted his teaching prerogatives, his bruised ego took it as the final insult.

> *The reality of his genius, of his immense discovery, of his powerful friends, of the truly mongrel nature of the Viennese intelligentsia, never overcame his greater sense of unworthiness.*

Five days later, without so much as saying good-bye to his friends and supporters, or telling them of his plans for the future, he fled Vienna.

Rokitansky, Skoda, Hebra, and the others were shocked. They had given him encouragement, support, and friendship. They had looked forward to his attaining positions of authority at the medical school. Rokitansky, years later, forgave, but Skoda never wrote, and, it is said, never spoke, the name of Semmelweis again. It was as though a trusted warrior had deserted in the midst of a decisive campaign.

It is tempting to call the flight of Ignac Semmelweis a great irony; to say, as many biographers have said, that just as victory was within grasp, he lost heart. Consider instead that it may not have been an irony at all, but an almost deliberate step on the inexorable journey that Semmelweis was taking toward self-destruction; furthermore, that victory and the attainment of a professorship at the hallowed Vienna Medical School were inconsistent with his unconscious prophecy for himself; that his self-image as a pitiable, bumbling outsider could not coexist with the imminent glare of the continuing open debate that would have been necessary against some of the outstanding non-Viennese obstetricians of the day; that in all likelihood he could not bring himself to put his provincial brand of German on paper next to the elegant writing of his peers; that he ran back to Hungary because it was safe, as one runs back to a mother; that he made himself believe in the fantasy of his rejection because it gave him the rationalization he needed to rush back into that mother's protecting arms.

Pest was not Vienna. In 1850 it was still an intellectual backwater. Whereas the revolutions of 1848 had brought some academic freedom to Vienna, they had only served as a warrant for the authorities to worsen the repression at the University of Pest. Semmelweis sought and won an unpaid appointment as Director of Obstetrics at the Rochus Hospital, where he achieved an impressively low maternal mortality figure of 0.85 percent. In 1855 he was elected Professor of Obstetrics at the university, a school so dominated by the politicians that its academic standards were mediocre at best.

For those who think of Ignac Semmelweis as a lonely figure, possessor of a great discovery that had

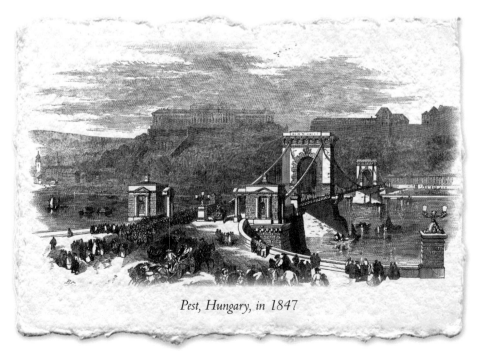

Pest, Hungary, in 1847

been suppressed and hidden by resentful colleagues, it is illuminating to read the description of him presented in a brochure to the voting faculty on the day of his election: "Ignac Semmelweis, age 36. . . . His well-known discovery has received the recognition of the Academy of Sciences in Vienna, and he is considered capable of further research."

As a professor, Semmelweis suddenly became a power to be dealt with. He involved himself in a whirlwind of activities—multiple faculty committees, multiple projects, multiple conflicts with colleagues. He was impetuous, he lacked tact, and he had a knack for alienating important people. Although his theory was never actively opposed in Hungary, it began to fade from view elsewhere, partly because of ignorance of the true basis of his work and partly because of the caliber of the opposition outside of Vienna.

It is part of the legend and myth of Ignac Semmelweis that his detractors were backward fools. This is no more true than the rest. Although there may indeed have been a few fools, the opposition to the Semmelweis doctrine included some of the most highly respected clinicians in Europe. Even so dominant and usually progressive a force in European medicine as the Berlin pathologist Rudolf Virchow was for years an opponent. It was as though, today, a new and inadequately described theory on the prevention of heart disease, promulgated but not yet published by a faculty member of a small state university, were opposed by Michael De Bakey, Surgeon General Everett Koop, and the director of the National Heart Institute.

There were valid reasons why acceptance of the theory was not widespread and enthusiastic. Conditions in Vienna for statistical analysis and clinicopathological studies were unique in the 1850s. Because Semmelweis had not published details of his observations and conclusions, only those who had watched them develop firsthand had good reason to accept them. He had done a few experiments on rabbits to support his thesis, but very few physicians knew of them. Moreover, his well-meaning friends had created some confusion by describing cadaver infection alone as the basis for his doctrine; their statements only skimmed the surface of his argument. In the absence of writings by Semmelweis himself, his friends could have clarified matters, but the Viennese scientists had become alienated by his desertion, and they in turn deserted him. In sum, then, Semmelweis' opponents had no access to all the facts and therefore could not fully comprehend the theory or accept the basis upon which it had been constructed.

The opposition fielded two major arguments against the Semmelweis doctrine. The first was that many of those who tried it could not duplicate his results. The reason was that most of the hospitals that made a trial of chlorine washes did so in an inconsistent and poorly supervised manner, with a predictably poor outcome. A generation later, this kind of half-hearted cleanliness would plague Joseph Lister's attempt to introduce antisepsis to the hospitals of Britain, leading to the disaffection of many potential converts.

The second argument against Semmelweis was, like Lumpe's, based on the apparent seasonal nature of the disease. Semmelweis was able to explain this by the simple method of observing the "coincidence" that the ups and downs attributed to seasons, as well as the comings and goings of the "epidemics" corresponded exactly to those times when, for various reasons, the number of corpse-dissecting students increased or fell. The arrival of each enthusiastic new student group elevated the mortality rate, which later dropped somewhat as they became less attentive to their autopsy duties. However, because he never published any of this until 1860, it was unknown to his critics.

Even had Semmelweis' explanation of seasonal variations been generally available, however, it is doubtful that it would have been accepted. No matter the progress that had by then been made in pathologic anatomy and physical diagnosis, Western medicine still lived with various stunted vestiges of ancient theories of disease etiology, like miasmas and vague constitutional imbalances. Concepts of single causative agents, which would enter the arena with the advent of the germ theory less than two decades later, were only barely construed, if at all. There was little precedent for a doctrine that invoked the direct action of invisible particles of putrid organic matter. To many critics, it would take a leap of faith which they were unable or unwilling to make.

Thus, to all these reasons for Semmelweis' failure must be added the factor of unfortunate timing. No one yet knew of the role of bacteria in infection. This meant that physicians, to accept the Semmelweis thesis, were required to believe in the noxiousness of particles they could neither see nor

> *Semmelweis' opponents had no access to all the facts and therefore could not fully comprehend the theory or accept the basis upon which it had been constructed.*

feel, but only smell. Still, this need not have been an insuperable obstacle. Many times in the history of clinical medicine, physicians have shown that they are not averse to taking up a method of treatment whose scientific basis has not yet been established, but which has worked out predictably well in the sickroom. Provided that the Hippocratic injunction to do no harm is not violated, much good can be accomplished during the period between a new therapy's introduction and its scientific validation. Had not Semmelweis been so ineffectual in his presentation, many otherwise reluctant physicians would certainly have joined willingly in his campaign. Some, better equipped perhaps to do it than Semmelweis, might have gone to the laboratory to attempt the transmission of puerperal fever from animal to animal. Had this occurred, there would have been proof, even without knowledge of bacteria, that such a thing was possible. But the few abortive experiments by Semmelweis himself were the only efforts in this direction.

The memory of Ignac Semmelweis soon died out in Vienna, except as an object of disparagement. It might be perceived as a great failing on the part of Rokitansky, Skoda, and Hebra that they did not follow up on the truth that had been shown to them by their quarrelsome departed colleague. And yet, how could they? Each of them was fully occupied in independent researches of his own, which he no doubt felt were more important than pursuing the Semmelweis doctrine, especially since none of them could yet perceive that it would have applicability to any field beyond obstetrics. Obstetrics at the Allgemeines Krankenhaus was in the forceful hands of Karl Braun, who had succeeded Semmelweis as Klein's assistant, and then become Chief on the older man's death in 1856. Braun wrote a book in 1855 listing thirty possible causes of childbed fever, of which # 28 was "cadaver infection," indicating that like so many others, he too misunderstood his antagonist.

Braun not only misunderstood Semmelweis, he disliked him intensely, to the point of attacking him at every opportunity. When one of Semmelweis' Budapest assistants published a paper on childbed fever in the *Vienna Medical Weekly* in 1856, it was probably Braun who supplied the editorial comment:

> *We had thought that this theory of chlorine disinfection perished long ago; the experience and the statistical evidence of most of the lying-in hospitals argue against the opinions expressed in this article: our readers should not allow themselves to be misled by this theory at the present time.*

Following the departure of Semmelweis, there had been a return to high mortality figures in Division I. Braun may have been an obstinate ox, but he was no murderer. When he became Chief he acted on a principle enunciated in his book: although cadaver particles were not the cause of childbed fever, no student whose hands smelled of a corpse would be permitted to examine a woman in labor. Thus did he circumvent the reality of the Semmelweis doctrine, and refuse to recognize the true basis of his own improved results.

It is difficult to know what made Ignac Semmelweis begin, finally, to speak out publicly and to write about his work. Perhaps he realized at last that until he himself clearly enunciated his observations and conclusions, broad understanding would never occur. In any event, almost eight years after his return to Hungary, he addressed the Medical Society of Pest-Buda on the topic "The Etiology of Puerperal Fever," and published his lecture in the Hungarian medical journal *Orvosi Hetilap*. It was his first written work on the discovery.

Over the next two years Semmelweis wrote letters to prominent obstetricians all over Europe asking their opinions of the theory. The responses he got rarely satisfied him, and caused increasing

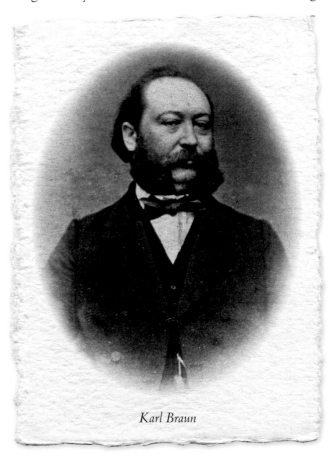

Karl Braun

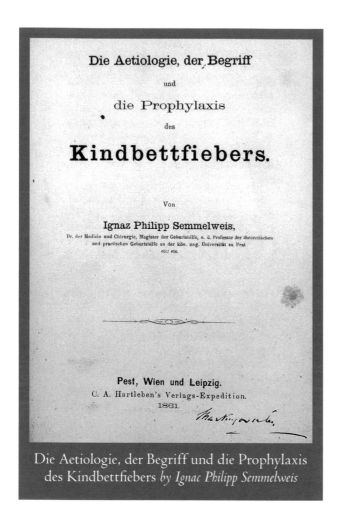

Die Aetiologie, der Begriff und die Prophylaxis des Kindbettfiebers *by Ignac Philipp Semmelweis*

I have been made responsible by Fate to reveal the truth which this book contains. . . . I must no longer think of my own peaceful disposition, but remember the lives that should be saved, depending on whether I or my adversaries win. . . . The many hours that I have spent in bitterness have not served as a warning; I have survived; my conscience will help me suffer whatever else may be in store for me.

The first part of the book deals, in a rambling, often repetitious fashion, with his theory. In the second part, in spite of his claim to have a peaceful disposition, Semmelweis delivers himself of a long polemic in which he not only answers all of his major detractors, but violently attacks most of them. His discussion is frequently interrupted by brief torrents of abuse. Some idea of the flavor of Semmelweis' writing is conveyed by Frank P. Murphy, who in 1941 undertook to accomplish the first English translation of the tortuous text:

From the translation we can see why the work has never before been published in English. The style is wordy and repetitious; the argument flows back and forth without progressing to any logical point; the author is egotistic and bellicose. We are conscious of signs of Semmelweis' mental aberration and feeling of persecution. Many have thought that the persecution complex was due to the hostile reception of the author's book but the book itself discloses the underlying paranoia. If Semmelweis had only spent more time in clearly stating his views and less in argument, his book would be twice as good and half as long! But that would not be Semmelweis as he really existed.

injury to the pride that had been so badly bruised in Vienna. The acceptance or rejection of the theory had always been deeply interwoven into his view of himself as accepted or rejected, and by 1860 his entire sense of self had apparently become indistinguishable from his theory. All of the frustrations came forth in the book he published in August of that year, *The Etiology, the Concept, and the Prevention of Puerperal Fever*, his *Hauptwerk*, his magnum opus, with which he meant to destroy his opposition. The following selection is from the brief introduction, and is characterized by an apparent humility interlarded with self-exalting ideation that suggests a drift toward madness.

The response of the medical world to the *Etiology* was either to ignore it or to attack it. The ignorers did so because the scientific section was so wordy and disjointed as to be almost impossible to wade through. Those who attacked it were enraged by the author's insults. But even more enraged was Ignac Semmelweis. A combination of rage and despair made him publish a series of open letters to some of the leaders of his opposition. The whirlwind of his passion became uncontrollable.

Some years ago, Ferenc Gyorgyey and I translated the open letters for publication by the Classics of Medicine Library. We were caught in the same dilemma that must have worried Frank Murphy. Should we convert Semmelweis' confusing circumlocutions into clear statements that would be comprehensible to American readers, or should we leave them as they were written, with their labored verbiage and wracking rhetoric, so that they might serve as a guide to the mental disarray of their author? We brought the problem one evening to a meeting of our colleagues at the Beaumont Medical Club, which is composed of amateur and a few professional medical historians whose good-natured approach to their subject is reminiscent of the way in which the old semipro baseball teams used to conduct their convivial recreations on the diamond. By the end of the discussion, the verdict was clear: only by absolute accuracy in reproducing every nuance of expression, every repetition, every verbosity, and every obfuscating departure from logical argumentation would our work be of any real value for the big-leaguers who might want to use it for scholarly study. In the introduction to the work we explained ourselves by using as a theme the words of John Millington Synge of the Abbey Theatre in Dublin: "A translation is no translation, unless it will give you the music of a poem along with the words of it."

With all of this as an introduction, herewith follow some examples of Semmelweis' impassioned insults, directed in his *Open Letters* of 1861 at several of the most highly respected obstetricians of the Germanic countries who had published in opposition to him. To Josef Spaeth, Professor of Obstetrics at the Josefs-Akademie of the University of Vienna, he wrote:

> *Herr Professor, you have convinced me that the Puerperal Sun which arose in Vienna in the year 1847 has not enlightened your mind even though it shone so near to you. . . . This arrogant ignoring of my doctrine, this arrogant boasting about errors, demands that I make the following declaration: Within myself, I bear the knowledge that since the year 1847 thousands and thousands of puerperal women and infants who have died would not have died had I not kept silent, instead of providing the necessary correction to every error that has been spread about puerperal fever. . . . And you, Herr Professor, have been a partner in this massacre. This murder must cease, and in order that the murder cease, I will keep watch, and anyone who dares to propagate dangerous errors about childbed fever will find in me an eager adversary. In order to put an end to these murders, I have no recourse but to mercilessly expose my adversaries.*

Likewise to Friedrich Scanzoni, Professor of Obstetrics at Würzburg, one of the most influential physicians of his time, a strongly worded missive was fired off. Some of the Semmelweis biographers consider Scanzoni the villain of their hero's life story, because of his particularly outspoken opposition to the *Lehre*, or theory. But he was neither evil nor stupid, only wrong. In spite of the many significant contributions he made to his specialty, history remembers him for his one serious error, his early resis-

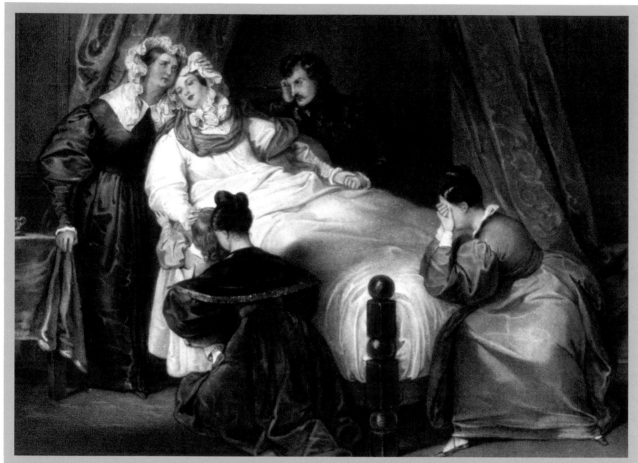

The death of a mother in childbirth, 1840

tance to the doctrine of hand-washing. Interestingly, in the fourth edition of his textbook, written long after his antagonist's death, he would give some grudging praise to Semmelweis, and even admit the validity of the basic principles of his theory. To Scanzoni, Semmelweis wrote:

> In order to put an end to the murders, I have seized the unshakable resolve to relentlessly oppose everyone who spreads errors about puerperal fever. . . . Your doctrine stamps the physician as a Turk, who in fatalistic, passive resignation allows this tragedy to engulf his puerperal women. . . . I have devoted 103 pages of my publication on childbed fever solely to the refutation of all of the errors and deceptions which hold you in their spell in regard to childbed fever. . . . I will publicly impart to you the necessary instruction. . . . Should you, Herr Professor, without having disproved my doctrine, continue to train your pupils in the doctrine of epidemic childbed fever, I declare before God and the world that you are a murderer and the "History of Childbed Fever" would not be unjust to you if it memorialized you as a medical Nero, in payment for having been the first to set himself against my lifesaving doctrine.

In a second letter to Scanzoni, Semmelweis added:

Herr Professor was right for thirteen years, because I was silent for thirteen years; now I have forsworn silence, and I will be right, and without doubt for as long as the human female shall give birth. To you Herr Professor, there remains nothing else but to adopt my doctrine, if you still want to salvage something of your reputation, whatever of it is still left to salvage. If you continue to adhere to the doctrine of epidemic childbed fever, advancing enlightenment will cause pseudo-epidemic childbed fever and your reputation to disappear from the face of the earth. . . . Herr Professor has proven that in spite of a new lying-in hospital, furnished with the best equipment, a great deal of homicide can be committed, if only one possesses the necessary talents.

Semmelweis then published a final open letter in 1862 containing similar statements, this time addressed to all professors of obstetrics. He was now taking on everybody.

During all of this literary *Sturm und Drang* it was becoming obvious to those around Semmelweis that his health, at least his physical health, was failing. By 1862, when he wrote the last open letter, he is described as having bouts of depression alternating with periods of elation. Although he could still carry out his professional duties, he was suffering from problems with his memory and from fits of bizarre behavior. Finally, in mid-July 1865, the obvious could no longer be denied—the Professor of Obstetrics at the University of Pest was uncontrollably psychotic.

Maria Semmelweis tried for two weeks to care for her husband at home, but finally gave up.

On July 31 she and a few others took him on the long train ride back to Vienna, where the kindly Hebra waited for his old and lost friend at the station. Immediately on arrival, Semmelweis was committed to a private asylum. The next day, when Frau Semmelweis came to visit, she was denied permission to see him, and sent away. Two weeks later, he was dead. Within forty-eight hours an autopsy and quick burial had taken place, the corpse having been taken from the asylum to the mortuary at the Vienna General Hospital, and then directly to the local Schmelz Cemetery. For the next twenty-five years, Ignac Semmelweis moldered in the foreign soil of Vienna, an alien even in death.

It has been traditional to say, and all of the major biographies without exception do say, that at his autopsy Semmelweis was found actually to have died of the same disease he had been fighting in mothers all of his professional life. A laceration sustained while examining one of his last patients is said to have become gangrenous, resulting in massive infection, with autopsy findings exactly like those of countless dead mothers and exactly like those of the martyred Kolletschka. It puts an ironic, poetic symmetry to the whole tragic story of the genius of puerperal fever. Unfortunately for the legend, this wounding, like so many other vital parts of the mythology, appears to be without firm basis in fact. The autopsy findings originally given out by the Austrians and the examination, photographs, and X-rays of the remains at their disinterment a century later are available, as are more recent disclosures. I have examined the pathological data carefully and shown them to several pathologists. These studies provide strong evidence that Ignac Semmelweis, like so many other violently psychotic patients of the time, was subjected to a beating at the hands of asylum personnel trying to restrain him shortly after his admission, and that it was from the injuries thus sustained that he died two weeks later.

Clearly, in his last years Semmelweis suffered from a progressive organic brain syndrome. From the available published materials, Dr. Elias E. Manuelidis, director of neuropathology at the Yale School of Medicine, feels sure that there is not sufficient evidence to indicate syphilis, the disease that has always been diagnosed by the Semmelweis biographers. He suggests that the organic condition may have been one not yet described in 1865: Alzheimer's presenile dementia; the clinicopathological picture of which is in many ways more consistent with the published descriptions and photographs of Semmelweis' symptoms and autopsy findings than syphilis.

Since 1978, when Dr. Manuelides made his diagnosis, it has been found that Alzheimer's occurs quite frequently in an older age group as well. In fact, most cases of this disease are now recognized in an elderly population. But the syndrome first described by Alois Alzheimer in 1907 was identified in patients in their middle years, and was hence dubbed "presenile." The clinical hallmarks of this type of the disease are deterioration of intellect, failure of memory, and a striking appearance of rapid aging in a patient in middle life, symptoms that become progressively more severe over a period of several years, and terminate in death. Among the prominent features of the syndrome are restlessness, hyperactivity, and defective judgment. All of the foregoing symptoms were frequently described in observations made during the period of Semmelweis' deterioration. While some of them occur also in certain cases of neurosyphilis, the memory loss, hyperactivity, and marked change in physical appearance that were prominent in Semmelweis' case are so characteristic of Alzheimer's disease that they argue convincingly in favor of that diagnosis.

The pathological changes in Semmelweis' brain also support this contention of presenile dementia, for they consist most prominently of

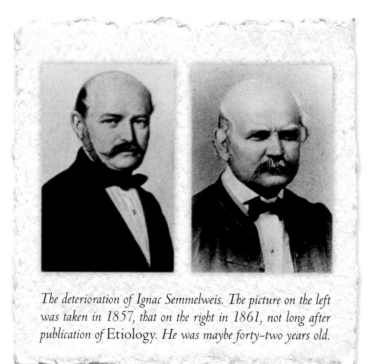

The deterioration of Ignac Semmelweis. The picture on the left was taken in 1857, that on the right in 1861, not long after publication of Etiology. *He was maybe forty-two years old.*

cerebral atrophy and a compensatory hydrocephalus, as seen with the naked eye. Although similar changes occur in many cases of syphilis, they are less likely to be as striking as in Alzheimer's disease.

I am not a psychoanalyst. A number of psychodynamically significant events occurred at crucial periods in Semmelweis' personal and family life, and much could doubtless be made of them. Some have been mentioned in a deliberately bare-bones manner in this chapter. Such factors will have to await investigation by other authors. My thesis can be summarized in a few paragraphs: Throughout his life Ignac Semmelweis saw himself as a graceless outsider, longingly looking in; the grocer's son from a backward province, coming with his clumsy dialect of German to the golden capital of the great Austrian Empire, a capital in which he felt that men of his background were looked down upon in both the professional and social spheres. By dint of hard work and a touch of genius he made a monumental discovery, and was embraced by some of the brightest stars of the rising new order in Austrian medicine. But they spoke well and wrote well, and were part of a select group of which he could never imagine himself a member; he felt unqualified to write or to speak in a public forum. Whereas more secure men might have tolerated criticism, Semmelweis saw every critique as a further personal rejection, and before long his theory and his sense of self became one and the same. Even when victory was at hand, his self-concept of being a defeated, clumsy outsider was too strong. He seized on a minor setback to flee the sunlit arena where just a little more debate and a little more time would have brought him recognition as one of Europe's outstanding clinical investigators. His friends and supporters were dumbfounded. But what seemed to them like disloyalty was merely insignificant little Naci Semmelweis, who could see himself only as a pride-injured, contentious outsider, never as a victorious professor in Vienna.

But flight to Pest did not solve his problem either. In the wave of Magyarization he wore Hungarian national costume and lectured in Hungarian, but he was still an outsider, perhaps telling himself that the Magyars looked on him as a German and the Germans as a second-class Hungarian. In spite of great success with the application of his theories in Pest, all criticism became intolerable, because it was further confirmation of his sense of the impossibility of acceptance and the inevitability of failure. And finally, in a fit of madness that was partially organic and partially the inexorable result of his almost conscious self-prophecy, he became Samson Agonistes, blind and raging, and tried to pull down the pillars of the temple of resistance to his theory, hoping to destroy those he saw as his enemies, even if it meant his own immolation. When it was all over, only Semmelweis was dead. The temple of resistance still stood.

And so Sophocles might have written it, with a Greek chorus of dying mothers—a great hero, a great truth, a great mission, and finally a mad flight of passionate arrogance resulting in destruction. The gods who were the professors of obstetrics did not bring it about; the state of mid-nineteenth-century science did not bring it about; the hero brought it upon himself.

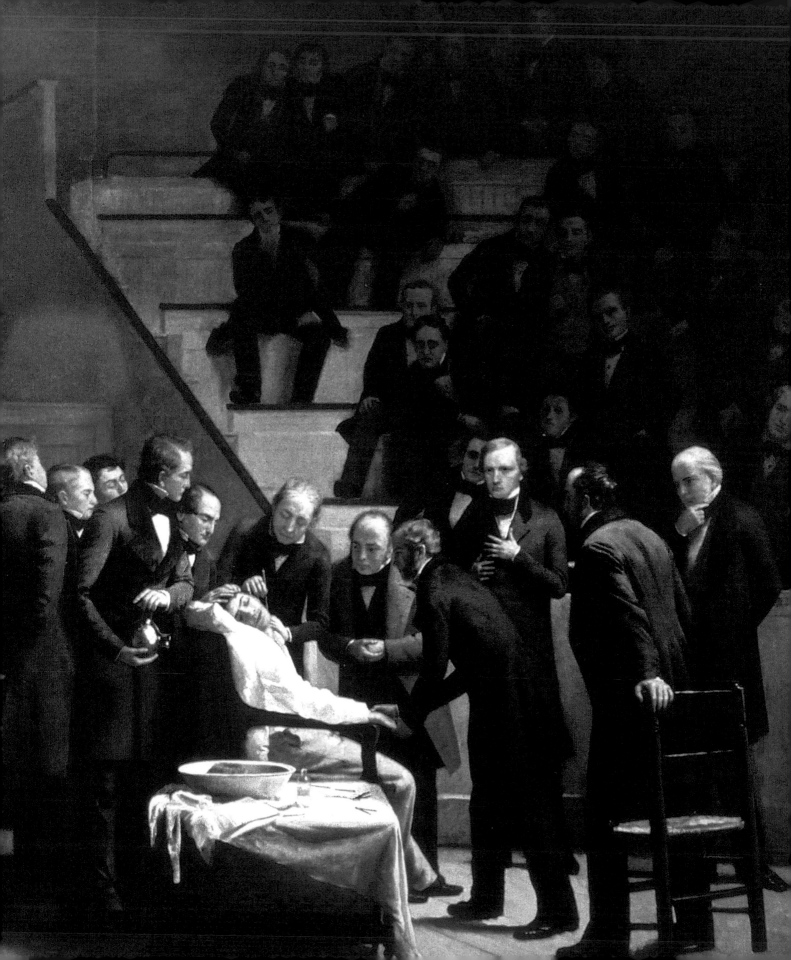

10

SURGERY WITHOUT PAIN

The Origins of General Anesthesia

While it does not appear to us that the discovery or, as some prefer to say, the invention of surgical anesthesia required any remarkable intellectual endowments or high scientific training, and it cannot be said that Long, Wells or Morton were possessed of these, it was the outcome of the spirit of inquiry, of keen observation, of boldness, of perseverance, of resourcefulness, of a search for means to improve a useful art, of interest in the practical rather than the theoretical, all traits more or less characteristic of the American mind, and I do not think that it was wholly an accident that our country should have given birth to the art of painless surgery. I find evidence of this view in the fact that not one but several Americans were working independently upon the same problem and that the solution of the problem is an exclusive achievement of our countrymen.

—William Henry Welch, Johns Hopkins Medical School

The invention of surgical anesthesia was the first major contribution that American medical science made to the world. To this day, it remains our greatest gift to the art of healing. None of the brilliant advances that have occurred in the twentieth century, none of our many Nobel laurels, eclipse the achievement of a small group of Americans almost 150 years ago. "Group" is not precisely the right word, because it implies a certain cohesiveness of effort, a certain partnership, a certain joining together of like-minded workers. Not only was there none of this kind of mutuality, but its very opposite was in fact the case. The various American actors in the drama of anesthesia's birth engaged each other in only one undertaking—a prolonged acrimonious battle over kudos and coin that still echoes down the corridors of time after a century and a half of debate.

Attempting to solve the problem of assigning credit for the discovery of inhalation anesthesia can be muddling to the mind and scrambling to the senses; the result is all too likely to be a confusing pandemonium of names, dates, claims, and pronouncements—and yet another literary monument to the human predisposition to contentiousness and rancor. Aiming to avoid this, I have chosen a simple star by which to steer my retelling: almost no one would deny that the crowning moment in the history of anesthesia occurred at the Massachusetts General Hospital on October 16, 1846, when William Thomas Green Morton demonstrated the effectiveness of ether. At that instant, surgical anesthesia began its existence; everything that led up to it was prologue, everything that was tangential to it was byplay, and everything that followed it was amplification. The purpose of this chapter is to relate the events surrounding that day—the prologue, the byplay, the ultimate dramatic moment, and the direct consequences to those who were involved. From that point on, the true infancy of the craft began, as physiological observations and pharmacological findings came forth, and as technology and instrumentation gradually created a sophisticated new specialty.

The concept of specialty is, in fact, a useful framework upon which to build the structure of the medical advances of the second half of the nineteenth century. The ancient art of healing became something quite new with the development of anesthesia, the advent of the germ theory, the recognition that tissues are made up of cells, and the introduction of modern pharmacology. Each of these fields was so demanding that it would require that researchers restrict their efforts to it alone. More and more, as the century progressed, the great physicians of the period are seen to be specialized either to the laboratory or the clinic, and more and more to highly focused areas within each. The greatest

clinicians would be those who best knew how to use the tools that others crafted in the laboratory to help them solve their patients' problems, while the greatest contributors to pure medical research would be those who were well acquainted with the diseases that most fearsomely challenged their colleagues on the wards.

The discovery, or rather the invention, of surgical anesthesia was the first of the four great movements in the process of transformation. Unlike the other three, it required no new vision to understand it and no casting off of old premises to accept it. Mankind had been waiting for it so long that its reception was predictably enthusiastic. Its advent was a forward step that was long overdue. The groundwork had been laid decades earlier, and if there is any wonderment that attaches to the final events, it should be directed to the fact that they occurred not because of the careful efforts of medical scientists, but rather out of a sequence of serendipity, salesmanship, and scheming.

The process by which anesthesia came into being was an aberration in the history of healing. As desperate as were the doctors of the early nineteenth century to prevent the intraoperative agony of their patients, they somehow failed to see, or rather to smell, the sleep-inducing agents that were as close to them as the ends of their noses. Until the fifth decade of the century, no trained physician took the single critical step toward pain-free surgery. The failure of vision was by those most qualified to see. Finally, it took resourcefulness rather than research, and a hunch rather than a hypothesis, to bring forth the nugget that had lain so long at the feet of medical science. The usual evolutionary machine of discovery had broken down and had to be repaired by a handful of alert artisans, almost all of whom were enterprising mechanics, but certainly not scientists.

One day general anesthesia did not exist, and the very next morning it was spreading its promise of salvation throughout the civilized world. Its appearance was like an act of God, but its messiah Morton was no saint. As quickly as the news of painless surgery permeated the awareness of eager believers, he began working to consolidate his primacy as its innovating archangel, and just as quickly did a clamor arise from at least four other claimants to priority or at least a share in the reward.

Individual historians differ in their assessments of the importance of the contributions made by the various participants in the saga. But no one who becomes at all familiar with this most dramatic of all journeys into medical progress can fail to grasp the unchallengeable truth that everything came to a focus on that October morning in 1846. Progress radiated from that place and time with a rapidity the like of which had never before resulted from any single scientific event. There was none of the skepticism that had greeted the work of Vesalius, or Harvey, or Laennec. There was only the happy relief that the agonies of yesteryear would be no more.

But long before Morton and long before what will be seen to be the ultimately tragic events that surrounded the birth of anesthesia, there was mystery and there was romance, and there were the magical adornments of literature. For ever since awareness first gleamed in the slowly awakening mind of man, he seems to have sought its opposite, either to produce a primeval painless unconsciousness or to find a world of fantasy more caressing than the often grim realities of daily life. Whether to induce senselessness in self or others, humankind has been entranced by the possibilities of slumber and its accompaniments.

In describing the earliest known attempts to induce sleep, I will write passages in which the fantastical seems to be mixed with the real, and the fictional with the documented. But the basic thread of the story and most of the details nevertheless do have a firm foundation in reality—the potions existed, much as they are described here, and if they did not always accomplish what was claimed for them, they and their chroniclers have

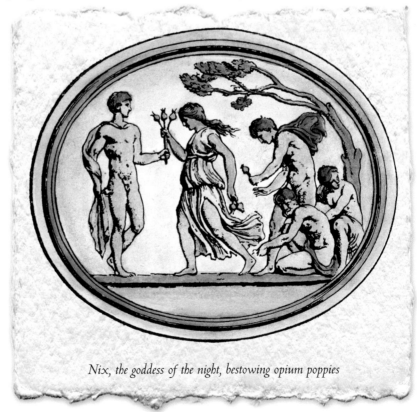

Nix, the goddess of the night, bestowing opium poppies

left us with a set of priceless images of flirtations with insensibility, and of dream worlds in which the historiographer and the poet dance to each other's most enchanting music.

We will begin with the poet, in fact with the Poet:

Not poppy, nor mandragora,
Nor all the drowsy syrups of the world,
Shall ever medicine thee to that sweet sleep
Which thou ow'dst yesterday.
—Othello, *Act III, scene iii*

The state of general obtundation that has been a practical necessity to all societies has been achieved, until relatively recent times, by methods that have been either herbal, psychological, or a combination of both. The physician-botanists of the seventeenth and eighteenth centuries were the heirs to a tradition as old as mankind itself, which reached its flower, so to speak, in the search for those plants that could be shown to affect the state of consciousness. Although the nature of the drugs producing the desired outcome had to await elucidation until the development of laboratory science, some of modern-day medicine's most commonly used narcotizing agents were well known to Greek and Roman healers. The principal anodynes of antiquity were derived from the poppy, the hyoscyamus, the mandragora, and of course the fermented flora that made alcohol. (The word "narcotic" itself is derived from *nark*, the Greek word for "stupor," as the word "anodyne" comes from a conjunction of *a* (n), meaning without, and *odyne*, meaning pain.)

Opium, called tears of poppy, came from the sap (tears, or *lacrimae*) obtained by cutting the unripe seed pod of the plant. The drops of milky juice were collected in a shell or dish and allowed to dry in the sun; the substance was well known in ancient times, and was utilized by many prominent physicians for centuries before our own. The writers of antiquity commonly used a word popularized by Virgil to refer to poppy-induced sleep: Letheon. Two thousand years later, that word would surface again, as the name given to ether by William Morton in an attempt to keep secret the true chemical nature of his formula.

From Aulus Cornelius Celsus we have a clear description of the use of tears of poppy and of one method of preparation. The works of Celsus, which date from the first century A.D., represent the oldest extant medical document after the Hippocratic Corpus; they were a compilation of treatises on medicine and other subjects, written for the aristocracy of his time. Because of the excellence of Celsus' literary style in Latin, his eight-volume *De Medicina* became one of the most widely read scientific works of the Renaissance revival of learning, and it has remained an excellent source of knowledge of Greek medicine, drawing heavily as it did upon Hippocratic and post-Hippocratic sources. Celsus writes:

Those pills which alleviate pain by causing sleep are called anodynes in Greek. It is bad practice to employ them except in cases of urgent necessity, for they are compounded of powerful drugs and are bad for the stomach. However, one may be used, which contains a denarius each of tears of poppy and galbanum, and two denarii each of myrrh, castoreum, and pepper. It is enough to swallow a piece the size of a bean.

Celsus also describes a method of pill preparation and several uses of the agent:

Take a handful of poppy when it is ripe for taking its tears, put it into a vessel, add enough water to cover it, and cook it. When it is well cooked, squeeze out the mass of poppy into the vessel before discarding it, and mix with the fluid an equal quantity of raisin wine. Boil it until it thickens, then cool it and make it into pills about the size of domestic beans.

They have many uses. They induce sleep, whether taken alone or dissolved in water. Added, in small quantity, to the juice of rue, or to raisin wine, they stop ear-ache. Dissolved in wine, they stop colic. Mixed with beeswax and attar of roses, and with a little saffron added, they cure inflammation of the vulva; and dissolved in water which is then applied to the forehead, they stop running of the eyes.

In the same way, if a painful vulva prevents sleep, take two denarii of saffron, one each of anise and myrrh, four of poppy tears, eight of hemlock seeds, and mix them into a paste by adding old wine. The dose is a piece the size of a lupin, dissolved in three glasses of water. But it is dangerous to administer when fever is present.

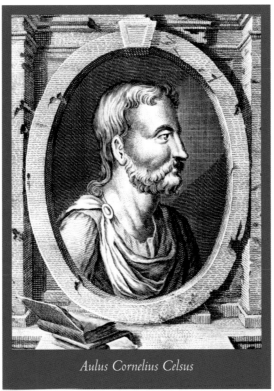

Aulus Cornelius Celsus

It has been theorized by some that the "drug which quenches pain and strife and brings forgetfulness of every ill" prepared by Helen, daughter of Zeus, in the *Odyssey*, was opium. Whether opium or some other anodyne, it is likely that Homer's reference to "such cunning drugs . . . drugs of

healing" was not fanciful, for the probability is high that even in those early times, the poppy was being used as a source of relief from physical and emotional pain.

Documentation of the use of mandrake (*Mandragora officinarum*) predates even Homer. Leah, wife of the Biblical patriarch Jacob, seems to have given her sister Rachel some mandrakes harvested by Leah's son Reuben, in return for which she was permitted to get their mutual husband back for the night of bliss during which Issachar was conceived. Because the plant was considered by many primitive societies to be both aphrodisiac and fecundative, it has been presumed by Old Testament scholars that Leah used it for these purposes, and successfully at that. The truth may perhaps lie in quite a different explanation, one based upon a pharmacological action of the drug that is real, unlike its supposed effects on virility. It is not impossible that Jacob's favors were bought with the bribe of narcotics, a situation replicated in modern life every day. In Genesis 30:16 we hear Leah saying to her husband, "Thou must come in unto me; for surely I have hired thee with my son's mandrakes."

The mandrake, or mandragora, is a member of the humble potato family. The plant has a short stem, with a root which is often forked, and a

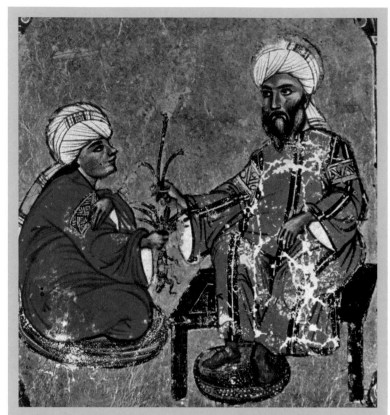

Dioscorides and student discuss the mandrake in an Arabic edition of De Materia Medica, *1229 A.D.*

Go and catch a falling star,
Get with child a mandrake root,
Tell me, where all past years are,
Or who cleft the Devil's foot.

Philemon Holland's translation of Pliny's *Historia Naturalis* (A.D. 77) contains the following statement: "It is an ordinarie thing to drinke it [juice of mandragora] . . . before the cutting, cauterizing, pricking or launcing of any member, to take away the sence and feeling of such extreme cures. And sufficient it is in some bodies to cast them into a sleep with the smell of Mandrage, against the time of such chirurgerie."

And in the first-century writings of Pedacius Dioscorides is to be found the following description of the use of mandrake:

berrylike orange fruit, sometimes referred to as the apple. The narcotic effect derives from the fact that one of a class of chemical compounds called belladona alkaloids can be extracted from the root, and to a lesser extent from the apple and the leaves. It is because the forked root can, with some imagination, be thought to have the appearance of the lower half of a curvaceous and full-figured human body that the plant was believed to be a love potion and an enhancer of fertility. John Donne alludes to the drug's powers and its presumed humanoid characteristics in his bitter outburst concerning the futility of seeking a steadfast love, which he illustrates by listing a few other tasks equally impossible:

But of ye male [mandragora] and white which some have called Norion, ye leaves are greater, white, broad, smooth as of the beet, and ye apples twice as big, drawing to saffron in ye colour, sweet smelling with a certain strongness which also ye shepherds eating are in a manner made asleep. . . . Using a Cyathus of it for such as cannot sleep, or are grievously pained, & upon whom being cut, or cauterized they wish to make a not-feeling pain. . . . For they do not apprehend the pain, because they are overborn with dead sleep, but the apples being smelled to, or eaten are soporiferous, & ye juice that is of them.

Dioscorides was a Greek surgeon in Nero's army, whose medical botany writings serve as an authoritative source for the first century A.D. Indeed, until the great medical advances of the sixteenth and seventeenth centuries, the works of Dioscorides were the foundation upon which the materia medica, the medical pharmacy, of western countries was based. His *De Materia Medica*, the source for almost all botanical knowledge for a millennium and a half, is one of the classics of medical literature; because of the beauty of the manuscripts into which it was variously translated, it is a classic of art history as well. Although it has been traditional to credit coinage of the word "anesthesia" to Oliver Wendell Holmes, it was actually Dioscorides who first used it. The word was revived by Quistorp in 1719 and was used by several practitioners of mesmerism in the nineteenth century, before Holmes finally made it stick by suggesting it to William Morton as the appropriate term for his new invention.

Henbane, *Hyoscyamus niger*, is another plant the tranquilizing or anesthetic properties of which are due to its being a source of belladonna alkaloid. Recognized as a very dangerous drug, it was often used to kill dogs and mice. Dioscorides described a method of burning it under a tree that resulted in narcotized birds falling to the ground, whereupon those still alive were easily caught and revived by distilling vinegar into their nostrils.

Dioscorides also writes of the use of various alcoholic potions to induce anesthesia. He recommends, for example, that a dose of two ounces of heavy wine be given to patients about to be cut for stone or cauterized. When amputation and other surgical procedures became more common in the sixteenth and seventeenth centuries, the drunken state was frequently relied upon to produce senselessness or decreased awareness. Other soporifics that had less general applicability were the juic-

es obtained from mulberries, from wild lettuce, and from the resinous and aromatic constituents of the hop plant even in an unfermented state. So closely did hops become associated in popular folklore with drowsiness that they were sometimes stuffed into pillows upon which anxious insomniacs were encouraged by lay healers to sleep.

The most popular method of inducing narcosis during the Middle Ages was the so-called soporific sponge, *Spongia somnifera*. Historians have found descriptions of it in manuscripts dating to the ninth century. In the twelfth century, Nicholas of Salerno described its ingredients as opium, hyoscyamus, mulberry juice, lettuce seed, hemlock, mandrake, and ivy. A fresh sea sponge was soaked in the mixture and allowed to dry "in the sun during the dog-days until all the liquid is

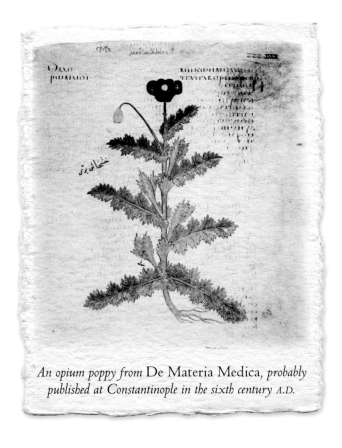

An opium poppy from De Materia Medica, *probably published at Constantinople in the sixth century A.D.*

consumed." When required for use, the concoction was reconstituted by dipping the sponge in water. Because the medieval manuscripts recommended applying the sponge to the subject's nostrils, it has been thought that this was meant to be a form of anesthesia by inhalation, but there is good evidence that the potion was usually administered as a drink. Reversal of the narcotizing effect was to be attained with the juice of fennel root or with vinegar.

The literature of the period abounds with references to soporific draughts. Thus, in one of the tales told in Boccaccio's *Decameron*, a gangrenous leg is operated upon under the influence of such a potion. *The Tragicall Historye of Romeus and Juliet*, written in 1562 by Arthur Brooke, contains the description by Friar Laurence to Juliet of a certain potent liquid:

> *Long since I did finde out, / and yet the way I know,*
> *Of certain rootes, and savory herbes / to make a kind of*
> *dowe, Which baked hard, and bet / into a powder fine,*
> *And drunk with conuite water, or / with any kynd of*
> *wine It doth in halfe an howre / astonne the taker so,*
> *And mastreth all his sences, that / he feeleth weale nor*
> *woe: And so it burieth vp / the sprite and liuing breath,*
> *That even the skilfull leche would say, / that he is slayne*
> *by death.*

Certainly, this poem was a source for Shakespeare's *Romeo and Juliet*. In Act IV, scene i, of that play, the Bard describes the result of a drink of "this distilling liquor," in terms so accurate that it is probable that he had personally witnessed its effects or at least heard a firsthand account. Marlowe, Middleton, and Donne are other English writers in whose works can be found references to the opiates of the time.

As in all other areas of scientific thought, the Middle Ages were indeed the dark ages when it came to advances in the pharmacology of anesthesia. In addition to all the well-known reasons for the intellectual stagnation of the period, there were two specific factors that militated against improvements in methods of narcosis. The first was the theological doctrine that pain serves God's purpose and therefore must not be alleviated; this is a concept that was to prove particularly significant during James Simpson's campaign to establish obstetrical anesthesia some centuries later. The second factor was simple ignorance of dosages, strengths, and even the nature of the active ingredients in the botanicals, because of which it was impossible to standardize results. The narcotics were accordingly regarded, and rightly so, as highly dangerous. After the Renaissance, the soporific sponges and similar hazardous draughts began to disappear from use; by the seventeenth century they were largely a thing of the past, although alcohol remained popular. One of the last English references to a narcotic mixture occurs in Act IV of Thomas Middleton's tragedy *Women Beware Women* (1657):

> *I'll imitate the pities of old surgeons*
> *To this lost limb, who, ere they show their art,*
> *Cast one asleep, then cut the diseased part.*

The final steps in the development of general anesthesia would require the introduction of methods that were based upon real science. Shortly before these steps were taken, however, a bit of false science was introduced upon the scene by a false messiah who claimed to cure disease and soothe the savage breast with a form of cosmic energy he called animal magnetism.

The name of the mountebank prophet was Anton Mesmer, and his artifice, known as mesmerism, amounted to a form of hypnosis that represents one of medicine's flirtations with the far peripheries of rational thought. His methods, extrascientific at best and crackpot at worst, seem to have entranced not only a large assortment of gullible patients, but also a few otherwise sensible researchers at University College Hospital in London. Led by John Elliotson, the college's Professor of Practical Medicine, an attempt was made to establish a firm basis upon which to experiment with mesmerism-induced painless surgery. The technique was used with varying degrees of success by its practitioners, but was finally abandoned as inefficient when ether was introduced by William Morton. Interestingly, several of the writers on medical hypnotism used the word "anesthesia" to refer to its effects.

(It should not be construed from the foregoing that I am scornful of the possibilities of hypnosis in medicine. Although there is much to ridicule in the origins of mesmerism, its legacy must be taken very seriously—from crackpot concepts may arise useful theories and useful tools. So it is proving to be with hypnosis.)

The real science that would lead to the birth of anesthesia involved the parallel and some-times interlacing development of two areas of study, namely the chemistry and physics of gases on the one hand and the physiology of respiration on the other. The list of major contributors to the needed research includes names which, although renowned for investigations in other areas of science, are not usually thought of in relation to clinical medicine; they are John Dalton, Joseph Priestley, Antoine Lavoisier, James Watt, Humphry Davy, and Michael Faraday.

The one responsible for the first modern chemical and physical studies of gases was Joseph Priestley (1733–1804), a politically controversial nonconformist minister whose contributions are made particularly noteworthy by the fact that he had never had so much as the rudiments of what

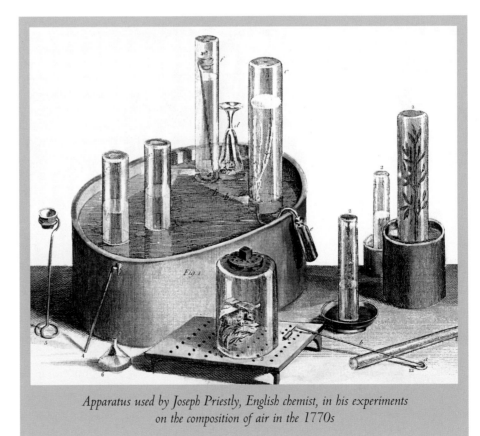

Apparatus used by Joseph Priestly, English chemist, in his experiments on the composition of air in the 1770s

passed, in eighteenth-century England, for a scientific education. Although his autodidactism resulted in some problems when dealing with theoretical concepts, it did not prevent him from describing nitrous oxide in 1772, isolating oxygen in 1774, and presenting the world with the incomparable gift of man-made soda water.

As Priestley's work with gases became known, and as Lavoisier made the signal contribution of elucidating the nature of oxygen and its function in respiration, visionary physicians began to look for ways in which the new knowledge could be used to treat disease, most particularly tuberculosis of the lungs; they could not know that the science of the time was not far enough advanced to convert their hopes into realities. The leading architect of this movement was Thomas Beddoes, whose interest in therapeutic inhalation resulted in the founding of the Pneumatic Medical Institution in Bristol, England, in 1798. The great James Watt prepared much of the apparatus for the Institution, no doubt to a large extent motivated by his own son's impending death of consumption, and twenty-year-old Humphry Davy was appointed as its first Superintendent of Experiments. It has been said that Davy, redeemed by his new employer from his indentured service to a surgeon-apothecary of Penzance, was Beddoes' greatest discovery. Within a year of assuming his duties at the Institution, he described the intoxicating effects of inhaling nitrous oxide, a study he had begun with self-experiments in 1795 when he was seventeen years old.

Not content with studying the effects of nitrous oxide on himself and upon animals, Davy began to use in his researches as extraordinary a group of experimental subjects as has ever been assembled, namely the leaders of the intellectual circle of Bristol, including Samuel Taylor Coleridge, Robert Southey, and Peter Roget. With such articulate experimentees to interview, as well as his own considerable powers of observation, Davy produced a book which has become a classic in the history of science, *Researches, Chemical and Philosophical; Chiefly Concerning Nitrous Oxide, or Dephlogisticated Nitrous Air, and Its Respiration.* The author was twenty-two years of age, and the publication of this volume in 1800 marks his first major contribution in what was to be a magnificently productive career. Davy was gifted with the ability to write clear and graphic descriptions and was a popular lecturer and a talented amateur poet; Coleridge said of him that if "he had not been the first chemist, he would have been the first poet of his age." Although that may have been the generous compliment of a good friend, the following sentences from *Researches* shed light not only upon his powers of observation, but on his gift of literary exposition as well. They describe the analgesia which Davy experienced as a consequence of breathing nitrous oxide:

In one instance, when I had a head-ache from indigestion, it was immediately removed by the effects of a large dose of gas; though it afterwards returned, but with much less violence. In a second instance, a slighter degree of head-ache was wholly removed by two doses of gas.

The power of the immediate operation of the gas in removing intense physical pain, I had a very good opportunity of ascertaining.

In cutting one of the unlucky teeth called dentes sapientiae, I experienced an extensive inflammation of the gum, accompanied with great pain which equally destroyed the power of repose, and of consistent action.

On the day when the inflammation was most trouble-some, I breathed three large doses of nitrous oxide. The pain always diminished after the first four or five inspirations; the thrilling came on as usual, and uneasiness was for a few minutes, swallowed up in pleasure. As the former state of mind however returned, the state of organ returned with it; and I once imagined that the pain was more severe after the experiment than before.

The possibility of using such an analgesic effect in surgery was not lost on the former surgeon's apprentice. In the section of the book devoted to "Conclusions," Davy permitted himself the following speculation:

As nitrous oxide in its extensive operation appears capable of destroying physical pain, it may probably be used with advantage during surgical operations in which no great effusion of blood takes place.

The caveat expressed in the final portion of the statement is explained by Davy's belief, unconfirmed by his own observation, that nitrous oxide increases the force of the circulation. It is an indication of his prescience that within a short time after anesthesia came into general use his apparently instinctive prediction was confirmed by the experience of surgeons, who still today grumble about the increased bloody ooze that sometimes moistens the operative field on those infrequent occasions when nitrous oxide is used. The gas seems to achieve this effect by raising the pressure in the peripheral veins just enough to make a small difference. I have often

seen a veteran anesthetist give a patient with tiny arm veins a few preparatory sniffs of the stuff in order to make his vessels bulge for the insertion of the intravenous needle.

Although Davy's was certainly the first reference to the possibility of using nitrous oxide as an inhalation anesthetic, neither he nor the contemporary scientific community recognized the implications of his conjecture, and he himself soon turned his attention away from pneumatic research, resigning his position at the Pneumatic Medical Institution in 1801 to become Director of the Chemical Laboratory of the recently established Royal Institution in London. His contri-

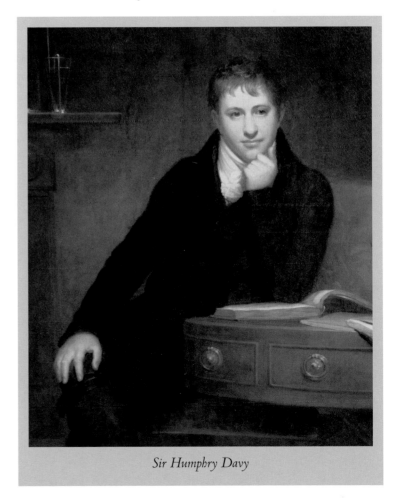

Sir Humphry Davy

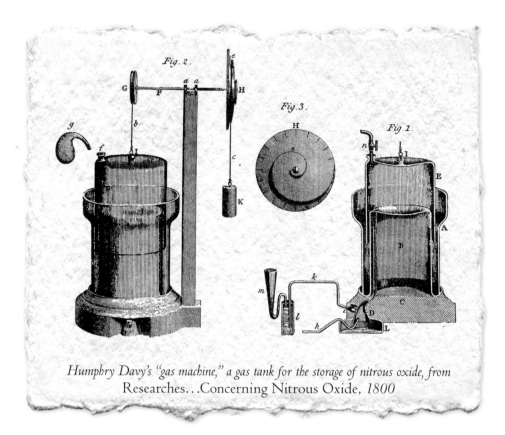

Humphry Davy's "gas machine," a gas tank for the storage of nitrous oxide, from Researches...Concerning Nitrous Oxide, *1800*

seems like good common-sense thinking can lead well-intentioned innocents into blind alleys, if their fuzzy concepts cannot yet be translated into terms with which contemporary science can deal. In Conant's words, "It is fortunate no one was killed; it is certain no one was cured. But Dr. Beddoes was no charlatan. In a charitable mood one may even claim he was a chemotherapist a hundred and fifty years ahead of his time and employing the wrong chemicals!"

butions from that point on were entirely in the realm of nonmedical chemistry and physics. Had he not directed his energies elsewhere, he might have taken that next critical step, and become the discoverer of inhalation anesthesia. The usual evolutionary process of medical science would thus have been maintained, and this chapter would have been much shorter, but also much less interesting.

As for Beddoes and his honest attempt to make a revolution in therapeutic methods, alas, nothing came of it. In spite of the brilliance of Watt and Davy, not a single therapy issued from the laboratory in Bristol. In his 1952 Bampton Lectures at Columbia University, James B. Conant used the story of the Pneumatic Medical Institution's brief life as an illustration of the way in which personal experience and what

The results of Davy's nitrous-oxide experiments did nevertheless have a profound, even if indirect, effect upon the history of anesthesia. For it was from the Pneumatic Institution that the word went out that the gas was indeed "a gas," to invoke the slang of the 1980s. Southey referred to the effects it had upon him as "a sensation perfectly new and delightful." The imaginative Coleridge, not yet ravaged by opium, found that inhaling the agent provided him "a highly pleasurable sensation of warmth over my whole frame" and the inclination to "laughing at those who were looking at me." Other visitors to the Institution were encouraged by Beddoes and Davy to try the vapor so that their experiences might be recorded. Before long, nitrous oxide, or laughing gas as it was soon to be called, was well known as an apparently harmless and often hilarious form of entertainment, and laughing gas parties had become common among university students and some segments of "liberated society."

Concurrently the same sort of thing was becoming known about ether. Because it is customary to regard laboratory chemistry as a development of the past two centuries, the fact that ether was first synthesized in 1540 may come as a surprise. It is to a twenty-five-year-old Prussian botanist, Valerius Cordus (1515–1544), doomed to a premature death at the age of twenty-nine, that the credit goes. Cordus distilled what was known as "sour oil of vitriol" (sulfuric acid) with "strong biting wine" (ethyl alcohol) to produce the "sweet vitriol" which, under the name of sulfuric ether (actually diethyl ether), was to change the course of medical history.

> *Before long, nitrous oxide, or laughing gas as it was soon to be called, was well known as an apparently harmless and often hilarious form of entertainment.*

Over the course of the next three centuries, a number of other workers synthesized sweet vitriol, including Robert Boyle in 1680, and even Isaac Newton in 1717. Johannes Augustus Siegmundus Frobenius, a German chemist who seems to have worked in Boyle's laboratory, gave the name "sulfuric ether" to the liquid, probably because of the extreme volatility that made it evaporate within moments of contact with air. Finally, in 1819, John Dalton published a definitive paper dealing with the compound's physical and chemical properties, "Memoir on Sulfuric Ether."

Apparently it was not until the early nineteenth century that observers began to note the lethargy and sleepiness that ether was capable of producing. As early as 1818 a note appeared in the *Quarterly Journal of Science and the Arts* describing the result that might be expected from inhaling its vapor, pointing out that "it produces effects very similar to those occasioned by nitrous oxide." This article, although published anonymously, is generally attributed to Michael Faraday, then twenty-six years of age. The effects of inhaling ether were also well known to Thomas Beddoes and to Humphry Davy, who themselves had had personal experience with it.

As with nitrous oxide, serious investigators were not the only ones to take note of the effects of ether vapor, and ether frolics like laughing-gas parties soon became popular forms of social escapism. Itinerant "professors" in horse-drawn wagons brought the charms of gaseous intoxication to the small towns of Europe and America, in the form of traveling demonstrations in which eager locals paid fees of various amounts to inhale a little laughing gas or sniff some ether, to the general amusement of their onlooking friends. Dollars or pounds or francs spent for a few bottles of nitrous oxide bought a bonanza of profits for the peripatetic "chemists" who demonstrated the vapory science for the enlightenment of their enthusiastic audiences.

Eventually, a few medical men must have caught on. It is hard to believe that the obvious

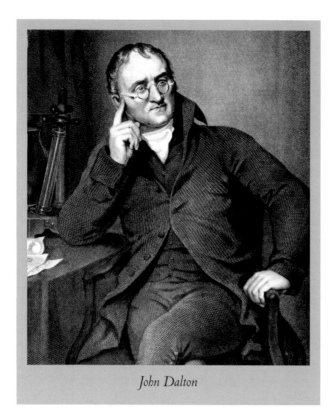
John Dalton

state of decreased sensibility they saw at such performances did not excite the minds of at least some rural physicians to the possibilities of surgical anesthesia. And yet, there seems to be no hard evidence that any but one man so much as gave a trial to either of the two gases. The mind of that man had been prepared by medical training so rigorous that it put him into the same category as the best-qualified practitioners in the United States, with the exception of those who had had the opportunity to study in Europe. He recognized an opportunity to try something new, and he took it.

There is a certain appropriateness in the fact that the professional training of Crawford Williamson Long (1815–1878) is an epitome of the entire range of medical education as it existed in the southern and western states of our country in the middle third of the nineteenth century. Although anyone calling himself a physician had to be licensed by the state in which he practiced, there was no requirement that the applicants for licensure have the M.D. degree. In fact, most of them did not. The majority of candidates who presented themselves for the oral qualifying examinations given by county medical societies had been trained by what was called the preceptor system, basically amounting to a four-year apprenticeship to a senior doctor in the community. If the student had attended lectures at one of the country's medical colleges, he was permitted to deduct a year from his indenture; only those few who had a formal American or European medical-school degree were privileged to go directly into practice.

The preceptor system was based on the ages-old principle by which artisans had learned their trades in all of the countries of the West. For a fee of approximately one hundred dollars a year, the student became, as a rule, a member of his preceptor's household, expected not only to carry out the routine professional duties of a medical assistant, but sometimes to do domestic chores as well. Over the period of training, he learned all that his teacher knew, which usually was not a great deal, considering the typical senior man's own inadequate education as well as the relatively primitive state of the profession in America at that time. In fact, to call it a profession at all is to stretch the definition of that august-sounding word to its limit. It was, in truth, little better than a line of work by which a farmer's son might provide some social mobility for himself, but certainly no drastic improvement in his financial prospects. Lester King, the historian of the American Medical Association, has referred to the practice of medicine in those days as being no more than "a superior sort of trade." Among the several reasons that the AMA was founded in 1846 was to elevate that trade to the status of a profession by raising its standards of education and ethics.

In 1835, Crawford Long graduated from Franklin College, now the University of Georgia, which had been chartered in Athens fifty years earlier. He taught school for a year in his hometown of Danielsville, and then apprenticed himself for a few months to Dr. George R. Grant, in the town of Jefferson. Although Long's brief period as a preceptee may have had its rewards, it is more likely to have been as described by Daniel Drake, the great physician and educator of the Mississippi Valley area, writing in 1832 about the apprenticeship system: "The physicians of the United States, are culpably inattentive to the studies of their pupils, and . . . this is one of the causes which retard the improvement, and arrest the elevation of the profession. Exceptions . . . are frequently met with, especially in the great cities; but they are still *only* exceptions."

Whatever may have been the quality of his brief experience with Dr. Grant, Long soon realized his need for more formal medical education, and set off on horseback to get it. His journey took him across the mountains of western North Carolina and eastern Tennessee, through forest lands that harbored not only isolated communities of backwoods settlers, but also the sometimes hostile Indian tribes that still lived in those areas. Finally, after several weeks, he arrived in Lexington, Kentucky, where he enrolled at the Medical Department of Transylvania University, at that time in the thirty-sixth year of its existence and thriving, with a roster of 262 students. But even

that foremost medical school in the South did not meet Long's requirements for a more scientific training, and in 1838 he traveled north to enter the University of Pennsylvania, America's oldest medical school, where the country's finest faculty had been assembled.

According to a biography written in 1928 by Long's daughter, Frances Long Taylor, it was during his student days in Philadelphia that her father first became acquainted with ether frolics and laughing-gas parties, having been introduced to the intoxicating effects of those two gases not in the classroom, but by the itinerant showmen who gave public lectures in what they grandly called chemistry. In writing this, however, she was underestimating the extent of her father's more formal knowledge of contemporary science. Under

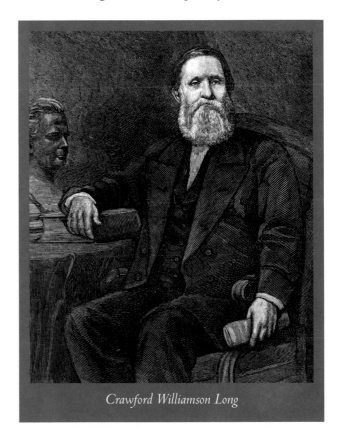

Crawford Williamson Long

the influence of the eminent practitioner and political figure Benjamin Rush, several members of the medical school's faculty had done work with pneumatic medicine, lecturing and writing about the properties of both nitrous oxide and ether. Nathaniel Chapman, Long's Professor of the Theory and Practice of Physic, had, in fact, written what is probably the best extant description of the pre-anesthetic clinical uses of ether, in his *Elements of Therapeutics and Materia Medica*, published in 1831.

After receiving his medical degree in 1839, the young physician "walked the wards" for eighteen months in New York, as so many of his northern colleagues had done in the great teaching hospitals of France and England. There were few southern physicians as well prepared for the highest quality of clinical work as was Crawford Long, and the temptation to return to Philadelphia to practice was great. But loyalty to his father brought him back to Jefferson, Georgia, where he bought the practice of his former preceptor, George Grant, in 1841. He was twenty-five years of age.

The course of Crawford Long's medical training has been reviewed not only because it characterized the type of educational pathway that could be taken by American physicians of his day, but also to point out that the great majority of practitioners departed from that track at any of several steps along the way, most commonly after the preceptorship. What we see in the education of Long is the best that the young country had to offer. He was not, as he has so often been characterized, a rural bumpkin of a doctor who chanced one day to use ether, but rather a highly trained physician with a strong background in clinical medicine and in the experimental methods of science, well prepared by education and by his own scientific inclinations to test his hunches by clinical trial. From the evidence of the quotation that opens this chapter, even the intellectually redoubtable William Henry Welch seems not to have appreciated the quality of Long's exposure to contemporary science.

The able and personable young physician soon became a popular figure in the community surrounding Jefferson, acquiring a circle of friends who brought to the area what they could of a worldly interest in things novel and intellectually adventurous. Not surprisingly, they became interested first in laughing gas, and then in ether. On several occasions during which Long and his friends used ether, he was able to make the same observation as had Faraday and Davy, namely that those who inhaled enough of the vapor "did not feel the least pain" when being struck a blow or falling down. There is no better example to be found of Pasteur's maxim "Where observation is concerned, chance favors only the prepared mind" than the use to which this highly trained physician put his experience.

In early spring of 1842, Long approached one of his patients with an appealing idea. The young

> *Those who inhaled enough of the vapor "did not feel the least pain" when being struck a blow or falling down.*

man, James Venable, had for some time been trying to work up the courage to have two cysts removed from the back of his neck, but had continued to procrastinate because of his fear of pain. Knowing that Venable was an experienced social sniffer of ether, his physician suggested that he undergo the operation while breathing through a towel onto which the volatile liquid was poured. The timorous patient was skeptical of the undertaking, but he agreed to go ahead with it provided that only one cyst was removed. Unwilling to give him the chance to change his mind, Long operated that very evening, March 30, 1842. So impressed was Venable with the simplicity of the whole business that he had the second cyst removed two months later.

Following these successes, Long amputated the diseased toe of a slave boy under ether, in July. Seven years later he wrote of having operated upon one or two etherized patients annually in the interval following these first procedures. He reported these cases in response to the controversy that had by then produced a storm of vituperative polemic over the when and who of anesthesia's invention. Unfortunately, he had waited until three years after hearing of William Morton's triumph in Boston. Even then, there was a characteristic reticence in his presentation, which he

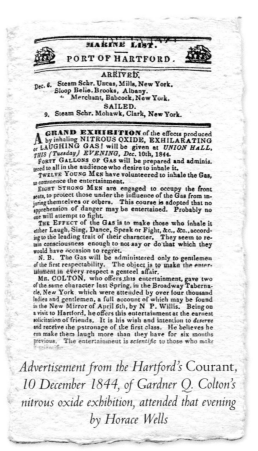

Advertisement from the Hartford's Courant, *10 December 1844, of Gardner Q. Colton's nitrous oxide exhibition, attended that evening by Horace Wells*

wrote only at the continued urging of friends who could not bear to see him silently suffer the injustice of being ignored as the true discoverer of surgical anesthesia. He could not be persuaded to publish until he had first traveled to the Medical College of Georgia in Augusta to describe before that faculty his experience with ether seven years earlier. Competitiveness was not Crawford Long's style. In the ensuing years of diatribe and invective, his exemplary behavior would be the only evidence of nobility on the filthy field of battle.

In later pages, Long's role in the anesthesia controversy will be described in more detail. For now, it is sufficient to point out that the undoubted fact of his priority does not mean that he should be considered to have introduced pain-free surgery to the world. His story remains tangential to the main line of the narrative. For, unlike the influence that Morton had, no one was ever emboldened to give surgical anesthesia because Long used it; medical science never learned from him that such a miracle was possible. All of this had to await William Thomas Green Morton and that portentous autumn morning in Boston.

Based on his training and his level of medical sophistication, Long was the ideal physician, albeit not in the ideal place, to have overcome the myopia of his fellows and launched the new era of pain-free surgery. Unfortunately, he dropped the ball. Had he persisted in his clinical work with ether, and had he published early, the story of anesthesia's birth might have reached its climax at this very point. The reasons for his lack of persistence are not clear, but whatever they were, they provided the occasion, as had Davy's defection to other projects, for another missed opportunity.

Long, of course, was only one of many physicians who became aware of the anesthetic effects of the two gases, and only one of the many customers of show-business purveyors of entertaining vapors. Among the most successful of the enterprising pitchmen was one Gardner Quincy Colton, a barnstorming lecturer who had some medical training and who, during the time when Long was using ether, was traveling about New England giving demonstrations of the wonders of electricity and the effects of nitrous oxide gas. He arrived in Hartford, Connecticut, on December 10, 1844, and promptly placed an advertisement in the local newspaper, the *Courant*.

That same evening, a successful young dentist of the city, Horace Wells, brought his wife, Elizabeth, to the laughing-gas show. During the course of the evening, one of the volunteers struck his leg on a wooden settee while under the influence of the agent. Although he had injured himself severely enough to cause bleeding, he was aware of no pain until the effects of the nitrous oxide had passed off. This did not escape the notice of Wells, who promptly at the conclusion of the performance approached Colton and asked him to take part in an experiment to see if a tooth might be painlessly extracted while the subject was thus sedated. They repaired to the dentist's office, where

a colleague named Riggs relieved Wells of one of his molars after sleep had been induced by a few whiffs of gas. Immediately on awakening from his painless nap, the single-minded Wells, who could think of nothing but the benefits that would accrue to his gum-sore patients, exclaimed jubilantly, "Ah, a new era in tooth-pulling!" Whether he was still slap-happy from the laughing gas or simply incapable of seeing the future beyond his own jaws, he seems not to have grasped the significance of the evening's events.

His tunnel vision did not last long. He learned how to prepare nitrous oxide from Colton, and then he and Riggs began to work with it. Within a month, he had successfully extracted teeth fifteen times without pain and felt that he was ready to introduce his method "into the hands of proper persons" who would know how to do appropriate experiments and make the best use of the new discovery.

In February 1845, Wells traveled to Boston, then as now one of the foremost centers of medical thought in America. With the aim of obtaining an introduction to the leading surgeons of that city, he sought the aid of a former student of his, William Thomas Green Morton, with whom he had had a brief period of professional partnership. Morton introduced Wells to Drs. George Hayward and John Collins Warren. Warren, the senior surgeon at the Massachusetts General Hospital, invited Wells to lecture to a class of Harvard medical students on the surgical possibilities of nitrous oxide and then to demonstrate its actual use in the case of a patient whose leg was to be amputated. The patient, perhaps preferring to take his chances with a few minutes of pain rather than putting his life into the hands of an unknown dentist with a bagful of mysterious vapors, demurred. After a few days of waiting, it was decided to reconvene the medical class and ask one of the students to volunteer to have a tooth pulled. What happened next is described in a letter that Wells wrote to the editor of the *Hartford Courant* almost two years later, on December 9, 1846, as his opening salvo in the battle over priority:

A large number of students, with several physicians, met to see the operation performed—one of their number to be the patient. Unfortunately for the experiment, the gas bag was by mistake withdrawn much too soon, and he was but partially under its influence when the tooth was extracted. He testified that he experienced some pain, but not as much as usually attends the operation. As there was no other patient present, that the experiment might be repeated, and as several expressed their opinion that it was a humbug affair (which in fact was all the thanks I got for this gratuitous service) I accordingly left the next morning for home.

"Several expressed their opinion that it was a humbug affair" was a supreme bit of understatement. What had actually happened was the first in a series of calamities that led eventually to the ruin of Horace Wells. At the very instant that he pulled out his volunteer's tooth, the young man jerked back his head and cried out in pain. Very likely, enough gas had not been administered by the impatient dentist, standing jittery and taut in the pit of an unfamiliar amphitheater, performing before skeptical onlookers who included some of the most distinguished physicians of Boston. But although, on full awakening, the subject of the extraction could remember but little pain, the damage had been done. Poor Wells retreated from the room amid the derisive hooting and hissing of the assembled onlookers. Of the epithets that assaulted his ears, "humbug" was among the least indelicate. He left Boston in defeat, in humiliation, and in his own eyes, in disgrace. The letter quoted above was not written by a man who was psychologically intact. The failure at the Massachusetts General Hospital had a devastating effect upon the spirit of Horace Wells. Immediately upon returning from Boston he put his house up for sale, and a few months later he sold his practice to Dr. Riggs.

Too depressed and agitated to practice the delicate work of dentistry, Wells turned his occasional bursts of nervous energy to several money-making projects, with indifferent success. The months dragged by, and still the anguish of his blighted hopes did not leave him. But through all of the tormented days, he still cherished a glim-

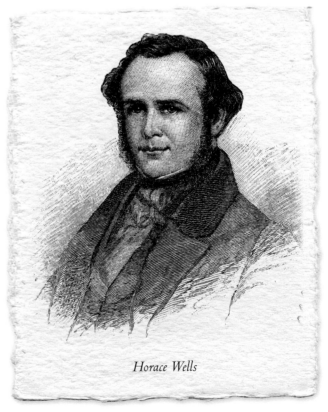

Horace Wells

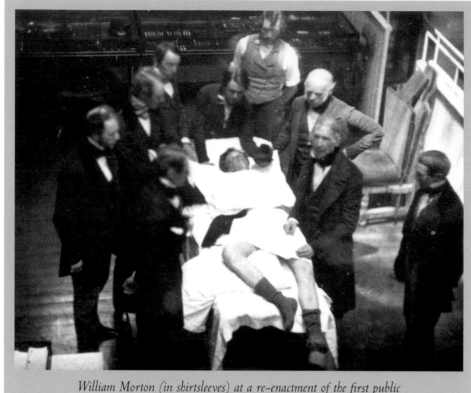

William Morton (in shirtsleeves) at a re-enactment of the first public demonstration of ether anesthesia in the operating room of the Massachusetts General Hospital, Boston, on October 16, 1846

remain asleep can be regulated at pleasure. While in this state, the severest surgical or dental operations may be performed, the patient not experiencing the slightest pain. I have perfected it, and am now about sending out agents to dispose of the right to use it. I will dispose of a right to an individual to use it in his own practice alone, or for a town, county or state. My object in writing to you is to know if you would not like to visit New York and the other cities, and dispose of rights upon shares. I have used the compound in more than a hundred and sixty cases in extracting teeth; and I have been invited to administer to patients in the Massachusetts General Hospital, and have succeeded in every case.

mer of optimism that something might yet come of his experiments with nitrous oxide; perhaps some other surgeon in some other place might recognize the contribution that Horace Wells could make to the art of medicine if only he was given another chance. And then, on a late-October morning in 1846, he received the devastating news that his dream would never come true. The message came in the form of a letter from William Morton:

Friend Wells. Dear Sir,—I write to inform you that I have discovered a preparation, by inhaling which a person is thrown into a sound sleep. The time required to produce sleep is only a few moments, and the time in which persons

The letter was dated October 19, 1846—three days after Morton had ushered in the era of surgical anesthesia by successfully etherizing a patient for an operation by John Collins Warren. In one stroke, Wells' prize had been stolen from him, and he had been offered the crumb of a subservient role by the very same ungrateful protégé to whom he himself had introduced the concept of pain-free surgery. His distress was made all the more bitter by Morton's having snatched away not only the glory but the gold as well, since it was obvious from the letter that he had already begun an active marketing campaign to peddle the rights to his invention.

There was no way in which Morton's devastating letter could be answered in a rational manner. His triumph was soon announced in an article by one of Warren's colleagues, which appeared on November 18 in the *Boston Medical and Surgical Journal*. Finally, on December 7, the *Hartford Courant* brought too close to home the news of Morton's acclaim. Wells, lacerated beyond recovery by his former assistant's public approbation, began his raging battle for recognition with that December 9 letter to the editor, ending his statement with a plaintive appeal: "I leave it for the public to decide to whom belongs the honor of this discovery."

The prologue is now complete. Everything that has been described up to this point is background and color for the ultimate dramatic act in the story of anesthesia, the successful operation by John Collins Warren upon a patient etherized by William Morton, on October 16, 1846.

It is difficult to make any sense of the emotional cacophony that came in the aftermath of that event without some concept of the personality of its leading player. What emerges from the various descriptions left to us by those who knew William Morton is perhaps best epitomized by a twentieth-century phrase: he was a young man in a hurry. Ambitious, in both the best and least-best senses of that word, he was hardworking, quick to grasp an opportunity, and very much aware of the financial rewards that can come with discovery. Whatever benefit he hoped to reap for mankind, he seems to have been driven far more by mercenary motives than by the love of science. In fact, he was not a scien-

tist in any sense—he was, pure and simple, an inventor looking for a bonanza.

Although practicing dentistry in Boston, Morton had never completed the studies he had undertaken in 1840 at the Baltimore College of Dental Surgery. But he did have every desire to improve his knowledge of technical matters, and accordingly attended two courses of lectures at the Massachusetts Medical College, during which he made the acquaintance of several members of the staff at the Massachusetts General Hospital. He studied chemistry privately with Charles T. Jackson, in whose house he was a boarder for a brief period. Jackson, a highly respected geologist, also directed a laboratory for research in analytical chemistry.

At the time we pick up the thread of Morton's life he had established himself in dental practice in Boston, after an unsuccessful partnership with Horace Wells in Hartford during 1842–1843. It was Morton who had been instrumental in arranging Wells' disastrous nitrous-oxide demonstration with John Collins Warren, and he had been a witness not only to its failure but also to some of his erstwhile associate's experiments. Whether Wells, as he later claimed, was also experimenting with ether in Morton's presence is uncertain.

By 1844, Morton was actively searching for some method of relieving the pain of dental extractions. He had developed a new kind of plate to hold false teeth in place, a plate that fit tightly against the gums. In the long run it offered the advantage of decreasing "denture breath" considerably, but to achieve the tight fit, the old roots and stumps of the patient's natural teeth had to be removed from the jaws. The process was so painful that Morton was losing patients to other dentists because of it. Thus, as an involved attorney, the forthright and by then famous Richard Henry Dana, Jr., stated several years later, "Dr. Morton had a direct pecuniary motive, bearing almost daily upon him, to alleviate or annihilate pain under his operations." There seems to have been a certain urgency about the entire undertaking, not only to accomplish it quickly, but to be the sole beneficiary of whatever financial rewards might come.

The chemist Jackson had told Morton two important things about ether: he had described the effect it had upon frolicking students, and he had suggested that the liquid applied directly on a patient's gum would numb the area around any tooth he wished to extract. Based on that advice, the young dentist had first used this method in July 1844, and had begun to ponder the possibility of using the compound or its vapors to induce some more general decrease in sensation. He knew from reading Jonathan Pereira's 1839 *Elements of Materia Medica* that inhaling the vapors of sulfuric ether would induce obtundation similar to what he had seen Wells produce with nitrous oxide, and he began, without telling Jackson, to seek out a safe method of using it.

Much of the summer of 1846 was spent in experiments with goldfish, caterpillars, insects, worms, and even a spaniel puppy. Morton finally tried the vapors on two of his dental apprentices, but could not convince himself that the results were predictable or satisfactory. All of his work was done in the greatest secrecy, for fear that his idea would fall into the hands of another. But the secrecy itself impeded his progress by preventing him from asking advice from appropriate sources. Since, in spite of his daring (or, as some thought, recklessness), he never did have a lot of faith in his own scientific knowledge, he eventually consulted his erstwhile chemistry mentor, Jackson. The older man recommended that Morton discard the use of the commercial product, and restrict himself to pure sulfuric ether so that there might be some consistency to his results. Jackson probably also encouraged him to try the inhalation technique on a patient named Eben Frost, who presented himself at Morton's office on the evening of September 30, 1846. The extraction of a tooth was accomplished on the sleeping, pain-free Frost, and Morton immediately made plans to go forward with a public

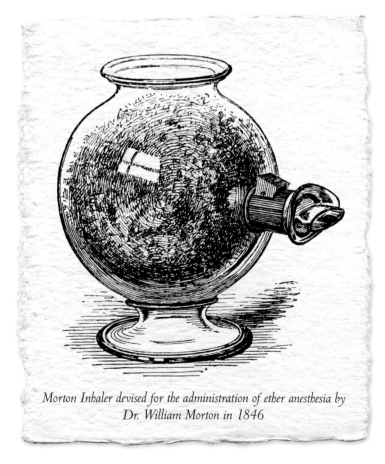

Morton Inhaler devised for the administration of ether anesthesia by Dr. William Morton in 1846

demonstration. But eager as he was to show the world that he had discovered a means of painless surgery, the pragmatic Morton first took the precaution of consulting a patent commissioner.

He took one other precaution as well, even before seeking advice on a patent—he contacted a newspaper. Although Morton claimed that he was not the source, it is hard to believe that anyone else could have been responsible for the notice which appeared in the *Boston Daily Journal* on October 1, 1846, the day after his operation on Frost:

> *Last evening, as we were informed by a gentleman who witnessed the operation, an ulcerated tooth was extracted from the mouth of an individual without giving the slightest pain. He was put into a kind of sleep, by inhaling a preparation, the effects of which lasted for about three quarters of a minute, just long enough to extract the tooth.*

With the ground thus prepared, Morton's next move was to pay a visit to John Collins Warren. In light of Warren's unhappy experience with the nitrous-oxide misadventure, the daring dentist was displaying, by this action, either considerable self-confidence or considerable foolhardiness—probably both. It certainly flew in the face of the principles of scientific restraint, in view of the fact that the twenty-seven-year-old tooth-puller's experience with the effects of ether on human beings was minimal, his knowledge of its hazards was nil, and he had not yet even bothered to do anything about designing an apparatus by which the gas could be administered to a real patient (the forty-five-second procedure on Frost had been done with an ether-soaked handkerchief). Warren had every reason to reject Morton's suggestion that ether be used for a surgical operation.

But here the character of John Collins Warren comes into play. An austere, highly skilled physician of considerable ambition, he had learned his operative techniques from the likes of Sir Astley Cooper and Baron Guillaume Dupuytren, the greatest European surgeons of their day. Although known for his prudence and good judgment, he was also renowned for his willingness to try new methods, having been a pioneer in certain orthopedic procedures, and the first surgeon in America to operate for strangulated hernia. He was Harvard's second Professor of Surgery, having succeeded his own father to that position in 1815. As one of the founders of the Massachusetts General Hospital and of the American Medical Association he was, at the time that Morton approached him, one of the young country's most revered senior physicians.

In 1846, Warren was sixty-eight years old, and within one year of relinquishing his professorship. His flint-faced, grizzled appearance belied the fact that in a lifetime of surgery he had never been able to inure himself to the horrors of the operating theater—even his devout Christian faith did not shield his conscience against the agonies to which he exposed those he was trying to heal. Perhaps it was his ineluctable destiny to be the medium through which in the words of his friend Oliver Wendell Holmes, "the fierce extremity of suffering has been steeped in the waters of forgetfulness, and the deepest furrow on the knotted brow of agony has been smoothed forever." He accepted Morton's proposition. The dentist received a short letter inviting him to come to the hospital within forty-eight hours "to administer to a patient who is then to be operated upon, the preparation which you have invented to diminish the sensibility to pain." So secretive had Morton been that even the operating surgeon did not know of what "the preparation" consisted.

With only two days' notice, Morton worked feverishly with an instrument maker to fashion a functional inhaling apparatus; it was completed so close to the last instant that he arrived at the operating theater fifteen minutes late on the appointed morning, just as Warren, despairing of his appearance, was poised to begin the operation without him. The seats of the amphitheater were filled with staff and students, many of them prepared to enjoy the humiliation of yet another dentist with a humbug remedy for surgical pain. The patient was a thin, tubercular young man, Gilbert Abbot, with a vascular tumor at the angle of his left jaw. After saying a few encouraging words to the proposed subject, Morton positioned the mouthpiece of the apparatus and told Abbot to breathe.

Within a few minutes, Gilbert Abbot was asleep. Morton looked over toward Warren and quietly said, "Sir, your patient is ready." The procedure began. The next events are best described in Warren's own words, in an article he wrote for the *Boston Medical and Surgical Journal* two months later:

I immediately made an incision about three inches long through the skin of the neck, and began a dissection among important nerves and blood-vessels without any expression of pain on the part of the patient. Soon after, he began to speak incoherently, and appeared to be in an agitated state during the remainder of the operation. Being asked immediately afterwards whether he had suffered much, he said that he had felt as if his neck had been scratched.

The virtually pain-free operation lasted twenty-five minutes. When it was over, John Collins Warren looked up at what had been, just moments before, a skeptical, even cynical audience, its members now hushed into an awed, reverential silence that must have come with the certain knowledge that they had been present at one of medicine's historic moments. They would have no use now for that derisive word which some of them had been waiting to hurl at the presumptuous dentist who now stood before them a hero. Warren contemplated his congregation for a moment, still thunderstruck at what had just been accomplished, and quietly announced the birth of anesthesia with an eloquently simple testimony: "Gentlemen, this is no humbug."

Several years later, when many more operations had been done under anesthesia, the now-retired old surgeon collected his thoughts and pondered the realization of his lifelong dream of surgery without pain. He told a new audience in that consecrated amphitheater, which has come to be called the Ether Dome:

A new era has opened on the operating surgeon. His visitations on the most delicate parts are performed, not only without the agonizing screams he has been accustomed to hear, but sometimes in a state of perfect insensibility, and, occasionally, even with an expression of pleasure on the part of the patient.

Who could have imagined that drawing a knife over the delicate skin of the face, might produce a sensation of unmixed delight? That the turning and twisting of instruments in the most sensitive bladder, might be accompanied by a delightful dream? That the contorting of anchylosed joints should coexist with a celestial vision?

If Ambroise Paré, and Louis, and Dessault, and Cheselden, and Hunter, and Cooper, could see what our eyes daily witness, how they would long to come among us, and perform their exploits once more.

And with what fresh vigor does the living surgeon, who is ready to resign his scalpel, grasp it, and wish again to go through his career under the new auspices.

As philanthropists we may well rejoice that we have had an agency, however slight, in conferring upon poor suffering humanity so precious a gift.

Unrestrained and free as God's own sunshine, it has gone forth to cheer and gladden the earth; it will awaken the gratitude of the present, and all coming generations. The student, who from distant lands or in distant ages, may visit this spot, will view it with increased interest, as he remembers that here was first demonstrated one of the most glorious truths of science.

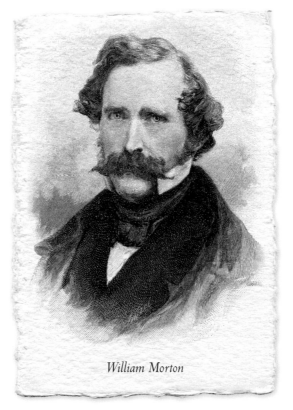

William Morton

In the weeks that followed his dramatic success, Morton persisted in refusing to disclose the nature of his invention. Optimistically afloat on a wave of acclaim from the hospital authorities, he continued to focus his thoughts on patents, profits, and capturing a worldwide market. His biographer, Nathan P. Rice, later estimated in his *Trials of a Public Benefactor* that Morton's share in the sale of rights to exclusive use of the gas in America alone would have been more than $350,000 over the fourteen-year period of a patent. The letter written to Wells on October 19 describes his planned approach (and provides a good example of the young entrepreneur's tendency to pad facts and distort events).

But two problems had arisen. The first was the intervention at this moment of Charles T. Jackson, whose visit to Morton on October 23 marked the beginning of a conflict that would become so acrimonious and finally so vicious that it did not end even long after both participants had been destroyed by its unremitting fury. To put the issue into its simplest terms, Jackson wanted a piece of the action. The patent commissioner Morton had consulted before the operation on Gilbert Abbot was R. H. Eddy, who, as it turned out, was one of the highly regarded Jackson's many admirers. Having concluded that it was probable that a patent on ether could be obtained, Eddy began to urge Morton to give the chemist a percentage of the profits that might be made. The two came to an agreement. On November 12, Letter Patent No. 4848 was issued to both Morton and Jackson, with the latter having agreed to assign his rights in return for 10 percent of the American profits; a similar patent was later taken out to cover foreign sales.

Although Charles Thomas Jackson has been portrayed up to this point as the accomplished and much-respected scientist that he was, it is necessary to describe another aspect of his character, without knowledge of which it is difficult to understand the foregoing and subsequent events. Jackson was a brilliant eccentric, in whom the seed of madness was firmly implanted, and by this time appears to have begun flourishing. Graduated in medicine from Harvard in 1829, he then studied in the hospitals of Paris for two years, at the same time developing an interest in geology and in analytical chemistry. On the return voyage from France, he made the acquaintance of Samuel F. B. Morse and showed him an electromagnet he was bringing back to Boston. As he scrutinized the instrument, Morse conceived of the idea that electricity might be the means by which information could be transmitted across long distances. On arriving home, he began a series of experiments which culminated in the invention of the telegraph. Charles Jackson did not hesitate to claim the credit for himself.

Nor was this the only example of his peculiar tendency to convert a suggestion or an incidental contribution into a claim that he was the originator of some scientific advance. When the army surgeon Captain William Beaumont was experimenting on a French Canadian trapper whose abdominal gunshot wound had healed in such a way as to leave an opening between his stomach and the outside world, he asked Jackson to do a chemical analysis of the digestive fluid that leaked out. Beaumont and the experimentee, Alexis St. Martin, were in Boston at the time, and when the gifted captain was ordered west by the army, Jackson attempted to prevent his reluctant subject's departure so that he could carry out some studies of his own. To cover his deception with an air of scientific necessity, he craftily obtained the signatures of two hundred congressmen on a petition describing the importance of his analysis to America and humanity. Had not the Secretary of War rejected the petition, Jackson might have claimed the credit we now give to William Beaumont as our country's first physiologist.

Replica of anaesthesia apparatus for administering ether

Even as recently as that very year of 1846, Charles Jackson was embroiled in another conflict that he was destined to lose, with Christian Schoenbein, over the German chemist's invention of guncotton. So Jackson rode into the arena of anesthesia controversy on an experienced charger, carrying a well-used lance. The fact that he had been knocked from his steed in every previous tournament only increased the fever of his obsessed determination to win this one.

Morton's second problem was the difficulty—indeed, the impossibility—of keeping the nature of his gas a secret. His addition of aromatic compounds to the mixture could not disguise its characteristic odor from physicians, and even his denial that ether was the active ingredient would only delay discovery for a short time. Moreover, in acquiring a patent, Morton had reckoned without the objections of the physicians of the Massachusetts General Hospital, and of the dental profession. Warren, in his own words, "checked by the information that an exclusive patent had been taken out, and that no application could be made without the permission of the proprietor," would not allow further use of the agent until the patent restrictions were relaxed. After a three-week moratorium, Morton grudgingly agreed to share his secret with the hospital, provided that all information was considered confidential. On November 7, etherization resumed with the first pain-free amputation. Two weeks later, the inventor met with two representatives of the hospital, Henry Jacob Bigelow and Oliver Wendell Holmes, and gave the name Letheon to sulfuric ether, in an attempt to keep up some semblance of concealment. The term was borrowed, at the suggestion of Holmes, from the writings of Virgil, who

had, as noted earlier, applied it to the restful sleep induced by the tears of the poppy plant.

The imprimatur of Boston culture was thus put on the new technique by none other than Holmes himself, thirty-seven years of age and about to be named Professor of Anatomy and Physiology at the Harvard Medical School. The discovery needed a name, even if its principal ingredient was to remain a secret. Holmes suggested that it be "anesthesia," with the adjective being "anesthetic." He pointed out in a letter to Morton that whatever name he chose, it *"will be repeated by the tongues of every civilized race of mankind"*—the emphasis is Holmes'.

(As noted earlier, the word "anesthesia" had originally been used by Dioscorides in the first century, and subsequently by some of the exponents of mesmerism. Although not to be found in Samuel Johnson's dictionary, it did appear in a lexicon written in 1721, and is also defined in Pan's medical dictionary of 1819. Its familiarity to the Autocrat of the Breakfast Table would seem to stem from its use in several of the texts of the time; he may have found it in his copy of John Mason Good's *Physiological System of Nosology*, published in 1823. So, although Dr. Holmes is often credited with coining the word, he would have been the first to acknowledge its ancient lineage.)

Even as the negotiations over rights and confidentiality were taking place, the Harvard physicians had been preparing to tell the news to America's scientific community. On November 3, a brief abstract of the events was read before the American Academy of Arts and Sciences, and then on November 9 a full paper was given at a meeting of the Boston Society of Medical Improvement, by Henry Jacob Bigelow. The paper was printed in the November 18 issue of the *Boston Medical and Surgical Journal*—now an expensive collector's item, because it carries the first formal published announcement of the discovery of surgical anesthesia. By then Bigelow, who was soon to replace John Collins Warren as the leading surgeon of New England, had carried out a number of experiments, and a few further clinical cases had been done.

The news of the great discovery spread quickly to Europe, in a way that was as common then as it is today. Henry Bigelow's proud father, Jacob, sent off a letter to his London friend Francis Boott, enclosing a clipping of his son's paper. Without wasting a moment after receiving the communication, Boott arranged for a dentist named Robinson to extract a tooth of one Miss Lonsdale in his study at home. Within a few minutes of the lady's having recovered from her slumber, Boott sent the news via messenger to his colleague Robert Liston, the dexterous and daring Professor of Surgery at University College, London. The day being Saturday, Liston waited only for the weekend to be over before carrying out Europe's first surgical operation under ether, on Monday, December 19. Before beginning to do the procedure, an amputation, he is reported to have told the assembled students and assistants, "We are going to try a Yankee dodge today, gentlemen, for making men insensible." When the final bits of bandaging had been completed, the great British surgeon, a member of the same medical faculty that had laughed at John Elliotson and the mesmerists only eight years before, proclaimed loudly to all who could hear his booming voice, "This Yankee dodge, gentlemen, beats mesmerism hollow." Sitting quietly among the onlookers was a nineteen-year-old undergraduate working toward his baccalaureate degree, Joseph Lister—of whom more will be said later.

To give ether the ultimate test, Liston next used it to pull out the nail of a patient's great toe, in his words "one of the most painful operations in surgery." He then wrote to Boott thanking him for his suggestion and describing his "most perfect and satisfactory results" in the two cases. Boott forwarded the letter and the copy of Bigelow's paper to the *Lancet*, already at that early date one of the world's most authoritative medical journals, which published both on January 2, 1847. Within three weeks, ether had been used at the Allgemeines Krankenhaus in Vienna and the University Surgical Hospital in Erlangen, Germany. On February 1, the eminent Parisian surgeon Alfred Velpeau of the Charité reported to the French Academy of Sciences that his experimental work with the gas had proved its usefulness beyond any doubt. In the summer of 1847, Peter Parker, a Yale–trained physician-missionary, began working with ether halfway around the world, in China, utilizing it in a series of operations performed in the small building he called the Canton Hospital.

As Morton was being extolled and his invention applauded by the world, the wily Jackson did not sit idly by, satisfied with only 10 percent of the forthcoming profits and very little of the glory. Just as in his petition to Congress he had played down the role of William Beaumont thirteen years earlier, he now planned to characterize Morton as someone who had merely acted as his agent in carrying out the technical aspects of the great invention. On November 13, and again on December 1, 1846, he wrote to a highly placed friend in Paris, claiming to be the discoverer of anesthesia, the usefulness of which had been amply demonstrated at the Massachusetts General Hospital in consequence of his request to "a dentist of this city" that he so carry out his, Jackson's, instructions. These letters were read before the French Academy of Sciences on January 18, 1847, a fact which soon became known to Morton. The alarmed dentist, realizing the craftiness of his opponent, rapidly set about collecting sworn statements of witnesses.

Meantime, Horace Wells had also determined to seek an audience in Paris, and traveled there to petition the Academy of Medicine and the Academy of Sciences. It is uncertain how extensively the two academies investigated his claims at that time, but both did publish extracts from his petitioning letter in their proceedings. It had not occurred to the unfortunate Wells to bring definite evidence with him in the form of testimonials, with the result that at the time he returned home in March

1847, the outlook for his recognition appeared bleak. Immediately on his ship arriving in Boston he began assembling sworn statements, and within a few days was back in Hartford to collect more.

With Wells' journey to Paris, and Jackson's apparently successful reception by the Academy of Sciences, Morton felt that his seeming advantage was in imminent danger of being lost. He could not anticipate that the supposedly sophisticated Jackson would proceed to advance not his own, but his rival's position, by outsmarting himself.

It came about in the following way. Edward Everett, president of Harvard College, and John Collins Warren, both wishing to put the new discovery and its historical evolution on firm scientific ground, suggested to their academic colleague in chemistry that he prepare a presentation for the American Academy of Sciences, of which Everett was then vice-president. Jackson saw in this an opportunity to legitimize his claims in what was then the outstanding Amer-

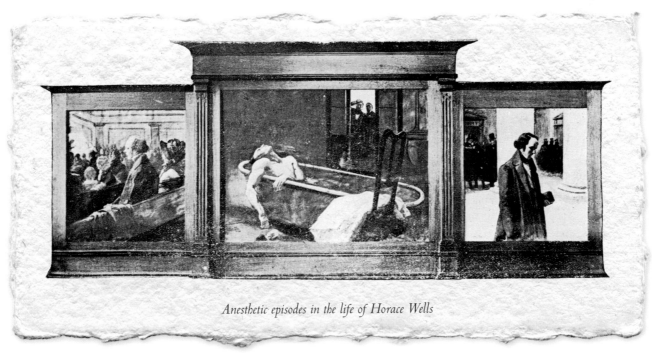

Anesthetic episodes in the life of Horace Wells

ican scientific body. He wrote his presentation in such a way that it not only proclaimed him as the inventor of anesthesia, but implied that he made this claim with the support of Everett and Warren and with the official sanction of the academy. He sent copies across the sea to Paris, and also to the aptly named *Boston Daily Advertiser*, which printed the text on March 1. Although this action made him look better abroad, it exploded in his face at home. Offended at having been used this way, the Academy of Sciences disavowed the statement, never had it read before one of its meetings, and refused to publish it in its *Transactions*. Jackson suddenly found himself under a cloud of suspicion in the very group he had most hoped to persuade, the American scientific community. Everett's distrust in particular was heightened by the fact that he had been the congressman who, thirteen years earlier, had allowed himself to be convinced to present Jackson's petition concerning St. Martin to the Secretary of War.

Now the hostilities had begun in earnest. The rest of Morton's life, and much of the rest of Jackson's, was taken up by a frenzied round of claims, petitions to Congress, crescendos of personal misery, and finally, for each of them, death under tragic circumstances. But at this point, an oasis of sanity somehow intruded itself briefly into the midst of the controversy's intellectually arid wasteland. Morton, perhaps made more secure in his position by the reverberations of his rival's misjudgment, managed to write a temperate and lucid brochure containing complete instructions for the administration of ether, which he published in September 1847. In addition to this, he prepared

a memoir which was presented to the French Academy of Sciences at its meeting of November 2, by which time the tide at home was strongly in his favor.

The selfsame tide that was lifting the fortunes of William Morton was drowning Horace Wells'. Only a week after disembarking from France, he published his only separate work on anesthesia, entitled *History of the Application of Nitrous Oxide Gas, Ether and Other Vapors*, containing the testimonials he had gathered. He sent the originals of the supporting letters to Paris to be reviewed by the academies. But neither the letters, nor the journey to Paris, nor the *History* reversed the inexorable downturn in his fortunes. In January 1848, leaving his wife and child behind in Hartford without funds for their support, Wells, by now crazed with the injustice of his fate, moved to New York, determined to continue his experiments with nitrous oxide, with ether, and with chloroform, which latter agent had meanwhile been introduced as an anesthetic by James Young Simpson in November 1847. In the January 17, 1848, edition of the *New York Evening Post*, an advertisement appeared in which the offer was made that "H. Wells, surgeon dentist, the discoveror of 'Letheon,' having removed to New York, will give gratuitous advice respecting the use of chloroform, nitrous oxide gas, and 'Letheon' as applied to the extraction of teeth from 10 o'clock A.M. until 3 o'clock P.M. Residence 120 Chambers St, West of Broadway."

Only four days later, on his thirty-third birthday, the man who had invented nitrous oxide anesthesia was thrown into the Tombs prison. The charge against him was that he had hurled sulfuric acid at some ladies of easy virtue walking their beat on Broadway. His degradation seemed to be complete.

But there was to be one final tragic act in the drama, and an epilogue the irony of which magnifies its ghastliness. On January 22, 1848, Horace Wells, whose experiments had made him a chloroform addict, inhaled just enough of a smuggled bottle of that compound to make himself partly insensible, and then ended his life by drawing a razor across the major artery in his left groin. This letter was found in his cell:

Sunday, evening, 7 o'clock I again take up pen to finish what I have to say. Great God! Has it come to this? Is it not all a dream? Before 12 o'clock tonight I am to pay the debt of nature. Yes, even if I was to go free tomorrow, I could not live and be called a villain. God knows I am not one. . . . Oh! my dear wife and child, whom I leave destitute of the means of support—I would still live and work for you, but I cannot—for if I were to live on, I should become a maniac. I feel that I am one already.

And now the epilogue. During Wells' frustrating visit to Paris, he had been befriended by an American dentist, C. Starr Brewster, who helped him to present his case to the two academies and also to the Paris Medical Society. Twelve days after his suicide, the following letter arrived for Wells from Brewster, and was opened by his disconsolate widow:

My Dear Wells:
    I have just returned from a meeting of the Paris Medical Society where they voted that to Horace Wells of Hartford, Connecticut, United States of America is *due the honor of having successfully discovered and successfully applied the first use of vapors or gases whereby surgical operations could be performed without pain. . . .*

And so, a martyr to the discovery of anesthesia, Horace Wells received a recognition that came too late to save his life or to give balm to his troubled mind.

Perhaps because of the death of Wells, the authorities at the Massachusetts General Hospital felt called upon to blow away some of the dismal clouds of confusion by preparing an official history of the controversy, in which the claims of all of the participants would be reviewed and evaluated. The report was written by Richard Henry Dana, Jr., and its conclusion was clear: the Board of Trustees of the hospital considered William Morton to be the true discoverer of ether anesthesia. With Morton's memoir to the French Academy of Sciences appended to it, the article was made available to the public in a periodical called *Littel's Living Age* on March 18, 1848.

The board went even further. Its members subscribed one thousand dollars to be given as an honorarium to the young man whom they had now decided was one of the great benefactors of mankind. The accompanying testimonial closed with the following words:

We also enclose the subscription book in a casket which accompanies this note. Among its signatures you will find names of not a few of those most distinguished among us for worth and intelligence; and it may be remembered that it is signed by every member of the Board of Trustees. You will, we are sure, highly value this first testimonial, slight as it is, of the gratitude of your fellow-citizens. That you may hereafter receive an adequate national reward is the sincere wish of your obedient servants.

That sincere wish was shared, of course, by William Morton. Although the hospital authorities were convinced of his claim, other interested parties were still unsure. For some time there had been more than honor at stake, as Congress was preparing to decide upon a bill awarding a purse of $100,000 to whoever they should decide deserved the distinction of priority. The legislators might not have embarked on their well-meant project had they been able to anticipate the series of disputed claims that would cause the decision-making process to drag on for years.

It was in response to the bill that Crawford Long was now prevailed upon to publish his report in the *Southern Medical and Surgical Journal* in December 1849. At the urging of friends, he also wrote to Senator William Crosby Dawson and to his congressman, Junius Hillyer, describing the work that he had done. Dawson, intent on investigating his fellow Georgian's claim, chose an unlikely agent to do it for him, the renowned Boston chemist Charles T. Jackson.

When Jackson arrived in Athens, Georgia, on March 8, 1854, he had already written a book three years earlier in which he gave his own version of the discovery of anesthesia, *Etherization of Animals and of Man*. And yet, when he studied Long's documents, he became convinced of the successful operations on James Venable and the others. He proposed to Long that the two of them prepare a joint claim to Congress, with Jackson being given credit for the discovery and Long for the first clinical use, thereby effectively shutting out the heirs of Horace Wells and also that *bête noire* of Jackson's, William Morton. Long saw no reason to share anything, not because he was stubborn or greedy, but because he felt the certainty of being right.

Jackson, whatever else may be said of him, was too honest, at least in this case, to falsify his report to Dawson. Of course, it is not necessary to point out that his honesty was encouraged by his hatred of Morton. On April 5, 1854, when the Senate was making its final judgment on the bill, Senator Dawson announced that he had a letter from Dr. Jackson acknowledging that the unfamiliar name of Dr. Crawford Williamson Long was the one to which should be assigned the honor of having been the first to use ether. Since the bill specified that the award was to be given either to Morton, Jackson, or the representatives of Wells, whichever was judged most fitting by the secretary of the treasury, the introduction of Long's name threw the entire proceeding into a parliamentary tailspin, from which it never recovered. The final version of the legislation, although passed by the Senate, was tabled by the House of Representatives, and died. The congressional battle was over, as was Crawford Long's involvement.

William Morton, whose victory had seemed at one point to be complete, now turned to the civil courts to try to prove his case for claiming a valid patent. But as he had early revealed the nature of Letheon to the physicians of the Hospital so that, at their insistence, it might be used by that institution and by other charitable facilities, and as the government of the United States had itself infringed its own patent by the free use of ether during the Mexican War (1846–1848), his legal rights had become unenforceable. With his monopoly thus destroyed, some of the licensees who had signed up with him for exclusive sales rights began legal suit. Such litigations were to prove futile for many reasons, not the least of which was that Morton had abandoned his dental practice in order to devote all of his energies, and also all of his money, to his claims. He was soon financially ruined, suing and being sued, and finally petitioning Congress for redress. Disappointed in the outcome of his entreaties to the government, he chose to institute an infringement suit against a charitable foundation, the New York Eye Infirmary. The 1863 verdict, which was later upheld by the United States Supreme Court, was unfavorable to him. The most crippling blow to his pride came the following year, when the medical establishment which had originally embraced him now signified that its patience with his contentiousness was at an end—at the instigation of the Eye Infirmary staff, he was censured, in scathing language, by the American Medical Association, on June 24, 1864:

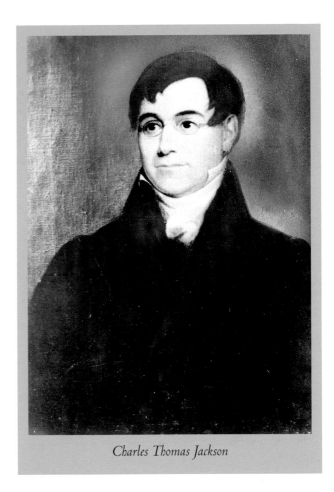

Charles Thomas Jackson

Whereas, The said Dr. Morton, by suits brought against charitable medical institutions for infringements of an alleged patent covering all anesthetic agents, not claiming sulfuric ether only, but the state of anesthesia, however produced, as his invention, has by this act put himself beyond the pale of an honorable profession and of true labors in the cause of science and humanity therefore

Resolved, That the American Medical Association enter their protest against any appropriation to Dr. Morton, on the ground of his unworthy conduct. . . .

That glorious tide that had so recently lifted him to fame had become a maelstrom that threatened to drown Morton's soul. An article in the June 1868 issue of the *Atlantic Monthly*, sup-porting Jackson's position, inflamed his resentment beyond reason. In July, he made yet one more fruitless journey to Washington, but the frustration of its disappointing outcome proved to be too much for him. He arrived back in New York in the midst of a stiflingly humid heat wave, feeling dejected and sick. On an impulse, he decided to take his wife, Elizabeth, on a cooling buggy ride through Central Park. Their little wagon was moving at a good clip along one of the lakeside roads when Morton suddenly and inexplicably jerked the horse to a stop, leaped out, and plunged his head downward into the tepid water. Obviously disturbed, he was urged by the distraught Elizabeth to climb back into the buggy, which he reluctantly agreed to do. They had driven only a short distance farther when he precipitously vaulted from the rig once more, threw his body over a nearby fence, and fell to the ground on the other side, unconscious. Several hours later, the tormented dentist whom William Henry Welch so rightfully called "the least heroic of great discoverers" was dead of a cerebral hemorrhage.

Charles Jackson fared no better. Never the most stable of personalities, he became more unbalanced as the years passed. One day in 1873, five years after William Morton's death, the aging provocateur came across his late antagonist's grave in Boston's Mount Auburn cemetery. It bore the epitaph:

> William T. G. Morton.
> Inventor and Revealer of Anesthetic Inhalation.
> By whom pain in surgery was averted and annulled.
> Before whom in all time surgery was agony.
> Since whom science has control of pain.

Reading the words on the stone broke what little was left of the fragile structure of Jackson's reason. He was admitted to the McLean Asylum in Belmont, Massachusetts, where he passed the last seven years of his life, completely psychotic. He died on August 28, 1880, at the age of seventy-five, his only triumph over his rivals being in longevity.

While none of the four contenders for the crown of discovery had an easy life after the controversies began, at least it can be said that Crawford Long's, though arduous and toilsome, did not end in tragedy. Not only was he unique among the four in not being destroyed by the

anesthesia dispute, but he was also the only one who emerged with honor. His contribution, forgotten in the din made by the others, was rediscovered in 1877 by the South Carolina gynecologist J. Marion Sims, who wrote a thorough discussion of its originality in the *Virginia Medical Monthly*. The article gave considerable emotional sustenance to the aging Long, by then beaten down by the burdens of caring for a large group of indigent patients in an area that had been impoverished by the ravages brought by the Civil War and a long Yankee occupation.

Even Crawford Long's death involved his own self-negation, and it involved anesthesia as well. On June 16, 1878, the sixty-two-year-old country practitioner had just completed the delivery of a child from an etherized mother when he felt a wave of unconsciousness coming over him. In the moment before being enveloped in darkness he managed to pass the infant into the arms of an attendant, with the admonition "Care for the mother and the child first." He fell across the patient's bed, and a few hours later was dead of a massive stroke.

Over the next few decades, posthumous recognition of Long came in the form of statues, plaques, portraits, and oratorical tributes. The most recognized and widely seen of the memorials stands in the Statuary Hall of the United States Capitol. Long and his Franklin College roommate, Alexander Stephens (who had gone on to become one of the South's foremost political figures), were chosen by the state legislature to be the two honored sons whose statues would represent the highest accomplishments of Georgia. It was a choice well made.

In the course of this narrative, allusion has been made to the youth of most of the significant contributors to the history of inhalation anesthesia. Not only is this not an isolated situation in the annals of scientific discovery, but it tends to be the case more often than not. Andreas Vesalius became the Professor of Anatomy at Padua on the day after his graduation from the medical school in 1537; by the age of twenty-eight he had produced his monumental *De Humani Corporis Fabrica* and changed forever the ways in which physicians evaluate scientific evidence. Three hundred years later, the landmark discoveries in anesthesia were made by a group of men so young that most had scarcely begun to pursue the pattern of their careers. The prolonged period that is required to train today's investigator in the sophisticated technology of modern research makes it unlikely that people in their twenties will ever again be the leaders of science. Here and there, now and then, a great contribution will be made by a man or woman whose training is not yet complete, but they will be unusual instances and unusual individuals.

No matter the prolongation of the apprenticeship, however, the fact that the ebullient minds of the young percolate with an exciting curiosity and aggressive aspirations will always mean that much of scientific progress will inevitably come from youthful workers in the first decade following their training. Our present-day Mortons and Davys are in their thirties, which is almost as good as being in their twenties. Although William Osler's half-serious recommendation to put men of forty out to pasture has been modified by time and good sense, the world of discovery is still very much the world of the young, and so it will always be.

Nevertheless, we should not dismiss the value of the rewarding leisure for contemplation that comes to many researchers as they reach the final years of their productivity. Experience, wisdom, and the carefully burnished ability to look back on a lifetime of evolving ideas brings a perspective and a philosophical point of view that will, from time to time, result in a concept that shakes the temple of science. In the very year that Vesalius changed the course of medical progress, the seventy-year-old Nicolaus Copernicus published *De Revolutionibus Orbium Coelestium*, and the world was never the same again. As we wonder about our emeritus professors or dwell pessimistically on the hurtling, albeit insidious, passage of the brightest years of our own professional lives, we would do well to conjure up in the mind's eye the hoary image of old Copernicus, receiving on his deathbed the first printed copy of one of the most significant books ever to be produced by the intellect of man. Science is for all seasons, and all seasons are for all of us.

> *The fact that the ebullient minds of the young percolate with an exciting curiosity and aggressive aspirations will always mean that much of scientific progress will inevitably come from youthful workers.*

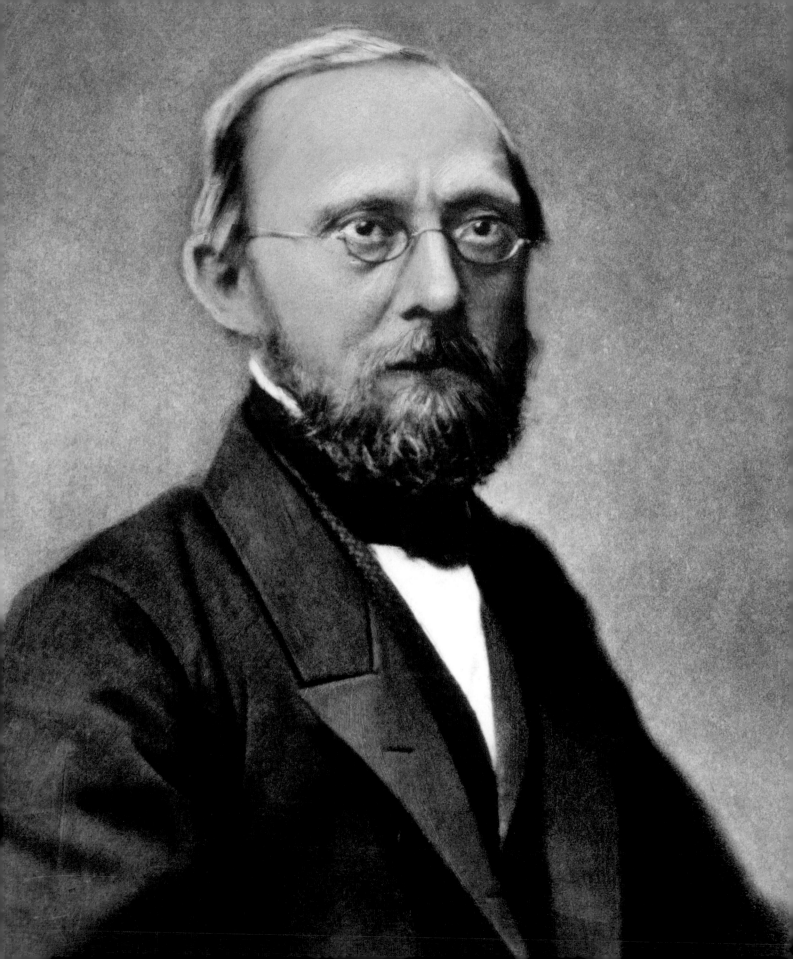

11

THE FUNDAMENTAL UNIT OF LIFE

Sick Cells, Microscopes, and Rudolf Virchow

Once we have recognized that disease is naught else than the process of life under altered conditions, the concept of healing expands to imply the maintenance or re-establishment of the normal conditions of existence.

—Rudolf Virchow

Metaphysicians, Idealists, Iatromechanics, Iatrochemists, Experimental Physiologists, Natural Philosophers, Mystics, Magnetizers, Exorcisers, Galenists, Modern Paracelsian Homunculi, Stahlianists, Humoral Pathologists, Gastricists, Infarct-Men, Broussaisists, Contrastimulists, Natural Historians, Physiatricists, Ideal-Pathologists, German Christian Theosophists, Schoenleinian Epigones, Pseudo-Schoenleinians, Homeobiotics, Homeopathists, Isopathists, Homeopathic Allopathists, Psorists and Scorists, Hydropathists, Electricity-Men, Physiologists after Hamberger, Heinrothians, Sachsians, Keiserians, Hegelians, Morisonians, Phrenologists, Iatrostatisticians.

You have just read a list, drawn up in 1840, of the various schools of thought into which medical theory was at that time divided. Each school had its own explanation for the still-unsolved puzzle of why it is that people get sick, and how best to go about curing them. The work of Morgagni, Bichat, Laennec, and the others had identified and even classified many of the visible alterations produced in tissues and organs by the process of disease, but no one yet knew what made the pathological events occur in the first place. Each philosophical school had its own system; each system had its own theory. In spite of them all, the phenomena of Nature-gone-awry remained cloaked in mystery.

Some of the systems-makers, the Exorcisers and Mystics, for example, plainly went beyond the constraints of orderly reason, but others, such as the Natural Philosophers and Humoral Pathologists, built their intellectual structure on objectively verifiable evidence that had been observed and studied by physicians for millennia. The members of the latter group were, in fact, heirs to the ancients' theory of the four humors, four humors now refined into a quasi-scientific formulation that sought the key to disease by postulating the existence of a set of hypothetical disordered body fluids. Although the nineteenth-century humoralists were possessed of far more facts than their long line of predecessors, they continued nevertheless to confound their interpretation of what they saw by using all the old errors of interpolation, extrapolation, and conjecture. Perhaps they were simply too impatient—in the absence of information to fill the gaps in their knowledge, they demanded to understand things before their science had yet wrested from Nature enough of her secrets. Among the believers in the systems of Natural Philosophy, Humoral Pathology, and several other of the sects were some of the century's most prominent students of biology and medicine. They were gifted, they were attentive, and they were genuine in intent—their error was in leaping before enough looking had made it possible to step safely from one verifiable point to the next.

A major element in the confusion was everyone's attempt to create some sense of order out of the burgeoning clutter of observations that scientific-minded investigators were then pouring into the increasingly chaotic storehouse of knowledge. The problem was addressed by the construction of the various systems of thought listed above, which were really nothing more than ways of looking at disease, ways that could be used as frameworks on which to hang the freshly acquired facts. The proponents of each system thought that theirs would prove to be the eventual edifice of healing, by which the storehouse of knowledge might become the stately mansion in which medical science would dwell.

Up to the present point in the narrative of this book, only the localizing and diagnosing of the sites of disease have been considered, as well as the sequence by which pathological processes evolve. Treatment has not been much discussed. No matter the sophistication of Laennec's method of physical examination or Hunter's understanding of inflammation and injury, neither of them had very effective therapy to offer the sick people who came to them for cure. When they chose weapons from their therapeutic arsenals, they had to fall back on vague concepts of humors, fluxes, and altered states of irritability. Much of what they offered was based on some uncertain attempt to restore an ill-understood balance that had become jangled. They bled their patients, and they puked them and purged them and blistered them as their professional forefathers had always done; they confused the metabolisms of the sick with dazzling combinations of botanicals whose real actions were only partially known, and often not known at all. They stimulated in cases whose cause was thought to be too little excitation, and they tried to introduce a touch of torpor when the opposite was the case. In short, except when the need for amputation or lancing was obvious, the healers didn't really know what they were doing.

There was a single simple reason for the ignorance: in spite of every philosophical system that had ever been constructed, no one, but no one, knew for sure what causes disease. The Greeks had taught that a person gets sick because a combination of factors has gone askew, involving an interplay between one's basic nature, one's environment, and a set of external stimuli. Effective treatment, therefore, should consist of removing the insalubrious stimuli, and restoring the balance between the various factors. By the logic of this system, an entire individual gets sick, not just a part of him and not just an organ. Then, after Morgagni, the sick man became a man within whom was a sick organ; after Bichat, he became a man within whom was a sick tissue. Although disease theory focused deeper and deeper into the hidden recesss of the whole patient (and, paradoxically, moved farther and farther away from him as a human being), it nevertheless drew no closer to an identification of the actual cause of sickness.

Still, as long as surroundings, personal habits, or an entire life situation were thought to be the primary causative factors in disease, doctors seemingly could offer something to cure an abnormality. When, with Morgagni, the focus began to fall on ever less accessible internal sites, the target of therapy also became increasingly inaccessible. Before a whole man could be cured, the smallest beginnings of his pathology had to be found. That had not yet happened. Until it did, the idea of truly specific treatment directed at the particular mechanism that had gone wrong would remain a fantasy.

> *In spite of every philosophical system that had ever been constructed, no one, but no one, knew for sure what causes disease.*

This was the underlying difficulty which the physicians of the mid-nineteenth century still faced. The ultimate seats, or sites, of disease had not yet been localized; in what elemental structure, whether solid or fluid, does the very first thing go wrong? How does that first thing result eventually in the visible abnormalities that the new generation of pathologic anatomists were describing in increasing numbers of autopsies? Only when that initiating site had been identified would research be able to turn its attention away from conjecture, and toward the problem of specific therapy for a specific process.

To one scientist goes the credit of tracking down that elusive focus, that basic unit in which disease begins. That focus is, of course, the cell, and it was the supreme accomplishment of the German pathologist Rudolf Virchow that he discovered not only that the cell is the basic unit of disease, but also that it is the basic unit of health, and of life itself.

Once the cell theory took hold, there was no longer any need to speculate about altered body fluids, over- or under-supplies of irritability, or the effects of ill-defined stimuli. After Virchow, it was time to study the events that go on in a cell by which it maintains healthy life—what is called its normal physiology. Once that was understood, the cell's alterations in disease, its *pathologic* physiology or pathophysiology, could be elucidated. Pathologic physiology, and therefore disease, becomes thus reducible to a set of disordered biochemical phenomena susceptible to correction by highly specific therapeutic agents, or by the extirpation of the groups of cells, tissues, or organs in which the pathological event is occurring. That is the basis of twentieth-century medicine. It is the legacy left to us by Rudolf Virchow.

There is a paradox in all of this. At the same time that Virchow was the scientist whose microscope traced the focus of disease to its finite chamber, he was his era's leading exponent of the thesis that a man is the product of his life situation. Environmental influences, occupation, heredity, even social class played as strong a role in his image of the sick patient as did the pathological changes he saw through his high-power lenses. Although a spokesman for the philosophy of the ancient Cnidians, he was also a spokesman for the philosophy of the Hippocratic Coans. He recognized, as do all modern healers, the primacy of understanding specific pathophysiological processes if one is to cure disease. But he recognized also the primacy of the whole person if disease is to be prevented. The best medicine is practiced when both concepts find their appropriate usefulness in both the prevention and the cure. Virchow deserves to be

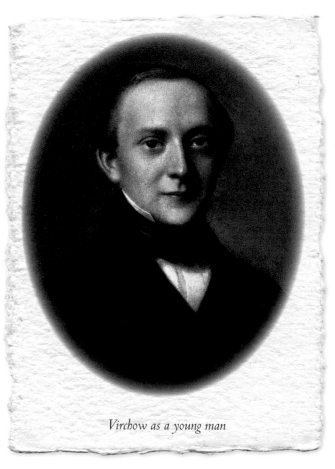

Virchow as a young man

the hero of those holistic thinkers of today who acknowledge the role of science, just as he is the hero of students of pathophysiology who understand the humanity of sick people.

Rudolf Ludwig Carl Virchow was born in Pomerania, the most northeastern of the provinces of Prussia, on October 13, 1821. The town of his birth lies some seventy-five miles inside Poland today, and goes by the name of Swidwin. But in 1821, that little town of Schivelbein was among the most Junker-influenced communities in all Germany, notwithstanding the doubtlessly Polish roots of some of its family trees, including that of the Virchows. Rudolf's father was a farmer who doubled as the treasurer of Schivelbein. One would hope that he handled the municipality's money better than his own, because he was often in financially straitened circumstances as the result of a succession of failed business ventures.

Rudolf studied at the community school, and took private lessons to prepare for the gymnasium, or high school, of Cöslin, the chief town of the district. By the time he came to Cöslin at the age of thirteen he had already mastered Latin; he embarked on an outstanding secondary-school career that saw him graduate at the head of his class in 1839. In the title of his graduation thesis there is a portent of things to come—it seems to foretell not only his attitude about his own career, but the emergence as well of a social conscience that exalted the labor of one's hands: "A Life Filled with Toil and Work Is No Burden, but a Blessing."

In the autumn of 1839, Rudolf enrolled at the Friedrich-Wilhelms Institut, a school whose purpose, as a unit of the University of Berlin, was to train medical officers for the Prussian army. Its appeal to the impecunious boy from the provinces lay in its free tuition; also appealing was the fact that, with German medicine beginning its ascent to the glorious heights it would later achieve, there were some outstanding teachers on the institute's faculty, including Europe's foremost physiologist, Johannes Müller. Müller was thirty-eight years old at the time, and had already done much of the work that would bring him recognition as the founder of scientific medical research in Germany. If there is one man to whose pupils all of the greatness of nineteenth-century middle-European medical accomplishment may be traced, it is Johannes Müller, a biologist, comparative anatomist, biochemist, pathologist, psychologist, and master teacher. His many disciples became the leaders of the next generation of medical progress; the greatest of them was Rudolf Virchow.

The Friedrich-Wilhelms Institut was in essence a military academy that served as a medical school. Life was spartan there. The curriculum, starched stiff with Prussian rigidity, left little opportunity for independent study. Fortified with the usual daily ration of sauerkraut, sausage, and beer, the students were forced to grind through sixty hours of classes each week, of which forty-eight were spent in the lecture hall. In a letter to his father, Rudolf wrote, "So it goes unceasingly every day from six in the morning to eleven at night except Sunday, and how rapidly the days and weeks fly you can see for yourselves. One becomes so tired that in the evening he sets his eyes toward the bed eagerly, from which he rises in the morning as tired as if he had slept in a half lethargy."

The overworked medical student nevertheless found the time to do some things on his own. He attended lectures on logic, on history, and on Arabic poetry. By then he could read Greek, Latin, and Hebrew, and he spoke several European languages fluently, including Italian, which he had taught himself during the summer between secondary school and the beginning of classes at the institute. He set out also to learn something about politics, and he developed a fascination with archaeology. When he had been in Berlin two years, he wrote home to his father that his aim was to acquire "no less than a universal knowledge of nature from the God-head down to the stone."

His father, Carl Christian Ludwig Virchow, did not approve of such a wide-ranging search for knowledge of so many things. To a failed entrepreneur whose fortunes rose and fell on the basis of his yearly potato crop, it was of paramount importance that his son be industrious in his classroom studies, so that he might make a good marriage and enter a thriving bourgeois medical practice. Security, comfort, and the trappings of upper-middle-class respectability were the eventual rewards Carl envisioned for the hardships his son was enduring in the Procrustean atmosphere of the Friedrich-Wilhelms Institut. He could not know how arid was the intellectual content of such a place, how stifling the daily routine and the uniformity of the students' expectations. Even had he heard them, he would not have understood that most of the lectures were without logic and those who suffered through them were memorizing without thought. His was not the kind of mind that could savor those precious few moments spent in the presence of men like Johannes Müller, who taught his pupils not the lucrative skills of the successful practitioner, but the excitement of researching into the basic truths of human biology. Mostly, Carl Christian Ludwig Virchow did not understand his son. He accused the boy of thinking himself too good for the ordinary curriculum, and so much wiser than his teachers that he could learn nothing from them. In February 1842, Rudolf wrote him the following letter:

My Dear Father,

You state that I am an egoist; that is possible. But you accuse me of having an overweening opinion of myself; that is far from being true. Genuine knowledge is conscious of its ignorance; how much and how painfully do I feel the gaps in my knowledge. It is for this reason that I do not stand still in any branch of science. I learn gladly, but I defend my opinions out of conviction. . . .

There is much that is uncertain and restless about me. . . . My future is too unsure. My circumstances for the present are very unfavorable, however much it may still appear that luck had accompanied me. They compel me to do what I would not like to do, and I can hardly hope to attain what I wish for. It was always thus. You wanted to make a fine society man out of me, something for which even now I care very little. In every school vacation you told me that all my knowledge was worthless without that. . . . My time is filled completely with hear-

ing, learning, and repeating things that are in part very insipid; for the things that really interest me, I can find time almost only at the expense of my health. Nevertheless, I occupy myself zealously with that which I do not desire and which I find unpleasant, because at some time it may well become the only means of my support. I will reconcile myself to it, and will even be able to renounce my favorite occupations. . . .

I want to say only this, that in me there is certainly much pride and egoism, even more than is good; also much that is phantastic and dreamy together with perhaps a little good. But you misunderstand me if you think my pride is based on my knowledge, the incompleteness of which I can see best; it is based on the consciousness that I want something better and greater, that I feel a more earnest striving for intellectual development than most other people.

Upon receiving his M.D. degree in 1843, Virchow was appointed to the equivalent of today's rotating internship at Berlin's Charité Hospital. Although the short, thin, blond-haired physician enjoyed his work on the wards, he found himself increasingly drawn to the research of the autopsy pathologist Robert Froriep, in whose laboratory he improved his ability to use the microscope. Because Froriep was coeditor of a journal that published summaries of foreign medical studies, Virchow soon made himself familiar with the latest work that was being done in the more advanced medical environments of France and England.

Within his first three years out of medical school, the enthusiastic young researcher made two of the three major discoveries that modern physicians associate with his name. The first was his discovery of leukemia in 1845, and the second was his demonstration in early 1846 of the true nature of the process by which blood clots cause thrombosis and embolism, terms which he introduced. The former contribution was made simultaneously by the Scottish physiologist John Hughes Bennett, who thought that what he was seeing in his microscope was a form of pyemia, or blood infection. Virchow, however, understood its true nature from the first, calling it "white blood" and later coining the word "leukemia."

Virchow's thrombosis-embolism research disproved a pet theory of the older generation of physicians. Because clots were so often found in blood vessels at autopsy, the French pathologist Jean Cruveilhier had preached the erroneous doctrine that phlebitis, inflammation of the veins, is the common denominator in all disease. *La phlébite domine toute la pathologie* was a motto he had made popular. When Virchow began his work with Froriep, he was assigned the project of studying the Frenchman's theory. He began by establishing criteria by which clots forming after death could be distinguished from those which occur as part of a disease process in the living patient. By his microscopic, chemical, and experimental animal studies, he identified two types of obstructing clots: the thrombus, which forms within a blood vessel at the site it is occluding, and the embolus, which is a thrombus that has detached itself from its point of origin and then traveled through the bloodstream to occlude some distant vessel. He solved a problem that had puzzled pathologists since Morgagni—the origin of the large clot that is so often found obstructing the major artery to the lungs of a patient who has died suddenly. In a paper he published in January 1846, "On the Occlusion of the Pulmonary Arteries," he demonstrated that such an embolus, usually from

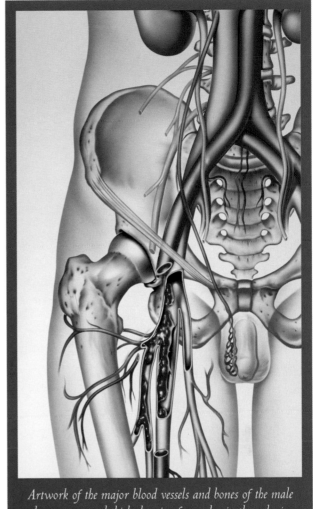

Artwork of the major blood vessels and bones of the male lower torso and thigh showing femoral vein thrombosis

veins in the legs or pelvis, is the cause of death in these patients. The doctrine of embolism—that a blood clot can travel long distances to obstruct a vessel in another part of the body—was the completely original idea of the twenty-four-year-old pathologist. It had never been considered by any previous investigator.

Cruveilhier was only the first medical icon to fall at the hands of Rudolf Virchow and his piercing scientific scrutiny. In his next episode of idol-smashing, an unfortunate impetuosity combined with his youthful self-righteousness to lead him to a bit of behavior that some of his contemporaries called ruthless. In the course of it, he demolished a speculative disease theory of Europe's most respected pathologist, Karl von Rokitansky of Vienna, with such devastating and calculated thoroughness that not a shred of it remained viable. Rokitansky's erroneous doctrine had originated in that never-never land where faulty reasoning is used to explain inaccurate observations. But although it deserved to be exploded, Virchow was so overly zealous in his attack that his assault had the effect of heaping ridicule on the head of the theory's promulgator, and his colleagues' disapproval on his own. The assault diminished, albeit temporarily, the esteem in which the older man was held throughout the medical community of Europe. It is a testament to Rokitansky's scientific honesty that he recognized his error and withdrew the theory; it is a testament to his dignified forbearance that not only his own reputation but his antagonist's survived the affair. Within a few years, a more mature Virchow would develop a far greater degree of sensible restraint.

Later in 1846, Virchow succeeded Froriep as Prosector in Pathology at the Charité. In the following year, in association with his friend Benno Reinhardt, he published the first volume of a journal which is still in existence today under the name *Virchow's Archive*. Its official title is a statement of the interrelationships of those aspects of human biology that its editor, for the rest of his life, would proclaim to be the trinity of scientific medicine: *The Archive of Pathological Anatomy and Physiology, and Clinical Medicine*. The basis of understanding disease, Virchow held, is the study of the way in which it distorts not only normal structure, but normal function as well.

The very first article in the *Archive* created an uproar among the physicians of Germany. In it, Virchow outlined his perception that disease is not an aberration engrafted onto a healthy organism, but is simply health disordered. The dominant theorists of his day viewed sickness as a condition quite foreign to the normal functioning of tissues, arising within the body or entering from without, living an enervating existence like some foreign parasite sucking out the strength of its unwilling host. To them, pathological tissues were produced *de novo* from a theoretical mother-substance gone wrong, or perhaps by deposition from the blood itself. By this formulation, diseased structures are so different from healthy ones that nothing can be learned about the one by studying the other, and it was this formulation that Virchow challenged in that first essay, "Points of View in Scientific Medicine," articulating his definition of that critical term "scientific medicine":

Scientific medicine has for its subject the changed conditions under which the diseased body or the particular ail-

> *Virchow outlined his perception that disease is not an aberration engrafted onto a healthy organism, but is simply health disordered.*

ing organs exist, the identifications of deviations in the phenomena of normal life which occur under specifically altered conditions, and, finally, the discovery of means for abolishing the abnormal conditions. This presupposes therefore a knowledge of the normal course of the phenomena of life and the conditions which make this normal course possible. Hence, the basis of scientific medicine is physiology. There are two parts to scientific medicine: pathology, which should provide information about altered conditions and altered physiology, and therapy, which seeks out the means of restoring or maintaining normal conditions. Essentially, clinical medicine is not scientific medicine, not even when practised by the greatest master; clinical medicine is the application of scientific medicine.

It must be recognized that this is not the time for systems, but the time for detailed investigations. . . . The final decision in these matters rests with a science which thus far exists only in its earliest beginnings and which appears destined to replace general pathology. I refer here to the science of pathologic physiology. . . . Pathologic anatomy is the doctrine of deranged structure; pathologic physiology is the doctrine of deranged function.

A science of pathologic physiology is necessary. . . . Pathologic physiology derives its questions in part from pathologic anatomy, in part from bedside medicine; it obtains its answers partly from observation at the sickbed . . . and partly from animal experiment. Experiment is the ultimate court of the science of pathologic physiology. . . .

Let us not deceive ourselves about the present state of medicine. It is undeniable that our spirits are exhausted by the innumerable hypothetical systems which are constantly being cast to the winds and replaced by new ones. A few more mishaps, however, and this time of disturbance will have passed by and it will be understood that only dispassionate, diligent, and steady work, true work of observation or experiment, has permanent value. The science of pathologic physiology will then gradually fulfill its promise, not as the creation of a few overheated heads, but from the cooperation of many painstaking investigators—a pathologic physiology which will be the stronghold of scientific medicine.

With this statement, the twenty-six-year-old researcher had laid out his credo for the medical world to see. He had also laid out the program for his life: alterations in structure provide clues to alterations in function; the key to understanding and treating sickness is to understand the ways in which normal function becomes abnormal. It is therefore in the study of pathophysiology that disease is to be conquered. Observation, experiment, hard work, and a steadfast disavowal of unjustifiable speculation—these were the intellectual weapons for the battle. They were inherited from Vesalius, and Harvey, and Hunter, and Laennec. Rudolf Virchow, an indefatigable student of medical history, acknowledged his debt to each of them.

The leading medical figures in Germany were not pleased to be admonished by a stripling that their adherence to various systems represented a misconception of the nature of science. But there was something about Virchow's supreme self-confidence that compelled them to continue listening. As he himself put it in a letter to his father:

I do not deceive myself. With real knowledge and forceful language, one can impress everyone today, even those in the highest ranks, because everything is empty and rotten up to the top. . . . Everywhere it is necessary to start again from scratch, and there is so much to be accomplished that sometimes one truly despairs. If I did not have the evidence before me that I am regarded at the Charité as an authority in scientific matters, and that *everyone believes what I say, I would surely have already given up. I, who have worked for such a short time, and who am ignorant of so much—I, an authority? It is ridiculous! Since I myself know so little, those who ask me must know even less.*

That was a fair statement of the situation. Some of the adherents of the various systems realized that they were groping in the dark, and were not unprepared to listen to a new voice that seemed so sure of itself. Because the new voice belonged to a young man who had, in his first few years out of medical school, made two major discoveries, they listened to it with particular interest. In addition, the incisive logic of Virchow's harsh debunking of Rokitansky, and the zeal with which he pursued it, had created an aura about him that made humbler minds hesitate to challenge his opinions thereafter. He was a scientific young Lochinvar, riding in to snatch the bride away from undeserving suitors. In this case, though, the prize was much greater than fair Ellen in a nuptial bower—what he sought was the soft hand of Nature herself, that he might better discover her closet secrets.

Virchow was also becoming interested in the relationships between disease and the environmental circumstances in which it occurred, and

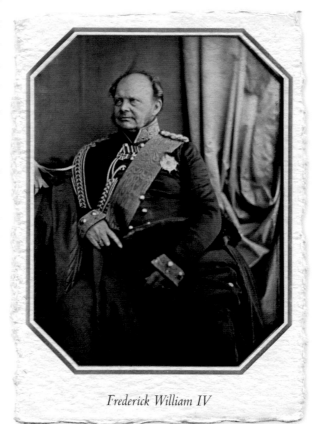

Frederick William IV

he did not hesitate to blame the contemporary social structure for some of the problems he saw. Early in 1848, word reached the capital of an epidemic of typhus among weavers in Upper Silesia, which, abetted by a concurrent famine and the failure of the local authorities to take action, was costing the lives of increasing numbers of the impoverished peasants in the region. In one of his letters to his father, he wrote, "This distress in Silesia is such a disgrace to the government that all their excuses cannot change it in the least. Nothing can mitigate the scandal which is created by the deaths of thousands. From the medical standpoint, the epidemic is so interesting that I have the strongest desire to see it close at hand."

The Berlin press badgered the Prussian ruler, Frederick William IV, to do something about the disaster. Finally, the public outcry forced the government to form a commission of investigation, under the direction of the Privy Councillor for Health. Rudolf Virchow's "strongest desire" was fulfilled when he was named medical officer to the commission. He arrived in Silesia on February 20, 1848, and spent almost three weeks studying not only the medical aspects of the epidemic but the environmental conditions in which it had originated. His report was a stinging rebuke to the authority of the crown and the way in which it dealt with its poorest subjects. The fact that he compounded his criticism by publishing it in the *Archive* did not endear him to the authorities.

Virchow wrote his report while the full fury of his wrath remained at its zenith. After a thorough description of the autopsy findings in the typhus victims, the kinds of treatments that had been used, and the epidemiological aspects of the outbreak, he left off the scientific discussion to engage his major thesis: misrule by the Prussian autocracy was the root cause of the Silesian calamity. It was a failure by the government to allow autonomous self-rule, to provide proper roads, agricultural improvements, and support of industry that had led to the present conditions. But the fundamental evil was Berlin's withholding of full democracy and universal education, which kept the peasants of Silesia in a state of moral degradation, personal filth, and indolence. As a physician, he felt his duty keenly: "Medicine is a social science and as the science of man, has a duty to perform in recognizing these problems as its own and in offering the means by which a solution may be reached." He offered the means, and he was willing to expend a great deal of the energies of his lifetime trying to implement them:

> *There is a simple and direct answer to the question of how similar conditions may be prevented in the future: Culture, with its daughters Freedom and Prosperity. Less simple, however is the practical solution of this great social problem. Without our realizing it, medicine has carried us into the social sphere, there to meet up with the great problems of our time. Let us be well aware that we are not concerned here with the treatment of a patient by means of medicinal remedies and the adjustment of his home environment. No, we are dealing with the entire culture of a million and a half of our fellow citizens who have been physically and morally degraded.*

A French medical philosopher of the late eighteenth century, Pierre Cabanis, had written, "Sickness is dependent upon the blunders of society." Virchow now became Europe's leading scientific exponent of that thesis. Many times during the course of his career he was able to demonstrate relationships between widespread diseases and social inequities. Not only typhus, but cholera, tuberculosis, scurvy, some mental diseases, and even cretinism were included in his list of those many maladies that result from the unequal distribution of civilization's advantages. He articulated again and again his conviction that the medical profession is responsible to do all in its power to abolish the social conditions that cause disease: "Physicians are the natural attorneys of the poor."

The ultimate power, however, is in the hands of rulers. In words his émigré countrymen Karl Marx and Friedrich Engels might have used (*The Communist Manifesto* was also published in 1848), Virchow stated in the conclusion of his report on Silesia, "Every individual has the right of existence and health, and the State is responsible for ensuring this." He wrote out a formidable agenda for his fellow physicians, but an even more demanding one for the processes of government. Already one of the rising young generals in the battle for scientific victory over disease, he now began his rapid rise in the ranks of those soldiers of social policy who had in their hands that most powerful of weapons, the making of laws. He entered the field of politics, in accordance with a statement he would write a few years later: "The improvement of medicine would eventually prolong human life, but improvement of social conditions could achieve this result more rapidly and more successfully."

Within a week of Virchow's return from Silesia, the popular uprisings that history has given the name Revolutions of 1848 exploded on the boulevards of Berlin. He and thousands of his fellow liberals threw up barricades in the streets against the government troops, in much the same manner as had been happening in the other capitals of Europe. The brief victory of the forces of democracy allowed the young firebrand to make violent speeches to large audiences of eager revolutionaries, with the result that he was elected to the new Prussian Diet. Being under the parliamentary age, he could not take his seat, but he created for himself a pulpit almost as bully as the one he was forced by his youth to relinquish—he founded a journal called *Medical Reform,* whose pages he filled with both his scientific and his political beliefs.

During this heady period of his life, there emerged a quality in Rudolf Virchow that was almost deliberately dangerous to his career. Not only were many of his political speeches overtly inflammatory, but he seemed at times to make a point of abrading the sensibilities of the conservative authorities in ways that he knew to be particularly offensive to them. In a community of the religiously orthodox, where loyalty to church was equated with loyalty to crown, he openly proclaimed his agnosticism. He fired off snidely clever anti-Hohenzollern jibes that were repeated many times with pleasure among his supporters, but provoked neck-reddening Prussian rage when they reached the ears of the royalists.

In fact, by openly thumbing his nose at the government in his writings and widely acclaimed speeches, Virchow was daring the authorities to revoke his appointment at the Charité. They took the dare. Not even his brilliant researches on leukemia, embolism, and thrombosis sufficed to save his job. He was ordered to resign.

The resignation lasted one week. Realizing that the forces of reaction were once more in the ascendancy, and that his radicalism would mean the end of his all-important research, Virchow became very pragmatic. When he was offered his job back in return for signing a statement promising to forgo the open expression of his political convictions, he agreed to sign.

The authorities, however, did not trust him, and began to look for ways to get him out of Berlin while still keeping him within the channel of German medicine's mainstream. The ideal op-

> "The improvement of medicine would eventually prolong human life, but improvement of social conditions could achieve this result more rapidly and more successfully."

portunity presented itself in the form of a specially created Chair of Pathology at the University of Würzburg. Würzburg's Professor of Obstetrics, Friedrich Scanzoni, who was a contemporary and an old friend, interceded with the government ministers to establish the post for Virchow, thus providing him with a warm and welcoming medical environment into which to be banished.

There was one item of great urgency to be attended to before the newly appointed professor left Berlin. Throughout his life he was known for his lack of attention to schedules, and for leaving or arriving at the last possible instant. Affairs of the heart were no exception. On the day of his departure for Würzburg, he became engaged to Rose, the seventeen-year-old daughter of his friend Carl Mayer. Mayer, although the most successful practicing obstetrician in Berlin, was a political progressive, whose home had become a salon in which liberal-thinking friends gathered several times each week for discussions and mutual support. To the selfless, worshipful Rose, the outspoken young doctor was a hero who was being made to suffer for his devotion to the cause of democracy. Of the romance and its culmination, her fiancé wrote with unaccustomed tenderness:

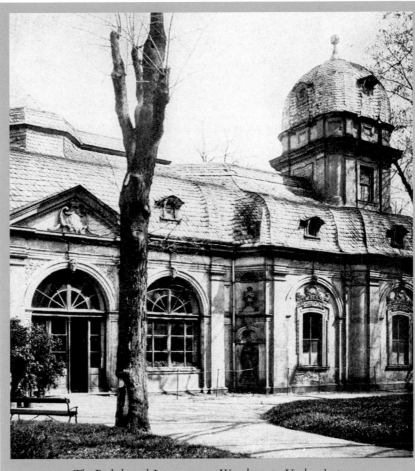

The Pathological Institution at Würzburg in Virchow's time

While listening to my conversations she grew so familiar with my thoughts, in a sense she was thus educated by me, so that I do not know anyone who could understand me better than she. And I, I became fond of her, I knew not how or when; but one fine day I became aware that unexpectedly she had taken possession of my heart. This happened at a very sad time. On the same day, the last day of March, when my little Rose was confirmed I received the official notification of my dismissal.

At that moment, I considered it more honorable to hide my feelings for Rose. . . . Thus I remained reserved, even after my appointment to Würzburg had come, and yet I was unable to leave Berlin. And when

I finally saw, how from day to day Rose was less able to hide her sadness, when I saw that she was suffering, and obviously on my account, I could not longer restrain myself. On Monday, I had come to say goodbye, but the afternoon already found us in each other's arms. Thus it happened.

As can be gathered from the foregoing paragraph, Rose considered her role to be that of helpmeet to the great man she had married. She nurtured no ambitions for herself, save to smooth the path for him. His brief description indicates, in fact, that he educated her for that kind of partnership. Very little has been written about her except that apparently no strains in her relationship with Virchow ever disturbed the serene course of their marriage, or the stable home in which their three sons and three daughters were raised.

When the new Professor of Pathology arrived in Würzburg, he found there a congenial atmosphere quite different from the bustling busyness of Berlin. Set among vineyards in the rolling Bavarian hills through which flows the Main River, the community of fifty thousand was one of those small gems of a university town for which Germany is noted. Throughout the nineteenth century, it attracted a superior medical faculty, whose leading lights at the time were, besides Virchow, Scanzoni and the embryologist and microscopic anatomist Albert von Kölliker. It was at this venerable institution that the Professor of Physics, Wilhelm Roentgen, would discover X-rays in 1895.

Virchow's arrival at the university must have intimidated some of his fellow faculty members. His abrasive knuckle-rapping of the revered Rokitansky, his solution of the fundamental puzzle of thrombosis and embolism, his discovery of

the entity of leukemia, all gave him an academic stature unmatched by that of any of his new colleagues, as well as the reputation of being a forceful defender of his own views. He was teaching himself English, which, with his ability to speak French, Italian, and Dutch, gave him a mastery of the five languages in which were written everything that was of any importance in contemporary science; his Greek, Latin, Hebrew, and Arabic were good enough to allow familiarity with older sources as well. Moreover, his volatile political reputation had preceded him. It was not without reason that the Bavarian ministry had resisted his appointment until the relentless pressure from Scanzoni and the bureaucrats in Berlin forced them to accede.

They need not have worried. Although Virchow continued some of his activities as a social reformer, he was neither revolutionary nor contentious during the Bavarian period. He had come too close to ruin in Berlin to be less than circumspect in Würzburg. He knew that if he was to realize his goal of reforming both the scientific and the sociological aspects of medicine, he must not continue on his incendiary path. He began his own reformation by allowing *Medical Reform* to die a quiet death. The next seven years were to be devoted to science.

Rudolf Virchow was only one of many chastened revolutionaries whose appetite for conflict was dulled by the ultimate failure of the Revolutions of 1848. All over Europe, idealistic young people became either discouraged or very practical or both, plunging themselves into work that had no political connections. The twenty-year-old German Ferdinand Cohn, later to become a pioneer bacteriologist, expressed the pessimism of the liberals in his diary note for September 25, 1849: "Germany dead; France dead; Italy dead; Hungary dead; only cholera and court-martials immortal. I have retired from this unfriendly outside world, buried myself in my books and studies; seeing few people, learning much, only inspired by nature."

Freed from political distractions, Virchow made his tenure in Würzburg the most productive period of his life. He was surrounded by a small group of able researchers, with whom he quickly proved his ability to work in harmony even though he had criticized the work of several of them prior to joining their company. He held the first Chair of Pathological Anatomy in Germany; he and Kölliker, who had come to the university only the year before, attracted a large number of students. In fact, some of Virchow's biographers opine that had he done nothing else, the galaxy of stars he trained during this time would have sufficed to establish him as one of the greatest teachers in the history of medicine.

The students had good reason to congregate in ever-increasing numbers. Not only was their professor a scholar of high attainment, but he was engaged in projects of the sort that fascinated the young physicians who had come to learn the new scientific medicine. In the space of the barely five years since Virchow had graduated from medical school, his work had transformed the curriculum, at least in Würzburg. What he taught was an epoch away from what he had learned in the lecture halls of the Friedrich-Wilhelms Institut. His researches embraced the subjects of inflammation, cancer, tuberculosis, typhoid fever, cysts of the liver, kidney disease, cholera, cretinism, amyloidosis, and the anatomy of the skin, nails, bone, cartilage, and connective tissue. He undertook, with others, the publication of a six-volume *Handbook of Special Pathology and Therapeutics,* and he collaborated on a manual of general pathology. In 1851, he and two of his colleagues began a *Yearbook of Achievements and Progress in Medicine,* which he continued to edit until his death,

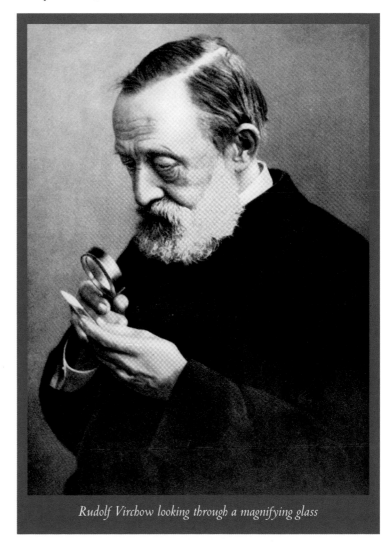

Rudolf Virchow looking through a magnifying glass

by which time it had long been known as *Virchow's Yearbook.*

During the Würzburg years, Virchow also developed some of the pedagogical methods he would use throughout his teaching career. Most memorable among them was his so-called table railroad, the moving track that passed the demonstration microscopes from student to student so that each might peruse the slides set up by their teacher. The rattling of the mounted instruments as they traveled along the conveyance system was frequently punctuated by Virchow's injunction "Learn to see microscopically."

To learn to see microscopically was to master the instrument by which medicine was beginning to magnify its view not only of the infinitely small processes of disease, but also of its ability to correct them. Improvements that had only recently been made in the technology of the lens systems set the stage, as it were, for the giant strides in medicine that were soon to be taken. More will be said about the vital importance to medical progress of those advances in microscope technique in the next chapter, but for now it is sufficient to point out that over the previous century and a half, no such advances had taken place.

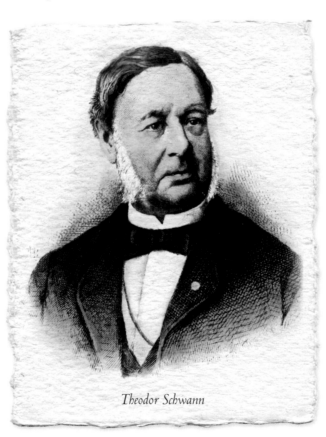
Theodor Schwann

Most of the material that Virchow mounted on the stages of his students' microscopes was used to demonstrate his rapidly evolving ideas about the structure of human tissues. It was in Würzburg that he developed his thesis that the fundamental unit of life is the cell. The word "cell" had been introduced into the vocabulary of science by the polymathic Robert Hooke in his book *Micrographia,* written in English in 1665, during that brief period when so many observations were being made with primitive microscopes. He wrote, "I took a good clear piece of cork, and with a pen-knife sharpened as keen as a razor, I cut a piece of it off, and thereby left the surface of it exceeding smooth, then examining it very diligently with a microscope, methought I could perceive it to be a little porous. These pores or cells were not very deep but consisted of a great many little boxes." Almost two hundred years later, those "great many little boxes" would be shown to be the building blocks of which all living organisms are constructed.

From time to time after Hooke's description, one investigator or another would make reference to cells, whether by that name or as "globules," or "vesicles," or "bladders," but their significance remained obscure for that century and a half until the researches of Giovanni Battista Amici and Joseph Jackson Lister resulted in the development of new lens systems, with which a wealth of observations began to be reported in the years after 1830. The first one of major importance was the discovery in 1831 by the English botanist Robert Brown that each plant cell contains within it a core structure he called a nucleus.

Brown reported his observation in the same year in which a twenty-seven-year-old German lawyer named Matthias Schleiden became so despondent over his inadequacies in the practice of his profession that he one day fired a bullet into his head. Fortunately for science, either his aim or his knowledge of anatomy was faulty, and he hit no vital part of his brain. Upon recovering, he took up the study of botany, which was a good thing, because he proved to be far more adept with plants than with plaintiffs or pistols. In 1838, he published what would prove to be a landmark paper describing experiments that supported his theory that all plant tissues consist of cells. Although he erred in stating that each cell develops spontaneously out of the material in its nucleus, he had, by his major step forward, established the beginning of a cell theory of life, and with it the foundation of the modern science of botany.

The next advance had its beginnings over coffee and cigars. Lingering one evening after a hearty meal with his friend Theodor Schwann, Schleiden discussed his findings at length. Schwann, who was one of Johannes Müller's favorite pupils, had already seen nucleated cells in animal tissues. Following his conversation with Schleiden, he set about to prove that what was true in botany was true also in zoology. In 1839

he published a book whose title told it all: *Microscopic Investigations of the Similarities in Structure and Development of Animals and Plants*. Schwann was sensitive to the fact that he was treading on ground that had been the subject of earnest debate for a score of centuries, not only among investigators, but among philosophers and theologians as well; his subject matter dealt with the very basis of life. Unlike Schleiden, who was a Jew, and Virchow, who recognized no authority higher than the top of his own cranium, the devoutly Catholic zoologist was willing to risk no possibility of an ecclesiastical rebuke. Before publishing his book, he submitted it to his bishop for approval.

Schwann was no Galileo, and his bishop was no Pope Paul V—his book was found not to violate any dogma. Coming so closely upon the heels of Schleiden's discovery, it proved to be the needed synthesis of all the significant findings that had been made in the microscopic study of cells since 1830. There had been such a confusion of new information produced by so many researchers that it had been growing impossible to see clearly through the profuse jumble of findings, or to separate valid experiments from misinterpreted observations. With Schleiden's work, and now Schwann's, the basic elements of the cell theory had been put forth. So linked are the names of those two scientists in the minds of present-day biologists that it is rare to hear one of them pronounced without the other; it would be like saying Gilbert without Sullivan or rock without roll. Schleiden and Schwann—the very euphony of it has been used as a mnemonic by freshman biology students for a hundred years.

There is a statement in Schwann's book that establishes the fundamental proposition of his theory: "There is one universal principle of development for the most elementary parts of organisms however they may differ, and that principle is the formation of the cells." It was to be understood that the cell itself is best described as a microscopic mass of protoplasm enclosed within a membrane, and endowed with a life of its own.

There remained the puzzle of where cells come from, and it is here that Schwann went astray. He believed that they arise not by generation from a parent cell but by a process analogous to crystallization within the organism, from a hypothetical mother liquor to which he gave the name "cytoblastema." Spontaneous generation, the concept that each new organism is newly produced from elementary substances or even nothingness, had been hotly debated since the beginnings of western civilization. Without entering into the theological implications of the argument, Louis Pasteur would usher it permanently off the stage of scientific consideration a few decades later, but for the moment it formed a major portion of Schwann's concept of cellular development.

It was Rudolf Virchow who prepared the way for its exit. The year in which Schwann's book appeared was also the year in which Virchow began his medical education at the Friedrich-Wilhelms Institut. The transfer of focus from tissues to cells, and then the clarification of the universality of the structure of all living things, stimulated ever more effective research. Virtually every medical phenomenon studied by Virchow after he began his career as an investigator was concerned in one way or another with cells. In an 1852 publication dealing with the cell as the basic unit of nutrition, he not only made no mention of the cytoblastema, but announced that his experiments led him to the be-

lief that a new cell can be produced only by the division into two of a cell already present. Two years later, he declared quite specifically, "There is no life except through direct succession." Finally, in 1855, he wrote an article in his own *Archive* in which he spoke of the pathology of the future, the pathology which would deal with events that occur within cells, events which maintain life when they go well and cause disease when they do not. It was in this paper that he used for the first time the aphorism which was to become the rallying cry of his disciples: *Omnis cellula a cellula,* every cell comes from a previously existing cell. Without equivocation, he affirmed the inevitability of his conclusion: "No matter how we twist and turn, we shall eventually come back to the cell."

Another inevitability was that the preeminence Rudolf Virchow had by this time attained in European science would ordain his being lured back to a professorship in Berlin. He had been sought out by other universities, but, happy and productive in the idyllic academia of Würzburg, he refused them all. The *gemütlich* collegiality of his fellow teachers and his separation from the prickles of politics calmed his natural pugnacity. He had three children and the most supportive of wives. In Würzburg, he had allowed himself to grow up. The Rudolf Virchow who in 1856 received the call to the Chair of Pathology in Berlin was a much wiser and more mature man than the fiery bridegroom whom the police of that city had tried to expel when he returned for his wedding six years earlier.

He agreed to accept the post that was now so entreatingly offered, but he laid down conditions. If the University of Berlin was to have him back, it was to be on his own terms. A pathological institute must be built for him, in which the practical work of research and hospital pathology would be done. The building was rapidly erected, and Virchow returned in triumph to be recognized as the most influential figure in German medicine. From this time on, a trend which had been increasingly evident over the course of the previous decade became a fact—captured by Rudolf Virchow, the baton of medical leadership passed from France to the German-speaking countries. There it would remain until the early part of the twentieth century, when it was wrenched away by war and the ascendancy of American science.

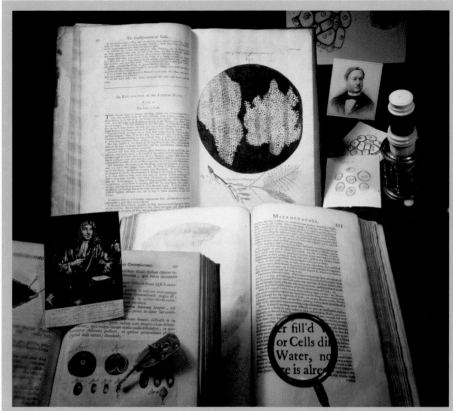

Composite photograph illustrating three major figures in the world of light microscopy. At bottom left is the Dutch naturalist Antoni van Leeuwenhoek (1632-1723), father of microscopy. Right is the contribution of Robert Hooke (1635-1703) who published the first book on microscopy, Micrographia. *Top right is Theodor Schwann (1810-1882), German physiologist, who showed that the cell is the basic unit of life.*

One of Virchow's first undertakings in Berlin was to acquaint the physicians of the city with the latest developments in the field of pathology, and with his own contributions. In order to present this material in a way that would be comprehensible to ordinary practitioners, he clarified it, organized it, and put it into the form of twenty consecutive lectures which he delivered at the new Pathological Institute biweekly between February and April of 1858. He hired a certain Herr Langenhaun to sit in the audience and take down

the lectures in shorthand exactly as he presented them. After what he describes as "but slight alterations," he published them as a book titled *Cellular Pathology* in the late summer. His intention, he wrote in the preface, was "to give a concise view of a comprehensive subject." So much interest was aroused by both the originality of the view and the importance of the subject that he was required, before a year had passed, to publish another edition. The first paragraph in the second edition's preface deserves to be reproduced here, because it says much about the scientist, his book,

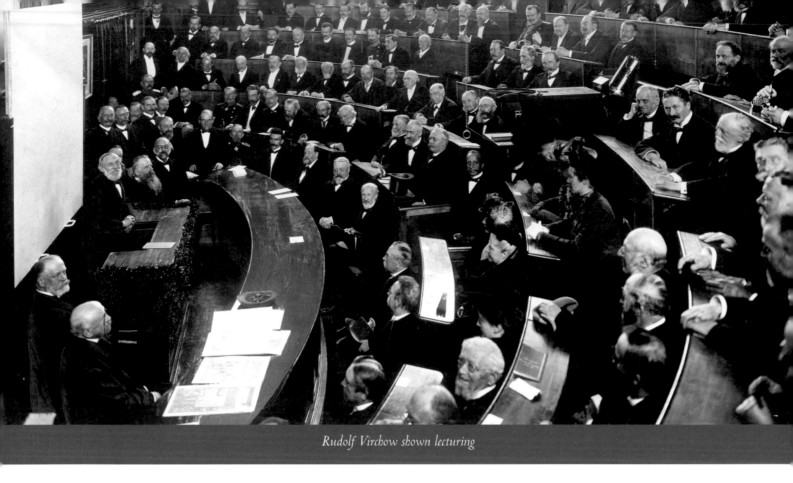

Rudolf Virchow shown lecturing

and the reception it aroused in the world community of medicine:

> *The present attempt to bring the results of my experience, which are at variance with what is ordinarily taught, before the notice of the medical public at large, in a connected form, has produced unexpected results; it has found many friends and vigorous opponents. Both of these results are certainly very desirable; for my friends will find in this book no arbitrary settlement of questions, nothing systematical or dogmatical, and my opponents will be compelled at length to abandon their fine phrases and to set to work and examine the matters for themselves. Both can only contribute to the impulsion and advancement of medical science.*

Virchow's contribution "to the impulsion and advancement of medical science" was incalcula-

ble. Almost a century later, Edward Krumbhaar, Professor of Pathology at the University of Pennsylvania and a distinguished historian of his field, wrote, "This book deserves to be placed with Vesalius' *Fabrica*, Harvey's *De Motu*, and Morgagni's *De Sedibus* . . . as the greatest tetrad of medical books since Hippocrates." In 1902, William Welch, who was considered at the time the dean of American medicine, wrote that the establishment by Virchow of the doctrine of cellular pathology marked the "greatest advance which scientific medicine had made since its beginning."

What Virchow accomplished in *Cellular Pathology* was nothing less than to enunciate the principles upon which medical research would be based for the next hundred years and more. In one sweeping declaration, he cleared the medical air of all residue of humors and humbug. The reliance on the evidence of one's senses demanded by Vesalius, the emphasis on experiment demanded by Harvey and Hunter, the painstaking search for primary seats of symptoms demanded by Morgagni, the meticulous correlation between the manifestations of disease and their anatomical basis demanded by Laennec—all found their point of focus in the work of Rudolf Virchow. In the slightly purplish prose of one of his pupils, the physician-writer Carl Ludwig Schleich, "His was an eagle's eye, that saw deep into the most secret reaction of the sick organism, and traced the grey footprints of death and disease over the flower-strewn fields of life. . . . He never rested in his efforts to trace the dragon of sickness to its remotest lair, and it was his unforgettable achievement to follow it to its final retreat in the mosaic caverns of the organism, the cells."

Schleich's lavender language may be overblown, but his description nevertheless underestimates the magnitude of Virchow's contribution. He did much more than merely track the dragon to its mosaic caverns; he discovered that even the finite structure of disordered anatomy is only a clue—the real cause of disease is to be found not in disorders of form but in disorders of function. It is not the way the sick cell *looks* that is the problem, but the way it *acts;* the key is therefore not the cell itself, but what goes on inside of it; it is not to pathological anatomy but to pathologic physiology that physicians must look to solve the fundamental riddles of sickness.

> *The very origins of life go down the bathroom drain hundreds of billions of times each day.*

And so, after *Cellular Pathology,* microscopic studies of healthy and diseased tissues began to be used to investigate the chemical and physical events that were occurring within cells. The research specialties of physiology and biochemistry expanded rapidly. Pharmacology immediately outgrew its image as some kind of medical botany and began to take on its rightful role in paving the pathways back to biochemical health. For the first time in the long history of cancer's destructiveness, the healers understood that malignancies arise from normal structures—a patient's first cancer cell is not an invading parasite or a nubbin left over from embryological development, but the offspring of a healthy parent in which some alteration has occurred.

That the healthy parent itself had a healthy parent was another of Virchow's propositions. Each cell has a sire and a grandsire and a great-grandsire and a direct line of ancestry that, were it somehow traceable, would lead inexorably back to the puddles of primordial ooze in which life first arose so many millions of years ago. A cell reproduces itself by dividing into two by a process called mitosis; there is no spontaneous generation, there are no rabbits in nature's hat. There is only a continuity from one cellular unit to its offspring. All the cells of all of us are cousins. More than one biology teacher has illustrated the consecutiveness of the process by pointing out to his class that each time we wash our hands, we destroy numberless thousands of skin cells, and thereby end a line that stretches back to the dimmest prehistory of our species. The very origins of life go down the bathroom drain hundreds of billions of times each day.

There was more. It is exactly because the cell is the center of all the inherited phenomena of life that it is critical to understand its relationship with its environment, meaning not only its fellow cells, but also the medium in which they exist together. That medium is called the extracellular fluid. The extracellular fluid not only brings nourishment to each cell, but at the same time provides it with a vehicle for the disposal of the wastes produced by its functioning. Twenty years after *Cellular Pathology,* the French physiologist Claude Bernard introduced the concept of the *milieu intérieur,* the internal environment in which the cells are bathed and from which they take the materials they need for life, returning to it the end products of their metabolism.

The cycle of William Harvey was thus completed: the circulating blood replenishes and sanitizes the extracellular fluid, which is basically a filtered product of itself. The materials brought by the blood to the extracellular fluid pass into the cell in exchange for those end products the cell no longer needs or those which it has produced to supply the needs of other cells, such as hormones and di-

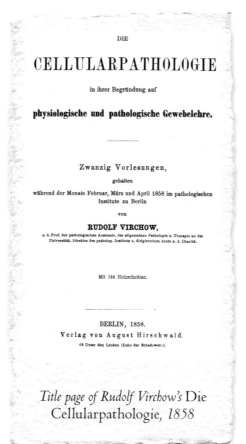

Title page of Rudolf Virchow's Die Cellularpathologie, *1858*

gestive enzymes. The process is called osmosis. When the philosophers of previous centuries had so blithely spoken of the balance of nature, and of the animal economy, they never really knew how to define those inexact terms, although they used them freely. The work of Rudolf Virchow ultimately led to the discovery of their meaning: the exquisite balance of nature that provides the mutually nourishing exchanges of which every cell partakes, in every living thing.

The animal or plant thus is to be viewed as a complex organism made up of an assemblage of simple microscopic organisms, the cells, in biochemical balance with the nourishing fluid in which they are bathed. Each of those individual cells makes its own highly specific contribution to the life of the animal or plant. Similar kinds of cells doing a similar type of job tend to be grouped together within the tissues that make up the organs of the body. A single human organ, such as the spleen or kidney, carries out multiple functions because it has multiple tissues and multiple kinds of cells within it.

Consider a short tubular length of upper intestine, with its various layers. There is an external coating of shiny, moist protective tissue whose flattened cells enable the gut to slither safely against its adjacent coils in the capacious recesses of the abdomen; just inside this is a layer of variously oriented muscle tissues that cause the gut to undulate and squeeze in such a way that it grinds up food and mixes it with intestinal juice so that it can peristalse its way onward; the inner-most layer is composed of absorp-tive tissue whose cells, in addition to secreting mucus, allow digested nutrients to pass through to enter the tiny capillaries of the blood-stream; the capillaries enter deeper vessels which course through yet another layer, which not only func-tions as a cushion between absorp-tive lining and muscle tissue but also contains clumps of lymphatic cells that filter filth and partake in as yet undiscovered mechanisms of immunity. There is more: the inner lining is bejeweled with tiny nests of hormone- and enzyme-producing cells, and who knows what else. The intestine, by the way, is a simple organ. Try the liver.

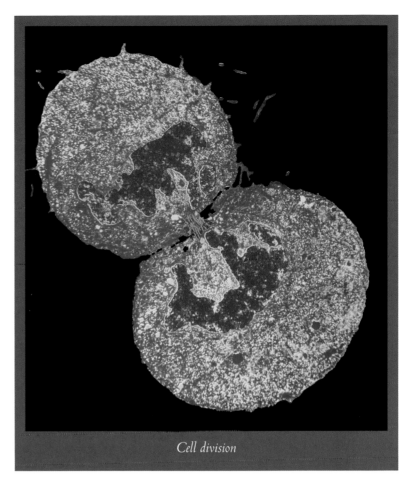

Cell division

It is not difficult to understand why a scientist as sociologically aware as Rudolf Virchow should have seen an analogy between the whole organism and the State. The State is, after all, made up of many individuals of different sorts, grouped into economic, social, and political or-ganizations that serve the common good in dis-tinct ways. Although the whole organism may be governed from a central station, its life is really the totality of the lives of each of the individual members. To quote from the first lecture of *Cel-lular Pathology:*

The structural composition of a body of considerable size, a so-called individual, always represents a kind of social arrangement of parts, an arrangement of a social kind, in which a number of individual existences are mutu-ally dependent, but in such a way, that every element has its own special action, and, even though it derives its stimulus to activity from other parts, yet alone effects the actual performance of its own duties.

The major principles set forth in *Cellular Pa-thology* remain the major principles of medical science today. Certainly, Virchow made errors in some of his formulations. Some of the errors were unavoidable because of the state of knowl-edge and technology of his time, and some were due to flawed reasoning that did not hold up against the evidence discovered by later workers. But he managed to disenfranchise the systematists and to build the true lasting framework whose blueprint had eluded all of his predecessors. He built it on the solid foundation of the scientific method.

Two months after Rudolf Virchow's birth in Pomerania, there had come into the world in the city of Rouen a French infant who was destined to write a book that would prove to be, like *Cellular Pathology,* another of those startling path-pointers to modern thought. One year before the publication of Virchow's text, the Frenchman's book appeared on the shelves of Parisian dealers. It was a scandalous novel called *Madame Bovary*. Its author,

Gustave Flaubert, and his publisher had survived a formal indictment on charges of immorality when the work had earlier been printed as a series in the *Revue de Paris*. At that time, the dispirited and pessimistic Flaubert had written to a friend: "This book is much more indicative of patience than of genius, of labor than of talent." Had he been asked, Rudolf Virchow would have said the same thing about *Cellular Pathology*, but for a different reason. Flaubert said it because he believed it. Virchow by then knew enough to hide his inherent immodesty, and so he too would have denied what was obvious to any clear-eyed reader—not only patience and labor, but also genius and talent are in abundant evidence on each page of both of the two masterworks.

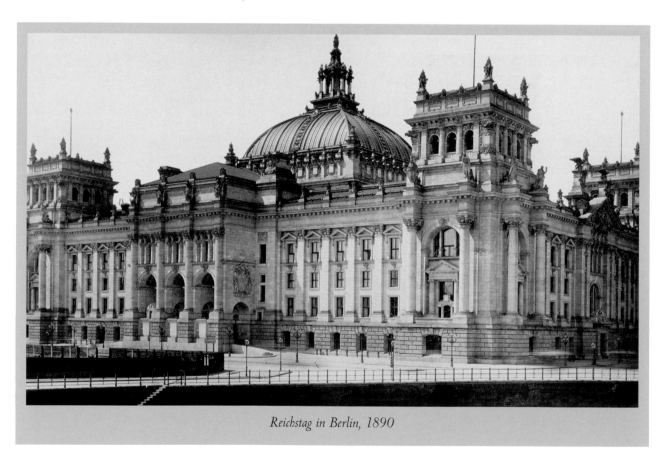

Reichstag in Berlin, 1890

Virchow had all of those qualities in abundance, and he did not spare their use, nor did he restrict it to the field of scientific research. His belief in the mutual dependence of the basic units of social organization extended itself to the body politic. Having returned to Berlin, he returned also to the insistent rumblings of his liberal conscience. In his later years he would become known as "the Pope of German medicine," but he was another kind of Pope as well, in his dedication to the English poet's proposition that the proper study of mankind is man.

There have been so many confused meanings of the word "humanism," especially in late-twentieth-century America, that it is refreshing to look back at its definition by the precise mind of Rudolf Virchow; he saw humanism as having evolved since the Renaissance to allow for the insights of science: "the scientific knowledge of the manifold and various relations of the thoughtful individual person to the ever-changing world." Such a definition included cells, psyche, and social status. It included the health of each organ, the health of the entire person, and the health of the society. Man was to be studied not only with the microscope, but with the macroscopic view that sees the universal vision of his humanity. To this end, it was necessary for Virchow to return to politics.

In 1859, Virchow was elected a member of the Berlin City Council, an office he would hold for forty-two years. This was followed in 1862 by his election to the Prussian House of Deputies, where he became one of the founders of the radical German Progressive Party. From 1880 to 1893, he was a member of the Reichstag. Most of his work on the City Council dealt with public health matters, largely in an attempt to solve the dreadful problems that existed at that time in the hospital system and in the sanitation of the municipality. Most Berliners had no indoor toilets or central water supply. The toilets that did exist emptied into deep gutters leading to the city's canals and the fouled depths of the sluggish Spree River. Some observers have called mid-nineteenth-century Berlin a city built on a sewer. Various foreign visitors have left accounts of the ever-present stench of human leavings that corrupted the air. The nostrils of the young Henry Adams, recently arrived from the pristine precincts of Boston, were particularly offended. In later years he wrote of the capital city of Germany that it was "dirty, uncivilized, and in most respects disquieting. . . . The condition of Germany was a scandal and nuisance to every earnest German, all of whose energies were turned to reforming it from top to bottom."

Among the most earnest, and certainly the most energetic, of the reformers was City Councillor Rudolf Virchow. Driven along by the vigor of his enthusiasms, the civic authorities adopted his programs for improving the sewage system, revamping the old ineffective hospital organization, and setting new criteria of hygiene for the public schools. He was responsible also for instituting stricter methods of food inspection and elevation of the standards for the training of nurses. During his four decades of service to the city, his influence wrought major changes in every area of public health. By the turn of the century, the individual units who were his fellow Berliners were surrounded in all aspects of their lives by an environment far more nourishing and sanitary than the milieu in which he found them when he took up his labors in 1859. The entire organism of Berlin was healthier by far. At his death in 1902, the

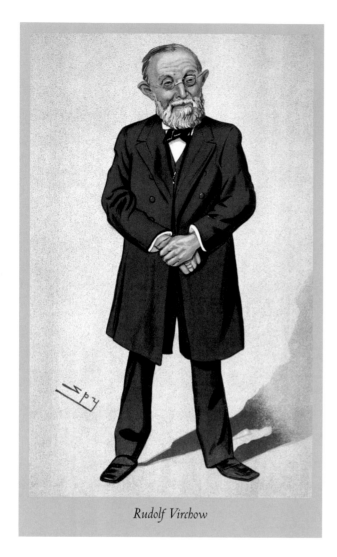

Rudolf Virchow

be directed by an aristocracy of princes and Prussian landowners. Although, paradoxically, a good many liberal and democratic gains were made during his tenure, they were meant only to blunt the demands of the progressives, to "steal the socialists' thunder," as Bismarck himself put it. The tone of his regime was set by a single sentence in the first speech he made after his appointment as prime minister: "The great questions of our day cannot be solved by speeches and majority votes—that was the great mistake of 1848 and 1849—but by blood and iron."

The year in which Bismarck was chosen to lead Germany was the year in which Rudolf Virchow was elected to the Abgeordentenhaus, or House of Deputies, which was the lower chamber of the Prussian Diet. The upper chamber was the Herrenhaus, or House of Lords. A concurrence of timing and a collision of temperament set the stage for a personal antipathy between the two strong-willed men that persisted until the end of the chancellor's career in 1890. Virchow was no longer a mere *provocateur* as he had been in 1848, but a mature political figure who spoke against the policies of the regime with logic and determination; he made the German Progressive Party, with himself as its chief goad, the constant antagonist of Bismarck's machinations.

Matters came to a head in 1865. Virchow, as chairman of the finance committee of the House of Deputies, defeated Bismarck's demand for an appropriation to expand the German navy. Seeking a pretext to rid himself for good of his irritating opponent, Bismarck accused the scrappy opposition leader of having called him a liar during the course of the debate. That Bismarck did plenty of lying is something that was never doubt-

British Medical Journal correctly pointed out: "It is not too much to say that modern Berlin is a splendid monument of his zeal in the service of his country." Virchow did for the physiology of his city what Christopher Wren did for the anatomy of London.

In matters strictly political, however, Virchow's labors were to be largely in vain. Junker-led in the person of Otto von Bismarck after 1862, Germany pursued a relentless course toward conservatism, chauvinism, and European supremacy. The Imperial Germany envisioned by Bismarck was to

ed by any of his contemporaries, and Virchow was certainly not the first opponent to call him on it. Nevertheless, the brawny, physically imposing Junker sent the slight, bespectacled professor a letter of challenge to a duel, naming the minister of war as his second. It was an act of cowardice on Bismarck's part; expert in the use of sword and pistol, skilled in all the questionable arts of the Prussian dueling class, he had stooped to a revenge that was laughable in its unseemliness. Virchow did, in fact, laugh. What gave him even more satisfaction was to make others laugh too, by offering to accept the challenge only if his opponent would agree to fighting it out with scalpels. His final derisive response was to point out that his life was too important to be offered up as a silly sacrifice to his challenger's honor. The duel never took place.

But after Bismarck had managed to manipulate Prussia into his much-desired war against Austria and the rest of Germany in 1866, the success of that venture increased his strength and split the opposition. Germany was now well on the way toward unification, an outcome so widely wished by its citizenry that even the liberals fell, for the most part, into the prime minister's bed. Virchow's power to lead a strong opposition was broken. No longer did he represent the majority viewpoint; he was thereafter the voice only of a small group of progressive thinkers. Though he was elected to the German Reichstag in 1880, he took little part in the debates of that parliamentary body.

If his political enemies had raised any questions about Virchow's physical courage in the wake of the aborted duel of 1865, they were answered by his service in the Franco-Prussian War of 1870–1871. With his two older sons as orderlies, he put himself in charge of the first hospital train that went to the front. He took an active role in caring for the wounded, most conspicuously in the fighting around Metz. Although both of his boys came down with typhus, from which they fortunately recovered, he continued his work to assure the proper treatment and transportation of the injured troops. Much impressed by the work done by American physicians during the Civil War, he used some of their methods of design in the building of military hospitals.

The Red Cross, which had been officially recognized only four years before, at the Geneva Conference of 1866, represented to Virchow the finest exemplification of the proper ideology-blind humanitarian instincts of the art of healing. He wrote:

The mission of medicine is above all to prepare for the era of peace. In the midst of the horrors of war, she and she alone is officially called upon to be present on the battlefield as the representative of humanity and peace among men. Without discriminating, she takes friend and foe alike into her helping arms, to heal the bleeding wound, to nurse the broken limb, to cool the thirsty lips. In the powder-smoke of battle, she unfurls the banner with the red cross on it, which all civilized nations have now recognized as the symbol of immunity. She erects a sacred asylum for the wounded, protecting them from further attack, and assuring them of skilled assistance. Wherever there is need, her simple tents and barracks are erected, as shelters of human love and compassion.

When the war ended, Virchow returned to science. But though he continued to make contributions to the literature of pathology, he spent his research energies increasingly with anthropology rather than with medicine, eventually producing a total of 1,180 publications in that field, including several books. The anthropological studies grew out of his never-ending search for the origins of life. Whether seeking man's essence in the protoplasm of his cells or in the structure of his skull, the quest was always the same—what is that essence, how did it get its start, by what path has it arrived where it is today, and what can be done to keep it in harmony with its fellows and its environment? For all time, those will remain the eternal questions, toward whose answers no one has ever taken greater steps than Rudolf Virchow.

The work in anthropology thus naturally extended itself into ethnology and archaeology, as Virchow sought to understand the nature and origins of races, cultures, and ancient civilizations. Always an active member of numerous medical organizations, he now became instrumental in the founding of the German Anthropological Society and the Berlin Society for Anthropology, Ethnology, and Primitive History. He edited several journals in these disciplines and he was a founder of the Museum of Ethnology in Berlin. Among the assistant curators who came under his influence at the museum, from 1883 to 1886, was a young man named Franz Boas, who later emigrated to the United States, where he became a major force in American anthropology. To many, Boas is best known as the teacher of Margaret Mead.

Virchow arranged the financing of any number of anthropological and archaeological expeditions, and he personally took part in several himself. Among them was the famous dig in which

Heinrich Schliemann discovered the ruins of ancient Troy. Several colleagues who accompanied Virchow on his Trojan journey have left reminiscences of his medical care of the impoverished local population of the area in which they were working. It was due to his friendship with the peripatetic Schliemann, who had become an American citizen, that the latter donated his discovered treasures to the Berlin Museum of Ethnology.

There were other digs, in the Caucasus and in Egypt. In each study, Virchow applied all of the tools of the emerging scientific technology to aid him in solving the riddles presented by his findings. When Conrad Roentgen discovered X-rays in 1895, Virchow, although seventy-four years old, was quick to put them to use in the analysis of his unearthed finds. The value of such studies, his leadership of societies and journals, and his major contributions to the theory of skull growth made Virchow one of the leaders of German anthropology. Indeed, so prominent a figure is he in the history of that discipline that many of its fraters have no idea that he held equal status in the field of medical science, or they assume that the founder of cellular pathology must be some other fellow with the same name.

Somehow, because of the popularized form of history that recalls the events of the past as a series of anecdotes, Rudolf Virchow is best remembered by more than a few as the disprover of one of his fatherland's most dangerous national myths, the theory of German racial purity. The pernicious fantasy of direct descent from some mighty Germanic *Volk* or bioethnic nation has been used to justify some of the most heinous crimes in the history of mankind. On a lesser scale of malice, that bogus belief has excluded some of the nation's greatest figures from being accepted as full members in the community of German-speaking peoples.

Part of the mythology that follows from the belief in an unadulterated *Volk* is the mischievous proposition that no one can be a German in the cultural sense unless he is also a German in the sense of stainless biology. The next malicious step from such an absurdity is to impugn the patriotism of everyone whose physical characteristics mark him as not directly descended from the fantasized tall, blond, blue-eyed warriors of days gone by. The reality around them of a great variety in the height, shape, and coloring of their ethnic fellows has never been permitted to interfere with the self-righteous cant of racists, be they German or anything else.

Little wonder, considering his own Slavic ancestry, that Virchow, as one of the greatest contributors to his country's culture, should scoff at this offense to both humanism and scientific reality. His detailed studies of the structure of tribal skulls dug up all over northern central Europe convinced him of the implausibility of there having been any archetypal Germanic progenitors. To prove his point further, he undertook in 1876 to conduct a survey of some 6,760,000 German schoolchildren to determine frequencies of

various combinations of eye, skin, and hair color. Researchers in Austria, Holland, Belgium, and Switzerland soon began similar studies of their own.

The results were as might have been expected by anyone who was not blind. Fewer than 32 percent of German children had the supposed coloring of their putative Teutonic ancestors, while more than 54 percent were a mongrelly mixture of color types. More than 14 percent were found

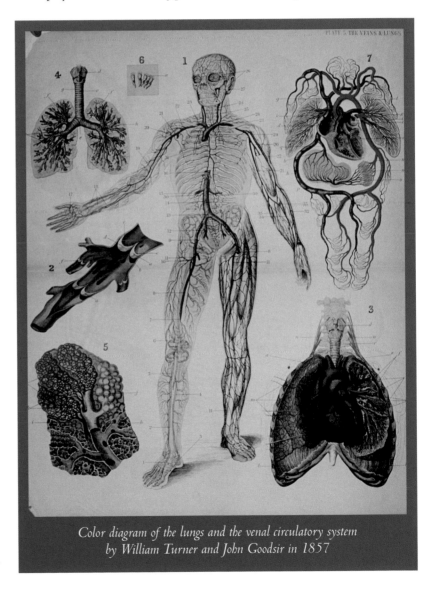

Color diagram of the lungs and the venal circulatory system by William Turner and John Goodsir in 1857

to be full "browns": brown eyes, brown hair, and brownish skin.

The census of the Jewish children of Germany was made separately, and its almost predictable outcome lent public support to Virchow's oft-pronounced rejection of the rising tide of German anti-Semitism. Although the Jewish group as a whole had a significantly higher proportion of "browns" at 42 percent, more than 11 percent had the perfect blond hair, blue eyes, and light skin of the idealized, albeit nonexistent, pure strain of Teutons. The remaining 47 percent demonstrated the same mongrel mix of hues as did the majority of their German classmates. The final results of the study were published in the *Archive of Pathology* in 1886, three years before the birth of Adolf Hitler. Of the many reasons invoked by the dictator to castigate Virchow's memory, the ethnic census ranked at the top of the list.

Virchow enjoyed nothing more than this kind of study, because it gave the lie to a popular misconception that seemed to have a basis in some authoritative source or accepted wisdom. To him, the first business of both science and politics was to expose the flimsy tissue of which an unsupported doctrine was woven, and then to undo its threads and cast them to the four winds. Once he had blown up an erroneous theory, he pursued the unsolved problem's solution like a sleuth, until he was able to replace the old error with a formulation that was in accordance with observable phenomena and verifiable experiments, and was susceptible of being proved true. But even this was usually not enough. Having arrived at the new doctrine, he considered it imperative that it be announced to the world in such an emphatic way that not only would it be accepted as a definitive

truth, but its author would be hailed as the sole discoverer of a new continent of thought.

It was in this latter aspect of his scientific quest that Virchow exposed himself all of his life to charges of self-promotion. Having made one of his surpassing contributions, he was reluctant to share the laurels with others whose work might in any way dim the luster of his own priority. No matter how independently he had reached his conclusions, there were always a few investigators whose efforts had paralleled his. But for accidents of timing and the vagaries of research, for example, we would today credit much of the cell theory to the German scientist Robert Remak or the Englishman John Goodsir. Virchow took his research just a little further than they took theirs, and put forth his scientific argument just a little better. As one of his biographers, Erwin Ackerknecht, has stated: "In addition to the fact that Virchow's findings were more meaningful, he propagated them with that tireless zeal and almost sinister energy in which nobody has ever excelled him."

In spite of Virchow's great popularity in England, a few of that country's scientists have not to this day forgiven him for failing to accord what they consider proper honor to Goodsir. As recently as 1958, Professor A. H. T. Robb-Smith of Oxford's Radcliffe Infirmary was provoked to write a letter to the *Lancet* in which he pointed out that the famous aphorism *Omnis cellula a cellula* had actually been first used by someone named Raspail in 1825. The occasion of Robb-Smith's letter was the ceremonial surrounding the centennial of *Cellular Pathology*, to which he replied in part that while "it is churlish to denigrate the commemoration of a great man's achievements... Virchow's great contribution to the concept of the continuity of cell life was not his originality of thought... but his propagandist ability to convince his colleagues of the absolute rightness of his views."

Of course, the accused propagandist would not have been so successful at his campaigns had he not himself been so completely convinced of his "absolute rightness," a conviction that was strengthened in every instance by the sheer volume of the documentation he provided for his opinions. He never presented an idea that was half-baked; though his theories, like those of all scientists, were neither perfect nor complete, they never lacked for supporting evidence. Self-aggrandizement was not his foremost motive, if indeed it was a motive at all. He wanted only to achieve recognition for the theories themselves, and it was to this end that he admittedly went out on the hustings. The hustings of science being regional meetings and scholarly journals, he was a prolific writer and a frequent presence at gatherings of his peers, as well as a leader in several prominent medical societies. In the following chapter there

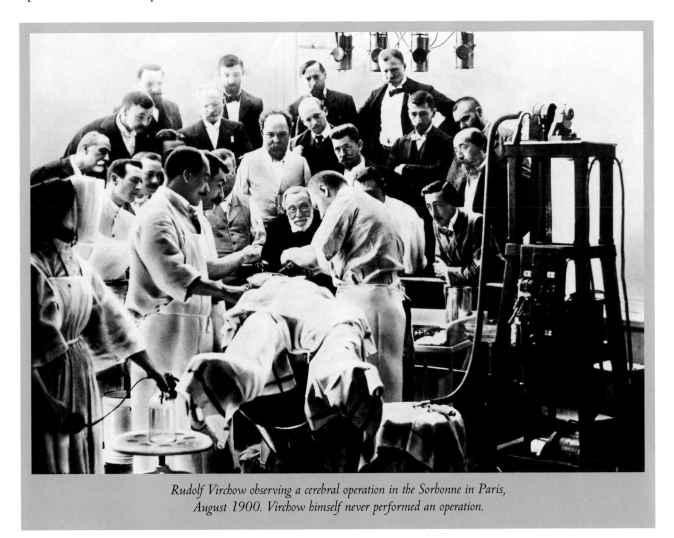

Rudolf Virchow observing a cerebral operation in the Sorbonne in Paris, August 1900. Virchow himself never performed an operation.

will be described the similar scientific evangelism of a much more self-effacing physician, Joseph Lister, who understood as well as his German colleague the pragmatic necessity of propagandizing for truth.

"Self-effacing" was not an adjective that has ever been used in relation to Rudolf Virchow. The brashness of the young agitator of 1848 matured into the certitude of the Pope of German medicine. In 1868, he wrote an accurate appraisal of the influence he knew he would have on the generations to come: "When they speak of the German School, it is me that they mean."

Such a man does not treat his students with kid-glove gentleness. He was a bit of a martinet, who was irresistibly given to dripping sarcastic acid on the intellectual fingers of fumbling assistants. Nevertheless, though they sometimes trembled in his presence, all who dealt with him knew that their professor was basically a kindly man, and his generosity of spirit earned him the loyalty of several generations of younger scientists; the success of many of them was due in no small part to his encouragement and his inculcation of meticulous patterns of thinking.

Carl Schleich was Virchow's assistant at the Charité for three years. In his autobiography, *Those Were Good Days*, he gives a vivid description of his first encounter with his chief, then sixty-two years old. The new assistants were dressed in the formal attire which was *de rigueur* on such occasions:

> We stood before the door in dress coats, white ties, gloves, and silk hats. . . . The door opened; the chief attendant, Hübner, Virchow's autocratic factotum, ushered us "medical apprentices," as he called all probationers, into the room, and we stood before the potentate: a little yel-low-skinned, owl-faced, spectacled man with peculiarly piercing yet slightly veiled eyes, which were conspicuously lacking in eyelashes. The eyelids were parchment-like and thin as paper. The nose was firmly chiselled, expressing the pride of its owner in its gracefully curving nostrils, which quivered, as though half scornfully, when he spoke. The lips were pale and bloodless, and the grey beard was thin. He was eating a roll and butter as we entered, and beside his plate stood a cup of café-au-lait. This was his lunch; his only refreshment between breakfast and dinner, though his day was spent in lecturing, receiving callers, examining candidates, recording the findings of the dissecting room, making anthropological measurements, attending the sessions of parliament, etc. His wife, who in her manners and way of speaking had acquired the very rhythm of her husband, and was entirely under the spell of his eminence, told me once that Virchow almost always worked until 1:00 A.M. and later at home, and was never in bed after 6:00 A.M. Nevertheless, during the six semesters which I spent in his Institute he was never once absent (apart from holidays and professional journeys).

Virchow was not an ascetic, but he did live a simple, unadorned life, without ostentation or any need for social deference from or to anyone. Distinctions, honors, and plaudits came to him aplenty, but they never changed the simplicity of his attitude toward himself. Pope he may have been, but he was a common man withal, free of pretension and free of class consciousness. At his death, a correspondent for the *Times* of London wrote:

> He was always the same, whether shaking hands with Royalty, accepting the respectful homage of an important deputation, packing up in his own house, or lecturing

to the most scientific gathering in the world—always the simple little grey man, sincere, kindly, unassuming, absorbed in his subject, not in himself, crammed with information, profound and penetrating in thought, plain in utterance, the embodiment of accurate knowledge and sound judgement, the true servant of truth.

It was said of Virchow by one of his students that the only reason he rode in the second-class railway carriage on his frequent excursions was that there was no third class. With friends he was a genial companion who loved to hoist a seidel of beer and sing a song once in a while. His children adored him, although the hours he spent with them were restricted to weekends and some vacations. As has been noted earlier, his wife created a living pattern in their home that was paced to his professional work.

The typical Virchow day was fully described by another former assistant, Sir Felix Semon, who had trained in Berlin before emigrating to England:

He would conduct an examination from 8 to 10, would superintend a microscopic class from 10 to 12, would lecture from 12 to 1, would be in the Reichstag from 2 to 5, in the Town Council from 5 to 6, in some

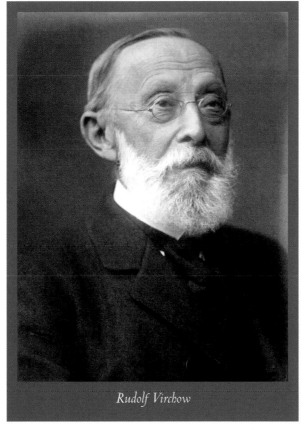

Rudolf Virchow

committee meeting of the Prussian Parliament from 6 to 7, and preside at the meeting of the Berlin Medical Society or at the Anthropological Society, or deliver some popular address, or again do committee work from 7 to 9. Well may I be asked, "But where did his meals come in? Where did all his enormous original and editorial literary work, his correspondence, his family life come in?" Well, that is the wonder of all who had the privilege of coming near him.

Virchow's hectic pace seemed to fuel his energy rather than diminish it. He wrote more than two thousand books and papers during his lifetime, and was the editor for many times that number, always scrutinizing every word of every manuscript so that no error might pass into one of the journals for whose contents he was the ever-vigilant concierge. In the growing internationalism of late-nineteenth-century medicine, he was a prime mover, in the most literal sense. A constantly sought-out presence at the International Medical Congress each time it met, he was a frequent participant on the program of various European scientific societies. At the age of eighty, his vacation trip took him on a tour of centers of research in London, Edinburgh, Transylvania, Breslau, and Switzerland. During the magnificent international celebration of his eightieth birthday, attended by notables from all over the world, of whom Lord Lister was one, he gave a two-hour address. Without reading from notes, he reviewed the development of medicine and his own role in its recent history.

In the end, it was the very force of Virchow's undiminished energies that did him in. On January 4, 1902, rushing to get to an appointment, he leaped from an electric streetcar and lost his footing on the roadway of the Leipziger Strasse. The neck of his femur was fractured. His strength was sapped by the months of physical idleness that were required by the slow healing process. Finally, he recovered enough of his old vigor to go off with Rose to spend the summer in the Harz Mountains, but he fell again and was reinjured. This time, cardiac problems supervened, and it was necessary to transport him back to Berlin, where he died on September 5.

Rudolf Virchow's funeral was a public celebration of his life. Throngs of his fellow citizens lined the sidewalks to pay him homage as the procession wended its way through the streets of the city for which he had accomplished so much. Wilhelm II sent a telegram of condolence to Rose Virchow. Had he been able to lean forward in his celestial seat and peer down at our planet through his steel-rimmed eyeglasses, the infidel deceased would surely have been amused to read that his country's ruler had invoked the Deity in behalf of those family members left behind. The cocky old skeptic, who put just about as much stock in the Kaiser's religious beliefs as he did in his politics, would nevertheless have applauded the perceptiveness of the rest of the message

telegraphed to his widow: "May the Lord God comfort you in your great sorrow, and may the thought console you that the great investigator, healer, and teacher whose life-work opened up new channels for medical science, is mourned in grateful recognition by his King and the whole educated world."

In one of the various encomiums that appeared in the lay press on succeeding days, it was noted that with Virchow's death, the people of Germany had lost not one, but four, great men—their leading pathologist, anthropologist, sanitarian, and liberal. In three of those fields, he had laid the groundwork upon which his successors built ever greater structures of achievement. Only his political efforts failed in the face of the overwhelming tide of reactionary nationalism that overtook his country after its unification. But the ideas he espoused, of democracy, culture, freedom, and prosperity, attained their ultimate triumph in a western Europe that stands today on the principles for which he fought.

To a great extent, Virchow's most important contribution, the cell theory of disease, is as much a philosophical as a scientific concept. It touches upon the very substance of the existence of each of us, and upon the substance of our relationships to our fellows. He enlarged his thesis of basic life units to include the social structure of mankind, and made it clear that though overall direction may come from some specially designated part of the organism, no person's contribution has more importance than another's.

Virchow taught his successors that the activities taking place within the cell are the vital processes of life for which man has been searching since dimmest prehistory. Together with the work of Claude Bernard, his teachings emphasized the interdependence of cells and their surrounding environment. Deriving from the work of the German Virchow and the Frenchman Bernard, modern scientists study ever more basic participating factors in the processes of existence. For the medical student of today, it is no longer sufficient to learn anatomy, physiology, biochemistry, and pathology. The curriculum bulletins of modern medical schools list courses in the biology of the cell and of the molecules within it and without it. The membrane that surrounds the basic unit, the forces of energy that affect it, and the secrets of its work and sustenance are subjected to scrutiny of the most minutely precise sort. The future of basic medical research is in the hands of such as the geneticists and immunologists and maybe even the psychobiologists. There are mathematicians, physicists, chemists, and engineers who have never set foot in a medical laboratory, and yet are investigating problems that will lead to the great advances in healing of the next century.

But there are also other subjects that modern medical students are required to master whose inclusion in the curriculum would warm the ectoplasm of Virchow's spirit, could he but know of them: epidemiology, biostatistics, public health, and behavioral sciences. The "normal condition of existence" interested Rudolf Virchow as much as the abnormal. He believed, and time has vindicated him, that it is by the maintenance, or restoration, of equity between the basic units of life and their surroundings that health is to be most successfully nurtured, whether of the individual or the entire organism. He was Hippocrates with a microscope.

In the nineteenth century, it was commonly believed that science would one day provide the means by which the happiness of humanity would be attained. That faith has proved to be naive; the discoveries of science can be just as destructive as they are vitalizing, just as enslaving as they are liberating. It is not science that will determine the future of our race, but the fickle nature of our ambivalence toward the uses to which we will put its bounties. Rudolf Virchow recognized that ambivalence, and he never lost hope that it could be overcome by goodwill among people and nations. When peace had returned following the Franco-Prussian War between his country and the country of Claude Bernard, he expressed his faith in the ability of individuals and nations to heal their disordered conditions and return to a state of health. Although history in this instance proved him wrong, perhaps his hope will yet be fulfilled in the life-times of our children's children, or our cells' cells:

With peace once more with us, may the entire world of science assert its influence to promote for all people the reconciliation of minds and hearts and insight into our community of interests. Then may all the citizens of each of the two nations recognize that their true purpose and life work can be realized only upon the foundation of their country's development; for that reason the soil must be free from foreign invasion. The development of nations must find its highest goal in a humane understanding, which raises the individual far above the narrow confines of nationalism to the highest realms of humanity. . . . May it remain for science to treasure and to bring to realization the beautiful motto: Peace on Earth.

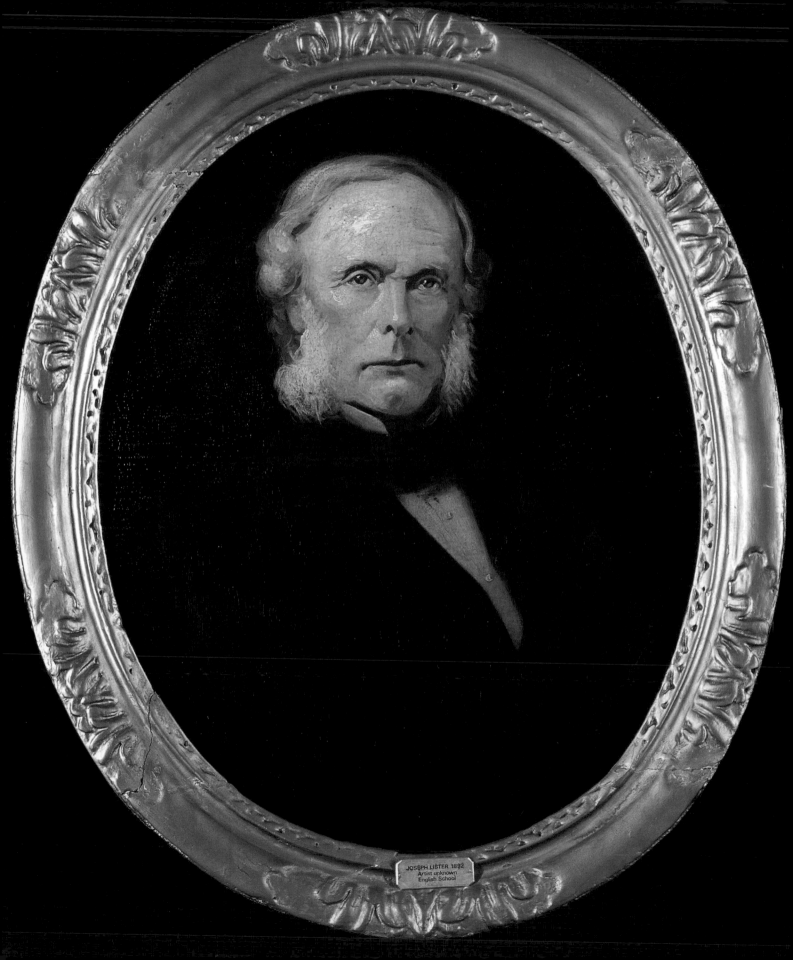

JOSEPH LISTER 1892
Artist unknown
English School

12

"To Tend the Fleshly Tabernacle of the Immortal Spirit"

Joseph Lister's Antiseptic Surgery

When George IV of England decided in 1821 that an unsightly cyst must be surgically excised from his scalp, he did not stop to consider that he would be risking his life by undergoing the simple operation. In George's time, a procedure of the type he proposed was accompanied by a mortality rate considerably higher than that of modern-day open-heart surgery. The great killer was postoperative infection. Its ever-looming specter haunted the conscience and walked the dreams of every surgeon each time he picked up his scalpel in an attempt to heal. To be a surgeon in those days was to have become inured not only to the shrieking struggles taking place in the operating theater but also to the nauseous stench of putrefying flesh that fouled the air of the postsurgical wards.

The king's chosen surgeon, Astley Cooper, was terrified by the prospect of making an incision on his sovereign's head. Of the various forms of infection he feared, it was the dreaded erysipelas that most worried him. "I was very averse from doing it," he later wrote. "I had always been successful,

and I saw that the operation, if it were followed by erysipelas, would destroy all of my happiness, and blast my reputation. . . . I was thunderstruck, and felt giddy at the idea of my fate hanging upon such an event."

Nowadays it is known that the rapidly infiltrating inflammation of erysipelas is caused by the toxic effects of chains of ball-shaped bacteria we call streptococci. In Cooper's time, only one thing about the disease was certain: it spread a furious redness through its victim's incised tissues with enormous rapidity, killing more often than not. Once the process got under way, nothing except an incomprehensible change of mind by Nature herself could make it cease from expanding. No one knew what initiated erysipelas in surgical wounds, no one knew how to prevent it, and no one knew how to throw up an effective roadblock against its breakneck progression.

Somehow, Cooper collected his courage, removed the cyst, and saw his patient through a providentially uneventful healing process. George expressed his gratitude in the time-honored way of royalty—he knighted his deliverer. A monarch's wen had been removed on a monarch's whim, fortune had smiled, and the sun shone on a new British knight.

From the safety of historical distance, it is perhaps too easy to underestimate what was a matter of frightening magnitude until scarcely a hundred years ago. The problem of postsurgical infections became increasingly troublesome with each passing decade of the nineteenth century. As the professional and economic opportunities for surgeons improved, more of them were trained, and more new techniques were developed, so that the numbers of operations began to multiply. The numbers of complications multiplied along with them. Wound infections were so common that patients and their doctors came to expect pus after every operation. An occasional wound would surprise its observers by healing cleanly without a bit of inflammation, but this was unusual and quite unexplainable. If a patient was lucky, his infection would localize itself to the immediate area of the incision. In such cases, a thick cream-colored odorless fluid would appear within five or six days, and then erupt through the incision to flow freely through its gaping edges, which then gradually filled in behind it with healthy young scar tissue. The appearance of this welcome effluvium was hailed as a sure sign that the wound would heal. The much-desired drainage was understandably called "laudable pus."

In later years, it would be discovered that laudable pus was produced by the action of staphylococci, spherical bacteria which group themselves in clumps and tend to go about their purulent business in a relatively localized fashion. When compared to some of the other microbial invaders

that frequently lurked in the depths of wounds, the staphylococci were friends of the nineteenth-century surgeon. The streptococcus, on the other hand, was not content to languish in walled-off pools of purulence; there was no way to drain its noxiousness into a bowl. It was a malign microbe that burned its way centrifugally like an uncontrolled brushfire, sending a toxic poison ahead of it into the bloodstream. Like a harbinger of death, the toxin made itself known by high fevers and teeth-rattling chills. Though the syndrome was known as erysipelas by the doctors, its victims had a better name for it—they called it St. Anthony's Fire.

Still, from the mischief of the streptococcus there was at least some hope that a patient might survive. But there was another form of infection that doomed every one of its victims to a horrible death. This was a foul-smelling disgusting mess of putridity that went by the name of hospital gangrene. The infection was the result of a mix of microbes, some of which we now call anaerobes, because they grow best in the absence of oxygen and therefore invade deeply into the tissues of their powerless host. Its loathsome progression took place at a rate far less rapid than did the hot blush of erysipelas, but there was a relentless deliberateness to its plodding drift, enabling it to digest every bit of involved tissue into a gray slough of oozing necrosis. It killed everything in its path, and did so in a ghastly nightmare of wet stench that choked the nostrils and permeated the clothes of European and American surgeons for generations. Every postoperative hospital ward stank with it.

To compound the problems of some patients, a cluster of any of the responsible organisms, or clots containing them, could enter the veins from an infected wound at any time, resulting in the types of blood poisoning called septicemia and pyemia. When either of these dreaded complications occurred, the blood vessels became highways of death, transporting the migrant bacteria to various parts of the body where they might settle, multiply, and destroy organs by creating abscesses within them. Erysipelas, septicemia, and pyemia arising from the infected postpartum uterus are said to have been the pestilences whereby childbed-fever patients fell victim to the ministrations of their unwashed accoucheurs. And as if all of this were not enough, there was also the ever-present danger of tetanus. Although more common in battle injuries and farm accidents, tetanus claimed many a patient whose only wound had been made within the walls of a big-city hospital.

Every form of bacterium could be introduced into lacerated protoplasm by any of several mechanisms, and not a single one of them was so much as guessed at by other than a handful of seers whose preachings went unheeded. Semmelweis, Holmes, and the others used logic to inform their clinical observations, but no one had yet shown that germs cause disease. Their precepts and those of the few other visionaries who wrote in the first half of the nineteenth century had been untimely ripped from the gestating womb of scientific investigation. Their theories came before they were ready to be born. What was required was a normal full-term pregnancy of research in which an idea could develop to a sufficient state of maturity that it was ready to be received by a welcoming world. That this delivery could take place was assured by a pregnancy of quite a different sort,

which would begin within a year of King George's operation—on December 27, 1822, in the small eastern French town of Dôle, Louis Pasteur was born.

The discoveries of Pasteur were to change medical science in many ways, but it was in the understanding of surgical wound infections that they had their most immediate impact. The first patients to benefit were those undergoing major amputations, the most common operation of the time. In an 1867 article titled *Hospitalism,* Sir James Simpson of Edinburgh, the inventor of chloroform anesthesia, provided some disheartening statistics for these procedures. He studied the results of more than two thousand in-hospital extremity amputations in Britain, and found that 41 percent of patients died if their operations were done in hospitals with more than three hundred beds; infection was by far the greatest cause of death. In another two hundred patients whose amputations were done out-of-hospital in country practice, only 11 percent died. Postoperative mortality figures were high in all of the hospitals of Europe, Paris reporting 60 percent, Zurich 46 percent, and Glasgow 34 percent, with equivalent figures coming from Berlin, Munich, Copenhagen, and other continental cities. America was not doing much better. The Massachusetts General Hospital had a mortality rate of 26 percent for amputations, and the Pennsylvania Hospital reported 24 percent. Simpson correctly warned, "The man laid on the operating table in one of our surgical hospitals, is exposed to more chances of death than the English soldier on the field of Waterloo." One result of the septic carnage was a movement in several European cities to raze the most dis-

1,098 were amputations, 237 were for breast cancer, and almost all the rest involved relatively superficial structures. The infection rate was high in every category, and so was the death rate.

Sir Frederick Treves, who was to become one of England's leading surgeons around the turn of the twentieth century, was training in London in the early 1870s. When he reached his mid-fifties, Treves retired from practice to devote himself to a pursuit in which his skills were as great as they were in the operating theater—he became a writer of books and essays, many of which dealt with his life as a surgeon and a world traveler. "The Elephant Man" is the product of his talented pen. The very next essay in the series of which that classic tale is a part is titled "The Old Receiving Room," in which we may read the words of this gifted writer describing the operating theater of the London Hospital as it was in the period just before Pasteur's teachings were accepted:

Treatment was very rough. The surgeon was rough. He had inherited that attitude from the days when operations were carried through without anaesthetics, and when he had need to be rough, strong and quick, as well as very indifferent to pain. Pain was with him a thing that had to be. It was a regrettable feature of disease. It had to be submitted to. . . .

In the [operating] theatre was a stove which was always kept alight, winter and summer, night and day. The object was to have a fire at all times ready whereat to heat the irons used for the arrest of bleeding as had been

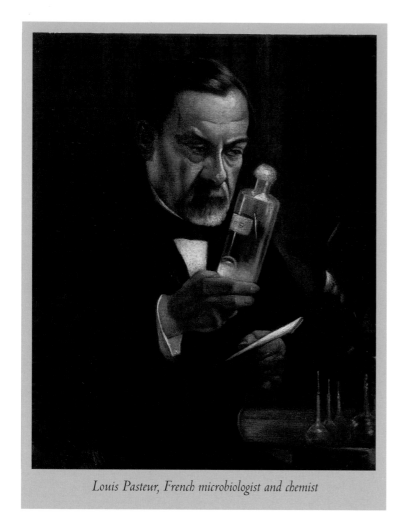

Louis Pasteur, French microbiologist and chemist

reputable of the offending institutions, and a few of them were torn down.

Because of the danger of sepsis, the discovery of anesthesia was prevented from having its anticipated effect upon the volume or nature of surgery that could be performed. The threat of infection made it impossible to operate within the body cavities except under the most unusual circumstances. Operations remained of necessity restricted to the amputation of extremities and the removal of tumors of the breast and body wall. Of 1,924 surgical procedures done at the Massachusetts General Hospital between 1847 and 1870,

the practice since the days of Elizabeth. Antiseptics were not yet in use. Sepsis was the prevailing condition in the wards. Practically all major wounds suppurated. Pus was the most common subject of converse, because it was the most prominent feature in the surgeon's work. It was classified according to degrees of vileness. "Laudable" pus was considered rather a fine thing, something to be proud of. "Sanious" pus was not only nasty in appearance but regrettable, while "ichorous" pus represented the most malignant depths to which matter could attain.

There was no object in being clean. Indeed, cleanliness was out of place. It was considered to be finicking and affected. An executioner might as well manicure his nails before chopping off a head. The surgeon operated in a slaughterhouse-suggesting frock coat of black cloth. It was stiff with the blood and the filth of years. The more sodden it was the more forcibly did it bear evidence to the surgeon's prowess. I, of course, commenced my surgical career in such a coat, of which I was quite proud. Wounds were dressed with "charpie" soaked in oil. Both oil and dressing were frankly and exultingly septic. Charpie was a species of cotton waste obtained from cast linen. It would probably now be discarded by a motor mechanic as being too dirty for use on a car.

Owing to the suppurating wounds the stench in the wards was of a kind not easily forgotten. I can recall it to this day with unappreciated ease. There was one sponge to a ward. With this putrid article and a basin of once-clear water all the wounds in the ward were washed in turn twice a day. By this ritual any chance that a patient had of recovery was eliminated. I remember a whole ward being decimated by hospital gangrene. The modern student has no knowledge of this disease. He has never seen it and, thank heaven, he never

will. People often say how wonderful it was that surgical patients lived in these days. As a matter of fact they did not live, or at least only a few of them did.

The attitude that the public assumed towards hospitals and their works at the time of which I write may be illustrated by the following incident. I was instructed by my surgeon to obtain a woman's permission for an operation on her daughter. The operation was one of no great magnitude. I interviewed the mother in the Receiving Room. I discussed the procedure with her in great detail and, I trust, in a sympathetic and hopeful man-

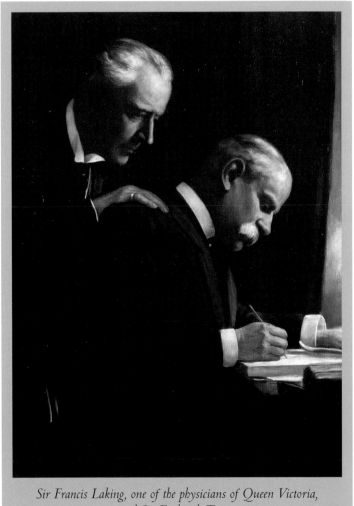

Sir Francis Laking, one of the physicians of Queen Victoria, and Sir Frederick Treves

ner. After I had finished my discourse I asked her if she would consent to the performance of the operation. She replied: "Oh! it is all very well to talk about consenting, but who is to pay for the funeral?"

That the world was delivered from all of this festering horror and its surgeons' machismo insouciance was the work of Joseph Lister, who accomplished it by bringing the fruits of Pasteur's pure science to the operating theaters and surgical wards of the hospitals of Europe. Like so many of the medical discoverers whose stories are told in this book, he was at first disbelieved by more than a few of his colleagues, who ridiculed and rejected his precepts. It took decades for his work to be so completely accepted that science, in a final fulfillment of John Hunter's example, could be brought as a full partner into the specialty of surgery. Ironically, the correctness of his views was finally recognized only after his methods were no longer needed to achieve the objective of preventing surgical infection. By then, better techniques had been found, all based on Lister's original insight that Louis Pasteur's discovery of germs in souring alcohol might be applied to identifying the cause of wound infections.

Pasteur found his putrefying bacteria in fermenting beer and wine; Lister found them in septic wounds. Thirty-five years later, America's ambassador to England, whose country had been among the last to embrace Lister's triumphant contribution, paid him a long-overdue honor on behalf of all mankind, when he greeted him with the words: "My lord, it is not a Profession, it is not a Nation, it is Humanity itself which, with uncovered head, salutes you."

The literary gifts of the surgeon who was also a sensitive writer must here again be called upon. Frederick Treves, who lived through the pre- and post-Listerian eras, called by some the B.C. and A.D. of surgery, one day wrote an assessment that epitomizes every critical analysis that has ever been made of Lister's work:

Lister created anew the ancient art of healing; he made a reality of the hope which had for all time sustained the surgeon's endeavors; he removed the impenetrable cloud which had stood for centuries between great principles and successful practice; and he rendered possible a treatment which had hitherto been but the vision of the dreamer. The nature of his discovery—like that of most great movements—was splendid in its simplicity and magnificent in its littleness. To the surgeon's craft it was but the 'one thing needful.' With it came the promise of a wondrous future; without it was the hopelessness of an impotent past.

Giovanni Morgagni had taught physicians to seek out the seats of their patients' symptoms within their organs. Lister, using the science of microscopy, now taught them to seek the primary causes of many of those organ derangements by looking into Pasteur's "world of the infinitely small." He was that great scientist's leading apostle in the English-speaking world, indeed in the non-French-speaking world.

A student of the life of Joseph Lister may spend months or years researching all that has been written about him by those with whom he worked, and find not a single word of anything but praise for his character. When so much has been recorded about an individual and every bit of it provides only further evidence of a kind of earthbound saintliness, biographers, especially those of the modern debunking kind, always assume that a great deal has gone unrecorded. They look at the available facts, at decisions made, at the possibility of motivations perhaps impure, and seem always to be able to come up with something that is at least raffish, a few shady involvements or questionable patterns of behavior. If nothing else, there should be a detectable touch of smugness about being so good.

Not so with Lister. There seems to have been a quality about him that was so warmly, serenely, gently strong that words like "dignity," "forbearance," "integrity," "sweetness," and "honor" only leave his biographers as beggared for description as they did his contemporaries. His opponents admired him, and even his most relentless antagonists, fulminate against his theories though they might, spoke not a harsh word about the man himself. There was a flavor of simple goodness in his life, flowing evenly from the philosophical spring of a distinctive faith that has nourished the spirit of more than a few of the moral leaders of the past three hundred years. The source of that spring is to be found in the ethical principles of the Religious Society of Friends.

The early Friends, who first began to organize themselves in Oliver Cromwell's mid-seventeenth-century Puritan England, were so filled with a sense of spiritual power that they were said to fairly quake with the fervor of their belief. Though the word "Quaker" was at first thrown at them in derision, they soon began to use it themselves, as something by which their commitment to a specific mission might be emphasized. The mission of the Quakers was simply stated by their founder, George Fox—it was "to wait upon the Lord," a concept derived from Isaiah 40:31: "But they that wait upon the Lord shall renew their strength; they shall mount up with wings as eagles; they shall run and not be weary; and they shall walk and not faint."

If waiting upon the Lord was their mission, the generative force that enabled Quakers to carry it out was the element they call the Inner Light, "that of God in every one." It is the essence of God within that makes a Friend rise to speak in a meeting for worship, and it is the essence of God within that leads him to do God's work on earth. No man is better than any other and no man is better than any woman. There is no hierarchy, no ritual. For Friends, there is no need for pride or pomp, there is only the need to do the kindnesses of friends. God's work on earth is to be done on earth—the world was not created to be set aside, it was created to be lived in. Worldly goods and worldly power are not to be renounced, for they provide the means to serve. A Friend in Lister's day was recognized by his plain Quaker-gray, almost black, clothes, by his earnest humility, and by a philanthropy

> *His opponents admired him, and even his most relentless antagonists, fulminate against his theories though they might, spoke not a harsh word about the man himself.*

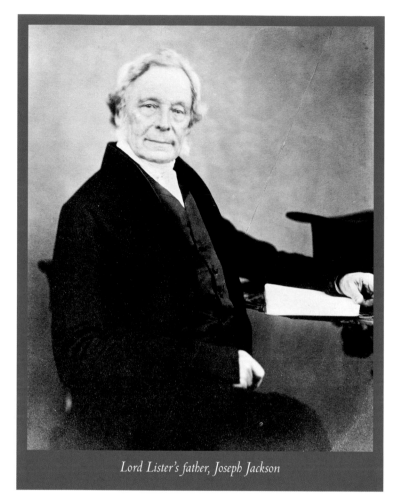

Lord Lister's father, Joseph Jackson

of its inhabitants. It was here that Joseph Lister was born on April 5, 1827, the family's fourth child and second son.

In those days, membership in the Society of Friends affected every aspect of life. Since Quakers would neither take an oath nor subscribe to the Thirty-nine Articles of the Episcopal faith, the great universities were closed to them, as were many of the better secondary schools. They did not dance, they did not hunt, and they had no music in their homes. They had no interest in sports or frolicsome diversions. Their worldly concerns were confined to business, education, and the life of the mind. It will not seem surprising, considering the directness and honesty of their world-view, that the Quaker intellect was often attracted to science. Self-taught in hours stolen from business, Quaker scientists in that era of the enlightened amateur made some important practical contributions. In the words of Rickman Godlee, Lister's nephew, "Even amongst those of moderate circumstances, it was common to find an intellectual man of high scientific attainments serving behind his own counter."

Among the most outstanding of the intellectual men of high scientific attainments was Lister *père*, Joseph Jackson. In spite of having left school at the age of fourteen to enter his father's wine-importing firm, he taught himself enough mathematics and optics to become a skilled microscopist. One of his closest friends was a shy young

whose charity was as quiet when giving money as it was when giving love.

In order to give, one had first to have. Nineteenth-century Quakers were hardworking in business and adept at investing. Consequently, many members of the Society became wealthy, and among them were the forebears of Joseph Lister. His father, Joseph Jackson Lister, was a wine merchant whose business had prospered so well that he was able to buy a beautiful Queen Anne house in Upton, at that time a country village far to the east of central London. Surrounded by its gardens and fields, Upton House was a mansion, no matter the plain way of life

Guy's Hospital doctor named Thomas Hodgkin, destined for posthumous renown for having described the disease that is called by his name. The two Friends undertook a study of the microscopic characteristics of the blood, with the result that they published observations demonstrating that red corpuscles are biconcave in shape. They showed also that under certain circumstances these disk-shaped structures tend to line up against each other like stacks of coins, formations called rouleaux.

The discovery of the true shape of red cells and their tendency to rouleaux formation was a significant contribution, but Joseph Jackson Lister later solved another problem, this one in optics, that was of even greater import to science. He discovered what optic physicists call the law of aplanatic foci, enabling him to devise a lens combination that overcame the technical difficulty called chromatic aberration that had plagued microscopists for a hundred and fifty years. For this he was elected a Fellow of the Royal Society.

Up until this time, the microscope had never been as useful to science as might have been hoped. Galileo's early-seventeenth-century account of using his microscope to see "flies which look as big as a lamb, covered all over with hair and very pointed nails" had impressed virtually no one. The great astronomer was himself too occupied with looking up to look down, and seems to have thought of microscopes as a source of amusement. Later in the century, Anton van Leeuwenhoek, using superior lenses of his own design and grinding, was able to see what he called animalcules and we now call bacteria, and a brief flurry of microscopic discovery followed,

including Marcello Malpighi's description of the capillaries in 1660. But throughout the eighteenth century, there were investigators, John Hunter among them, who considered the microscope to be a tool of dangerous deception. The reason for this skepticism was the distorted image produced by the relatively primitive magnification systems of the time. Visual aberrations resulted from the spherical shape of the lenses and their tendency to disperse ordinary light into the various colors of its spectrum—aberrations that were greatly increased by increasing the magnifying power of the microscopes. The practice of making observations with such distorting lenses, and using the full glare of the sun as the source of light, resulted in images in which could be seen all sorts of objects that were not really there. Astute observers recognized this, and stayed away from any but simple hand-held glasses.

Once the importance of pathological anatomy was established following the work of Giovanni Battista Morgagni and his successors, however, efforts were undertaken by several investigators to find a method of reducing aberration so that useful methods of high magnification might be made available. The result was that after 150 years of inactivity, the major problems were solved in the short span of four years. The first step was the invention in 1826 by the Italian Giovanni Battista Amici of the water-immersion lens, which made use of the principle that passing light through media of different refracting powers reduces aberration in the same way as does the human eye. The second, building on Amici's contribution, was Joseph Jackson Lister's.

In his 1900 Huxley Lecture, Joseph Lister spoke of "my father, whose labours had raised the compound microscope from little better than a scientific toy to the powerful engine for investigation." A contemporary referred to the elder Lister as "the pillar and source of all the microscopy of the age." In the next generation, the instrument would reach its ultimate usefulness in the hands of Louis Pasteur, whose studies led in turn to those of Joseph Jackson's own son, a young man whose scientific teeth were figuratively cut on the barrels of his father's finest microscopes.

Young Joseph Lister thus grew up in a home devoted to God and to science. His mother, prior to her marriage, was the director of reading and writing for girls at the Ackworth Friends School, and a devoted teacher of her children during their early years. Young Joseph proved from the very beginning of his education to be an excellent scholar. He seems to have become fascinated with nature at an early age, and particularly with medicine. Even before his teens, he announced his intention to become a surgeon, a decision greeted with some surprise by a family none of whose members had ever chosen a professional career.

Having excelled at the Quaker schools to which he was sent, Joseph enrolled at the age of sixteen at University College in London. Founded eighteen years earlier, "the godless college," as it was called by friends and detractors alike, was intended to be an Oxbridge for everyone, regardless of social rank or religious belief. Joseph Jackson counseled his son about the importance of a general education prior to embarking on a career in medicine, advice even more important

today than it was in 1844. The boy enrolled in the B.A. program, a course of study requiring three years.

In 1847, young Lister began his matriculation at the medical school of University College. After such long anticipation, his first year was a grave disappointment. He made the mistake of taking lodgings with an elderly Quaker whose rigidly conducted household was far more gloomy than his own home, and he applied himself so diligently to his studies that he took little time to rest, and soon lost his usual air of optimistic cheerfulness. In his first year also he had an attack of a mild form of smallpox and attempted to return to classes before he had fully recovered. The result was an episode that was diagnosed as a nervous breakdown.

After trying to fight off depression and a state of uncontrollable introspection for some months, in early 1848 he was finally prevailed upon to drop out of school and take a long holiday; after some rest, followed by a bit of traveling in Ireland, he was ready to resume his studies. At the time, his father wrote him a letter to which he may have had many an occasion to refer during the difficult later years when he was trying to convince his surgical brethren about the validity of the germ theory of disease:

Believe us, my tenderly beloved son, that thy proper part now is to cherish a pious cheerful spirit, open to see and to enjoy the bounties and the beauties spread around us:—not to give way to turning thy thoughts upon thyself nor even at present to dwell long on serious things. Thou wilt remember how strongly Dr. Hodgkin cautioned thee on these points, as dangerous to thy mental as well as bodily health.

With purpose renewed, in late 1848 Joseph returned to the University College medical school for the winter session, determined to live by his father's counsel. The fortitude of his Quaker upbringing had returned to him. He knew what had to be done.

Joseph Jackson's counsel and his example were not the only gifts he gave to his son. One of his best microscopes accompanied the boy to the medical school, and it was put to good use. Already an accomplished *aficionado* of the instrument, Joseph spent a great deal of his free time continuing his observations and sharing his knowledge. He presented two papers on his own work before the Hospital Medical Society, which proved to be strikingly predictable of the course he would take in his professional career. One was titled "Gangrene," and the other was "Use of the Microscope in Medicine," a subject of particular interest to his fellows because the school provided no formal teaching in the subject. He also did some original research on certain microscopic muscles, those of the iris and those that erect the tiny hair shafts in the skin to make goose bumps. Even with all of this extra work, he found time to apply himself so effectively to his studies that he received his degree with Honors in 1852.

Lister served a term as house physician, and then spent nine months as a house surgeon, forms of indenture roughly equivalent to the modern American internship. By the end of this time, he was twenty-seven years old

and he had completed his formal training. There was no need, thanks to his family's comfortable circumstances, to rush out into practice. During his school years he had been particularly close to the Professor of Physiology, William Sharpey, who now suggested that he spend some time visiting other clinics, in order to broaden his view of surgery. Sharpey was a friend of James Syme, the Professor of Clinical Surgery at Edinburgh, and it was to that institution that the physiologist recommended his young protégé travel prior to a tour of the European hospitals.

Within days of his arrival in Edinburgh in September 1853, the young surgeon realized

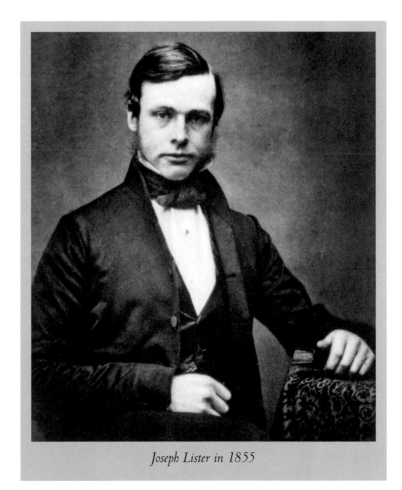

Joseph Lister in 1855

that he had found a second father in his new mentor, though their natures, even their appearances, could not have been more at variance. Lister, just under six feet in height, gave the impression, with his powerful chest and handsome head, of being a much larger man than he actually was. He was reserved and modest, with a friendly eye and a quietly twinkling sense of generous humor that seemed to betoken a total lack of competitiveness. In spite of his unostentatious Quaker ways, he possessed a cultured mind and could speak fluent French and German. Altogether, he conveyed an air of urbanity completely lacking in the outspoken, combative little professor with whom he had come to study. Syme's face was plain—some called him homely and even a little sour-looking. Fifty-four years old at the time, he was generally considered to be the best technical surgeon in the British Isles, and his razor-sharp mind and his obstinate self-assurance made him a formidable opponent in medical disputation. It was as though each of the men saw a submerged part of his own personality in the other, and allowed a secret admiration for his unconscious alter ego to forge a deep friendship.

An enthusiast, Syme inspired Lister with an excitement that made him decide to remain in Edinburgh after his month's visit was over. Lawson Tait, the prominent Birmingham surgeon of a generation later, was a student at the time, and has left a graphic description of the type of operating extravaganza that was to be witnessed when the professor took up his scalpel to carry out one of the procedures that even he rarely dared in the 1850s. Reading Tait's account of one such display, one does not find it difficult to understand why a young man in training would unhesitatingly give up any other plan in order to throw in his lot with the colorful performer:

The operating theatre of the old infirmary was crowded; every seat, even of the top gallery, was occupied. There were probably seven or eight hundred spectators, for Syme was to operate on a gluteal aneurysm. He was then in the zenith of his fame and in the very best of his powers, his hand as steady and his eye as true as it had ever been—incomparably the greatest surgeon I have ever seen. He entered the theatre with the recognized procession of assistants, house surgeon, and dressers, and was greeted with a subdued murmur of applause. The spectators included men of all ages and ranks in the profession, very many who had come from great distances to see the great feat—like Bickersteth, of Liverpool, who came specially to assist, if I remember rightly, and of course there were many boys like myself from fifteen upward. The patient was put to sleep, Syme buttoned up his dress-coat, turned up his sleeve, I saw a rush of blood, and in a few minutes the placing of the patient in the carrying-basket, and a round of applause, announced the end of the operation.

When the professor offered him an official post as his house surgeon, young Lister fairly leaped at the opportunity. If he had ever had any doubts about his suitability for a surgical career, the period spent with Syme surely dispelled them. Though there were horrible sights to be seen in the operating theater and frightful tragedies unfolded before his eyes each day, Lister had fallen in thrall to that peculiar form of enchantment that comes to embrace every surgeon who is any good at his work. It enveloped me when I was a twenty-two-year-old student in New Haven, as it has enveloped other thousands of young men and now young women too, in different times and different places. It is independent of those other forces by which so many doctors are gripped—the sense of mission or obligation, the driving need to be of service to one's fellow creatures. It is even independent of the intense intellectual satisfaction of the specialty. Although each of these factors must coexist with it, what I refer to here is the sheer enjoyment of being a surgeon, an enjoyment made all the more seductive by an awareness that there is a touch of aberrance in it. In a letter to his father, Lister wrote of that feeling of exhilaration:

If the love of surgery is a proof of a person's being adapted for it, then certainly I am fitted to be a surgeon: for thou canst hardly conceive what a high degree of enjoyment I am from day to day experiencing in this bloody and butcherly department of the healing art. I am more and more delighted with my profession, and sometimes almost question whether it is possible such a delightful pursuit can continue. My only wonder is that persons who really love Surgery for its own sake are rare.

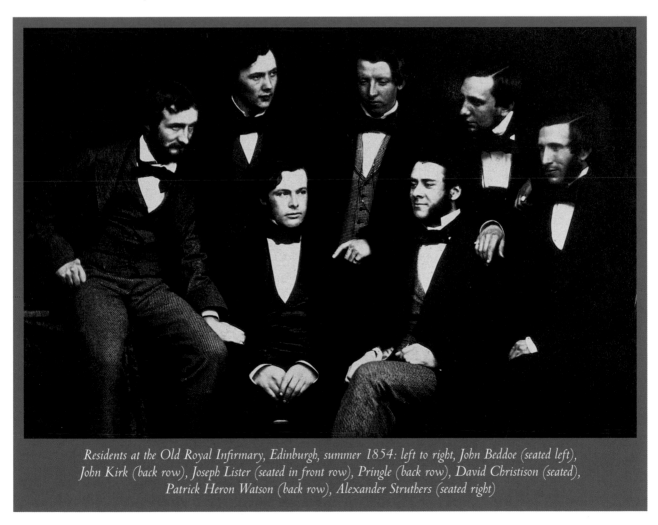

Residents at the Old Royal Infirmary, Edinburgh, summer 1854: left to right, John Beddoe (seated left), John Kirk (back row), Joseph Lister (seated in front row), Pringle (back row), David Christison (seated), Patrick Heron Watson (back row), Alexander Struthers (seated right)

Lister planned to return to London when his training appointment ended in February 1855, but a few months before he was due to leave, news came of the death in the Crimean War of one of the Edinburgh staff surgeons. He hastened to apply for the vacant post, and by April of 1855 he was installed as Assistant Surgeon to the Edinburgh Royal Infirmary and Lecturer in Surgery to the Royal College of Surgeons of Edinburgh.

Surgery had not been the only object of Lister's fascination during his almost two years in Scotland. A frequent visitor to Syme's hospitable home, he had early begun to spend increasing amounts of time in the company of his chief's eldest daughter, Agnes. Syme, undoubtedly of the opinion that his young assistant was tailor-made for his daughter, approved; Joseph Lister *père*, though much impressed with everything he heard about Agnes, was less sanguine, for it was in those days the rule that a Quaker who married out of the faith must either resign from the Society of Friends or be disowned. Eventually, though, he came to terms with his son's inevitable decision. Perhaps he took comfort in an epistle published by the Society of Friends only a year before: "True religion stands neither in forms nor in the formal absence of forms." And although Agnes Syme Lister's new husband now became a member of the Church of England, his outlook remained that of a Friend. Neither better nor worse than his fellows, he chose to be just a little different; neither remoteness nor aloofness set him apart from other men, just the fact of remaining as singular as his now discontinued thee-thou form of address. Though he stopped wearing the somber outward adornments of a Quaker, he never changed the inner adornments of his character.

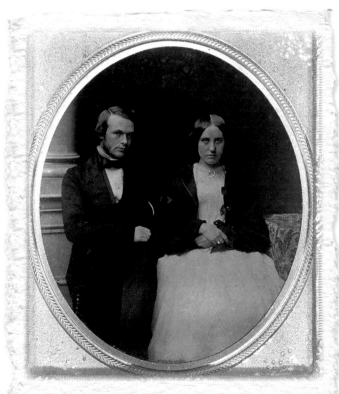

Joseph Lister and his wife, Agnes Lister, seated, within oval frame

The young Listers took a working honeymoon. After four weeks in the English Lake Country, they began a three-month tour of the continent. Except in Paris, whose hospitals Joseph had seen the previous year, they visited the clinics of almost all of the cities to which they traveled. They went to Padua and Bologna, and then on to the Allgemeines Krankenhaus in Vienna, considered to be the most important of the hospitals on their itinerary. Karl von Rokitansky had been a dinner guest at Upton House fourteen years earlier, and the renowned pathologist now spent a good deal of time entertaining his former host's son. For obvious reasons, this 1856 visit has been the cause of much speculation among scholars concerning possible conversations that might have taken place on the subject of Semmelweis. There are two reasons to doubt that such communications occurred. First, Lister later wrote that he had never known the work of the tortured Hungarian until long after his own discovery that germs cause infections. Second, even if there were reason to doubt the word of a man whose every other statement has proved to be unimpeachable, there is the well-known fact that the genius of puerperal fever was not often spoken about in Vienna after his flight to Budapest in 1850. There is no evidence of a Semmelweis influence at work in Lister's development of antisepsis.

After stopping at hospitals in Prague, Berlin, Würzburg, and other German cities, the newlyweds returned home via Paris, moving into a house on Rutland Street only a few doors from Syme's consulting rooms and a fifteen-minute walk from the University and the Edinburgh Royal Infirmary. With home, hospital, and school all within a comfortably small venue, Joseph Lister now set out in earnest on his life's work.

It was a hectic life of clinical surgery and research upon which he was embarking. As a surgical consultant and as Syme's first assistant he was subject to urgent calls at any time of day or night. Though he had only a small private practice of his own, there was a busy schedule of rounds and clinics at the infirmary and the constant attention to his teaching obligations, which included the preparation of lectures. There was no such thing as a biological supply company in those days; he

had to gather organs from the slaughterhouse and small animals from the streams and fields. He read constantly in the French and German literature of physiology and surgery.

From the very first, Agnes was Joseph's research assistant, amanuensis, and the most critical reader of his manuscripts. They converted the back kitchen of their new home into a laboratory where Lister, with his wife's help, began a wide-ranging series of investigations. His skill at microscopy soon enabled him to make contributions to the understanding of the structure and functioning of nerve and muscle fibers, blood coagulation, lymph flow, and that most persistently fascinating topic, inflammation. Experiment after experiment was carried out in the kitchen laboratory. Every investigation was recorded, as were his lecture notes and his later manuscripts, in the easily legible script of his associate, Agnes.

A letter Lister wrote to his father sometime before his marriage illustrates the zeal with which he went about his experiments:

> I have long wished to see the process of inflammation in the frog's foot, and, as I think I once told thee, felt that the early stages of that process had not been traced as they might be. . . . Accordingly . . . having gotten a frog from Duddington Loch . . . I proceeded last evening to the investigation . . . and a most glorious night I had of it.

Of Lister's early experiments, those that were to have most influence on his thinking were the studies of blood clotting and inflammation. The final result of his researches was to convince him that in order for coagulation to take place, the blood must be put into contact with some type of extraneous foreign material. In

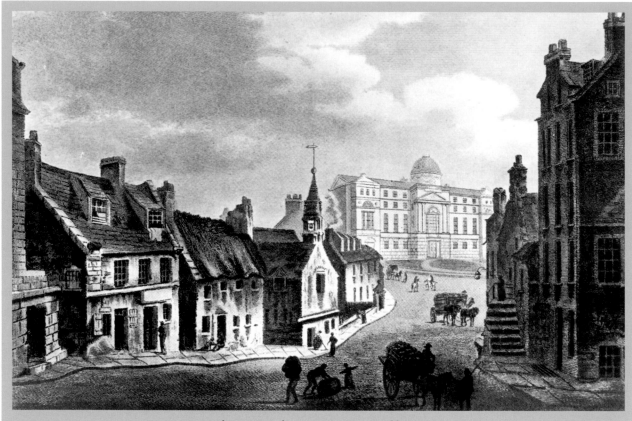

Glasgow Royal Infirmary, from an old print

other words, something active must be done to it in order to make it clot. Accepted nowadays as axiomatic, Lister's observations solved one of the mysteries of the time—why does blood remain in a fluid state in the arteries and veins? As long as flow continues in an intact vessel, no coagulation can occur in normal blood. If the lining of the vessel is injured or disrupted, or if the blood comes into contact with something other than the inner coat of its vessels, it promptly clots. This observation put Lister in a frame of mind to consider that other alterations of physiology must also require some foreign intervention. He could easily prove this to be true in the case of inflammation. Studies of the inflamma-tory process served also to acquaint him with the microscopic changes exhibited by putrefying infected tissues.

Lister's reputation as a researcher and teacher grew rapidly. When the Professor of Surgery at the University of Glasgow announced his retirement in 1859, Syme was contacted to determine whether he would use his influence to convince his son-in-law to accept the chair and to consider an appointment as Surgeon to the Glasgow Infirmary. Not much convincing was needed. By March of 1860, Joseph and Agnes had settled in that city, which, with a population of slightly less than 400,000, was twice the size of Edinburgh.

After a preliminary summer session, the real business of the school year began in the fall. In those days, an Inaugural Lecture was an event of momentous significance; this one in Glasgow was to set the tone not only for Lister's tenure, but for his entire career as well. As he went off to the lecture hall with an entourage of his new colleagues just before noon on the appointed day, his anxious young wife, so much a participant in his career's success, tried to calm her nervousness by writing a letter to her mother-in-law in Upton. She began by describing the appearance of the amphitheater, whose refurbishing she and Joseph had supervised for the new term. She went on to set the scene as she visualized it in her mind's eye, and then heightened the drama even as her own feelings of worried suspense were increasing:

> *Now it is just about 12. Oh! I trust he may be blessed, and believe he will be. His gown will be going on for the first time except when I saw it tried on here. About 5 minutes past! he will be beginning! and how is he getting on?*

She need not have worried. Blessed he had always been, and blessed he would be on this day as well. His warm good nature made itself immediately apparent to the students, who took to his lecturing style as though they had been waiting for it all their lives. He made a few witty quips to lighten their mood, and then said some very serious things which, although meant to be about surgery, declared the ethos of his own professional life. Among them was the aphorism of Ambroise Paré: "I dressed him, God healed him." He told them of his belief that there are two great requisites for a healer: "First, a warm, loving heart; and secondly, truth in an earnest spirit." There is no full record of his remarks that afternoon, but he must have conveyed his view of medicine in similar terms to those he used in a graduation address almost two decades later:

> *If we had nothing but pecuniary rewards and worldly honors to look to, our profession would not be one to be desired. But in its practice you will find it to be attended with peculiar privileges, second to none in intense interest and pure pleasure. It is our proud office to tend the fleshly tabernacle of the immortal spirit, and our path, if rightly followed, will be guided by unfettered truth and love unfeigned. In pursuit of this noble and holy calling I wish you all God-speed.*

To tend the fleshly tabernacle of the immortal spirit was all the work of all the days of Joseph Lister's time on earth. Everything he did became part of that obligation. It was not in a spirit of sacrifice that he and his wife renounced worldly pleasures—it was rather in a spirit of exaltation that they had been given the talents and the opportunity to serve their Lord by serving mankind. It was, of course, not a privilege reserved to Quakers or even to the devout of any stripe. Many an atheist has borne it with nobility.

From the moment of that Inaugural Lecture, Lister became a favorite with the students. They made him Honorary President of their Medical Society, and 161 of them joined together at the end of his first academic year to address a petition to him in which they proclaimed "your eminent ability as a teacher of Surgery."

So new was the academic discipline of surgery that Lister was only the third occupant of the chair at Glasgow since its founding in 1815, and he was the first to devote full time to his specialty rather than to carry out its duties as part of a general practice. His research during the first years was a continuation of the earlier studies on inflammation and clotting. So well did these progress that he was invited to give the 1863 Croonian Lecture of the Royal Society of London. He chose as his topic "The Coagulation of the Blood."

Like all surgeons, Lister was distressed by the fact that virtually every surgical incision became infected. So universal was the presence of purulent drainage from wounds that most surgeons considered it an inevitable, natural course of events, as long as the pus was laudable. Lister refused to accept that point of view. His studies of inflammation had convinced him that normal healing should take place without tissue destruction and without infection, yet the specialty of surgery remained enmired in a sea of pus. It was not as though no one had thought up a theory, or even several, to explain putrefaction. The predominant theory was simple to understand, and made still simpler by the fact that there was no possibility, given the technology of the time, either to prove it or to disprove it. The cause of putrefaction was said to be the oxygen in the air. On entering the surgical wound, it was thought to oxidize or break down the molecules of unstable organic material, thus destroying the tissues and turning them into pus. There being no way to prevent oxygen from entering a wound, there was no way to prevent infection. It was an explanation as laudable as the pus it was meant

to justify, because it got everyone off the hook: if the omnipresent villain was oxygen—no surgeon could blame himself for being the cause of sepsis. That some infectious agent could be introduced into a wound by the operating team seems not to have been considered by anyone, except the scorned and now forgotten Semmelweis and the few others who had written of its role in the etiology of childbed fever.

The concept of oxygen-induced putrefaction made no sense to Lister, however. If it were tenable, healthy flesh should become infected spontaneously, since the normal blood flow carries oxygen to the tissues constantly. Moreover, it was rare in his experience to encounter a chest infection when a fractured rib released air into a bruised wound by puncturing a lung. No—there had to be some other explanation, and, Lister believed, it had to come from some foreign substance entering the incision.

His supposition that the cause of putrefaction was an as yet undiscovered foreign substance was based on his studies of coagulation and inflammation. In each case, the presence of some irritative or injuring agent was required to set the process going. Arguing by analogy, he found himself, although he would not know it until many years later, thinking along the same lines as had Semmelweis: there must be some *thing* that enters a wound to cause infection. Semmelweis imagined it to be carried in on the hands of the doctors. Lister imagined it to fall in from the air in which it lived. All that remained was to identify that invisible *thing*, and then to figure out a way to destroy it.

At this point, the scene must shift southward to the French city of Lille, and the laboratory of the thirty-four-year-old Professor of Chemistry who was also the Dean of the Faculty of Sciences, Louis Pasteur. We will have to go just a bit backward in time as well, to 1856, when a local manufacturer of beet-root alcohol had come to the professor to tell him of a mysterious catastrophe that was destroying his business and that of his colleagues in the local beer and wine industries: without any visible cause, a great deal of each batch of fermenting alcohol was spontaneously spoiling into a slimy juice of useless sour ooze. At that time, fermentation was thought by everyone to be a chemical process (this was why the distraught manufacturer had brought his problem to a chemist), but a few experiments with his microscope convinced Pasteur that sugar is fermented into alcohol not by some lifeless compound but by the yeasts which he found to be growing in it. In that portion of the manufacturer's batch which was spoiled, he identified not only the yeasts, but also great numbers of rod-shaped microbes. With this one series of observations he had discovered that the cause of normal fermentation is the action of yeasts, and that the cause

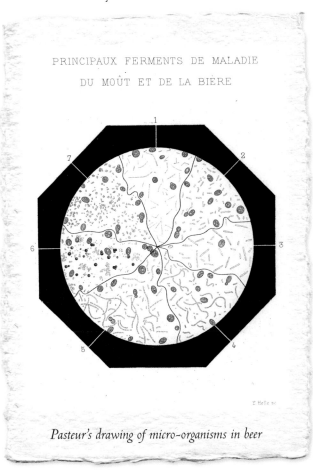

PRINCIPAUX FERMENTS DE MALADIE
DU MOÛT ET DE LA BIÈRE

Pasteur's drawing of micro-organisms in beer

of souring is the action of bacteria. He had entered what he later came to call "the world of the infinitely small."

Of course, Pasteur was not the first explorer of that world. Since ancient times, there had been occasional writers who theorized that some day a *contagium animatum* would be found, which would explain disease. One Girolamo Fracastoro had gone so far as to write about it in 1546, predicting the discovery of what he called *seminaria*, the still-unseen germs by which he thought some diseases were spread. Then, over one hundred years later, in a series of letters written to the Royal Society of London beginning in 1676, Anton van Leeuwenhoek described the microscopic "animalcules" which he found in water, water-soaked organic materials, and finally in scrapings from his own back teeth, and identified the bacteria we know today as streptococci, bacilli, and spirilla. However, somehow in all the years that came after that no one took the trouble to seek such bacteria in the effluvia of disease; no one related Leeuwenhoek's animalcules to Fracastoro's *seminaria*.

Then, in the span of a few years, Louis Pasteur not only made the correlation but proved by ex-

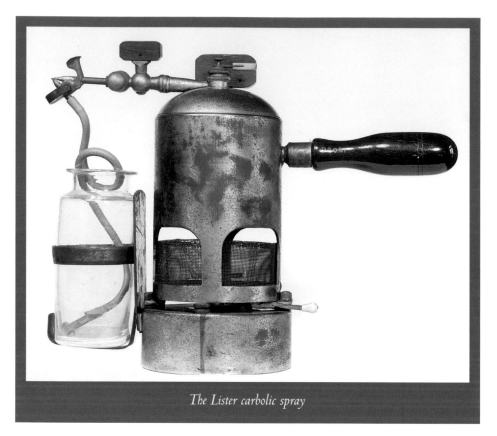

The Lister carbolic spray

tor, that statement has no better example than the way in which Joseph Lister would use Pasteur's discovery of bacterial putrefaction to explain wound infection.

Pasteur published the results of his fermentation experiments in 1857 and 1859, with follow-up studies later, in the French scientific journal *Compte Rendu de l'Académie des Sciences*. They were read in 1865 by Glasgow's Professor of Chemistry, Thomas Anderson, who, knowing of Lister's determination to solve the problem of surgical sepsis, called them to his colleague's attention. Lister's "prepared mind" recognized immediately that the French chemist had demonstrated the *thing* he was seeking, the cause of decomposition of organic matter, the perfect explanation for the occurrence of wound infections.

periment that these germs do not arise *de novo* by a process of spontaneous generation as so many had believed; instead they are present because they have reproduced themselves from the original organisms that intruded into the material being studied. And he demonstrated that a liquid rendered germfree by boiling would stay unputrefied so long as no new germs were allowed to enter the flask in which it was kept.

At its inaugural assembly on December 7, 1854, Pasteur had addressed the Lille Faculty of Science. One of the sentences he uttered on that day has since become a maxim well known to all researchers: *Dans les champs de l'observation, le hasard ne favorise que les esprits préparés,* "Where observation is concerned, chance favors only the prepared mind." Certainly true of the career of its origina-

Lister read Pasteur's articles over and over, and he and Agnes repeated every one of the experiments in their home laboratory. He came to the same conclusions as had the Frenchman: fermentation and putrefaction in previously sterilized solutions of sugar or protein are always caused by the introduction of microscopic organisms from outside. Like Pasteur, he considered the primary source of contamination to be invisible germ-laden dust particles falling from the air. Since air could not be kept from a wound, to prevent infection, a way must be found to destroy the bacteria that were constantly dropping onto the open cut surface of an operative incision. In his words, "If the wound could be treated with some substance which without doing serious mischief to the human tissues, would kill the microbes already contained in it, and prevent the further access of others in the living state, putrefaction might be prevented however freely the air with its oxygen should enter." He later put the problem in even simpler terms: "When I read Pasteur's original paper I said to myself, 'Just as we may destroy lice on the head of a child who has pediculi, by poisonous applications which will not injure the scalp, so, I believe, we can use poisons on wounds to destroy bacteria without injuring the soft tissues of the patient.'"

The next step would obviously be to find the proper poison to disinfect wounds without causing irreversible damage. Lister decided upon carbolic acid, again because of his prepared mind. The elders of the nearby community of Carlisle had successfully used small quantities of that chemical to destroy the foul odors of their urban refuse; in the process, they had also rendered odorless the nearby pastures that were irrigated with the waste's liquid content. A secondary unanticipated gain had been the destruction of the protozoan parasites with which the local cattle had been becoming infected when they grazed on these lands. It seemed obvious to Lister that the carbolic acid was killing the organisms that decomposed the refuse and gave it its characteristic odor of putrefaction. The proper disinfectant poison was thus at hand.

Lister decided to try the carbolic-acid method first in the treatment of compound fractures, injuries in which the sharp edge of the splintered bone could be seen through the crushed skin laceration. Such wounds had a high rate of infection, often requiring amputations, which in turn became filled with pus within days. On August 12, 1865, ironically one day following the obscure death of Ignac Semmelweis in a Vienna madhouse, an eleven-year-old boy named James Greenlees was run over by the wheel of a horse-drawn cart. On being brought to the Glasgow Royal Infirmary he was found to have a fractured tibia exposed through a wound an inch and a half long and three quarters of an inch wide. It was the ideal injury, not too dirty and not too extensive, upon which to use the new technique. Lister dressed the area with a lint bandage dipped in carbolic acid. The leg was then splinted, and allowed to remain untouched for four days. Afterward, the dressing was changed periodically until complete healing was found to have taken place. The process took six weeks. Lister's first clinical experiment was a success.

In the succeeding months, one patient after another was treated in much the same way. Ten more cases of compound fracture were seen, of whom eight recovered without untoward event. One of the remaining two developed hospital gangrene

> *"Where observation is concerned, chance favors only the prepared mind."*

and required amputation while Lister was away for a few weeks; the other bled to death when a sharp bone fragment pierced a major artery after several weeks of good recovery. Carbolic-acid antisepsis, as the new concept of disinfecting a wound was to be called, was obviously worth further study.

Lister next turned his attention to a condition called psoas abscess. This fearsome complication of spinal tuberculosis took the form of a large collection of pus lying on one of the long muscles in the back of the abdominal cavity. Such abscesses grew very large, eventually coming to protrude into the groin. When they were incised for the necessary drainage, the resulting open wound often became invaded by the organisms of hospital gangrene, erysipelas, or the others, with death as the usual consequence. Lister developed a technique of disinfecting the skin around the incision with carbolic acid and then dressing the drained cavity with a puttylike substance of which the disinfectant solution was a major constituent. Again, results were excellent, compared to what had been before.

When he was sufficiently encouraged by his treatment of psoas abscess, Lister felt justified in applying his new method to amputations. The results were so gratifying that in 1867 he published a series of five papers in the *Lancet*, announcing the invention of antisepsis. The title was a long one, because it was meant to convey the importance of the text: *The Antiseptic System: On a New Method of Treating Compound Fracture, Abscess, etc.; with Observations on the Conditions of Suppuration.*

As Lister's experience grew, he modified his techniques to take advantage of his increasing store of knowledge. Every innovation was car-

ried out with meticulous care; it seemed to some onlookers as though the ritual were as important as the theory behind it. Not only were the wounds exposed to carbolic acid during the operation, but also all instruments as well as the hands of the surgical team. And yet, Lister's operating-theater attire was not different from that in which his nonantiseptic colleagues customarily worked. He rarely removed his coat, preferring to roll his sleeves back in the manner of the day, and then to turn up the collar of his frock coat to protect the white starched shirt collar he always wore, so that it would not become sodden from the cloud of antiseptic spray which he later introduced. He dipped his hands in carbolic, applied soaked towels to the skin around the planned incision, and went to work, stopping frequently to rerinse wound, hands, and instruments with the disinfectant.

Postoperative management consisted of periodic dressing changes during which everything touching the incision was again disinfected, in an atmosphere heavy with spray-filled air. By late 1869, a large enough experience with amputations had been accumulated that the results could be submitted to the *Lancet* for publication. Although Lister acknowledged that the numbers were still too small for proper statistical analysis, he correctly pointed out that when "the details are considered, they are highly valuable with reference to the question we are considering." The summary figures follow, exactly as they appeared in the issue of the *Lancet* for January 8, 1870. They speak for themselves:

Before the antiseptic period, 16 deaths in 35 cases; or 1 death in every 2½ cases.

Not included in the statistics were the many wounds treated antiseptically which were thereby made to heal so well that amputation was avoided. Without carbolic acid, many of them would have resulted in infection and death. The paper stated, "If the history of all the contused wounds of the hands and feet that have been treated in my wards during the last three years were recorded, including many compound fractures not reckoned as such in our classification and several compound dislocations, it would be enough to convince the most sceptical of the advantages of the antiseptic system."

The publication of his results on amputation was the culmination of Lister's work in Glasgow. The term of office of the Surgeon to the Glasgow Infirmary, limited to ten years and non-renewable, came to an end in 1870, and Lister had no wish to stay on at the university once his clinical appointment was ended. For several years he had been seeking a longer-lasting post elsewhere, applying for those that held any interest for him as they came up. He was not successful when a professor-

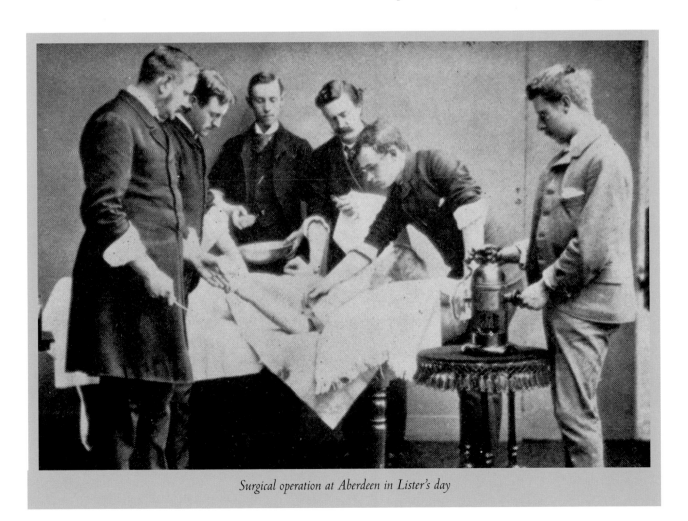

Surgical operation at Aberdeen in Lister's day

ship became vacant at Edinburgh in 1864, or at his *alma mater*, University College, in 1866. He had begun to despair as his Glasgow term drew to a close, when a cerebral thrombosis suffered by his father-in-law proved, quite literally, to be a stroke of good fortune for him. When the partially paralyzed Syme resigned his Chair of Clinical Surgery, a group of 127 Edinburgh students wrote to Lister begging him to become a candidate. Their letter stated, in part, "We feel sure that if you are appointed to this Chair, the benevolence of your character and the urbanity of your manners, will speedily draw around you a large band of attached and devoted followers." He was appointed to the post in August of 1869, and by October he and Agnes were once again settled in Edinburgh. He was forty-two years old. The happiest years of his life were about to begin.

Although Lister's benevolence and urbanity may have been well known to the Edinburgh student body, the news of his introduction of antiseptic surgery does not seem to have thus far reached them. His methods were receiving a warm reception at some of the continental hospitals, but no British surgeons outside of Glasgow had yet been converted either to antisepsis or to the principle upon which it was based, the theory that microbes can be the cause of certain diseases and of decomposition in tissues. Even at this early stage, debates were beginning to be heard about the significance of finding bacteria in infected wounds. There were those who believed that they were secondary invaders that entered after putrefaction had begun, rather than being the source of the infection. There were other skeptics who considered the germs to be harmless contaminants, refusing to believe that they played any role in the process of infection and unconvinced by Lister's improved results in the treatment of compound fractures and abscesses, or by his still-small series of amputations. In addition, there were several alternate theories, now best consigned to the abstruse researches of medical historians (oxidation of tissues, mentioned above, was the least speculative), which purported to explain suppuration and contagion by mechanisms other than marauding microbes.

Such was the state of affairs when the Listers moved into their large new home at 9 Charlotte Square in Edinburgh. During the next eight years, as heated discussions raged in every major center of medical thought about what was coming to be called the germ theory of disease, Lister became one of the best known and most controversial scientists in the world. His practice and his clinic population grew large enough to enable him to test his techniques in a wide variety of operations, and his spreading fame brought increasing numbers of foreign visitors who wished to learn them. Once again, he and Agnes put together a kitchen laboratory and set to work on a series of investigations of wound infection.

To his students, it seemed puzzling that a surgeon would interest himself in such things as test tubes and microscopes. They flocked to him because of his quiet goodness and because he could teach them how to avoid infection; the theory behind it was of little interest to them. Here is the description written by one of them, J. R. Leeson, who came to visit his professor at home soon after his arrival in Edinburgh:

I felt instinctively that I was in the presence of a very unusual personality: such a combination of refinement, ability, benevolence, and sweetness of disposition as I had never before met; he seemed the embodiment of high purpose; an emanation of goodness radiated from him. . . .

He led me to the windows before which on a long table were several rows of test-tubes covered with glass shades, half full of various liquids, and in the mouth of each was a plug of cotton wool.

It was a curious assemblage such as I had never seen, nor could I form the least conjecture as to what they were or why they should be plugged with cotton wool; my experience of test-tubes was an open mouth, and I never remember having seen them closed.

With the greatest care and pride he picked out one here and there, held it up to the light and seemed inexplicably pleased at its condition: this was clear, this was turbid, and this was mouldy. Of course I tried to show an intelligent interest, but had not the faintest idea as to what it was all about and wondered what connection they could have with my visit or with any branch of surgery; and I remember thinking it strange that so eminent a surgeon should be interested in such an unusual subject and could find time to study such irrelevant and out-of-the-way matters.

At Edinburgh, the new Professor of Clinical Surgery lectured twice a week in that large amphitheater described by Lawson Tait. He

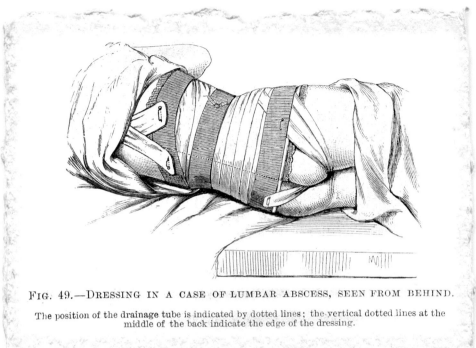

FIG. 49.—DRESSING IN A CASE OF LUMBAR ABSCESS, SEEN FROM BEHIND.

The position of the drainage tube is indicated by dotted lines; the vertical dotted lines at the middle of the back indicate the edge of the dressing.

Dressing in a case of lumbar abscess, from behind

discoursed on the physiology and bacteriology upon which his practical teachings were based, and he demonstrated the increasingly more complex methodology of his carbolic-acid technique. He had discovered the nature of sepsis, and his mission was to explain its prevention. He imagined the air to be swarming with microscopic organisms and every wound therefore to be by its very nature already contaminated from the instant of incision. His aim was to decontaminate everything that came into contact with exposed flesh, and he used carbolic solutions of varying strengths to do it, even going so far as to design a machine that sprayed a fine mist of the material, through which he operated heedless of its effect on his own lungs and those of his assistants.

Although Lister successively decreased the concentration of the carbolic in order to lessen skin irritation, everything else about Listerism, as the antiseptic technique became known, gradually grew more complicated. In its final form, it required that an inner crust of blood and carbolic be covered with a layer of waterproof silk upon which were wrapped exactly eight layers of carbolized muslin between the outer two of which was a sheet of gutta percha. The whole pungent mass was drenched with liquid resin and paraffin; it was then covered over with waxed taffeta soaked in more carbolic. Lister believed that any variation in the method might lead to failure.

And the results of compulsive adherence to Listerism were impressive. In his last three years in Glasgow, its inventor had had only one case of wound erysipelas. Hospital gangrene, on those few occasions when it occurred, did so in a mild form. Such improvements continued in Edinburgh. The number of wound infections remained low, Lister's mortality figures allowed him to dare more complicated operations, and the periods of recuperation of his patients were significantly shorter than those of his colleagues' patients in the same hospital. Needless to say, so were the lists of his dead patients.

Nevertheless, he continued to have few converts among the local surgeons. Books have been written about why it was that the entire surgical world did not immediately embrace Lister's teachings. One of the reasons is obvious: it was a great deal easier not to believe in them. Imagine a fifty-year-old surgeon at the height of his career, accustomed to striding into his amphitheater, changing into his old frock coat stained with the dried pus and blood of many a gory encounter, and then commencing to operate without the inconvenience of so much as a pre-

liminary hand-wash; with his patient hastily etherized, he slam-bangs his way through the usual ten-minute operation and prepares for the next. Not since medical school, and even then only a few times if at all, has he looked down the barrel of a microscope. One day, he attends a lecture delivered by a professor who is surrounded by a distinctly nonsurgical array of flasks, lenses, and small glass-covered dishes, during which he is told that little invisible creatures are his real enemy, and that in order to defeat them he must soak to the wrist in a corrosive solution, operate through a spray of acrid vapor, interrupt the blinding speed of his procedure numerous times to irrigate the wound and all of his instruments with a chemical disinfectant, laboriously apply a complicated sharp-smelling dressing in a meticulously ritualistic way, and then follow very specific rules about dressing changes in the postoperative period. Then imagine that same surgeon at his club in the evening, lifting a glass of port to his lips with red, puffy hands chapped by the corrosive fluid in which they have soaked during the day.

And finally, imagine the worst thing of all. Imagine what it must have felt like for such a surgeon to accept a theory that confronts him with the intolerable fact that for the previous fifteen years of his career he has been killing his patients by allowing into their wounds microbes which he should have been destroying.

For such reasons, many a surgeon at the height of his career found the premises of Listerism unacceptable. Some few tried just enough elements of the ritual to feel themselves encumbered by it but not enough to make it work— their breaks in technique prevented success, and so they abandoned its directives all too willingly as being worthless. Lister himself did not expect early universal acceptance of his principles. He predicted that it would take a generation for them and for the germ theory to become part of medical practice. There are theologians who believe that the ancient Israelites were made to wander forty years in the wilderness in order that the slave mentality should die out and a new liberated post-Egypt generation be born. Perhaps it was similar reasoning that made Lister realize that the promised land of safe surgery would be vouchsafed only unto a newly born tribe of believers.

In 1874, Lister wrote the first in a series of letters exchanged with Louis Pasteur, to thank him for furnishing the key with which the secrets of wound sepsis had been unlocked. It was the British professor's use of that key that gave the clue to the French chemist that his own discovery of the alcohol-souring microbes could be applied to seeking the causes of disease. In later years his studies along this Listerian line of thinking would result, as noted earlier, in the identification of the specific bacterial agents of certain infections and, through use of an attenuated strain of the anthrax bacillus, in the innoculation of patients to produce immunity. Thus it was by a process that went from Pasteur to Lister and back again to Pasteur that the so-called germ theory of disease was eventually to be proved in practice.

> *Lister himself did not expect early universal acceptance of his principles. He predicted that it would take a generation for them and for the germ theory to become part of medical practice.*

But not yet. Even in the late 1880s there continued to be debates published in our own American surgical literature concerning the validity of the germ theory. J. Collins Warren, the grandson of the first American to operate under ether anesthesia, visited Lister in Glasgow in 1869. He later wrote that when he returned to Boston and tried to be an evangelist of antisepsis at the Massachusetts General Hospital, he was "coldly informed that the carbolic acid treatment had been discarded." An imperfect trial had failed, and no more were to be attempted.

Articles on the germ theory appeared only infrequently in the American medical journals of the time. According to this country's physicians, the question of whether bacteria cause disease still awaited a definitive answer. Science was not yet a significant factor in medical thinking on this side of the Atlantic—anything that came out of a laboratory smacked of dubious foreign influences. Among those who opposed antisepsis and refused to accept the germ theory were some of the leaders of American surgery. Dr. Samuel Gross of Philadelphia, whose surgical textbook was the most popular in the country, was unconvinced that antisepsis did any good. He refused to use it. In 1876, as part of a review of the development of medicine on the hundredth anniversary of the independence of the United States, he noted that the surgeons of his native land did not believe in Listerism. He has been immortalized by Thomas Eakins in the famous painting called *The Gross Clinic*, in which he is shown operating in the traditional frock coat without an iota of antisepsis in sight. The patient's mother is depicted cringing a few feet behind his bare and bloody scalpel-wielding hand. The canvas was painted in 1875, nine long years after Joseph Lister had first described his doctrine in the most widely read medical journal in the English language.

In the same year during which Gross wrote his article, Joseph Lister was invited by the Cen-tennial Medical Commission of Philadelphia to attend the congress which was part of America's hundredth-anniversary celebration. The president of the Commission was the nonbelieving Philadelphia professor, who nevertheless graciously asked his English colleague to be the chairman of the Section of Surgery, an honor eagerly accepted as an opportunity to preach the antisepsis doctrine to the as yet unaccepting Americans.

The reception that greeted Lister himself was far more enthusiastic, however, than the one accorded the three-hour oration in which he attempted to convert his audience. His convictions, as eloquently expressed as they were, did not suffice to accomplish any major changes in attitude, especially when he demonstrated the complicated nature of his dressings. His personality and determination were admired much more than his antimicrobial technique. An observer for the *Boston Medical and Surgical Journal* caught the Americans' reaction: "He has a laughing face, but his firm mouth and bright eye give it character. Modesty is stamped upon his every act and word, but he *does* believe in antiseptic surgery."

Things were different, however, on the continent of Europe. For reasons that

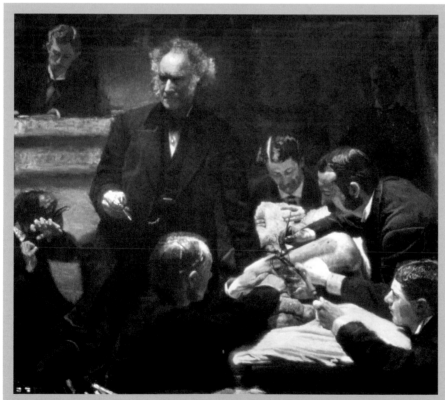

Thomas Eakins' 1875 painting of an operation by America's leading surgeon, Dr. Samuel Gross, a determined opponent of Joseph Lister and antisepsis

will be discussed more fully a few pages onward, continental and particularly German-speaking surgeons were far more prepared than the Americans to believe in the concept that infection is caused by microbes. Once the germ theory was accepted, the use of antisepsis or an equivalent technique was a natural consequence. Among the pioneers was Ritter von Nussbaum of Munich, who wrote Lister describing the way in which "We experienced one surprise after another. . . . Not another case of hospital gangrene appeared. . . . Our results became better and better, the time of healing shorter, and the pyemia and erysipelas completely disappeared." Nussbaum expressed the feelings of many of Lister's continental disciples when he added, "I hold that next to that of chloroform-narcosis your discovery is the greatest and most blessed in our Science. God reward you for it, and grant you a long and happy life."

As has so often happened in the history of science, it had taken the tragedy of war to provide a setting in which innovation could emerge. In the brief but ferocious Franco-Prussian War of 1870–1871, the few surgeons who used Lister's methods had been able to demonstrate mortality statistics that were much better than those of the great majority of their colleagues. The postoperative carnage among the patients of Georg Friedrich Louis Stromeyer, surgeon general successively of the Schleswig-Holstein and Hanoverian armies, was thirty-six deaths following thirty-six amputations through the knee joint. What made this statistic all the more depressing was that Stromeyer was no incompetent—Fielding Garrison has called him "the father of modern military surgery in Germany." Neither were the French statistics any cause for acclaim; of 13,173 amputations of all sorts done in the military hospitals of France, including fingers and toes, 10,006 ended in death.

After the war, German surgeons, prepared by the growing scientific spirit at home, began to travel to Edinburgh to learn about antisepsis. Close on their heels came the French, and then representatives of other continental countries as well. By the time of the 1875 German Surgical Congress, many enthusiastic disciples had been won over. One of the most outspoken was Ritter von Nussbaum, who exhorted his audience, "Look at my sick wards recently ravaged by death. I can only say that my assistants and my nurses and I are overwhelmed with joy. It is with the greatest zeal that we undergo all the extra pains required by the treatment." Nussbaum also wrote a short book on antisepsis. Translated into French, Italian, and Greek, it led to the rapid continental spread of Listerism.

Among the most beholden of the Germans was Stromeyer, who went so far as to write a laudatory poem titled "Lister." He undertook the translation himself, and it should be read mindful of the caveat that his good intentions are somewhat marred by the fractured quality of his Teutonized English. Here is the first stanza, sounding as though it were written as a send-up for a senior-class show at some modern American medical school. No significance should be attached to the fact that the personal pronoun referring to the author of antisepsis is capitalized as though he were also the Author of us all. Although this does give the poem somewhat the quality of a paean to God, it should be remembered that the Germans treat their nouns and pronouns this way as a matter of course:

Mankind looks grateful now on Thee
For what Thou didst in Surgery.
And Death must often go amiss,
By smelling antiseptik Bliss.

Some weeks after the German Surgical Congress, Joseph and Agnes Lister, with his brother's family of four, went on a tour of the continent, part of which was planned as a visit to the German hospitals to evaluate the success of antisepsis. After traveling through France and Italy, they journeyed to Munich, Leipzig, Berlin, Halle, and several other cities. Having been embraced by Nussbaum in Munich, they were treated to what their hosts called a "Lister-Banquet" in Leipzig, attended by some 350 professors, physicians, and students. There were many light, bright moments that evening. The guest of honor was entertained by humorous songs written for him, among which was one titled "The Carbolic Acid Tingle-Tangle." Unfortunately for posterity, its lyrics seem not to have been preserved. Professor Karl Thiersch proposed the honoree's health, and pointed out that antisepsis, like so many other great inventions, was in the midst of passing through what he called the three usual stages of discovery: "The first, when the world smiles and shakes its

> *"The first, when the world smiles and shakes its head and says, 'It's all nonsense'; the second with a shrug of the shoulders and a look of contempt, 'It's the merest humbug'; and finally, 'Oh, that's an old story, we knew that long ago.'"*

head and says, 'It's all nonsense'; the second with a shrug of the shoulders and a look of contempt, 'It's the merest humbug'; and finally, 'Oh, that's an old story, we knew that long ago.'"

The *Lancet* of June 19, 1875, described the German visit in a way that was incomprehensible to the still-skeptical surgeons of the English-speaking countries: "The progress of Professor Lister through the University towns of Germany, which he is visiting chiefly, we believe, with a view to inquire into the mode in which the antiseptic treatment is carried out in the Continent, has assumed the character of a triumphal march." A similar reception awaited him four years later when he attended the International Congress of Medicine in Amsterdam. He was greeted, according to the *British Medical Journal,* with "an enthusiasm that knew no bounds," a prolonged standing ovation, and the encomium of the president, Professor Donders: "It is not only our admiration that we offer you, it is our gratitude, and that of the nations to which we belong."

Nevertheless, Lister's own countrymen remained fixated, like most Americans, at Thiersch's second stage. Although increasing numbers of younger British surgeons were beginning to accept antisepsis, most of the senior professors at the great London teaching hospitals stood stolidly opposed. As long as they remained so, Lister felt that he had not been successful with the group whose endorsement he valued most highly. And then, in 1877, an opportunity presented itself by which the situation might be turned around. Upon the death of its incumbent, Joseph Lister was offered the Chair of Surgery at the Medical School of King's College, London.

At first, it seemed inconceivable to his colleagues that he would leave one of the most prestigious schools in the world, as Edinburgh then was, to go to an institution of a decidedly lower caliber. Not only would he be taking a backward step academically, but he would have to give up a thriving private practice, the ample clinical opportunities for patient study at the Royal Infirmary, and his scores of devoted students. In return, he would enter an environment hostile to his teachings and resentful of his ever-growing international fame. When his students learned that their beloved teacher was giving serious consideration to the offer, they presented him with a petition of seven hundred signatures, begging him to remain.

There was a lot to leave behind in Edinburgh that was the stuff of happiness and the reward of the appreciative love in which Joseph Lister was enveloped wherever he went in that city. A student, John Stewart, has left us with one of the many moving descriptions that were in later years written by his pupils to portray their mentor as he was seen by them and by his patients. The quotes within the text are taken from a poem by William Ernest Henley, who is best known as the author of "Invictus," written while he was Lister's surgical patient at the Edinburgh Royal Infirmary:

Among the happiest recollections of those Edinburgh days are those of the Sunday afternoon hospital visits. This was one of Lister's ways of keeping the Sabbath Day. The coachman and the horses had a rest. Lister came to the Infirmary on foot. The picture is plain before me now. . . . Someone suddenly says, "Here comes the Chief!" and we see our hero enter through the little side-gate, pass down the slope, with his easy rapid stride, a light cane in his hand, and on his handsome face a look of happy meditation. The house-surgeon meets him at the main door, and in a few minutes they enter the ward. Students come to attention, patients' faces beam. I wonder if there were anywhere else in the world a surgeon whose pupils held him in more reverent admiration, whose patients so trusted him, loved and positively adored him. He cannot be unconscious of this feeling, the "soft lines of tranquil thought" grow softer, that "face at once benign and proud and shy" is suffused with the unaffected pleasure of this modest and simple-minded great man as he begins his tour of the ward.

But his friends and his students reckoned without the deeply ingrained Quaker sense of mission. As there is a fundamental strain of mysticism in the Inner Light concept of the Society of Friends, there is also a deep commitment to evangelicism.

For Lister, transfer to King's College was an inevitable part of his mission to carry the message of the germ theory to every doubting doctor who still disbelieved it. There was never any question in his mind but that he must accept the London offer. By October of 1877, Agnes and he had moved into a spacious house at 12 Park Crescent, near enough to Regent's Park so that they could stroll through its beautiful gardens. The professor brought four skilled assistants to London, to help him set up his new teaching program and to be his fellow missionaries. To the childless Listers, they were like surrogate sons. Among them was John Stewart.

Lister's Inaugural Lecture at King's was as well attended as had been its counterpart at Glasgow. The members of his audience, having come prepared to listen to a description of surgical operations, were chagrined to hear their new Professor launch into a learned scientific disquisition. Standing behind a laboratory table covered with tubes, flasks, and various other of the paraphernalia of bacteriology, he spoke about things of which they knew nothing and cared nothing. The polite applause at the lecture's end lulled Lister and his four disciples into thinking that they had made a good beginning. They soon learned otherwise. As Stewart described it, "The next few weeks were to us of his staff the abomination of desolation. There seemed to be a colossal apathy, an inconceivable indifference to the light which, to our minds, shone so brightly, a monstrous inertia to the force of new ideas."

Lister did not make much progress with his campaign during those early years at King's College. The attendance at his lectures dwindled down to ten or twenty semi-interested souls, in contrast to the three or four hundred enthusiasts who had crowded the hall each time he spoke in Edinburgh. The students soon learned that he taught nothing that was of use in the examinations of the Royal College of Surgeons, since those inquisitions were conducted by clinicians to whom the germ theory, and anything to do with science, was anathema.

Distressed and disappointed though he certainly was, Lister never betrayed a whit of antagonism or impatience with those who ignored him or those who maligned his doctrine. His assistants became accustomed to the quiet sigh of resignation with which he responded to the criticisms of lesser men. Sometimes a transient look of sadness could be seen crossing his face, but nothing beyond that momentary alteration ever revealed his pain. Long used to having their own occasional lapses treated by the Chief with merely a gentle word of admonition, his Edinburgh lads now saw more clearly than ever the majesty of which some are capable even when their greatest work is mocked. They strengthened themselves with the words from the Book of Proverbs which their professor so often used as the final sentences in a lecture, both in Scotland and here in England: "Let not mercy and truth forsake thee; bind them about thy neck."

If only a few English converts appeared among Lister's sparse audiences, continental visitors again began to fill many of the empty seats in the lecture hall and to appear on the wards, as they had done in Edinburgh. Leading European surgeons sent their protégés to learn his methods. In the memoirs of Sir St. Clair Thomson, one of the house surgeons at the time, is recorded that it was necessary to post the hospital's no-smoking sign in French and German for the benefit of the foreigners. On some days, the scene in the auditorium epitomized the scene in the greater medical world: as many as sixty continental surgeons occupied the front seats, intermingling with no more than ten English students. Not infrequently, the professor delivered half his lecture in one of the languages of the no-smoking sign.

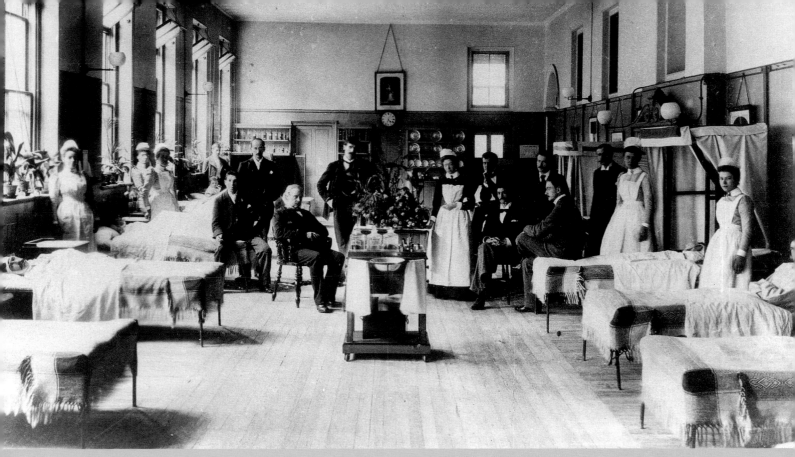

Baron Lister (seated) with his staff, Victoria ward, King's College Hospital, Lincoln's Inn Fields, 1893

Lister was thus a prophet not without honor save in his own country among his own countrymen, especially if those countrymen were surgeons. (Many pathologists, being trained to understand the ways of science, quickly accepted the germ theory and Listerism, as did other physicians who had some experience with research in physiology.) Still, he was confident the truth would win out, one way or another. Thomson describes standing beside his Chief on the steps of the hospital one day, after a particularly vigorous sally had been directed against his doctrine by a stubborn colleague. The year was 1883, and the fifty-six-year-old professor had heard just about every argument that could possibly be thrown at him, and each of them many times. Wearily and with a quiet certitude, he predict-

ed to his young pupil that the day must surely come when his principles would be universally utilized. Then, casting off his usual soft tone of serenity, he raised his voice just a bit to declare with a barely perceptible trace of sternness, "If the profession does not recognize them, the public will learn of them and the law will insist on them."

There were several reasons why the English were so slow to accept, or even to understand, antisepsis. Among them, of course, was the fact that Lister had made his techniques so complicated that they taxed the patience of those who would try them. But the overriding problem had to do with science, or rather its generally low condition of advancement in England even three quarters of a century after the death of John Hunter.

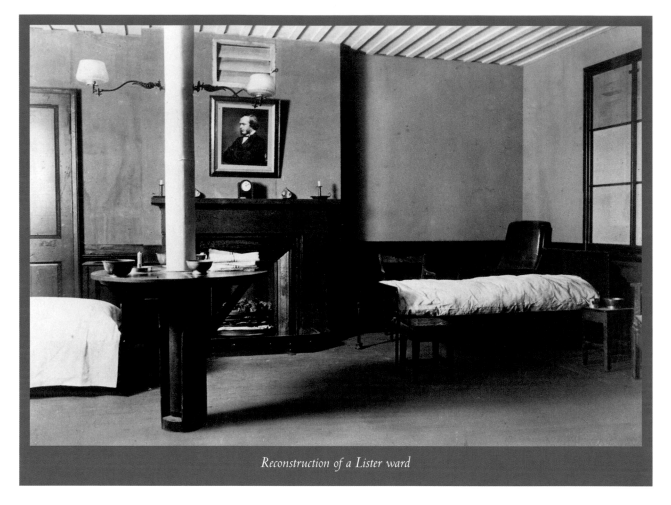

Reconstruction of a Lister ward

Hunter's legacy had become a bit like Galen's, its most important principles being honored only in the breach. The state of affairs is explicated by a perceptive editor who made the following observation in an issue of the *Lancet* in early 1878:

> *The truth is, that this is a question in science rather than in surgery, and hence, while eagerly adopted by the scientific Germans, and a little grudgingly by the semi-scientific Scotch, the antiseptic doctrine has never been in any degree appreciated or understood by the plodding and practical English surgeon. Happily for his patients, he has for a long time been to a considerable extent practising a partially antiseptic system, thanks to his cleanly English instincts; but it has been like the lady who talked prose without knowing it.*

The situation described by the *Lancet* editor is illustrated by the example of the aforementioned Lawson Tait, who had an enviably low rate of infections in his own series of gynecological operations, none of which had been done using the lessons of the germ theory, or so he thought. In his 1887 presidential address to the Birmingham and Midland Counties Branch of the British Medical Association he denied the validity of the germ theory of disease with the memorable words "To apply the conclusions derived from beef-tea in the flasks of the chemist's laboratory to the phenomena of living tissue is nonsense," and "I care not a fig for the germs." He scoffed at Listerism, and had only contempt for the principles of bacterial putrefaction upon which it was based: "It is when Lister comes in with his royal road to surgical success, still more when his German disciples, full of enthusiasm and quite empty of discrimination, appear on the scene, that I am in doubt, and equally in fear." On more than one occasion he offered to pack his wounds with dry germs, just to give the lie to Lister. He attributed his own salutary statistics to the liberal use of drainage tubes and absorbent dressings, as well as to his own "cleanly English instincts." The latter were in fact far more important than the former—Tait was known for his careful preoperative hand-washing and for his advocacy of plenty of soap and hot water on equipment and instruments. Though he may not have believed that germs cause putrefaction, he was nevertheless willy-nilly killing them before they got into his surgical wounds. He was unwittingly practicing a form of prophylaxis that would later become known as asepsis. He would one day be chagrined to discover that his results gave strong support for the very theory he sought to deride.

There was one other major factor in the foot-dragging of the English and of the Americans as well: they were resisting a powerful and ultimately overwhelming movement which was already beginning to permeate the atmosphere of German surgery. By this I mean the new order of things, in which the careful, meticulously executed operations permitted by antisepsis and anesthesia were replacing the old emphasis on speed and dazzling dexterity. The judiciously painstak-

ing operative technique of Lister himself was an example of what was on the horizon. The day of the spectacular *tour de force* was drawing to a close. No longer would it be necessary to amputate a leg in thirty seconds, as did Robert Liston, before oxygen could enter the wound to putrefy it, and before the struggling patient could break free of the staunch grip in which he was being held by muscular assistants.

A new type of man was entering the specialty of surgery, a prudent scientific technician who treated human tissues with delicacy and thoughtfulness rather than brute force and blinding speed. He was exemplified in England by Frederick Treves, and in America by William Stewart Halsted. As their teachings became more and more a part of daily medical practice, so did the germ theory and so did science. The old surgeon was more a theatrical performer than a student of disordered physiology. Certainly he was no man of science. The Listerian methods made many a senior operator an anachronism, superannuated by young men with a totally different set of talents from those by which their own teachers had achieved their success. The old surgeon's hour upon the stage was ending, but he was determined to delay his departure as long as he could.

Nevertheless, even at King's College Hospital, by the end of the 1870s there were a few signs that the resistance to antisepsis, although still formidable, was beginning to crumble in the face of Lister's scientific truth. The senior professor John Wood visited the Chief's wards and was so impressed with what he saw that in November 1878 he asked Lister to help him use the antiseptic technique in operations on two cases, one a goiter and the other an ovarian tumor. Both patients recovered without complication. Although Wood was three years older than Lister and too fixed in his operating habits to change them, he became a convert, at least in theory. This was all the more remarkable because he was the man who had been generally expected to be appointed to the chair now occupied by his rival, and he had been one of Lister's most ardent opponents. In the circumstances, one might, perhaps, forgive his grudging disclaimer, namely that the Germans needed antisepsis because "the Germans are dirty people . . . it is not really necessary in England."

Like Wood, however, other leading London surgeons finally began to see the merit not only in the practical application of Listerism, but in the entire set of principles that followed from the germ theory. At a meeting held at St. Thomas' Hospital in December 1879, Lister was hailed by some of the very men who had once been his adversaries. In 1883, Alexander Ogston, an early disciple from Aberdeen, wrote him a letter that might well have been composed by any of the increasing number of his followers: "You have changed Surgery, especially operative Surgery, from being a hazardous lottery into a safe and soundly-based science; you are the leader of the modern generation of scientific surgeons, and every wise and good man in our profession—especially in Scotland—looks up to you with respect and attachment as few men receive." Soon after this, Lister was knighted by Queen Victoria. Ironically, it was the same year in which he stood on the steps of King's College with Thomson, and

came close to losing his patience at the world's slowness to comprehend his message.

From that point on, the tide turned inexorably in his favor, or rather in favor of science. Tributes were showered on the newly dubbed Sir Joseph from all directions. He was made a Knight of the Prussian Order, and a Knight Commander of the Order of Denmark; he received medals and honorary degrees. Among them were doctorates from both Oxford and Cambridge, schools which his Quaker faith had made him ineligible to attend forty years earlier. He was awarded France's Boudet Prize for his application of Pasteur's discoveries to medicine, and he received Prussia's Order of Merit. Medical societies all over the world rushed to make him an honorary member.

As Lister's precepts became more and more a part of daily medical practice, so did the germ theory. Not only was Pasteur's continuing research providing ever more convincing evidence that microbes are the inciting cause of infectious disorders, but in 1876 a thirty-four-year-old German bacteriologist named Robert Koch had identified for the first time a specific bacterium as the cause of a specific disease, demonstrating in a simple, clear set of experiments that the bacillus found in the blood of animals suffering from anthrax was the direct agent that produced the pathological changes of that sickness when it was introduced in pure culture into other animals. The results of Koch's investigations were soon confirmed by Pasteur, who, as noted earlier, was able to develop a method to immunize against anthrax by using a bacillus of weakened virulence. In 1878, the final missing piece of evidence was supplied to Lister's original Pasteur-inspired thesis when Koch produced his monumental paper "Investigations Concerning the Etiology of Wound Infections," in which he was able to link six different kinds of surgical infections to six distinct bacteria. The scientific basis for the germ theory had been proved beyond question. It remained only for the nonscientists and the Lawson Taits to come to grips with it.

A medical paradox was making its presence felt during this time. It began to be realized, and Lister himself was one of the realizers, that air swarms with far fewer microbes than had been thought. This affected Sir Joseph only insofar as he decided that it was safe to abandon his pungent carbolic spray. But some of the younger students of the germ theory interpreted this perception in a much more far-reaching way. To them it meant that the organisms that contaminate surgical wounds must of necessity be carried into them by means other than particles falling from the atmosphere; the body seems to have defenses that make it immune to the small doses of bacte-

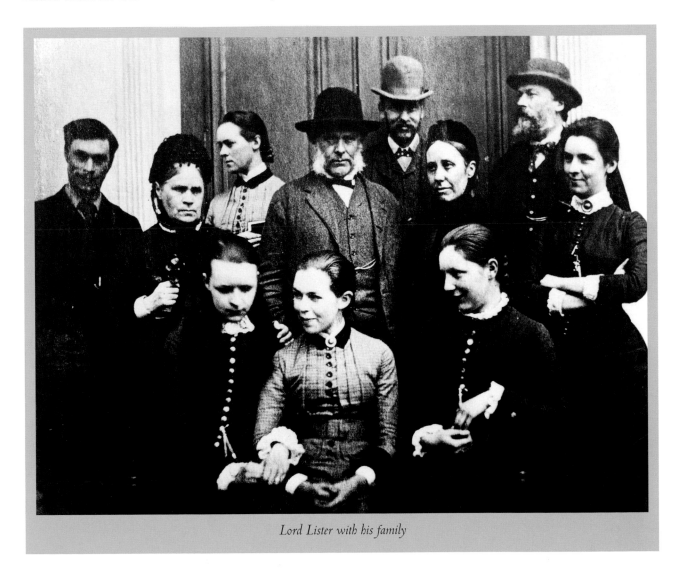

Lord Lister with his family

ria that reach it from the air. The obvious sources of major contamination were thus the hands and the instruments of medical personnel—the doctors and nurses. Wound infection was another of those "we have met the enemy and it is us" phenomena that have sojourned on this earth since long before Walt Kelly and Pogo.

It follows from the preceding that it is not the wound that requires disinfecting as Lister had thought, but rather every foreign germ-laden object with which it comes into contact. The doctrine of asepsis was born.

Antisepsis aimed to disinfect the wound itself, since it was considered to be already contaminated from the air. Asepsis requires the scrupulous sterilizing of everything that will touch the area of operation. Its proponents declared, quite correctly, that an incision made through uninfected tissues remains uninfected unless germ-carrying objects enter it. The surgeon's hands must be scrubbed, his instruments must be boiled, and the wound drapes must be rendered germ-free. The sterile incision can be made by the sterile knife held in the sterile hand only after the patient's skin has been made sterile by a disinfectant, whether carbolic acid or some equally effective agent. The disease-stained old frock coat must give way to the freshly laundered sterile gown. Thus was the insight of Ignac Semmelweis the Hungarian reborn, in an era which, thanks to the work of Pasteur the Frenchman, Lister the Englishman, and Koch the German, was ready to receive it and bid it warm welcome.

It now became Joseph Lister's turn to be superannuated. The very germ theory upon which Listerism was founded demanded that aseptic methods should replace antisepsis. In effect, asepsis is prophylaxis, while antisepsis is therapy. Better to prevent the cause of infection from entering a wound than to treat it once it has settled itself in place. Except for wounds that were already dirty, antisepsis began to become less useful even as its underlying theoretical framework was achieving universal recognition and its innovator was being hailed as a surgical savior. In 1883, Gustav Neuber of Kiel built a private hospital based on the aseptic principle that germs should be destroyed before, rather than after, they come into contact with patients. He designed a dust-free ventilating system, and he was the first to operate in surgical cap and gown. William Stewart Halsted of Baltimore popularized the use of rubber gloves in 1889. The Russian-born Ernst von Bergmann, Professor of Surgery in Berlin, introduced steam sterilization in 1886, and established the basic steps in our modern aseptic ritual in 1891.

In the final analysis, Listerism must be seen as a transitional phase. The excellent results obtained by its practitioners confirmed the practical validity of the germ theory and established the dictum that surgeons must apply the teachings of science in their daily hospital routines. But once the bacterial basis of infection had become firmly established in the laboratories of Pasteur and Koch, Listerism's shining hour came to an end. Ultimately, Joseph Lister deserved the encomiums of a grateful humanity not because of his methods, but because he awakened his fellow surgeons to the real cause of putrefaction in wounds and led them into scientific patterns of thought by which it could be prevented.

There was, however, one contribution of Joseph Lister that lives virtually in its original form to this very day. I refer to his perfection of the catgut suture so that it could safely be used in surgical operations. Because I have been unwilling to sidetrack the narrative of antigerm warfare with anything that might detract from its intensity, I have omitted, up to this point, one of the most practical innovations ever made in technical surgery.

Since the days of classical Greece, the strings of musical instruments have been made from the intestinal lining of sheep and other animals. Some ancient authors described the use of such strings to tie blood vessels; under the name *graciliu chordaru*, catgut was used by Galen for this purpose. Its great virtue was that it dissolved in the healing tissues and could be absorbed by them. But the tying off of blood vessels went in and out of fashion; every few hundred years it needed to be rediscovered, as by Ambroise Paré. In Joseph Lister's day, catgut was in use only for stringing instruments, and perhaps rackets of various sorts. In fact, the material had gotten its name as a bastardization of *kit-gut*, the kit being a small fiddle customarily favored by dancing masters. Both *kit* and *gut* seem to be derived from the Greek *kithara*, which was a lyre, a harp, or a lute.

When Lister began his work on antisepsis, it was the practice to tie off large blood vessels with nonabsorbable threads or metal wires pulled from a handful suspended through the buttonhole of the surgeon's bespattered frock coat. The ends of these ligatures were left long enough so that they hung out of the incision. In this way, they could be withdrawn through the soft decomposing tissues when infection occurred, an act which sometimes resulted in alarming hemorrhage from the lacerated vessels, and all too frequently in death. In wounds treated by the antiseptic method there were far fewer infections, which meant that there was no way, without re-opening the wound, to remove the foreign bodies which the long ties had become.

In seeking a suture material that would be dissolved and absorbed, Lister remembered catgut. Beginning in 1868, he carried out a long series of experiments with the material until he had arrived at the perfect way to prepare it for surgery, and to sterilize it in carbolic acid. He found that it would dissolve in the body in about a week, but could be given much longer life by permeating it with salts of chromic acid. Although various synthetic absorbable sutures have been invented in the past decade, there is not an operating room in the world where a goodly percentage of surgeons do not use plain and so-called chromic catgut as their preferred ligatures in certain types of tissues.

Lister's years at King's College were more leisurely than had been his tenures at Glasgow and Edinburgh. Although he was at first vexed by having so few patients, he soon came to appreciate the freedom this gave him for unhurried laboratory work and occasional recreation. Even when his London private practice eventually expanded, he remained free of many of the administrative and teaching obligations that had occupied so much of his time in Scotland. He became much sought after as a lecturer at British medical societies, and he accepted every invitation that he could fit into his schedule, with the same evangelical zeal that had brought him to King's in the first place. At the Seventh International Medical Congress, held in London in 1881, he had the richly deserved pleasure of introducing Louis Pasteur to Robert Koch, and receiving the brotherly praise of both of them.

Most important, Joseph and Agnes Lister began to take longer and more frequent holidays. He taught himself fly-fishing, not because he was an enthusiast, but because it gave him the opportunity to get out into the country and allowed a peaceful respite alone with his wife, who joined him on these expeditions. Together, they became expert bird-watchers, a hobby to which they applied themselves with the same excitement that had characterized all of their years of partnership in scientific study. In Sir Rickman Godlee's biography of his uncle Joseph, there is reproduced a typical page from the diary the couple kept on their birding expeditions. In every way, it reproduces the mutuality of their lifelong comradeship in the laboratory. A sketch appears of the bird they studied on the excerpted day, April 23, 1891. The sketch and its description are by Sir Joseph himself, while the remainder of the text on the page is by Lady Lister.

Although Lister attended many medical congresses and meetings, the most dramatic of them all was the grand celebration of Louis Pasteur's seventieth birthday, held at the Sorbonne on December 27, 1892. Sir Joseph had retired from King's the previous July, at the mandatory age of sixty-five. He now came to France not only as the representative of both the London and the Edinburgh Royal Societies, but also as the central personality in the dissemination of Pasteur's teachings. He delivered an eloquent address in French,

through the final portion of which he looked directly at the great scientist whose genius he was acclaiming. As he concluded, Pasteur, enfeebled by a stroke from which he was not fully recovered, rose slowly to his feet, made his way with difficulty toward the rostrum, and, clasping Lister to him with both arms, kissed him on each cheek. It was a historic moment, made all the more moving by its spontaneity.

The following March, the Listers left the cold of London to seek the earliest touches of spring warmth at Rapallo on the Italian Riviera. While there, Lady Lister developed pneumonia. In less than a week, the most devoted of companions was dead. Something died in her husband as well on that day. A man whose life has been so closely intertwined with that of another, whose every worldly accomplishment has really been the accomplishment of both, is not likely to say farewell to thirty-seven years of communion without a great piece of himself having been torn away. Joseph Lister never stopped mourning his best friend. Though he would live nineteen more years, it was without the same optimism of spirit that he had shared with Agnes. He continued to receive the honors that should come to the great as they age their way toward immortality, but without Agnes they were rewards empty of promise. In 1895 he was elected president of the Royal Society; in 1897 he was elevated to the peerage. Joseph, Baron Lister, was the first medical man to bear such a title. At his eightieth birthday in 1907, celebrated all over the world, a special "Lister Meeting" was held by the Surgical Institute in Vienna, at which the audience of five hundred rose and broke into a loud ovation when his portrait was projected above the platform. He accepted the world's gratitude humbly, and alone.

Baron Lister continued to write and to publish until the creeping fingers of infirmity began to clutch at his strength. As late as 1909, a letter of his, dealing with the catgut ligature, was published in both the *Lancet* and the *British Medical Journal*. But his sight and hearing were beginning to fail him. Rickman Godlee describes the sadness of going to visit his uncle during the last year of his life: "He looked wistfully at us and told us he had 'so much to say.' But alas, he was not able to give expression to these last thoughts."

Imperceptibly, the architect of germ-free surgery lapsed into unconsciousness. He died on the morning of February 10, 1912. A great public funeral was held in Westminster Abbey, but Baron Lister had left specific instructions that he was not to be buried there. He lies in the West Hampstead Cemetery, alongside his beloved Agnes.

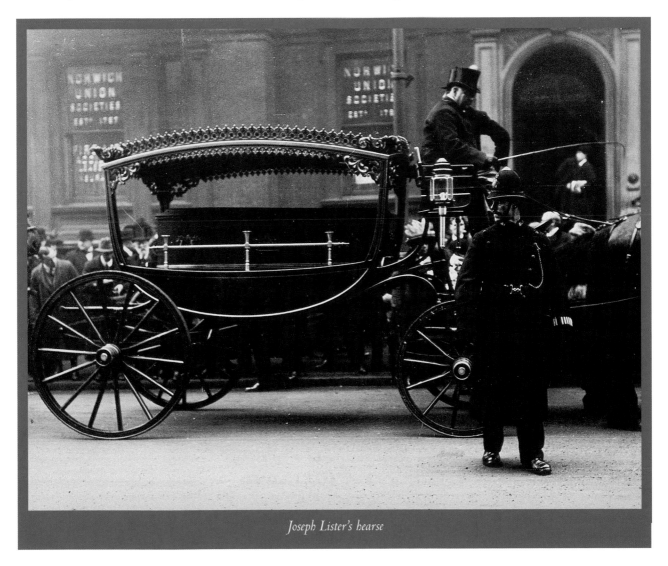

Joseph Lister's hearse

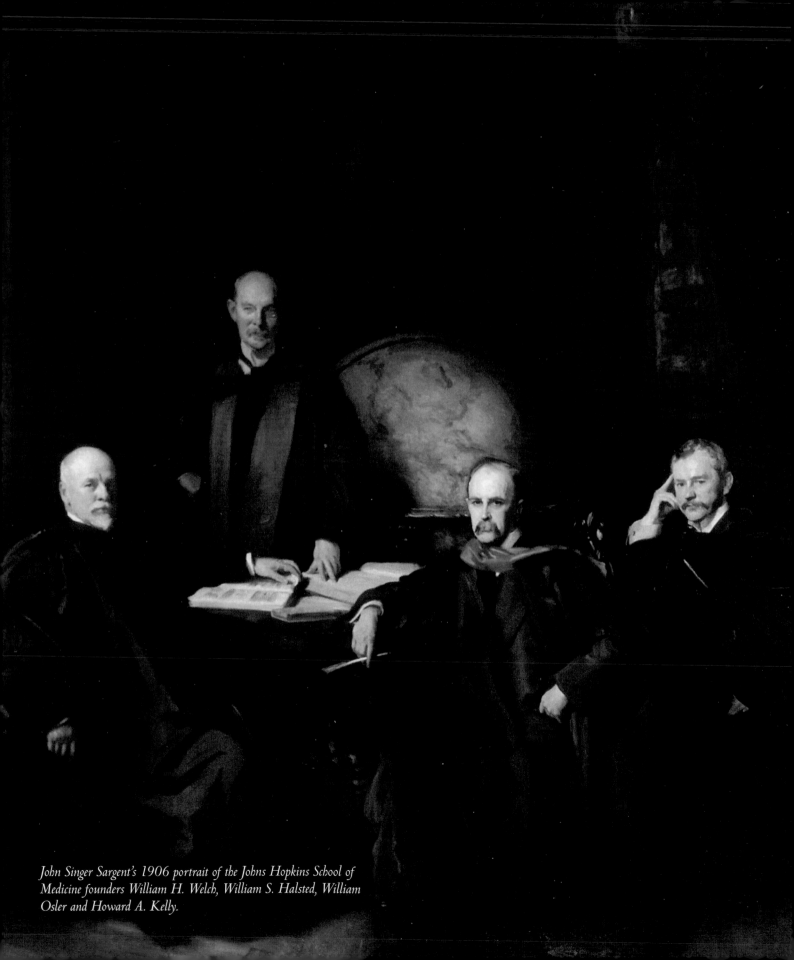

John Singer Sargent's 1906 portrait of the Johns Hopkins School of Medicine founders William H. Welch, William S. Halsted, William Osler and Howard A. Kelly.

13

MEDICAL SCIENCE COMES TO AMERICA

William Stewart Halsted
of Johns Hopkins

Late on the afternoon of the third Friday in November 1983, a busload of muscular Harvard undergraduates journeyed to New Haven, Connecticut, to engage an equivalent number of Yale stalwarts in a game of football the following day. This being the hundredth encounter between two schools whose gridiron rivalry has been so instrumental in the growth of American collegiate athletics, the accompanying hullabaloo was often deafening to listen to and blinding to read about. For days beforehand, the names of legendary stars, captains, and coaches of yesteryear filled the sports columns of newspapers in most cities of the Northeast. Even Handsome Dan, the Yale bulldog, was biographed in all of his incarnations. Monetary pledges were made by alumni, toasts were drunk (actually, more alumni were drunk than toasts), and each discoverable datum of the contesting between the ancient rivals was celebrated in every way that it is possible to commemorate such things. No name of any football luminary of either institution, no matter

how limited his candlepower, failed to appear in print.

Except one. On December 6, 1873, two years before that much-sung inaugural contest, Yale had fielded this country's first eleven-man football team, against a pickup group of Englishmen who called themselves Eton College. The modern gridiron sport that transfixes millions of Americans every autumn weekend has evolved from the rules used in that encounter. Forgotten in the festivities of a century later was the name of the captain of the victorious Yale eleven. He was William Stewart Halsted, a twenty-one-year-old senior from New York City.

The sturdily built young athlete was an indifferent student; his scholastic achievements would be magnified if they were called ordinary. After much searching, one of his biographers was forced to conclude, "The Yale Library has no record of his having borrowed any books." Having prepared at Andover in the same desultory way, Halsted was, like so many of his cronies, interested in athletics to the exclusion of the more cerebral activities which were meant to characterize Ivy League student life. Football was not his only sport. He was shortstop on the baseball team of the Class of '74, as well as being a member of the class crew; he was enough of a gymnast to have taken part in an exhibition to raise funds for his boating club. Photographs taken of him at that time show a faultlessly tailored, handsome (albeit somewhat jug-eared) dandy, looking every bit the rich man's son that he was.

The father of this combination of Beau Brummel and Frank Merriwell was the president of Halsted, Haines and Co., a family-owned textile-importing firm founded near the turn of the nineteenth century. The elder Halsted was descended from an ancestor who had settled in Hempstead, Long Island, in 1660. For a marriage partner, he had chosen his cousin, Mary Louisa Haines, herself descended from impeccable ancestors. The Halsteds lived in a town house at Fifth Avenue and 14th Street in Manhattan and a country house in Irvington, New York. It was in this constellation of the quintessential American aristocracy that the newborn star of William Stewart Halsted first shone on September 23, 1852.

Some species of medical magi must surely have journeyed to the distinctly unmangerlike precincts of the Halsted mansion, there to deliver to the silver-spooned babe the delayed-action gifts that would be unwrapped only after the completion of his unedifying years at Yale. If ever a deep-rooted plant bloomed late, it was this white-spatted, bowlered, cravated flower of the Ivy League, whose do-not-open-till-medical-school talents were never so much as suspected until almost too late. To pursue the botanical metaphor to a logi-

cally florid, but quite accurate, end point, when the petals of his intellect finally opened, they exposed pollen enough to inseminate the entire fallow field which was then American surgery. What grew thereafter was a new spirit, a new technique, and a completely original sense of leadership. An adjective was coined to describe it: it was called Halstedian.

Halsted reached manhood at a particularly propitious time in the history of American medicine. The majority of homegrown physicians were still obtaining most of their education in the old apprenticeship system, with the usual addition of a three-to-four-month session during each of two years at one of the predominantly doctor-owned medical schools. Those few students who could afford more advanced training went off to Europe in the time-honored way. In the young Halsted's day, it was usually in Germany and Austria that they found their efforts best rewarded. Even the rudiments of scientific medicine remained unfamiliar to most aspiring physicians who missed the European experience. The only exceptions were those who could pick it up secondhand from colleagues or journals.

As long as this state of affairs continued, America would remain in many respects a medical backwater. Science was the basis of everything that was new in the ancient art of healing, and science was focused in the laboratory. In the 1870s, the medical schools of our country were virtually without laboratories. In order to transform the American profession, a new generation of physicians would have to be trained in the methods of interpreting the increasingly vast amounts of technology and information. They would require the kinds of teaching that were then available only in Europe, and the exposure to scientists and facilities of a caliber rarely found at home. For this to take place, American medical education had to have a change of venue—out of the doctor-owned proprietary schools and into the scholarly atmosphere of the universities.

The model was to be the German system, and its prototype in the United States would be the Johns Hopkins Medical School in Baltimore. It was the destiny of William Halsted that he would become the first Professor of Surgery at this first American college of medicine that was truly a university graduate school. That the opportunity came to him was the shiny lining of a dark cloud, the consequence of a series of events that skimmed the cusp of personal tragedy like a tangent, and then soared off toward that tiny greensward reserved for the immortals of medical history. The William Stewart Halsted so luxuriously swaddled in his family's Manhattan town house on that late September morning in 1852 survived a fall from grace in his mid-thirties that brought him to near-ruin. He regenerated himself to become the man rightfully remembered as the father of American surgery.

There was a hint of the career that was to come later, in a statement Halsted wrote years afterward, concerning his life at Yale: "Devoted myself solely to athletics in college. In senior year purchased *Gray's Anatomy* and "Dalton's Physiology" and studied them with interest; attended a few clinics at the Yale Medical School." These were probably the clinics that were held at the New Haven Dispensary, an outpatient facility staffed by medical-school faculty. The dispensary was required for instruction because the senior staff at the New Haven Hospital were not willing to provide unlimited access on their wards to either faculty or students of the school. Having opened in 1871, it soon required more spacious facilities and was located during Halsted's senior year on Crown Street, only a few blocks from the undergraduate campus. It is appropriate to wonder whether the nonscholarly young athlete would have bothered to attend the clinic had it been situated closer to the hospital across town rather than in such close proximity to his own lodgings. For, although Halsted's uncle was a physician, there seems no evidence from his earlier years that medicine held any attraction for him. Thus an accident of municipal geography may have determined his choice of career. More likely, however, it was his fascination with "Dalton's Physiology" that was the major contributing factor.

Whatever may have been the stimulus, in the autumn of 1874 William Halsted enrolled as a medical student at the College of Physicians and Surgeons in New York, where his influential father was a member of the board of trustees. Although officially designated as the Medical Department of Columbia University, the school was in reality a completely autonomous institution. It was, in fact, owned by members of its faculty, as were all of the eight medical schools in New York at that time.

According to the rules of the college, each student, of whom there were 550 in 1874, matriculated as the preceptee of a faculty member. Halsted's preceptor was Professor of Anatomy Henry B. Sands, who, in 1879, was to become Professor of the Practice of Surgery. As fortunate as was his choice of preceptor, Halsted was blessed with an additional bit of luck by becoming student assistant to the author of his physiology text, John

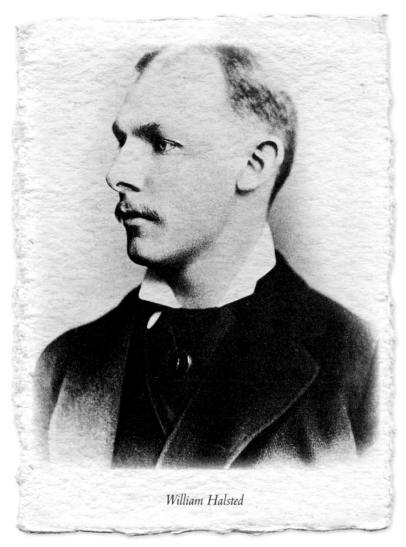

William Halsted

Internship in those days could be embarked upon before the formal granting of the doctorate. Halsted's, at Bellevue Hospital, began in October 1876 and continued for an eighteen-month period. Subsequently, he served as house physician to the New York Hospital from July to October 1878.

The transformation that had begun during his senior year at Yale was now complete. The gladiator-dandy who had strolled, almost offhandedly, a few blocks to observe at the New Haven Dispensary had become the serious student of medicine. The next step, especially since the financial means were available, was inevitable. When his service at the New York Hospital ended, Halsted embarked on a steamer for a two-year period of study in Europe. On November 4, 1878, the young physician arrived in Vienna, where he studied until the following spring. Most of his two years were spent visiting and working at the great German-speaking clinics, the world's leading centers of medical science.

There were good reasons that these institutions, in the latter half of the nineteenth century and until World War I, were the focus of much of the world's medical progress and medical education. Their preeminence had mainly to do with the organization of the universities. Much of the intellectual support for the Revolutions of 1848 had come from students and junior faculty members seeking to overthrow the

C. Dalton. He not only completed the three-year course, but apparently underwent a scholastic metamorphosis as well: he was awarded the M.D. degree with honors. He was among the top ten men in his class, that distinction being based upon his performance in the oral examinations and his thesis, entitled "Contraindications to Operations." Being one of the ten highest-ranking graduates made him eligible to compete in a written examination for a prize of one hundred dollars, which he won.

death grasp in which the higher education of the day was held by government ministries and the sinecures they provided for conservative older professors. And though, politically, the revolutions failed, major changes had occurred in the academic arena. Freedom of teaching and freedom of learning (*Lehrfreiheit und Lernfreiheit*) were established, and resulted in an atmosphere of more liberal study. Faculty positions were filled by a process of nominating several highly qualified candidates, from among whom the government could choose. This free and wide-open competition, as well as the existence of a goodly number of well-supported state universities, encouraged young graduates to be productive and popular teachers. Research thrived, as investigative opportunities multiplied and each new discovery opened up even more avenues in the laboratory and clinic. As French and English medicine fell from their previous positions of leadership, and with American medicine still in its relative infancy, young physicians flocked from all over the western world and parts of Asia to study in Germany, Austria, Switzerland, and Czechoslovakia.

Since prerevolutionary days Americans had gone to Europe to study and "walk the wards" in England and France; now every American graduate who could afford it went to a German city, lived with a family long enough to pick up the language, and then set out on his journey from center to center. For general practitioners it was a luxury; for any young man wishing to pursue a specialty it was an absolute necessity.

In his valuable study of this phenomenon, *American Doctors and German Universities*, Thomas Bonner estimates that at least 40 to 50 percent of the leading physicians of the United States born between 1850 and 1890 studied in Germany. In a chapter entitled "The German Magnet," he states that "no fewer than ten thousand Americans took some kind of formal medical study at Vienna between 1870 and 1914." The imperial city of Austria-Hungary was, in the words of William Henry Welch, the "Mecca of American Practitioners." Of Vienna's many medical attractions, the most celebrated was the director of the university's 2nd Surgical Clinic, Professor Theodor Billroth.

Halsted attended Billroth's lectures and operations, and worked closely in the laboratory with one of his assistants, Anton Wölfler, with whom he became close friends. At the same time, he devoted himself to the study of anatomy, becoming skillful in the use of the microscope. His European travels included periods at Würzburg (where he studied with Kölliker), Leipzig, Berlin, Kiel, Halle, and Hamburg, and another session in Vienna during the winter of 1879–1880. By the time he returned home, he had worked with a number of those men who are now recognized as having been the pioneers of modern medical science and clinical patient care. Under their guidance he pursued his interests in pathology, medicine, anatomy, embryology, and surgery. Though his contact with Rudolf Virchow seems to have been minimal, he absorbed the theoretical basis of the teachings of "the Pope of German medicine" from those who had been influenced by him.

The great laboratory studies that were being made by German workers in the fields of microscopic anatomy, pathology, bacteriology, physiology, and chemistry were starting to be reflected in the clinical beginnings of asepsis and surgical technology. It was a yeasty time for researchers, and the atmosphere of the German hospitals was a ferment of possibilities. As we read Halsted's descriptions of his two European years, it is apparent that they formed the foundation of the approach that he would take to clinical investigation for the rest of his life. Although he would found a distinctly American school of surgery, he remained German-influenced to the end of his days, or as his colleague William Osler put it, "very much *verdeutsched*."

Halsted returned to New York in September 1880. The depth and variety of his European experiences, as well as his own obvious abilities, combined to make him one of the most highly regarded young surgeons in the city. In recognition of his talents, his enthusiasms, and, it must be admitted, his connections, numerous opportunities came his way. He seems to have refused none of them. Looking back on the record of the succeeding four years, it is hard to imagine how he managed to accomplish all that he did. The very fever of his activities during that time lifted his career skyward with a velocity that could not be maintained without terrible cost.

The capable young surgeon became Demonstrator of Anatomy at the College of Physicians and Surgeons. He accepted Dr. Sands' offer of an association with him in surgical practice at the Roosevelt Hospital, where he later founded the Outpatient Department. Perhaps in doing so he was influenced by his Yale experience in the New Haven Dispensary, which had been established not only to provide patient care, but to substitute for the hospital as the primary locus for the instruction of medical students. In a letter to William Welch written many years later, Halsted stated that he spent every morning at the Department, including Sundays, until the spring of 1884, a period of three years. This makes even more remarkable the volume and extent of his other activities, all of which consequently were carried out in the afternoons and evenings.

In 1881, he was appointed Visiting Physician to the Charity Hospital, a large public institution on Blackwell's Island. Although his rounds were intended to be medical, the hospital's interns were so taken with his skills that whenever they could do so they declared waiting elective surgical procedures to be emergencies so that they could assist him in the operating room during his evening visits. In 1883, he added to his duties the position of Consulting Surgeon to the New York State Emigrant Hospital on Ward's Island, another obligation reserved for evenings. In that same year he became Visiting Surgeon to Bellevue Hospital, where he formed a strong bond of friendship with his fellow Yale alumnus the German-trained pathologist William Welch. He was also named Attending Surgeon at the Chambers Street Hospital, an institution reserved for the treatment of emergencies.

> *It was a yeasty time for researchers, and the atmosphere of the German hospitals was a ferment of possibilities.*

To this long list he added, toward the end of his New York period, the title of Visiting Surgeon to the Presbyterian Hospital. He was busy, he seemed happy, and he quickly acquired a reputation as an exciting and venturesome surgeon and a leader in the medical life of New York City.

Those who worked with William Halsted in Baltimore have remembered him as a methodical, almost unapproachable, and most emphatically reserved Professor of Surgery. The exuberant pace of his professional life in New York stood in distinct contrast to that later austere image, but even more striking was his reticence in matters social in Baltimore compared to the vivacity of his household in New York. He shared office and home with Dr. Thomas McBride, a successful physician a few years older than himself. Located on 25th Street, between Madison and Fourth Avenues, the bachelor ménage seems to have been conducted like a perpetual open house, where dinner parties and musical events were graced by a group of well-off young men from various professions and businesses. The house was located just around the corner from the University Club at 26th and Madison, and the Halsted-McBride movable feast encompassed both buildings. The rising young surgeon was known as a cheerful host, a good companion, and a star of the University Club bowling alley.

The verve and pace of the New York period was destined to falter in thickening quicksand within a few short years. But before that happened, a great deal was accomplished that foreshadowed the major contributions to research and to education for which Halsted would later become renowned. One episode in particular epitomized Halsted's role in promulgating the doctrine of germ-free surgery among his reluctant colleagues. Like most American physicians, the surgeons of New York were skeptical of Listerian principles, and of the theory that wound infections are caused by bacteria. Soon after he accepted his appointment to Bellevue Hospital, it became apparent to Halsted that proper sterile technique was an impossibility in the institution's operating rooms. Having become convinced by his European experience of the need for asepsis, he refused to do surgery under less than perfect circumstances. With help from some of his many friends, he raised $10,000 to erect in an enclosure on the hospital grounds a huge tent to serve as his personal operating pavilion. The tent was supplied with gas and hot water, had a finely laid maple floor, and was perforated with portholes for ventilation and light. In this controlled atmosphere, Halsted could practice the aseptic methods he had learned abroad—almost twenty years after the first writings of Joseph Lister.

During the New York years of 1883–1886, Halsted published or presented a total of twenty-one scientific papers, on a variety of topics. His first publication already revealed a certain prescience. Titled "Refusion in the Treatment of Carbonic Oxide Poisoning," it is significant also because it has been all but forgotten among Halsted's later great contributions that he was one of the earliest proponents of direct blood transfusion. In the article, he describes his rescue of a man brought into the Chambers Street Hospital near death of carbon-monoxide poisoning. He removed blood from the patient's arm, rid it of its fibrin clotting factor by gently stirring it, which also brought it into contact with the air, and then transfused it back into the patient in combination with a small quantity of donor blood. In the same publication, he describes a successful donor transfusion (from "a stout philanthropic German") in a case of septicemia, and the resuscitation of an eleven-year-old boy who was in shock following an injury. In this latter case he used salt solution instead of blood. The use of autotransfusion and the effective emergency treatment of hemorrhage by the intravenous infusion of salt solution are techniques that had to be rediscovered almost a century after Halsted's forgotten descriptions of them.

The cases reported in this publication did not represent Halsted's first use of blood transfusion. That event had taken place several years earlier, and was quite unplanned. In 1881, he had traveled to Albany, New York, to visit his sister, arriving at her home just as she was giving birth. Shortly thereafter, he was summoned in haste to her bedside, where he found her pale and pulseless due to a massive postpartum hemorrhage. In a note written years later he described his response to the situation: "After checking the hemorrhage, I transfused my sister with blood drawn into a syringe from one of my veins and injected immediately into one of hers. This was taking a great risk but she was so nearly moribund that I ventured it and with prompt result." This took place twenty years before transfusion was finally made safe by the discovery of blood groups by Karl Landsteiner of Vienna in 1901.

And now, to the fall—or rather, to the phoenix. The legendary Egyptian phoenix was a male bird of exceptionally gorgeous plumage, a characteristic shared by the subject of our story. By himself, this bird is said to have built and set fire to the funeral pyre upon which he then died, and from whose ashes he later arose reborn. The tale of the phoenix is the stuff of the classic resurrection story, found in mythol-

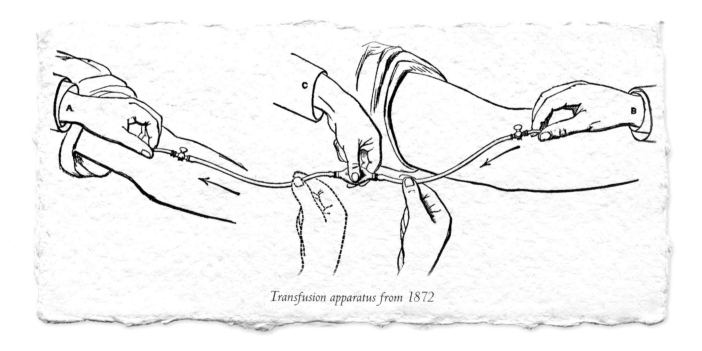

Transfusion apparatus from 1872

ogy, scripture, and in the biographies of men and women every day. It has many variations, ranging from the rebirth of nations to a modified modern pop form in which it is called the midlife crisis. In the case of William Halsted, the funeral pyre was powdered with cocaine.

Cocaine too is the subject of legends. The story of its first applications to the art of healing, in fact, has been embellished to the point where the accuracy of each detail has now or then been questioned. What follows is a brief outline of what is thought to be true.

In spite of so many newspaper headlines to the contrary, there are few sudden breakthroughs in the progress of medical science. Rarely can a single date be pointed out as the distinct time of origin of anything. And yet, as uncommon as such landmark scientific birthdays have been, the history of anesthesia claims two of them. The first occurred on October 16, 1846, when William Thomas Green Morton induced the first ether surgical sleep at the Massachusetts General Hospital. The second took place on September 15, 1884, when at the Heidelberg meeting of the German Ophthalmological Society, Dr. Josef Brettauer read a paper by a twenty-six-year-old junior faculty member of the Vienna Medical School who could not afford the costs of traveling personally to present his own work. The impecunious researcher was Dr. Karl Koller, and his startling paper described a brief series of experiments done during several weeks that summer, in which it was demon-

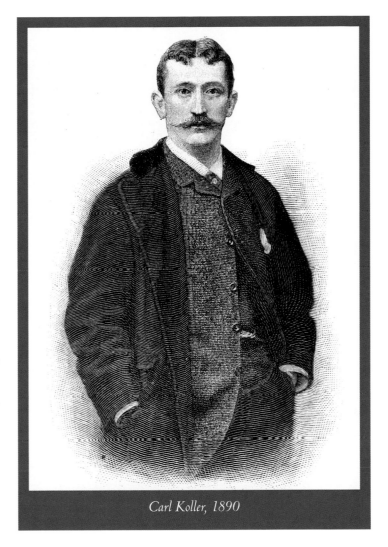

Carl Koller, 1890

strated that the surface of the eye could be anesthetized by the application of a few drops of cocaine, an alkaloid extracted from the American coca leaf, *Erythroxylon coca*. Since 1862, the drug had been known to produce numbing of the oral mucous membrane (of course, the Peruvian Indians had been aware of this for centuries), but no real work had been done with it for almost two decades. Then a twenty-eight-year-old neurologist in Vienna, one Sigmund Freud, began some experiments to determine its effect on the central nervous system. It was at Freud's suggestion that his friend Koller began his own cocaine study.

The news of the discovery of cocaine's local anesthetic effects was hailed throughout the surgical world, and experiments were immediately begun in a number of the great European centers. In Koller's own hospital, Halsted's old friend Anton Wölfler undertook an investigation to determine the drug's usefulness in general surgery. Whether by personal correspondence or by a report of the Heidelberg meeting that appeared in the *Medical Record* of October 11, 1884, Halsted was influenced to begin his own series of experiments. He enlisted a small group of his colleagues, as well as a number of medical students, and did work on local infiltration techniques as well as methods of blocking major nerve trunks. The group's experimental subjects were themselves and each other.

In the course of their work, the young researchers became aware of the exhilarating effects of the drug. Innocent of its addictive qualities, which were as yet unknown, some of them took to sniffing cocaine powder to enhance social experiences. With a few snorts, the most boring evening at the theater became a histrionic extravaganza. Friends were invited home for demonstrations; would-be participants in the research had to be turned away.

Halsted and his associates held high hopes, in more ways than one, for their investigations, but the personal cost soon became obvious. Several of them became addicted, including their leader. In spite of having accumulated a great deal of data, Halsted published only one paper on cocaine, a short article in the *New York Medical Journal* in September 1885. Written while his addiction was at its worst, it contrasts markedly, and frighteningly, with the clarity and precision of all of his other writing. A glance at the first sentence will illustrate the degree to which he had deteriorated, and also explains why no further cocaine publications were forthcoming:

Neither indifferent as to which of how many possibilities may best explain, nor yet at a loss to comprehend, why surgeons have, and that so many, quite without discredit, could have exhibited scarcely any interest in what, as a local anaesthetic, had been supposed, if not declared, by most so very sure to prove, especially to them, attractive, still I do not think that this circumstance, or some sense of obligation to rescue fragmentary reputation for surgeons rather than the belief that an opportunity existed for assisting others to an appreciable extent, induced me, several months ago, to write on the subject in hand the greater part of a somewhat comprehensible paper, which poor health disinclined me to complete.

Of the small group of young physicians who became cocaine-addicted, all but Halsted were eventually destroyed by it, professionally and personally. Even his roommate, Thomas McBride, who did not take part in the research, seems to have been bedeviled by the drug. He died under suspicious circumstances less than a year after the foregoing paper was published, aboard ship while returning from Europe after what was meant to be a health-restoring journey following some unnamed illness. The ship's doctor had been giving him injections of either cocaine or morphine solution from a bottle which he himself had brought on board. The concentration of narcotic in the solution was unknown, except to McBride.

For Halsted, the onset of cocaine dependency began a lifelong battle against despair and ruin that threatened the disintegration of his career as long as he drew breath. Every one of the golden blocks of accomplishment that made up the monument of his later fame was put into place while he was under a spell, first of cocaine and then of morphine.

Although he was never able to unfetter himself of his dependency on drugs, Halsted did manage to loosen the stranglehold in which they at first gripped him. He eventually became sufficiently free that he was able to work, to think clearly almost always, and to appear to unknowing associates as more a complicated eccentric than a furtive fugitive from an ever-lurking need. In this sense, he won out over his addiction. After his move to Baltimore, even those who were aware of his New York collapse seem to have believed that its effects were long behind him. Those who knew better kept his secret; they did not even speak of it among themselves. White lies were told, explaining away as the idiosyncrasies of a brilliant introvert his frequent bits of inappropriate behavior, his solitary annual trips to small European hotels, and his many episodes of either leaving the hospital abruptly in the midst of an urgent schedule or absenting himself entirely. What remained unspoken was the most obvious fact of all: an intrepid, even audacious young surgeon, whose career had hurtled relentlessly along the high road of personal and professional success in New York, arrived in Baltimore metamorphosed into a remote, ploddingly cautious, compulsive researcher whose earlier exhilarating instruction of students had turned lackluster, and whose greatest satisfaction seemed to come from the slow, meticulous accumulation of scientific evidence in the laboratory.

Even beyond the grave, the few loyal friends who knew the full magnitude of Halsted's secret strove zealously to guard it from disclosure. In trying to save his reputation, however, those well-meaning advocates actually did him a disservice. After the full truth became known, almost half a century after his death, Halsted's name shone more brightly than ever as an example of indomitable courage and the strength that can sometimes be marshaled by the human spirit.

For much of the information on Halsted's habit that appears in the following paragraphs, I am indebted to the excellent studies of Professor Peter Olch of the Armed Forces University of the Health Sciences. I found some of the rest of what I am about to describe in Yale's collection of the unpublished papers of Harvey Cushing, founder of the specialty of neurosurgery and Halsted's most celebrated disciple. The remainder was extracted from the contents of a small locked black book, written by the first Professor of Medicine at Johns Hopkins, William Osler, and not opened until 1969. Osler, not only the finest teacher of

> *For Halsted, the onset of cocaine dependency began a lifelong battle against despair and ruin that threatened the disintegration of his career as long as he drew breath.*

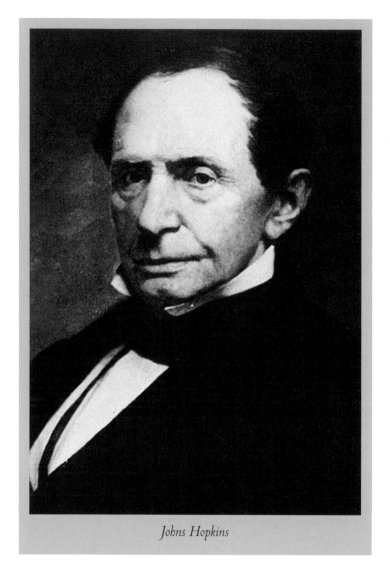

Johns Hopkins

The proneness to seclusion, the slight peculiarities amounting to eccentricities at times (which to his old friends in New York seemed more strange than to us), were the only outward traces of the daily battle through which this brave fellow lived for years. When we recommended him as full surgeon to the Hospital in 1890, I believed, and Welch did too, that he was no longer addicted to morphia. He had worked so well and so energetically that it did not seem possible that he could take the drug and do so much.

About six months after the full position had been given, I saw him in a severe chill, and this was the first intimation I had that he was still taking morphia. Subsequently I had many talks about it and gained his full confidence. He had never been able to reduce the amount to less than three grains daily; on this he could do his work comfortably and maintain his excellent physical vigor (for he was a very muscular fellow). I do not think that anyone suspected him, not even Welch.

medicine this continent has ever produced but also one of its most talented chroniclers, titled a part of the book "The Inner History of the Johns Hopkins Hospital." In it he revealed how he discovered, soon after Halsted's appointment to the Hopkins Chair of Surgery, that his colleague was taking large amounts of morphine. Very probably, he had begun using it during his attempts to break the cocaine habit; at least it interfered less disastrously with his life than did cocaine. Here is Osler:

It was due to the efforts of William Welch, in fact, that Halsted was able to reconstitute the fragments of his career. By the time of Halsted's collapse, the Bellevue pathologist had moved to Baltimore to take part in the final planning for the opening of the Johns Hopkins Hospital, as will presently be described. When he realized how disabled his friend was, he went back to New York, convinced him to go off on what he hoped would be a therapeutic sailing trip to the Windward Isles, and personally hired a schooner for the purpose. The cruise, taken during February and March of 1886, was a disaster. Among Cushing's collected letters in the Yale library there is a brief note dated December 5, 1930, by John Fulton describing a conversation he had had that day with the by then retired neurosurgeon. Cushing told him that Halsted took with him "enough cocaine to last him for all but the last two weeks of voyage." Fulton's note continues:

Could he break his addiction? No. He broke into the ship's drug store and continued the habit until the end of his life. . . . Harvey Cushing also told me this today, said that in fifteen years he was with Halsted (in his home only twice in that time!) he never suspected the cocaine habit, and only with difficulty was he led to accredit it many years later.

When Halsted returned home, he forced himself to come to grips with the fact that he would never break his addiction without some form of treatment, and admitted himself to the Butler Hospital, a private psychiatric facility in Providence, to attempt a cure. When he was discharged in November 1886, he acceded to Welch's wish that he come to Baltimore so that he could remain under his nurturing care as well as his watchful eye. Arriving at Hopkins the following month, he began to work in the laboratory with the anatomist Franklin P. Mall on an experimental study of intestinal suture methods. However well those researches may have gone, it became clear by early spring that Halsted's attempts at recovery were once again failing. On April 5, 1887, he was readmitted to Butler Hospital, where he remained un-

til he returned to the laboratory in January 1888. It was almost certainly during one of his Butler admissions that he began to use morphine, but it is only conjectural whether it was begun as part of his treatment or whether he bribed someone to smuggle it in to him.

Thus, though he was probably cocaine-free after settling in Baltimore, Halsted remained mor-

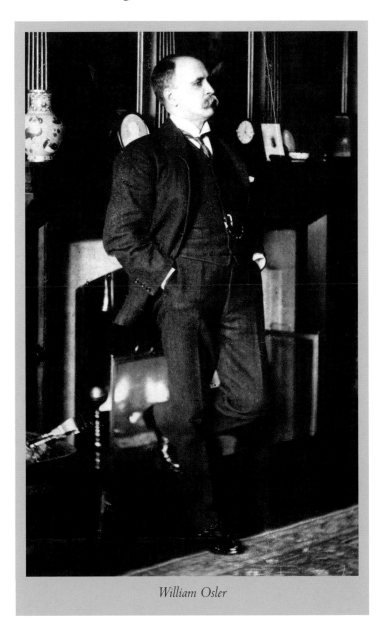

William Osler

phine-addicted the rest of his life. He was brought to Hopkins not to become a Professor of Surgery, but rather to pull together the shattered bits of his life. It was Welch's intention that he begin in the laboratory, and that he not stray from his own supervisory big-brother eye. The convalescent moved into the boardinghouse in which Welch rented rooms, and started on his research, which Peter Olch most appropriately calls "a form of occupational therapy" and most certainly not an academic appointment.

At this point, it is well to bring ourselves up to date about the remarkable new temple of healing into whose inner recesses the redeemed surgeon was now entering. At his death in 1874, the Baltimore merchant and banker Johns Hopkins had willed that half of his $7 million estate should be used to found a university, and the other half to found a hospital. In a letter written in 1873 to the trustees of the latter institution, he made a statement that indicates that he had sought out excellent advice concerning the contemporary deficiencies in American medical education and the ways in which they might be overcome: "You will bear in mind in all your work in relation to the hospital that it is my desire and purpose that this institution shall be a part of the medical school of the university for which I have amply provided in my will." There is no single factor that has been more instrumental in the rapid rise of American medicine to its present world preeminence than the principle enunciated by Hopkins: each medical school must not only be part of a university environment, but must be so closely affiliated with an excellent hospital that the two are for all intents and purposes part of the same tripartite endeavor of healing, teaching, and research.

The key to the success of the Johns Hopkins Medical School and its hospital was the choice of advisers and administrators made at first by its founder and later by the trustees he appointed. A goodly (read "goodly" in both the quantitative and the moral sense) number of the original trustees were, like Hopkins himself, members of the Religious Society of Friends, whose devotion to the principles of healing and education were as much a matter of faith as they were a civic responsibility. Moreover, and in this too they resembled the benefactor, they knew how to watch a dollar and squeeze every penny of value out of it. The Quaker reputation for philanthropy is matched only by the Quaker reputation for thrift.

The task was begun by inviting three university presidents to Baltimore in the summer of 1874 to give their guidance. They were Angell of Michigan, Eliot of Harvard, and White of Cornell. When they had completed their assignment and returned home, each of them received a letter asking his recommendation of a leader for the fledgling school. Without consulting one another, all three independently named the same man, Daniel Coit Gilman, the forty-year-old president of the University of California and the former secretary to the governing board of Yale's Sheffield Scientific School. Much has been written about Gilman's heroic contributions to Johns Hopkins and to American medical education, but for our purposes one sentence will suffice: he proved to be the right man in the right place at the right time.

An equally exemplary choice for chief adviser to the hospital was made by appointing Dr. John Shaw Billings, the principal founder of the Library of the United States Surgeon General's Office, now grown into the National Library of

Medicine. In later years he would become famous for two more remarkable achievements: the founding and original planning of the New York Public Library, and his immense service to the Johns Hopkins Hospital.

Setting about their great work, Gilman and Billings consulted with medical and scientific leaders throughout the world, and in 1876, Billings toured Europe, visiting major institutions and seeking out every possible source of information on hospital design and planning. Such was the commitment of our country's organized medical establishment to the Hopkins experiment that he was accompanied by Dr. E. M. Hunt, the president of the Section of Public Hygiene of the American Medical Association. Gradually plans were formulated, and a faculty and hospital staff gathered from all parts of the land and from Europe. On April 7, 1884, William Welch was named Professor of Pathology. In the words of Alan M. Chesney, who was dean of the school in the mid-twentieth century, "That appointment unquestionably constituted one of the most important single events in the history of both the School and the Hospital."

Like Gilman and Billings, Welch knew what had to be done. Making good use of his wide range of laboratory training in Germany, as well as an equally wide acquaintance with the most prominent of the new medical scientists of America, he was in an excellent position to help with curriculum and planning. The list of names of the original Johns Hopkins Medical School Fac-

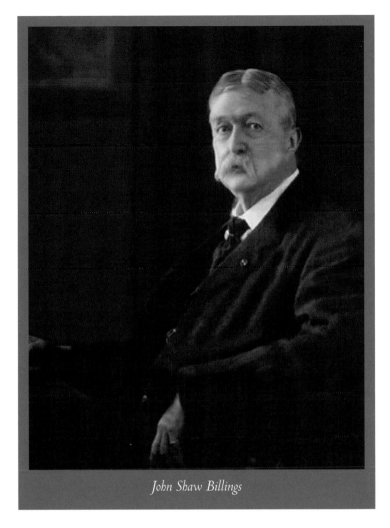

John Shaw Billings

ulty reads like an honor roll of the founders of medical science in the United States: Franklin P. Mall in anatomy, John Jacob Abel in pharmacology, William Howell in physiology, Ira Remsen in chemistry, William Welch in pathology, Howard Kelly in gynecology, and William Osler in medicine. They were all caught up in what one commentator called "the contagious companionship of excellence."

A word about Osler. Born in a small town in Ontario, and educated in medicine at McGill, he had been called to the University of Pennsylvania in 1884 to be Professor of Medicine at the age of thirty-five. Although he had studied in Berlin and Vienna, he was not quite so *verdeutscht* as were Welch and Halsted. Witty, urbane, gifted with a flair for the nuances of the English language, warmhearted almost to a fault, devoted to the education of young physicians to an even greater degree, if it can be imagined, than Welch, he became the leading light of the Hopkins faculty. He was the greatest clinical teacher of his day, not only for his own students, but also for the countless thousands who read his *Principles and Practice of Medicine,* the most popular such text in America, destined to outlive its author through the sixteenth edition of 1947. The magnetism of his sparkling personality and the breadth of his learning, medical and otherwise, in time made him the most sought-after speaker and the most famous doctor in the world. The fact that English began gradually to replace German as the international language of medicine was due more to his writings and speeches than to the works of any other man. American medical science needed a herald to proclaim its birth—that was to be one of the many roles of William Osler at Johns Hopkins.

The opening ceremonies of the hospital took place on May 7, 1889. The medical school's inaugural, however, was delayed by an unforeseen obstacle having to do with money. Of the $3.5 million the university had received by the terms of Mr. Hopkins' will, $1.5 million was invested in B&O Railroad common stock. Perhaps partly because of controls imposed on railroads by the Interstate Commerce Commission, newly created by an Act of Congress in 1887, the B&O was finding itself in serious financial straits, resulting in considerable loss of income to the school. Not

only its date of opening but its very future was in doubt.

In the end, the institution's financial problems resulted in a double benison for American medical education. Not only did their solving bring about the reversal of a historic inequity, but it resulted also in the admission of a caliber of student even higher than the faculty had anticipated. For that happy outcome, posterity is in debt to a quartet of young Baltimore women, all of whom were daughters of university trustees, the Misses M. Carey Thomas, Mary Elizabeth Garrett, Mary Gwinn, and Elizabeth King.

The motive of the Baltimore Four was quite simple and eminently appropriate, especially in consideration of the high-minded ideals expressed in the will of Mr. Hopkins. They demanded that women should share in the opportunity to obtain this new form of medical education, which promised to be the best in the United States. Their efforts resulted in the formation of the Women's Fund Committee, whose purpose was to raise enough money to open the school, but only on the condition that women be admitted on the same basis as men. Branch committees were formed in various cities, that in Washington being chaired by the wife of President Benjamin Harrison. By the autumn of 1890, $100,000 had been raised, which was offered to the trustees as the first payment on the total of $500,000 that was needed. The offer was accepted, and the trustees set about to raise the rest of the money in conjunction with the women. Although the committee continued to do its part, the total effort fell short. In December 1892, Mary Garrett, who had already donated a large percentage of the original gift, offered

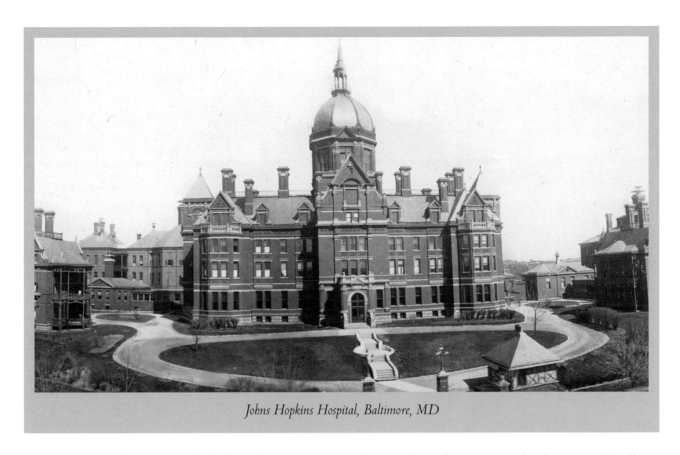

Johns Hopkins Hospital, Baltimore, MD

to contribute what was still lacking, but she attached some additional conditions: admission requirements should be set up such as to guarantee that the medical school would always remain a graduate school; college preparation was to be required in biology, chemistry, and physics, and the applicants were to be able to demonstrate a reading knowledge of German and French. In essence, therefore, only college graduates were to be admitted as medical students at Johns Hopkins.

Gilman was skeptical of these terms, as were some members of the faculty, who feared that they were so exacting and so much more advanced than those required for any other school in the country that few students would be willing to meet them. Attempts were made to dissuade Miss

Garrett, but she remained adamant. Finally, a compromise was reached allowing for the admission of students who, if they did not formally have an undergraduate degree, could give evidence by examination that they fulfilled the requirements that such a degree implies. Osler wrote in a letter to Welch that if the two of them had had to meet such rigorous standards, they would never have been admitted.

On the basis of the compromise, which was really a victory for Mary Garrett, the school opened in October 1893. Her total gift amounted to more than $350,000, but she gave even more. She commissioned John Singer Sargent to paint the most renowned of American medical portraits, of Welch, Halsted, Osler, and Kelly. That painting, *The Four Doctors*, now hangs in the medical school's

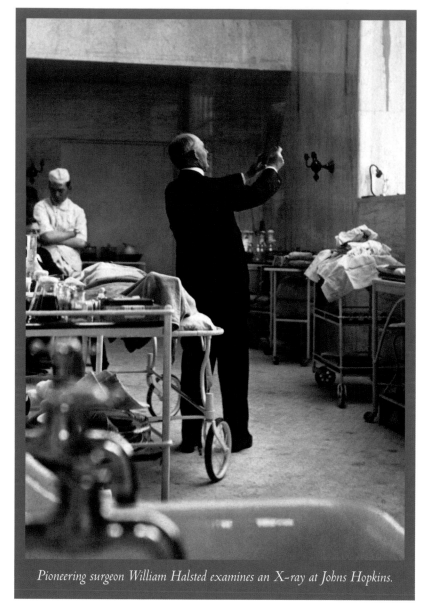

Pioneering surgeon William Halsted examines an X-ray at Johns Hopkins.

anywhere. They were thrown in with a young faculty who had been figuratively pawing the ground in anticipation of their arrival. The country's first complete medical laboratory courses awaited them, and a spirit of excitement not only permeated the atmosphere around the university, but spread out to the entire community of medical educators everywhere. American medicine was ready to start on its ascent; the great experiment was about to begin.

The books that record the research advances made by the Hopkins group during its first decades continue to be written today. Even the Germans soon found that they could not keep up with the work of those brilliant young professors in the fields of physiology, biochemistry, pharmacology, anatomy, embryology, pathology, bacteriology, and the clinical sciences. Most remarkable was that almost all of them were just starting out at the same time on the most productive period of their lives. At the opening of the hospital in 1889, Welch and Osler were thirty-nine, Halsted thirty-six, Kelly thirty-one, Abel thirty-two, and Mall twenty-seven; when Howell arrived in 1893, he was thirty-three.

The thirty Hopkins years surrounding the turn of the twentieth century surely rank with even the glorious decades of the Paris and Vien-

Welch Memorial Library, along with Sargent's portrait of the donor herself. In the words of Chesney, "To this lady, more than to any other single person, save only Johns Hopkins himself, does the School of Medicine owe its being."

The fifteen men and three women who made up the entering class of the medical school fulfilled the most rigorous requirements that had ever been asked of any entering medical students

na schools as the most fertile periods for progress that medical history has yet seen. But Hopkins had one advantage not shared by the other two: it was a completely new environment, and its faculty were allowed not only virtually total freedom to innovate, but a gigantic empty space in which to do it. It was for the best of reasons that the school and hospital would serve as the models by which the rest of American medical education and practice might transform itself, and as an index against which it could be measured.

Halsted settled permanently in Baltimore in January of 1888. Things began simply enough. He worked in Welch's laboratory, and soon started up a private practice. Before long, it became obvious to those who knew of his work in the various Baltimore hospitals that he was a highly skilled surgeon. William Macewen of Glasgow having refused the offer of a professorship, the hospital approached its opening without a chief of surgery. Taking a chance, almost certainly at the strong urging of Welch and Mall, the trustees appointed Halsted surgeon *pro tempore* in February 1889, and Surgeon-in-Chief to the outpatient clinic. Shortly thereafter, he was made an associate professor at the medical school. In March 1890, Osler wrote to Gilman (who by this time had already achieved so much that he was in England to receive honorary degrees from both Oxford and Cambridge), "Halsted is doing remarkable work in Surgery & I feel that his appointment to the University and the Hospital would be quite safe." The correctness of his judgment was verified two years later when Halsted was named Professor of Surgery and Surgeon-in-Chief to the Johns Hopkins Hospital.

What Halsted accomplished during his thirty-year tenure may be seen as a series of contributions that developed along three lines, each of which was a replacement of an outmoded approach. The first was a new method of training surgeons that replaced the old haphazardness of assisting a professor for endless years, putting in its stead a graduated system of increasingly complex responsibility; the second was an approach to surgical operations that replaced the flashiness of his predecessors' smash-and-grab technique with caution, gentleness, and accurate anatomical dissection; the third was the introduction of a group of new operations that replaced the mere carving away of the intrusive invading disease with procedures that were based on the principle of restoring normal physiology.

The method by which Halsted taught is the basis upon which we still design our postgraduate surgical education today, based in a general way on the German system. Briefly, Halsted was in charge of the surgical group at all times, and was, in fact, the only senior staff surgeon. Except for his occasional private patients and those few others upon whom he chose to operate personally, all beds were occupied by patients cared for by the house surgeon, equivalent to the present-day chief resident. Responsible to the house surgeon was a group of what we would today call assistant residents, who had been chosen to take part in the line of his succession over the subsequent years. Not only was there no guarantee that the members of this group would not lose their places along the way, but they all knew that only one of them would survive the pyramid of training to reach the pinnacle of house surgeon. Junior to these assistant residents was a group of interns, each chosen for a one-year period. At each level, the young surgeons were responsible for the training and supervision of those junior to them. The house surgeons averaged two years in that position, and going through the entire process took an average of eight years, although senior men from elsewhere could be appointed at any step along the pathway.

Thus was born the residency training program of this country. The effect on American surgery was like a transmutation from dross to gold within a generation. Of all the great teachers of the chirurgeon's art, only one, Theodor Billroth, founded a more illustrious school or left a more accomplished heritage of professional progeny. Halsted trained seventeen house surgeons, eleven of whom went on to institute university-type residencies similar to their mentor's at other institutions; from these, 166 chief residents graduated. As pointed out earlier, Halsted pollinated the country, with the result that the methods and techniques of what we call Halstedian surgery were the methods and techniques by which most American surgeons have been trained up to the present generation. The gentle, meticulous "Surgery of Safety" thus introduced became the distinctly American approach to operative craftsmanship. It is a source of pride to thousands of our country's surgical specialists that we trace our professional lineage directly to the master. Even after almost thirty years of being a surgeon, my own occasional flutterings of self-doubt in the operating room can always be stilled by reminding myself that my professor was Gustaf Lindskog, whose professor was Samuel Harvey, whose professor was Harvey Cushing, whose professor was William Halsted. The process of remembering is instantaneous, and the quiverings are gone in the wink of an eye.

In summing up William Halsted's career, at the conclusion of his 1930 biography, W. G. McCallum describes what so many of us who consider ourselves Halstedians have thought to be the primary lesson we have taken from our training: "It seems that his greatest service was that he worked out an attitude in operating upon the human body which must forever be the proper attitude of a surgeon. It was simply the recognition of the normal or physiological condition of the tissues which one should attempt to restore, realizing thoroughly their natural defenses and the reasons for their vulnerability." After Halsted, all properly trained American surgeons were practicing applied physiology each time they entered the operating room. The

> *Halsted pollinated the country, with the result that the methods and techniques of what we call Halstedian surgery were the methods and techniques by which most American surgeons have been trained up to the present generation.*

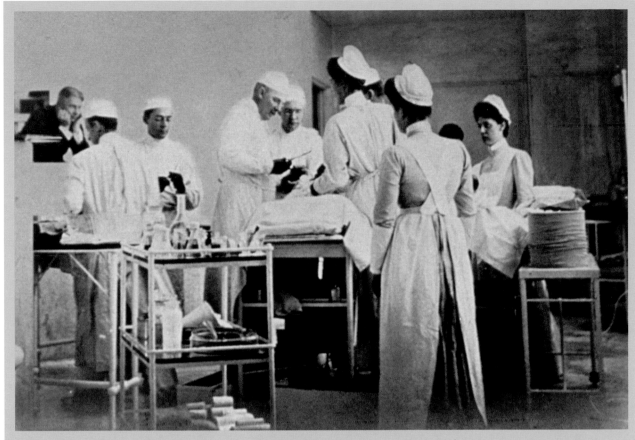

Dr. Cushing, Dr. Halsted, and Dr. Young in the operating theater

clock-conscious, often futile mayhem of an earlier era disappeared from the scene in this country, as surgeons began to understand his message that tissues treated with kindness respond better than tissues treated with haste.

In any consideration of Halsted's philosophy in matters of surgical technique, his work on groin or inguinal hernia must be described. When he began his studies of the tissue layers of the groin, while still in New York, recurrence rates were high and not a few people died after the operation. When he came to Baltimore, he carried out microscopic investigations to learn more about the way in which wounds heal. It was large-

ly as a result of such studies as these and the experiments on intestinal suture that he developed the essential concepts upon which his newly devised operative methods were based, such as absolute control of even the most minor bleeding, avoidance of unclosed pockets in the depths of wounds, gentle care of tissues, and their perfect approximation without excessive tightness or interference with blood supply. Prior to his innovations, technique was gross, hemostatic clamps were few, control of bleeding was careless, speed was paramount, and complications in healing were numerous. Even this cavalcade of hazards does not include those problems, so often lethal, that were the consequence of America's foot-dragging attitude toward asepsis.

Conceived on the careful application of his concepts, and utilizing his knowledge of both visible and microscopic anatomy, Halsted devised a hernia repair whose basic principles remain those used by all surgeons today. By restoring normal anatomy in a way that is consistent with the physiology of the affected groin tissues, he introduced the first reliable method of operating on a hernia. Until his work, the appearance of a nonreducible groin bulge signaled the onset of one of the most lethal of afflictions. He converted a previously insoluble problem into a straightforward, simple exercise in surgical technique, and thereby ended forever the reign of terror that the disease had visited upon mankind since time immemorial. The so-called Halsted II procedure today remains the gold standard, in that it is not only the most common approach to the repair of groin hernias, but the one against whose excellent results all others are measured. In his first series of almost twenty-five hundred patients, the recurrence rate was under 7 percent. Even today, with improved asepsis, instrumentation, and suture materials, commonly reported figures in the United States are only a bit better than that.

One of the tantalizing rewards that comes with reading old medical texts is the little peek of insight they occasionally provide into the daily hospital life of earlier times. In a paper read at the annual meeting of the Medico-Chirurgical Faculty of Maryland on November 17, 1892, Halsted described a twenty-year-old patient who had to be "discharged for insubordination." His offense was that, wishing to get his sluggish bowels moving, he violated the dictum of strict bed rest by getting up to take a laxative without permission on the seventh postoperative day. Hospital rules may not have been the only thing he broke, because it is recorded that he reappeared three years later with a recurrence of his hernia. Knowing what we now do about the safety of early postoperative activity, it is safe to say that his new hernia was very likely more a matter of coincidence than of stress-by-mischief. That does not, of course, rule out the possibility of inscrutable workings of some divine judgment visited upon those who failed to obey the surgical sachems of those days.

It has taken us until the waning decades of the twentieth century to realize that surgery can be done for people with groin hernia on an outpatient basis or with only a few days of hospitalization. Ironically, many patients have their operations done under local nerveblock anesthesia, utilizing methods pioneered by Halsted during his New York period; although he never experimented with cocaine blocks after his near-tragic experience, others took up the cause, developing techniques that are safe and effective.

Halsted made many advances in surgery of the thyroid, bile ducts, intestine, and aneurysms of the arteries. Like all surgeons of his time, and all surgeons of today, he considered his most fearsome enemy to be cancer, particularly cancer of the breast. Even people who know very little else about modern scientific medicine seem to have heard of the Halsted radical mastectomy, and to have an opinion about it.

It is a historical irony that William Halsted's great contribution to the treatment of what is essentially a women's disease should be the source of the castigation to which his memory has been subjected by some of the very beneficiaries of his work. On two occasions I have been handed the precarious responsibility of refereeing angry articles submitted to medical journals attacking Halsted, surgical attitudes in general, and the radical mastectomy in particular. On each occasion, it was difficult to tell whether the author had deliberately sacrificed fact on the altar of ideology, or whether ignorance was the main fuel of the diatribe. The authors of both articles, and of several others that somehow slipped through the reviewing process and into the pages of otherwise excellent journals, seem not to understand clinical science well enough to interpret medical literature or history well enough to appreciate the background against which Halsted's work was done.

This is not the forum in which to discuss the recent reevaluations of the proper therapy for breast cancer. It is sufficient to point out that almost no American surgeons still do the radical operation as Halsted described it, having abandoned it in the 1960s in favor of the modified procedure which leaves the chest-wall muscles intact. Moreover, we have come to realize that breast cancer is a systemic disease from the moment of its inception, which means that it has the capability of af-

fecting distant parts of the body quite early in its course. Surgery is therefore only one of the weapons that may be used against it. Radiation, chemotherapy, hormonal manipulation, and even (at least in the near future) immunotherapy may play a major role in individual situations. Treatment is today tailor-made for each patient.

Furthermore, it has been proved to the satisfaction of almost all physicians who treat this disease that early-stage breast cancer, which at present is the status of approximately one-third of patients, is treated as well with local excision and radiotherapy as it is with more extensive procedures. This is as far as our studies have taken us. American surgeons have demonstrated their willingness, in fact their enthusiasm, for changing a methodology when valid studies give them reason. Every one of us looks with hope to the future.

Nothing in the foregoing should take away from an appreciation of the impressive changes

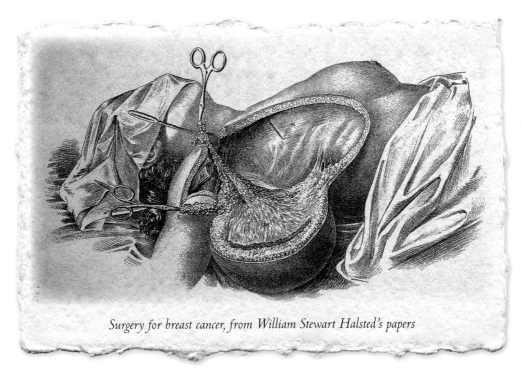

Surgery for breast cancer, from William Stewart Halsted's papers

that Halsted's operation produced in the results of breast-cancer treatment in the decades after its introduction. Because women soon began to find out that cure was, for the first time, a real possibility, many felt encouraged to seek treatment. Most victims of the feared disease had previously thought operation to be futile, as did so many of their physicians. Doomed to ulcerations, foul discharges, and disgusting odors, a large proportion of patients spent their last months alone, cut off by wretched choice from their closest associations.

With reference to cure rates, the situation at the time is best described by Halsted himself, in an 1894 publication dealing with mastectomy:

> Most of us heard our teachers in surgery admit that they have never cured a case of cancer of the breast. The younger Gross [died 1899] did not save one case in his first hundred. Hayes Agnew [died 1892] stated in a lecture a very short time before his death that he operated on breast cancers solely for the moral effect on the patients, that he believed the operation shortened rather than prolonged life. . . . I sometimes ask physicians who regularly consult us why they never send us cancers of the breast. They reply, as a rule, that they see many such cases but supposed they were incurable. We rarely meet a physician or surgeon who can testify to a single instance of a positive cure of breast cancer.

A serious problem associated with the pre-Halsted operations was local recurrence in the months following surgery. The wide excisions that were being done by the leading European surgeons did not prevent most of their patients from developing early return of tumor growth in the chest wall, even when survival had been prolonged. The most favorable statistics reported from the German clinics were those of Richard Volkmann of Leipzig, of whose 131 patients only 40 percent were free of such regrowths in less than four years. Billroth's figure was only 18 percent.

This, then, was the grim outlook for women with breast cancer when Halsted first began to consider the problem during his years of practice in New York. When he had visited the clinics of Billroth and Volkmann and the others in the years 1878–1880 he began to develop his theory that only by increasing the area of excision could there be any hope of providing cures or at least preventing early local recurrence. He noted that Volkmann's results improved after he began to remove the fibrous covering that lay on the surface of the chest-wall muscles. A few surgeons also were claiming that their patients did better when they excised the lymph glands from the nearby armpit that seemed to be involved with tumor, and at least one operator was cleaning out all of those glands.

In 1882, Halsted took the best features of all previous approaches and went one step further. His operation not only dissected away all of the armpit contents, but excised the chest-wall muscles as well, the entire specimen being removed in one large block so as to avoid the possibility of cutting across microscopic tumor. In 1894, he was able to present markedly improved statistics at a meeting of the Clinical Society of Maryland. The paper was a triumph of his ability to evaluate the work of others and extract the best of each of his predecessors, synthesizing all into a logical clinical approach. The success of his method depended not only upon its basis in pathological anatomy, but also upon the meticulous operative technique he had devised.

It was at the 1898 meeting of the American Surgical Association in New Orleans that Halsted's mastectomy became established, as had his hernia operation, as the standard against which to measure all other methods of treatment. He presented a series of 133 patients, seventy-six of whom were more than three years post-operative. Fifty-two percent of them were disease-free, which is particularly impressive considering the advanced state at which most women presented themselves in those days. Perhaps of equal importance was the fact noted by one of the discussants that Halsted had brought "hopefulness of prognosis as compared with former despair." The comment continued:

I have heard noted members of this association describe that a cancer patient will sooner or later die of cancer, whatever operation is done, unless she is fortunate enough to be killed by some intercurrent infection. One surgeon of prominence has pronounced operations for cancer to be utterly useless. In Dr. Halsted's series are included cases once regarded as absolutely unfit for operation, and even in these life has been prolonged by surgical interference and rendered more comfortable. Best of all, in some very serious cases the disease has not returned after a lapse of years. The distinguished author of this paper deserves and has our grateful acknowledgements for the brilliant light which he has thrown upon these dark places of surgery.

Although it is proper that most attention should be focused upon the role of any operation in curing disease, its secondary func-tion is always to alleviate the distress caused by that ailment, the so-called palliative effect. Even when cure is not possible, a surgical procedure may often relieve symptoms and provide physical comfort and a greater degree of tranquillity than would be possible without it. Over the years, critics and supporters alike have focused so much attention on cure rates that not enough emphasis has been placed on the strictly palliative effect that came with the introduction of the radical operation. Breast cancer has always been and is still a horrible disease. But after Halsted's contribution, at least there was no longer any need for women to suffer the emotionally crippling effects of living with masses of decaying draining tumor inadequately treated or not treated at all. The fact that some of Halsted's suppositions were wrong or that his operation may eventually become unnecessary should not detract from the magnitude of the change in prognosis that occurred after its introduction. (Halsted's work, although the most thorough and convincing, was not the only contribution being made to the treatment of mammary cancer at about the same time. Willy Meyer of New York, William Watson Cheyne of London, and others introduced similar operations. Each in his own way became a propagandist for the procedure, with the result that a huge leap forward took place in treatment. The results, as noted earlier, become even more impressive when we consider how far advanced were most of the tumors that were being treated.)

As we consider the many advantages that accrue to women who today are candidates for lesser procedures, we know that awareness of such a possibility brings patients to their physicians at an earlier stage of disease, thereby in itself saving many lives. We should not forget that at the time the radical mastectomy was devised, one of its most important by-products was to bring previously hopeless women to medical attention, because the word had gotten out that cure was possible and good palliation was virtually certain.

Because of their lucid narrative style, all of Halsted's papers read like literature. The 1920 publication in which he recounted the history of thyroid-gland surgery, including the evolution of his own operative methods, is a masterwork of medical communication. That monograph, *The Operative Story of Goitre,* is the one piece of scientific literature I know of that can be read around the campfire. It is an enthralling chronicle, as the narrator takes his readers from antiquity to 1920, interweaving the later stages of the history of thyroid surgery with the unfolding of his own interest in the field. He reviews ancient and medieval case reports and goes on to describe in detail the often harrowing operative adventures of earlier nineteenth-century surgeons who attempted to extirpate the gland. The reader comes to feel as though he were standing shoulder to shoulder with the boldest surgeons of an earlier time as they battled sudden massive hemorrhage, asphyxia, air bubbles sucked into major veins, and the nameless terror that this type of operating induced in surgeon and patient alike in those far-off days be-

Because of their lucid narrative style, all of Halsted's papers read like literature.

fore anesthesia. Finally, he brings his readers to the operations he himself had witnessed on his visits to Billroth in Vienna and Theodor Kocher in Berne. Correctly, he states, "Greater advance was made in the operative treatment of goitre in the decade from 1873 to 1883 than in all the foregoing years." In 1909, Kocher became the first of only a few surgeons to win a Nobel Prize, based on his contribution to the understanding of thyroid physiology and the treatment of its diseases.

Kocher and Billroth were major influences on William Halsted in all areas of surgical endeavor, but in none was this more true than in the investigation of the physiology and surgery of the thyroid. He had begun to study the gland's structure as early in his career as the Vienna days of 1879 and 1880. During subsequent visits to the Germanic clinics he had the opportunity to observe the progress that was being made there and in Berne. His Swiss sojourns brought him particular pleasure, since he found in Kocher a kindred spirit who valued careful technique, bloodless operating, and gentle handling of tissues as much as he himself did. This was entirely different from the performances of Billroth, whose rapid, dramatic surgical methods did not allow for much attention to minute detail.

For each of the two surgical giants there was one particular complication of his own thyroid surgery that he found depressing to contemplate and puzzling to explain. For Kocher it was myxedema, that condition of physical and mental torpor that results when a patient produces little or no thyroid hormone. For Billroth it was death from decreased levels of calcium in the blood due to inaction of the tiny glands called parathyroids that lie close to the thyroid itself. In time, the reason for each of the two problems became clear. It was as Halsted later wrote:

I have pondered this question for many years and conclude that the explanation probably lies in the operative methods of the two illustrious surgeons. Kocher, neat and precise, operating in a relatively bloodless manner, scrupulously removed the entire thyroid gland, doing little damage outside of its capsule. Billroth, operating more rapidly and, as I recall his manner (1879 and 1880), with less regard for the tissues and less concern for hemorrhage, might easily have removed the parathyroids or at least have interfered with their blood supply, and have left remnants of the thyroid.

Obviously, it was the Kocher brand of surgery that appealed to Halsted's meticulously precise nature. His operative methods paralleled those of the Swiss surgeon so exactly that what was influence seemed almost imitation. Not surprisingly, the only prominent predecessor in so painstaking an approach was Lister, although even he seemed somewhat hasty when compared to his two fastidious colleagues of succeeding generations. In commenting upon the conscientious gentleness that Halsted and Kocher taught to their disciples, one of its leading exponents of still the next generation, Harvey Cushing, said the following to the International Medical Congress at its 1913 meeting in London:

The accurate and detailed methods, in the use of which Kocher and Halsted were for so long the notable examples, have spread into all clinics—at least into those clinics where you or I would wish to entrust ourselves for operation. Observers no longer expect to be thrilled in an operating room; the spectacular public performances of the past, no longer condoned, are replaced by the quiet, rather tedious procedures which few beyond the operator, his assistants, and the immediate bystander can profitably see. The patient on the table, like the passenger in a car, runs greater risks if he have a loquacious driver, or one who takes close corners, exceeds the speed limit, or rides to admiration.

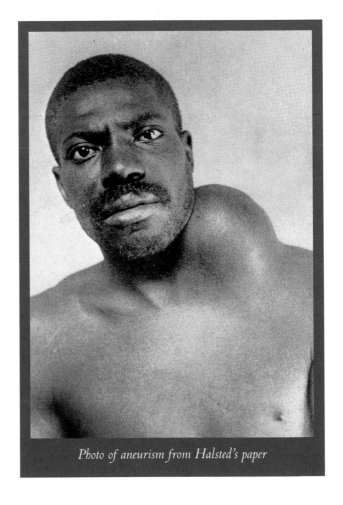

Photo of aneurism from Halsted's paper

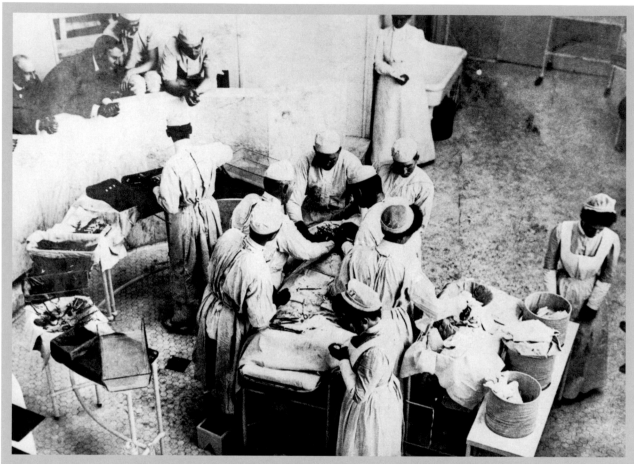

Dr. Halsted operates at Johns Hopkins, with assistants Cushing and Finney.

Surgery had come a long way since the spectacular exhibitions of such surgical headliners as James Syme and Robert Liston, he of the thirty-second amputation. Utilizing the principles of an absolutely bloodless operative field, anatomically perfect dissection of each structure, rigid sterility, and accurate closure with fine silk stitches of every layer of tissue, Halsted developed a technique of thyroidectomy that represented, and still does, the acme of the surgeon's art. His report of 650 operated cases of hyperthyroidism marked the beginning of effective therapy for that disorder in the United States, a path of clinical progress soon to be widened by such subsequent leaders of American surgery as Charles Mayo, George Crile, and Frank Lahey.

Sprinkled, albeit sparsely, throughout Halsted's writings are vignettes of personal experiences that give hints about his own life. In 1881, when the twenty-nine-year-old surgeon was in his second year of practice in New York, he operated on his own mother:

I was summoned to Albany one evening to see my mother, who for two years or more had been ill with an undiagnosed affection. . . . I found her very ill, slightly jaundiced, with tumefaction and great tenderness in the region of the gallbladder. So at 2 a.m. I operated, incised the gallbladder which was distended with pus and extracted seven stones. This was, I think, one of the earliest operations for gallstones in the country. My mother died about 2 years after my operation.

Another personal story, this one of far more lasting impact on the world of surgery, is told in a 1913 review article on surgical technique. The following paragraph, dealing with the irritative effects of sterilizing solutions, appears midway through the paper:

In the winter of 1889 and 1890—I cannot recall the month—the nurse in charge of my operating-room complained that the solutions of mercuric chloride produced a dermatitis of her arms and hands. As she was an unusually efficient woman, I gave the matter my consideration and one day in New York requested the Goodyear Rubber Company to make as an experiment two pair of thin rubber gloves with gauntlets. On trial these proved to be so satisfactory that additional gloves were ordered. In the autumn, on my return to town, an assistant who passed the instruments and threaded the needles was also provided with rubber gloves to wear at the operations. At first the operator wore them only when exploratory incisions into joints were made. After a time the assistants became so accustomed to working in gloves that they also wore them as operators and would remark that they seemed to be less expert with the bare hands than with the gloved hands.

This is very likely the most famous paragraph ever printed in the literature of surgery, not only for its description of the introduction of rubber operating gloves, but also because it is the only instance of the beginning of a researcher's love affair being recorded in a medical journal. That "unusually efficient woman" whose chemical rash had led to the use of surgical gloves was Caroline Hampton, who on June 4, 1890, became Mrs. William Stewart Halsted. It was a secure, mutually devoted marriage. Osler, with the literary twinkle in the eye so often found in his comments, later described his first awareness that the two were slipping into each other's affections, not to say arms. He walked into a room in the pathology laboratory one day and came upon the usually reticent surgeon demonstrating the anatomy of a dried fibula to the Director of Surgical Nursing. Their engagement was announced a week later. In *The Inner History of the Johns Hopkins Hospital*, Osler wrote of his colleague's marriage: "He married a woman after his own heart and, like himself . . . a little odd. They cared nothing for society, but were devoted to their dogs and horses."

The oddness of Caroline and William Halsted was not restricted to slight peculiarities—their childless marriage was a singular example of two people discovering common ground in being so uncommon. It would be hard to find a couple whose tranquil union depended so completely on their mutual ability each to let the other go off in any suitable direction unaccompanied, physically or emotionally. It was a strange form of congeniality, and an even stranger form of love. Nevertheless, it suited them both—and it worked.

In Harvey Cushing's Yale collection of letters between himself and Halsted, there is a twenty-page typewritten reminiscence of the man he always called "the professor." It includes this description of Caroline Halsted and the three-story brick house she shared with her husband at 1201 Eutaw Place. They had separate apartments, his on the second floor, hers on the third. They often had dinner together, but never breakfasted in each other's company:

The house, as I say, was cold and gloomy—a sort of Bleak House, with the high ceilings of the old Baltimore block residences. The furnace was never used and he would have only an open wood fire in his room. . . . His books and his study were on the second floor. On the third floor lived Mrs. Halsted and the pack of dachshunds. She was a strange, unadorned woman dressed in black who affected a masculine garb of the plainest sort; wore flat-heeled, mannish shoes and had her hair brushed straight back and fastened in a bun. Such a contrast to her husband! She was one of the early nurses at the J.H.H. . . . Having been put in charge of the operating room it was, I presume, a case of propinquity. They were a devoted couple though so far as I can recall I never saw them together but once in company. . . . Heuer and Mont Reid, I believe one summer after the war paid a visit at High Hampton which must have been delightful. Mrs. Halsted who was a daughter of General Wade Hampton ruled the mountaineers in her demesne with an iron hand, while the "Professor" devoted himself chiefly to his dahlias in which he specialized and of which he had a remarkable collection.

High Hampton was Caroline's two-thousand-acre family estate (she too was of the American aristocracy, southern-style) in North Carolina. At the end of each academic year, the Halsteds would leave Baltimore for the summer. After a month in the cool mountain air at High Hampton, cultivating his dahlias and peering heavenward through his telescope, the professor would go off to Europe alone, secluding himself in expensive hotels for long periods, seeing no one. We will never know whether morphine was his roommate, but it is hard to believe otherwise.

One of the unhidden things Halsted did while on his annual trips abroad was to have himself outfitted in London and Paris. In respect to matters sartorial, he had not changed from his younger days. He dressed to perfection, and no American tailor satisfied him. George Heuer, one of his house surgeons who later became Professor of Surgery at Cincinnati and Cornell, wrote of him that he was "a well-nigh perfectly appointed man. His black derby hat always looked new and was without fleck of dust, his dark blue suit was well-fitting, of fine material and faultlessly pressed, his linen was always immaculate, the cravat modest in coloring and expensive, his gloves absolutely unsoiled and his shoes shining with surpassing brilliance." Cushing's notes comment that even in the early days, when he rode to the hospital in a Baltimore streetcar, "he was usually in a top hat and frock coat with its accessories of stick, gloves, and a copy of the latest German surgical periodical."

Cushing, who was a bit of a dandy himself, wrote that although Halsted's suits were tailored in London, his kid shoes were narrow in the French style "with a pointed although truncated toe." He personally selected the place on the hide from which the leather was to be cut, and ordered six pairs at a time from his Paris bootmaker. Any pair with which he was dissatisfied was discarded on arrival. His dress shirts were sent to a Paris laundry, Halsted claiming that he could find not a single shop in America that knew how to handle them properly. I am surely not the only person who has wondered whether the boxes of returned shirts also contained hidden vials of narcotic.

Halsted's *boulevardier* image belied his behavior. He was anything but jaunty; in this apparent *bon vivant* there was very little *bon* and even less *vivant*. Words like "animated," "lively," and their synonyms would be misplaced in any description of his Baltimore personality. He was diffident, distant, and almost inaccessible under ordinary daily circumstances. It was as though he had made a moat around himself which he kept filled with a cool mixture of aloofness and a tinge of sarcasm. Secure within his isolating emotional buffer, he went about his day's work protected if not by a moat then by some encircling life preserver of detachment. When necessary, he could fend off an attack on his privacy with a perfectly aimed acid-soaked dart.

Halsted's penchant for sarcasm was so well known that medical students sometimes became inarticulate in his presence. It really made no difference that they did, because he was not much interested in teaching junior people. In fact, he did very little direct teaching in any event, except to his house surgeon. It is remarkable that the man who founded America's foremost school of surgery, who taught so much to so many generations of his successors, had no real interest in the personal instruction of those who came to learn from him. And yet, in any accurate assessment, he would have to be called a great teacher, whose

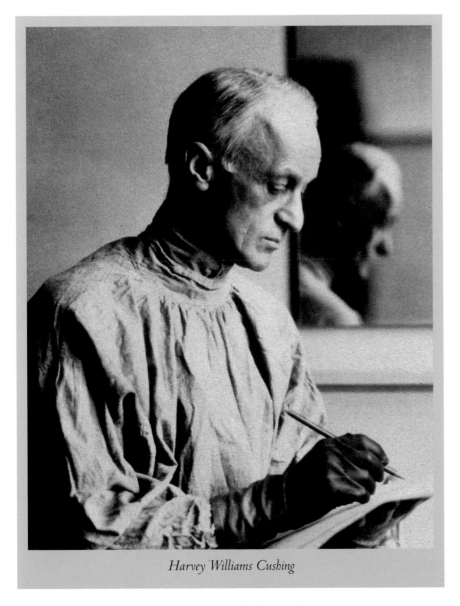

Harvey Williams Cushing

talent lay in his example rather than in his words. To be privileged to be part of his scrupulously executed laboratory experiments, to watch him examine a patient on the ward, to assist him in one of his meticulous operations, to observe the way in which he scrutinized the extirpated tissues postoperatively and then under the microscope, was to see a man creating the criteria by which American surgeons would judge themselves and each other forever after. It was impossible not to come away a better doctor after contact with such a man.

Of course, his diffidence was a multistructured thing. Though it made him seem a recluse, it also manifested itself in the form of a personal modesty that was in fact quite disarming. He was embarrassed by compliments, avoided all but a few of the honors that came his way, and is one of those unusual contributors to clinical medicine who was generous in sharing and even acceding priority to other investigators. On many occasions, he appeared actually to be more shy than reclusive, more insecure than distant.

In spite of all, Halsted somehow preserved just a trace of his buoyant prenarcotic personality, which he demonstrated in rare moments and only with certain close friends. He was capable of bursts of extroverted good fellowship and sudden displays of a hilarious sense of humor when he was in the company of Welch or one of his other few intimates. The truth was that even his sarcasm was meant only to defend against those slings and arrows that are imagined by such shy men. It was one of his distance-expanders; everyone who became at all familiar with him knew that. Deliberate unkindness was not in his nature.

The moat, a certain furtiveness that overcame him in times of narcotic-need, his towering inter-national eminence—all of these enlarged the space by which he stood separated from most other people. Those who were able to get closer felt a gentle warmth they could not have predicted, but they were few indeed. Heuer and several others have left touching descriptions of the acts of enormous kindness he demonstrated toward them, and of a brotherly affection that came from within a lonely man who in truth must have begged himself in vain for less rigidity and more love.

Amateur (and even professional) psychiatrists have had a half century of field days playing around with theoretical interpretations of Halsted's emotional life. You can imagine some of the things they have said. Consider only his peculiar marriage, his relationship with Welch, his addiction, his lifesaving interventions for both sister and mother, his apparent personality change between New York and Baltimore, and even his choice of surgery as a career, not to add the compulsiveness with which he carried it out. The list is very long, and quite irresistible. Fortunately for my credibility, there are space restraints on these chapters. Otherwise, I should be tempted like so many others to play psychohistorian, and become ridiculous. It is safer to proceed to more solid ground.

I know of no example that epitomizes more clearly the difference between pre- and post-Halstedian surgery than a description of Harvey Cushing's first day at Johns Hopkins as an assistant resident. After matriculating at Yale, Cushing had gone on to the Harvard Medical School, graduating in 1895. Following a year as house pupil at the Massachusetts General Hospital, he was accepted by Halsted for surgical training. Although he came to Baltimore from one of the leading medical centers of America, the transition to Hopkins was a passage out of the bruising bombast of nineteenth-century surgery and into the physiological serenity of the twentieth. Cushing remembered:

The surroundings at the J.H.H. were strange enough after what I had been through at the Massachusetts General. The talk was of pathology and bacteriology of which I knew so little that much of my time the first few months was passed alone at night in the room devoted to surgical pathology in the old pathological building looking at specimens with a German textbook at hand. . . . It was most disconcerting to me, after the hurly-burly of the M.G.H., to have my new Chief come, as it were apologetically, some day into Ward G; ask if he might be allowed to examine a particular patient; to have him spend an hour fiddling over a patient with cancer of the breast who had recently been admitted; and then to have him depart saying he was tired and would be able to do nothing more that day. If he were sufficiently interested he might ask that he be permitted to do the operation; and if he came and did operate, so soon as the breast was removed, leaving the huge closure and skin graft to Bloodgood [one of Halsted's residents], he would depart with the tissues. These he would study and ruminate over for an interminable time, meanwhile tagging innumerable areas which he wished to have [microscopically] sectioned.

Cushing later joined the Hopkins faculty, where he went from triumph to triumph as a surgeon, a researcher, and a teacher. Given responsibility by Halsted for all patients with brain tumors, he established through his research the basic principles upon which the specialty of neurosurgery is founded. After refusing professorships at several leading universities, he accepted Harvard's offer to be the first chief at the new Peter Bent Brigham Hospital, where he established a training program and an atmosphere that were patterned on the Hopkins model. When he retired in 1933, he was succeeded by Elliot Cutler. The following is a description of Cushing's initiation into the new world of Hopkins surgery, as he told it to Cutler many years later:

Being a newcomer he was not allowed in the operating room his first day there, though a patient from his ward was to be operated upon. It was with great misgiving that the young Cushing watched two and even three hours go by, while the great master [Halsted] took such exquisite care with each cell that there would be no injury to the patient. Finally when the patient returned to the ward after some four and one-half hours in the operating room, young Cushing was ready with restoratives and the customary medication that he had been ordered to give to surgical patients when a pupil at the Massachusetts General Hospital. When he was about to administer these medicaments, for he recalled from his days as a pupil at the Massachusetts General Hospital how ill those who returned from the operating room were even after a hurried procedure of minutes, not hours, Dr. Halsted entered the ward.

Dr. Cushing spoke up and said, "I am carrying out the usual procedure."

Noting the Trendelenburg position [used in the treatment of shock], Dr. Halsted said, "Is my patient ill? This is unusual. Let us examine her." Examination revealed a normal pulse rate and normal respiration. He then noted the hypodermic and said, "What is in the syringe?"

"Strychnine," said Cushing. "It will do the patient good."

Dr. Halsted asked a third question. "What do you think strychnine will do for the patient?" Having been educated in a school where memory and orders were the rule, Cushing did not know. He was then informed by Dr. Halsted that he should read up on strychnine. "If your reading convinces you that strychnine is good for the patient, by all means use it," said Halsted. Young Cushing never gave the strychnine, and he learned a great lesson—never do anything to a patient without understanding the why and wherefore.

It was the tracking down of the why and wherefore that linked William Stewart Halsted to the distinguished line of his predecessors in scientific medicine. Beginning with the Hippocratic physicians, the advances of medical science have resulted from a mixture of curiosity and the pragmatic need to know, in order that the sick may be healed. The lesson learned by Cushing in his first day in Baltimore was a lesson that William Halsted, by his example of a lifetime of seeking, taught to every American surgeon who followed him.

Throughout that lifetime, Halsted was frequently felled by minor illnesses of one sort or another. Certainly some of his periodic absences from the hospital were related to his addiction, but others were the result of a susceptibility to respiratory and other problems. He developed a bronchitis in 1919 that kept him confined to his home during the months of February and March. However, it became obvious in the spring that he was not fully recovered, and even a full summer in the much-beloved hills of High Hampton did not suffice to restore his strength. Then, still weakened by his bronchial condition, he began to have symptoms that he recognized as being due to stones in his bile duct; he returned to Baltimore at the end of August, quite sick. On September 2, he was operated upon by one of his former house surgeons, Richard Follis, who extracted the stones and removed the gall bladder. Healing was slow, being complicated by drainage of bile from the wound, but this finally cleared up and the patient gradually recovered.

Halsted returned to work. In 1920, he published *The Operative Story of Goitre,* and he remained active in the laboratory, continuing his intestinal suture experiments. But after a while he began to have episodes of what seemed to be a recurrence of stone, gradually increasing in frequency and severity. During the second and third weeks of August 1922, while at High Hampton, he again became very ill, with persistent fever, pain, and jaundice. He arrived in Baltimore by train on August 23, bringing with him his own supply of morphine,

> *The lesson learned by Cushing in his first day in Baltimore was a lesson that William Halsted, by his example of a lifetime of seeking, taught to every American surgeon who followed him.*

and a daily record of the amounts he had taken during the pain-racked summer.

No one seems to have given a second thought, at that time or since, to the concentration of the narcotic in Halsted's solution. On arrival in Baltimore, he told his medical attendants that it was made up in the proportion of one grain of morphine to 160 drops of water, which they accepted, having no clear reason to question it, and they even remarked on the small quantities required by their stoic professor to control his pain. Remembering the circumstances of Thomas McBride's death, and knowing of the contents of *The Inner History of the Johns Hopkins Hospital*, it seems not farfetched to suggest that the morphine concentration in Halsted's little bottle was quite a bit higher than his physicians were led to believe.

Two of his former house surgeons for whom Halsted had the highest regard, Heuer and Mont Reid, were summoned from Cincinnati, where they had recently gone to lead a newly organized department of surgery. On the morning of August 25, they explored their professor's bile duct and removed the single stone that was obstructing it. They closed the duct using a technique that had been invented by their patient. The postoperative course was stormy—on the afternoon of September 3, a gastrointestinal hemorrhage occurred. In spite of blood transfusions, the situation worsened, and on the morning of Thursday, September 7, 1922, Heuer and Reid lost their revered mentor to a postoperative pneumonia.

After autopsy, the cremated remains of the world's foremost surgeon were brought back to New York, to be buried in Greenwood Cemetery in Brooklyn. In that five-hundred-acre tract of gently rolling hills and luxuriant foliage, William Halsted's resting place is to be found across New York Bay overlooking lower Manhattan, where his early surgical triumphs had taken place, and his travail. Not far from his grave lie such leading figures in America's history as Horace Greeley, Henry Ward Beecher, Peter Cooper, and Samuel F. B. Morse. They are worthy company for the greatest surgical scholar our country has ever produced.

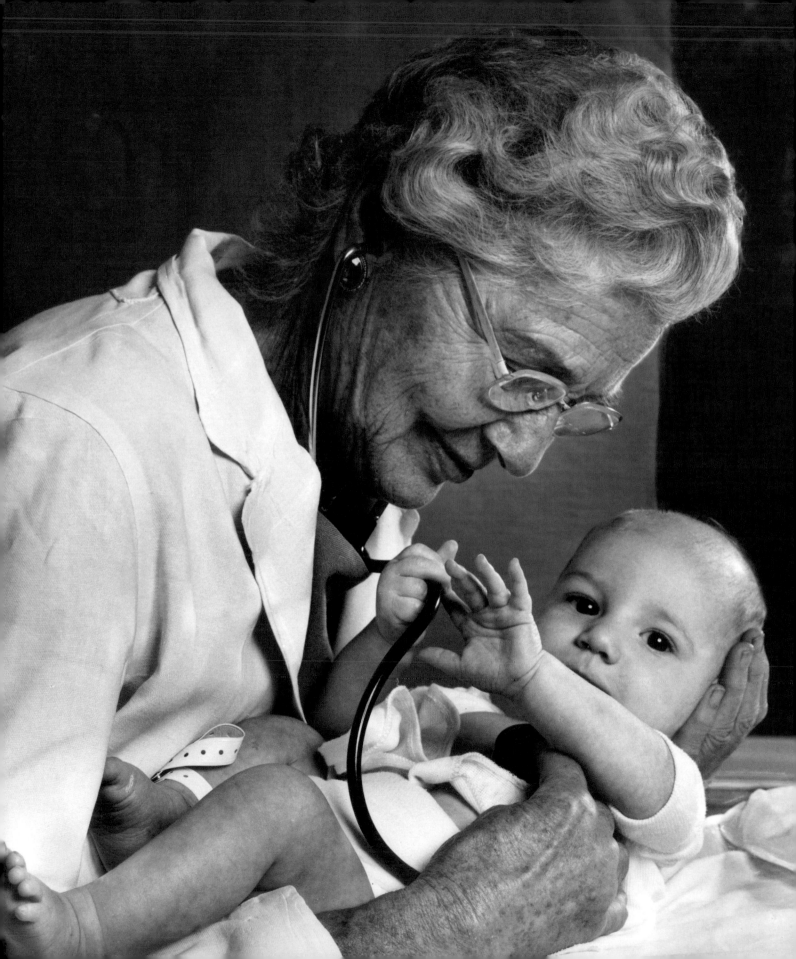

14

A Triumph of Twentieth-Century Medicine

Helen Taussig and the Blue-Baby Operation

*I*t was impossible for the great Johns Hopkins experiment in medical education to fail. The foundation was laid on a solid financial basis by a group of idealists whose aims, although visionary, were not unrealistic. The combination of vision and funding, when it is guided by an acute perception of rational goals, is a force of irresistible dynamism. The creation of Hopkins between 1876 and 1893 was due, as one observer put it, to "an angelic conjunction of men, money, and circumstances." The result was a new paradigm of a university, whose medical school and hospital would generate the energy and manpower by which the entire American system of training doctors transmuted itself from slag to silver.

The very year of the Hopkins inaugural was filled with portent. The centennial of our nation's birth was marked by two contrasting medical events, one in Germany and one in America, that epitomized the young country's adolescent reluctance to accept the new science it so desperately needed for its continuing development: in Breslau, Robert Koch demonstrated for the first time that a specific bacterium causes a specific disease; in Philadelphia, Joseph Lister was met with a cool reception when he tried to elucidate the scientific basis of antisepsis to a skeptical audience of eminent surgeons. Koch's work with the anthrax bacillus effectively proved the germ theory, but only to those who were ready to heed the message that science must be brought to the bedsides of the sick. The role of the Johns Hopkins Medical School was clear—it would set an example to convince America's physicians and educators that there could be no advancement in the art of healing without a major infusion of medical science; it would be the fountainhead from which that new branch of science would spread to the hospitals and universities of North America; it would bring the germ theory across the Atlantic.

The founders of Hopkins were well aware of their exemplary mission. From the very beginning, training assistantships and fellowships were set up in the laboratories to match the internship and residency opportunities that existed in the clinical specialties of medicine, surgery, and pediatrics. Like scholars from the rest of the university, Hopkins-trained medical researchers were sought after and fought over by schools all over the country, at least as much for their specific skills as for the resuscitating academic promise they breathed into many a flagging faculty beset by institutional inertia.

One of the most fundamental of the first educational innovations was to take the teaching of anatomy, physiology, pathology, and pharmacology out of the hands of local practitioners. The chairs in those subjects were made full-time, which meant that the university paid a salary to professors who devoted all of their efforts to teaching and research, without the distractions of private patient care. Within the first two decades, this system of remuneration became standard for the clinical departments as well, with all patient fees reverting to the school. The very fact that the salaries were much lower than the teachers might have earned from practice proved to be an advantage, since it attracted scholars dedicated enough to sacrifice income for the opportunity to do research and to educate young physicians.

Such an arrangement does have certain built-in problems, among which is its restriction of academia to those who can afford the financial penalty that comes with the professor's chair. But, for its time, it was an effective solution to the age-old problem of how best to discourage teachers from sacrificing their duties in the in-

terests of Mammon. At Hopkins, and at each of the schools that adopted it, the full-time system resulted in the recruitment of a cadre of men and women consecrated to a life of medical scholarship. The deliberate unworldliness of these people allowed a concentration on their pedagogical and research interests that was almost cloister-like in its single-minded pursuit of excellence in academic science.

It must be understood that the new institution was not arising *de novo* as a shining tower in the midst of a desolate morass of medical backwardness. The Hopkins created by Gilman, Billings, and the others is best understood as a response to the rumblings of a process that was already getting under way when the Baltimore school came along to accelerate it to a rate exceeding anyone's most fervent expectation. America was indeed far behind most European countries both in education and in the quality of medical care, but a beginning had been made, mostly on the individual initiative of young physicans themselves, to alter the situation. Thousands, like William Halsted, had sought advanced training abroad, especially in the laboratory sciences. When the American Physiological Society was founded in 1887, twenty of its twenty-eight members had studied in Europe, sixteen of them in Germany. Many ambitious young people had gone so far as to begin their process of self-improvement even before starting the formal study of medicine, spending several years in college, although most medical schools required no more than a high school degree, and it was common to waive even this criterion on the flimsiest of excuses. Some highly motivated students even had undergraduate degrees long before Hopkins made them mandatory.

All of this improvement, however, was based on the efforts of individual seekers. No organized effort got under way until that fateful year of 1876, when representatives of twenty-two medical schools met to form the American Medical College Association, which, although unsuccessful at first, reorganized itself in 1890 as the Association of American Medical Colleges. From then on, the pace of improvement picked up. By 1896, a third of the nation's 155 medical schools were abiding by the higher standards promulgated by the organization. Gradually, the association began to involve itself in cooperative efforts with the American Medical Association, with the aim of seeking solutions to national educational, research, and clinical needs. The inauguration of the Johns Hopkins Medical School in 1893 provided a focus for the highest aims of the reformers.

Once Hopkins had opened, medical educators found placed before them a solid edifice of evidence that the ills of American medicine could be solved. All that remained was to hold the disabilities up to the scrutiny of proper authorities, and then to mandate change. If change could not be mandated, it could, at the very least, be so forcefully encouraged as to make it irresistible. As in the case of Hopkins, it would take a combination of vision and funding, this time on a grand scale.

What was needed was a roving detective-gadfly who could study the debilities of the nation's system of medical education and then prescribe the process by which they might be resolved.

What was needed was a roving detective-gadfly who could study the debilities of the nation's system of medical education and then prescribe the process by which they might be resolved. This was not a job for a committee; it could only be done by a single individual of such proven ability that his conclusions would be trusted and his recommendations unhesitatingly instituted. At the critical moment, the critical individual appeared, in the person of Abraham Flexner.

Not surprisingly, Flexner was a product of the undergraduate program at Johns Hopkins University. The son of German-Jewish refugees from the post-1848 repressions, he had sped through college in two years, propelled by a combination of good brains and empty pockets. After graduation in 1886, he returned to his hometown of Louisville, Kentucky, to teach secondary school, and then in 1890 opened a private academy of his own. After fifteen years of considerable success, he closed the school because he wanted more training in psychology and philosophy, which he obtained at Harvard. He and his wife next spent a year of study in Germany, which resulted in the publication of his first book, *The American College*, in 1908. This stern critique of the educational methods of Harvard and the other established colleges came to the attention of a prominent educator, Henry

S. Pritchett. Pritchett had recently convinced Andrew Carnegie to endow an organization to make the profession of teaching more attractive to young people. When the resultant Carnegie Foundation for the Advancement of Teaching was founded in 1906, Pritchett left his post as the head of the Massachusetts Institute of Technology to become its president. As one of its first major projects, the foundation was planning a much-needed study of medical education in the United States and Canada. Pritchett in 1908 asked the forty-two-year-old Flexner to conduct the entire operation.

Over the next year, Flexner visited 155 schools in the two countries. He used the same criteria to evaluate each one: entrance requirements, size and training of faculty, financial condition of the school, quality of the laboratories, and the relationship between each school and the hospital in which its students and teachers worked. He was appalled at what he found. Even the better schools were none too good. Standards for admission were low, faculty were inadequately trained, most schools were privately owned purse-lining enterprises of their professors, laboratories were nominally equipped or filthy or both, and it was rare to find an institution whose students and teachers had free access to a good hospital. Hopkins was the one exception. As Flexner later wrote, "All honor to Gilman, Welch, Mall, Halsted, and their colleagues and students who hitched their wagon to a star and never flinched!"

Flexner's scathing indictment of American medical education was published in 1910 as Bulletin Number Four of the foundation. Although its official title was *Medical Education in the United States and Canada*, it soon became known as "the Flexner Report," and it was a sensation from the first day it appeared as front-page news. It passed devastating judgment on all but five schools, and even those fell well below the Hopkins standard. Intended to be more than a critique, it was also a program for reform. One of its recommendations was based on the excessive quantity and small quality of the schools: there should be a nationwide reorganization, eliminating 120 of them. In his 1960 autobiography, Flexner described the response:

The medical profession and the faculties of the medical schools, as well as the state boards of examiners, were absolutely flabbergasted by the pitiless exposure. We were threatened with lawsuits, and in one instance actually sued for libel for $150,000. I received anonymous letters warning me that I should be shot if I showed myself in Chicago, whereupon I went there to make a speech before a meeting called by the [American Medical Association] Council on Medical Education and returned unharmed. . . . Such a rattling of dead bones has never been heard in this country before or since. Schools collapsed to the right and left, usually without a murmur. A number of them pooled their resources. The seven schools of my native city, which . . . I had described with the same candor employed elsewhere, were reduced to one. The fifteen schools in Chicago, which I had called "the plague spot of the country in respect to medical education," were shortly consolidated into three.

In 1913, Flexner was invited to become a member of the General Education Board, founded by John D. Rockefeller, Jr., in 1902 to raise educational standards in the United States. He was entrusted with the mission of disbursing $50 million of Rockefeller money in such a way as to spread the successful results of the Hopkins experience to those medical schools that he judged to be worth saving. With a figurative blank checkbook, he began again to travel from one academic center to another, outlining to deans and faculties the measures that would be required to elevate their institutions to the desired levels of accomplishment. In each place his message was the same; it was based on his original criteria of evaluation: better laboratories, better students, better (full-time) faculty, and closer relationships with hospitals that served as the major teaching arenas for the clinical aspects of medical education. The models were to be Johns Hopkins and the German universities. Those schools that accepted the proposals were given the funds to implement them and were assisted in raising more funds on their own. The plan was so obviously the proper remedy that Rockefeller's original donation stimulated large contributions from other sources. The total grew to $600 million. With this enormous financial fertilizer, Abraham Flexner oversaw the emergence, to use his own words, of "American medical education from the lowest status to the highest in the civilized world."

The principles of the new system were not restricted to the instruction of medical students only. They included advanced training in the form of internships and residency appointments, and the encouragement of all trainees to do research, whether they had yet achieved the M.D. degree or not. The parent university was considered fundamental as a scholarly background in which to learn medicine; to this end, close ties were to be maintained between the academy and the clinic. Close ties were also basic to the relationship be-

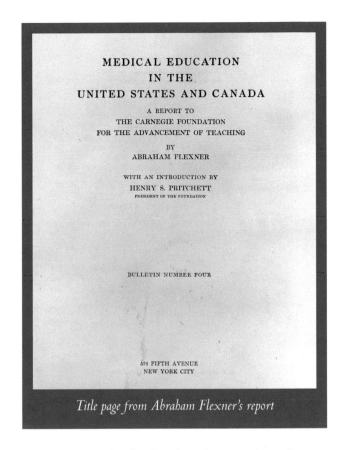

MEDICAL EDUCATION
IN THE
UNITED STATES AND CANADA
A REPORT TO
THE CARNEGIE FOUNDATION
FOR THE ADVANCEMENT OF TEACHING
BY
ABRAHAM FLEXNER

WITH AN INTRODUCTION BY
HENRY S. PRITCHETT
PRESIDENT OF THE FOUNDATION

BULLETIN NUMBER FOUR

576 FIFTH AVENUE
NEW YORK CITY

Title page from Abraham Flexner's report

tween the medical school and its teaching hospital, with the various departmental chairmen being chiefs of service on the hospital staff. Thus, the university's professor of surgery, for example, becomes the hospital's director of surgical services. In this capacity, he controls the appointments of all staff surgeons to assure competence and teaching ability.

Starting with high admission prerequisites for its students, and encompassing such matters as research and quality control of staff doctors, the new type of medical school was as much a state of mind as it was an institution for training healers. It began its influence on a doctor's life in the first hour of college and did not end it until the day of retirement. In such an academic atmosphere, the most advanced attainments of medical science were not only taught to young people, but were brought to the bedsides of the sick by a new type of healer who shared his hopes, his ideals, and even his lunch with his colleague of the laboratory. Everyone in such a place is a perpetual student of medicine.

The Flexner Report and the Rockefeller dollars changed the patterns of American philanthropy as much as they did the patterns of education. From that time onward, medical institutions became the beneficiaries of monies that had hitherto gone elsewhere, primarily to schools of theology. The situation seemed to reflect some vast change in the country's priorities. Once this direction had been established, it did not change, with the result that the newly restructured or newly created medical schools and hospitals continued to be prime recipients of public giving for the rest of the century.

The first institutions to benefit from the largess and counsel of the General Education Board were the universities of Chicago, Colorado, Iowa, Oregon, Rochester, Virginia, and Washington in St. Louis, as well as Columbia, Cornell, Duke, Harvard, McGill, Tulane, Vanderbilt, Western Reserve, and Yale. Hopkins, too, was reinfused with a large sum. Not only did these other schools structure themselves on the Baltimore model, but they developed sufficient academic strength that some of them began to attract Hopkins-trained faculty, thus reinforcing the structure upon which they were building. The long-range result was well described in 1970 by the medical historian John Field of UCLA: "So successful has been the work of her eminent sons and their colleagues that today Hopkins is but one of a number of outstanding medical schools in the United States—an outcome that would surely have delighted President Gil-

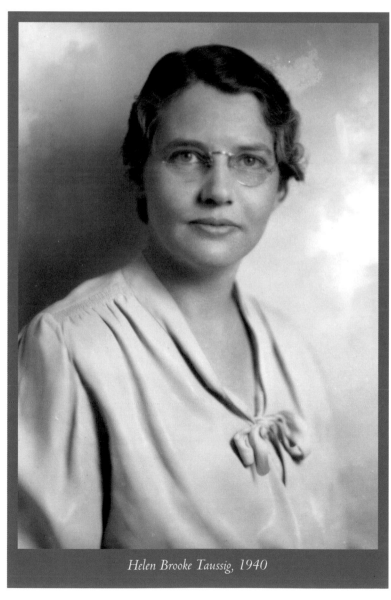

Helen Brooke Taussig, 1940

man and Doctors Welch, Osler, Halsted, and Kelly."

While the other schools were building, Johns Hopkins continued its patterns of excellence. Each year, major accomplishments in research and clinical care were reported in large numbers by its faculty. No matter the contributions of other American schools, none has remained more consistently in the forefront of progress than has Hopkins. Even in the face of today's abundance of superb institutions of medical science, Hopkins continues to be properly regarded among the finest. In seeking out a major figure whose contributions epitomize the emergence of twentieth-century American medical achievement, thoughts necessarily turn toward that first of our country's true universities, and one of the most dramatic advances that has ever been made there, the development of the "blue-baby operation" by Helen Taussig and Alfred Blalock.

Of the two, it is Taussig whose life seems to me the more representative of the story being told in this book. There is a continuing thread that is never lost in medical history, beginning with the Coan focus on man himself as the object of the healers' scrutiny. It was in the nature of man and everything that affects him that the Hippocratic physician sought to understand disease. His Cnidian colleague disagreed, and taught that the main focus must be on the sickness and the internal organ from which it arises, rather than on the whole patient in whom it makes its home, and it was via this reductionist approach of the Cnidians that science entered medicine. Until symptoms could be traced to their organs of origin, and then to their cells and molecules, classification and specific treat-

ment of disordered life processes would remain an impossibility. Therein lay the great advances that began to accelerate after Giovanni Morgagni, finally reaching their apotheosis in the superscientific medicine and the subspecialization of the latter decades of our own century. Having achieved an apotheosis, the ancient art of healing now needs an epiphany.

The epiphany is coming, and it is the Helen Taussigs that are its heralds. It is probably no coincidence that the advent of equality for women physicians should be accompanied by a reawakening of a sense of our original mission, the healing of our fellows. In an era when we sloganize so glibly of raising our consciousness about this or that, physicians are raising their sights, albeit still ever so slowly, up from the electron microscopes and ultrafiltration chambers into the pleading eyes of the sick. Hippocratism is returning to the practice of medicine, and it will bring with it the promise of fulfillment of the charge which we have been privileged since antiquity to undertake. Medicine is not a science, but an art that uses science to explore what William Harvey called Nature's closet secrets, that we may better minister to her children. We will remove the crackpot theories that have crept into holism, even as we humanize the detached indifference of reductionism, and thereby become the doctors we were always meant to be. Society will be the better for it, our patients will be the better for it, and we will be the better for it.

In the first chapter of this book, I quoted the Reverend William Sloane Coffin on the subject of the psychology of patients. On another occasion, I heard him say something that has taught me, although he meant it in another context, something about the psychology of doctors, as well. In discussing the women's liberation movement in America, he said, "The woman who most needs liberating is the woman who lives inside of each man." This, I think, is the great awareness that the increasing influence of female physicians has brought about. During my years of hospital training, we residents thought of ourselves as so many intrepid Spitfire pilots, roaring skyward in our efficient fighter planes to do battle with the forces of disease. The disease was the enemy, the cure was the victory, and the patient, I am ashamed to say, was too often merely the environment in which the encounter was fought. We had been taught to see it that way. It was necessary to learn the lesson well, in order to protect ourselves against the pain of others, and to abort any insidious tendency to identify with their sorrow. Our teachers believed in the interdiction against the enervating perils of what was called "emotional involvement." This is not to say that we were unkind to our patients, merely that we kept our distance. We treated them with respect and even with a kind of formalized dignity. We were as gentle as we knew how to be. But we were men apart—we towered over the sick as an adult towers over a child.

> *We have been shown, and it is to a great extent women physicians who have shown us, that our teachers were wrong—not only are we not compromised by allowing ourselves to feel what a patient feels, but we are often strengthened by it.*

Now something within us is being liberated. It is the thing that Bill Coffin spoke about. We have been shown, and it is to a great extent women physicians who have shown us, that our teachers were wrong—not only are we not compromised by allowing ourselves to feel what a patient feels, but we are often strengthened by it. A patient's life, the setting of his illness, the rending of his soul, the anguish of his family, the hope that lies in his recovery, have all become as much a part of his care as has a knowledge of the level of sodium ion in his blood. We are better nurturers now. The thing that is being liberated from inside ourselves is something that society has always seen as a feminine quality. To our astonishment, we are proud of it.

There is a different atmosphere around us these days. Women physicians have muted the boastful bugles that for too many centuries were used to proclaim medical conquest. They have made us less like centurions of cure and more like shepherds of sustenance for those who come to us for help. They have shown the reluctant among us that it is not necessary to be reticent in our personal devotion to our patients. Even ward rounds are different than they used to be; residents have more empathy, with their patients and with each other. Medicine is much more the healer's art than it has been since it first threw in its lot with science. I do not agree with those critics of my profession who say that our junior physicians are becoming ever more detached technocrats. The critics have not prowled the wards as I have, and they have not seen the changes of the past few years. Our young men are learning from our young women; our juniors are teaching their elders. We are no longer afraid to nurture. In nurturing our patients we nurture ourselves and make ourselves better doctors.

Nurturing, of course, is not new to us. Some of it has always gone on. Even the most diffident and distant of us have sometimes given much more than physical sustenance to our patients. Not enough of us, however, have given it *all of the time*. It is in the *all of the time* that Helen Taussig's greatness lies. It seems appropriate that in recounting the life of a mid-twentieth-century physician whose contributions represent the best of Cnidian reductionism we are able to describe one whose career embodied Hippocratic holism as well. Helen Taussig brought a combination of pure science and human empathy to bear on one of the oldest problems of pathological anatomy, and found a solution that was recognized as the acme of the healer's art.

Only ten years after the 1761 publication of *De Sedibus*, the Dutch physician Eduard Sandifort wrote a Morgagni-like treatise, *Observationes Anatomico-Pathologicae*, based upon his postmortem dissections of patients whose clinical care he had closely followed until the time of death. Although Sandifort's four-volume work included descriptions of many previously un-

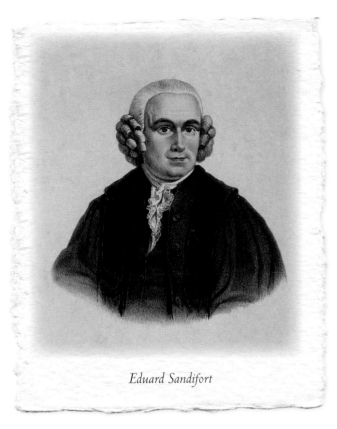

Eduard Sandifort

described entities, it has been best remembered for the case report of a child who "was perfectly normal at birth and throughout the first year of life, and then and then only, did a dusky color develop." Gradually, the child became more bluegray in appearance, especially with exertion. He developed increasing shortness of breath. When he was bled in an attempt to improve his breathing, the blood was found to be bluish in color and very thick. So well was Sandifort known for being able to elucidate pathology at autopsy that the boy's family requested that he dissect the body of their son when he died at the age of twelve. Because he had been normal at birth, it was expected that evidence would be found of some condition that was acquired from the surrounding environment, perhaps the fumes of the family's coal

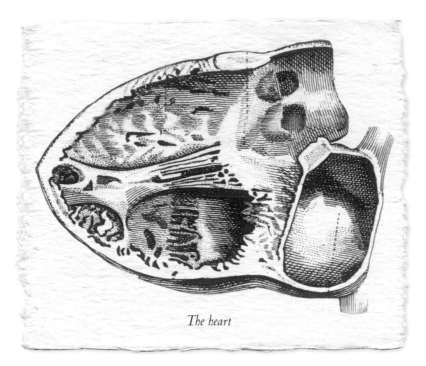

The heart

er is the ventricle. The right side of the heart receives blood returning from the periphery of the body and pumps it on out via the pulmonary artery to the lungs, to be replenished with oxygen. From there, the pulmonary veins return it to the left side, whence it is pumped out into the aorta to go back out to nourish the tissues. The heart is thus seen as two separate pumps working in a coordinated rhythm to do two separate jobs; the right-sided pump drives blood to the lungs, and the left-sided pump drives it to the rest of the body. Because the left side has to pump much harder to do its job, the pressure within it is considerably higher than within the right side.

The result of the boy's congenital anomaly was that a great deal of the blood returning from the body never reached the lungs to be replenished with oxygen. Instead, it had passed through the defect in the interventricular septum (that central shared wall) and been pumped right back out again, bypassing the lungs completely. The cause of the blueness, or cyanosis, was clear: a large proportion of the boy's circulating blood volume, since it was short-circuited past the lungs, never had the opportunity to become resaturated with oxygen. The reason the symptoms worsened with age was simply that the tiny pulmonary outflow tract did not significantly enlarge as the child grew bigger and as his body required more oxygen. Therefore a proportionally larger volume of bluish blood went unrefreshed to the tissues, and the symptoms of oxygen deprivation worsened.

stove. Sandifort, on opening the chest, was surprised to see that the pulmonary artery, which carries blood from the right side of the heart to the lungs, was abnormally small and tight. There was a hole in the muscular wall that separates the main right pumping chamber, the right ventricle, from the left. This meant that blood was so obstructed in its passage to the lungs that a considerable portion of it backed up into the right ventricle with each heartbeat, and passed unoxygenated through the defect in the wall, or septum, directly into the left ventricle, and from there on out into the general circulation via the aorta.

A brief review of anatomy is probably in order at this point. It is best to think of the heart as two distinct organs, lying on opposite sides of a central shared wall, the septum. Each of the two parts has an upper chamber which receives blood, and a lower chamber that pumps it out again. The upper chamber is called the atrium and the low-

In 1888, the Professor of Anatomical Pathology at Marseilles, Étienne-Louis Fallot, recognized that the condition described by Sandifort has four anatomical components: tightness, or stenosis, of the pulmonary outflow tract; interventricular septal defect; a thick-walled right ventricle caused by the effort of pumping against the obstruction; and an aorta displaced so much to the right side that blood easily enters it directly from the right ventricle as well as through the septal defect. The congenital heart disease he described was named for him; it is called the tetralogy of Fallot.

The tetralogy of Fallot soon became a source of fascination to physicians, who appreciated that Fallot was correct when he pointed out that 75 percent of cyanotic children, the so-called blue babies, would be found at autopsy to have its anatomical abnormalities, with the remainder having a variety of other sorts of congenital defects, some of which were individual components of the full unlucky package. Using the various methods of physical examination as they became more sophisticated in the late nineteenth century, premortem diagnosis of the anomaly became gradually less difficult to make. Based on clinical history, the murmur heard through the stethoscope, and heart size and motion as determined by the techniques of palpation and percussion, a number of cases were described over the course of the next half century. Nevertheless, most cyanotic children defied the efforts of even the most skilled examiners to solve the diagnostic puzzles presented by their array of findings. It was enough to grapple with the tragic reality that nothing could be done for them.

The study of the tetralogy led to an awareness of the various other forms of congenital heart disease as well, and the problems posed by them. Before any thought of effective treatment could be entertained, it was necessary to find some method of differentiating the anatomical defects of each type from all of the others, and to classify the several major anomalies in such a way as to simplify the chaotic confusion of disordered physiologies they presented. This major task was accomplished by a Canadian physician named Maude Abbott.

Maude Abbott's career began in the very earliest of the days when women were entering the medical profession. Having graduated in 1890 from the Arts Faculty at Montreal's McGill University in only the third class to accept women, she tried in vain to be admitted to the institution's men-only Medical Faculty. She put up a prodigious struggle, enlisting friends, newspapers, and public opinion in her favor. Although debates and discussions became heated, between the physicians of Montreal and the school, she was finally turned away, receiving her notification from the registrar with the statement that McGill "could not see its way to undertaking the medical education of women."

On the corner of Ontario and Mance streets, in the middle of bustling downtown Montreal, was a small building that housed the medical school of the University of Bishop's College. That university having decided to accept women, Maude Abbott was invited to join the medical school's first class. Bishop's was no McGill, but Abbott eagerly accepted the offer; she graduated with the Senior Anatomy Prize and the Chancellor's Prize for academic achievement.

The next step was to learn German and travel to Zurich, where she matriculated at the medical school in the winter term of 1894. She then spent two years at the University of Vienna. In 1897 she returned to Montreal and opened a general practice.

But the private practice of medicine was not for Maude Abbott. Like so many other physicians whose appointment book is slow to fill, she volunteered to do some academic work. Although the authorities at McGill had not wanted her as a student, they gladly gave the able young woman an unpaid post as assistant curator of the school's museum of pathology. Constantly trying to improve her knowledge, she traveled to various medical centers to study their museum methods. In 1898, in Baltimore, she met William Osler, who pointed out to her that the McGill museum contained as yet untapped treasures that could be used in the classification of disease and in developing more accurate methods of diagnosis. She returned home with renewed purpose. The following year she consulted Osler about a specimen of cor triloculare, a three-chambered heart, and with his encouragement began to study congenital cardiac defects. In a lifetime of work, she became the world's foremost authority not only on the anatomical cardiac derangements but also on the disordered physiology produced by their effects. Abbott's work reached its culmination in 1936, with the publication of her *Atlas of Congenital Cardiac Disease*, a compendium of a thousand cases which she had personally dissected. It became the veritable bible for anyone who wished to learn about the pathologic anatomy and pathophysiology of inborn defects of the heart.

Helen Taussig's path to medical education was a great deal easier than Abbott's, but made tortuous nevertheless by her being female and being born too soon, in 1898. She was the daughter of a Harvard professor of economics, and she attended Radcliffe for two years, after which she transferred to Berkeley to get out of the shadow of being Professor Taussig's daughter. When she told her father on graduation in 1921 that she wanted to go into medicine, he suggested public health instead; "That's a very good field for women," he said. The dean of Harvard's School of Public Health, however, very politely told her that she could enroll in the four-year course, but that no woman would be granted a degree. Equally politely, she turned down the opportunity.

Refusing to be discouraged, Taussig determined to prepare to enter medical school by a less circuitous route. The Harvard Medical School did not accept women (and would not until 1945), but she did obtain permission to study histology there and anatomy at Boston University. At the suggestion of BU Professor of Anatomy Alexander Begg, she undertook an investigation of the muscle of the heart. Begg, who was also dean of the university's medical school, encouraged her to apply to Johns Hopkins, in order that she might make the most of her obvious talents. In later years she wrote a brief autobiographical piece in which she described her decision to take Begg's advice, and the opportunities that came her way in Baltimore. Its title reveals much about why she made her career as a pediatric cardiologist: "Little Choice and a Stimulating Environment."

Helen Taussig's understanding of the functioning of heart muscle was put to good use when she was given a job at the Hopkins Heart Station, where she worked during her four years at the school. Although there were ten women in her 1923 class of seventy students, the medical service offered an internship to only one of them at graduation, according to a long-standing custom probably based on a well-meaning conception of proportional representation. This most coveted of appointments went to her classmate Vivian Tappan, who outranked her by 0.2 point. To compensate her for that, her supervisor at the Heart Station, Edward Carter, gave her a fellowship in cardiology.

During the course of that year, a new chairman of pediatrics, Edwards A. Park, came down from Yale and instituted a Pediatric Cardiac Clinic, to which Taussig was one of the assigned physicians. Park was extremely kind to all of his trainees, and just the sort of guiding spirit the young cardiologist needed at this point in her career. Not only was he one of the most outspoken proponents of women in medicine, but he had no patience with discrimination of any kind. In later years, Taussig recalled an episode in which he was asked by another institution to recommend a candidate to fill an academic post. Among the listed qualifications was that the person be neither female nor Jewish. Park's reply wasted no words: "I could recommend no one for any place where women and Jews were excluded because Jews and women have contributed so much to the Harriet Lane Home and to the Johns Hopkins Hospital." That sentence, written at a period when bigotry toward both groups was an accepted fact of university life, was a courageous statement of principle that would not have been made by many of Park's colleagues. It is not difficult to understand why Helen Taussig immediately felt a commonality of spirit with such a man.

Having thus discovered a mentor, and a good friend as well, Taussig chose to spend the next year and a half as an intern in his department. Upon completing her service in 1930, she was appointed an assistant in pediatrics at the Johns Hopkins Hospital. In spite of her low level on the academic ladder, Park expressed his confidence in his young protégée by naming her Physician-in-Charge of the Pediatric Cardiac Clinic, located in the Harriet Lane Home, the Hopkins children's division. The field of pediatric cardiology and Helen Taussig's career both benefited from starting off together. She began her academic life when

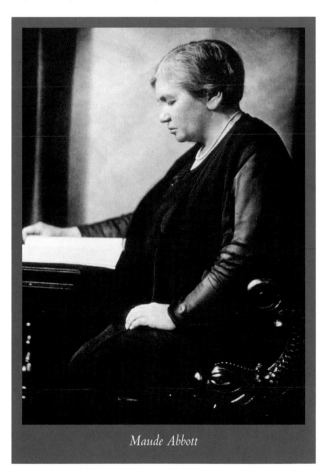

Maude Abbott

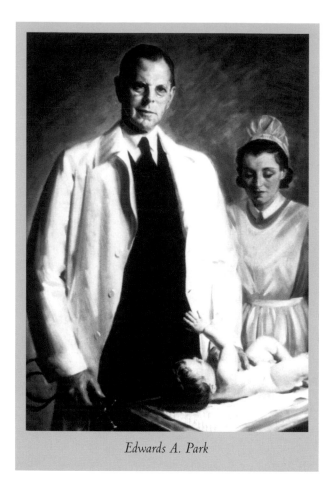

Edwards A. Park

medicine was just beginning to recognize that the heart diseases of children required the scrupulous attention that they would only get if a cohort of physicians was willing to dedicate itself completely to their study. So closely did Taussig's life become intertwined with the life of the new specialty that it became impossible, in later years, to speak of the latter without describing the contributions of the former.

Park was as generous as he could be with his newly born clinic, but his departmental budget had other urgent claims on it as well. Every one of the several new projects he had initiated required financing, and each of them therefore received a somewhat smaller slice than might have

been wished. To the Pediatric Cardiac Clinic, he gave an electrocardiograph, a new fluoroscope, a technician-secretary, a social worker, four thousand dollars, and Helen Taussig. The four thousand dollars paid all of the expenses, including the salary of the Physician-in-Charge. Fortunately, the other personnel were on the regular hospital payroll.

When Taussig began her work, she assumed that all of her time would be devoted to the treatment of patients whose hearts had been damaged by rheumatic fever, which was then a leading killer of young children. At least half of those who recovered from its acute phase were left with serious abnormalities of the heart valves. Previously assigned to the regular adult medical clinic, these children now came in large numbers to the new pediatric facility, and it was all the Physician-in-Charge could do to keep up with the work of supervising their care. But Park had other ideas—he was determined that a study of congenital heart disease should be undertaken. Except for Abbott's ongoing work in pathophysiological classification, nothing had really been accomplished after the descriptions of Fallot and a few others.

Because she trusted the wisdom of her mentor, and because she had "little choice and a stimulating environment," Taussig now started off on a study of a group of children whose underlying diseases were obscure and completely untreatable. First, she practiced with her fluoroscope until she became skilled in its use. She was using what was then considered a great technological advance, and she had no idea where it would take her. By passing X-ray beams through the body, the machine projected onto a fluorescent screen a pellucid image of the lungs, and of the heart and great vessels as they pulsated within the chest. When word got out of her interest, she did not lack for patients. As has so often happened when a facility is set up for the care of an incurable medical condition, physicians gladly referred all of their problem cases to the new clinic in the hope that something could be done for them.

At first, Taussig could do nothing more than try to make some sense out of the subtle differences between the findings in individual children: some were cyanotic and some were not; most of the cyanotics had tetralogy, but some had other, more obscure, reasons for inadequate blood flow to the lungs; some had valve problems, some had holes in the septum between right and left sides, some had hearts that had not completed their embryological development, and some had hearts so ineffectual that they failed shortly after birth. Diagnosis was possible only for the more common problems, such as tetralogy, and even then it was not infrequently proved wrong at autopsy.

An afternoon spent in the Pediatric Cardiology Clinic was a test for even the most stoic of physicians. Underdeveloped children, so short of breath that they had spells of unconsciousness with the most minimal exertion, came in large numbers. With noses, ears, extremities, and sometimes entire bodies ink-blue with cyanosis, they squatted on the floor or lay still on the examining tables so as not to worsen their air-hunger. As time went on, certain children appeared more frequently, as symptoms progressed and parents became more desperate for help. Attachments between Helen Taussig and some of her patients, indeed their entire families, grew stronger and stronger. The young unmarried doctor became another aunt to the kids and a sister to their parents. She never made any attempt to control the depth of her concern for every aspect of each family's life. As the kindly Edwards Park was her own sheet anchor in a sea of troubles, she became a stabilizing force for many a troubled couple struggling to cope with the reality of evolving hopelessness.

Gradually, in the fluttering light of her fluoroscope, Taussig began to recognize patterns. Turning her little patients every which way in front of her machine's luminosity, letting its penetrating rays make their bodies virtually transparent, she watched with awe as maldeveloped hearts struggled in forceful desperation to push blood past nature's obstructions; she gazed daily on sights that no one had ever before witnessed; she recorded images that previously could only be guessed at, or seen in the autopsy room when it was too late. She remembered it this way: "Soon I realized that changes in the size and shape of the heart and great vessels in cyanotic infants were of great diagnostic value. By studying the heart in all positions—anterior, posterior and in the left and right anterior oblique positions—one could determine which chambers were enlarged and which were small or absent."

When she had learned enough to know what questions to ask, Taussig visited Maude Abbott at McGill. The year was 1938, and she had by this time spent many hours dissecting the hearts of her own deceased patients in Baltimore. She now needed to see a collection of every congenital defect thus far discovered and to develop some comprehension of how Abbott had classified them. On her return, she was much better able to correlate pathological anatomy with the evidence

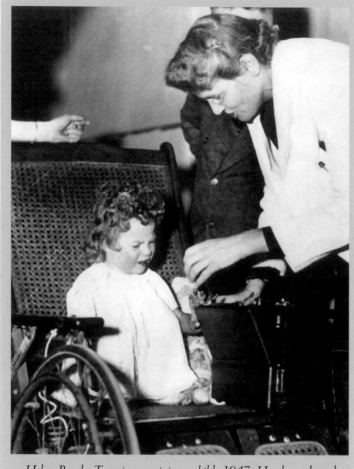

Helen Brooke Taussig examining a child, 1947. Her large, boxed hearing aid is next to the child.

distinctive quality of its particular way of heaving. Using the clues available to her hands, her eyes, and the rhythmic waves of the electrocardiogram, she could usually predict what her trainees with normal hearing would hear through their stethoscopes.

But diagnosis, no matter its rapidly developing expertness, did not help one bit when it came to treatment. Taussig was in exactly the same position with respect to congenital heart defects as her colleagues of a century earlier had been with most of the diseases they saw: a diagnosis might be made, symptoms might be alleviated, but no cure was possible. A few patients whose anomalies involved the large vessels outside the heart had by this time undergone successful operations. Intrepid surgeons had excised coarctations, which are narrowings of the aorta. The short narrowing could be cut out, and the two wide-open ends sewn together using newly developed techniques of blood-vessel suture. The results were excellent. But there seemed to be no way to improve the status of children whose problems were within the heart itself.

One other major cardiac anomaly that had been successfully cured was the persistent ductus arteriosus. During embryonic life, the blood of the fetus gets its oxygen from the mother, since the lungs cannot be used. In order for the circulation to bypass the lungs, nature has provided a duct, the ductus arteriosus, which shunts the blood from the pulmonary artery directly into the aorta. At birth, the ductus, no longer needed,

of her fluoroscope, her electrocardiograph, and her increasingly productive methods of physical examination.

It was in the use of this latter technique, the physical examination, that one of Taussig's greatest talents lay. Left somewhat deafened by a childhood attack of whooping cough, she was not able to hear murmurs very well. Consequently, she developed her powers of observation and her sense of touch to such an acuteness that she was able to obtain a great deal of information by looking at a child's chest and putting her hand on it to feel the

closes as the infant takes its first breaths. Occasionally, for reasons not yet clear, the vessel remains open. When this happens, the flow within it is usually reversed, because the pressure in the aorta of the newborn has become so much higher than that in the pulmonary artery. Accordingly, the lungs get too much blood at too high a pressure, a condition called pulmonary hypertension. The treatment is an operation to tie off the open ductus, which must be done before the child's lungs have been irreversibly damaged by years of accommodating more blood than they can handle. By the early 1940s the operation had been successfully performed in a number of children.

Because a person with one congenital anomaly not infrequently has others, some of Taussig's children with tetralogy of Fallot also had a persistent ductus. As she studied these patients in her clinic and followed several of them to the autopsy table, she began to appreciate the fact that children with both a persistent ductus and a tetralogy did reasonably well, but would begin to deteriorate if the ductus spontaneously closed later in childhood. Obviously, the ductus was serving to accomplish the opposite of what it did in the embryo: it allowed blood to pass from the high-pressure aorta into the low-pressure pulmonary artery beyond the obstruction. By shunting the circulation around the obstructed pulmonary outflow tract, it provided a bypass that markedly increased flow to the lungs. The logical solution for patients with tetralogy, then, was to surgically build a ductus. To Helen Taussig, the building of a ductus seemed a straightforward matter of plumbing— put a length of pipe in the right place, and thereby divert the blue blood around the narrowed pul-

monary artery and into the lungs so that it can be oxygenated.

Of course, the pediatric cardiologist had no idea of how to go about this, but she knew exactly the right plumbers to consult. They were Alfred Blalock and Vivian Thomas.

At the time when Helen Taussig came up with her plan, Blalock was forty-four years old and had been chairman of the Hopkins Department of Surgery for two years. Born in Culloden, Georgia, the son of a successful merchant, he was a graduate of the University of Georgia and the Johns Hopkins Medical School. He had begun his training as house officer in urology after failing to get one of William Halsted's coveted internships. However, he did so well on the urology service that Halsted, shortly before his death in 1922, appointed him assistant resident in surgery. In 1925, not having survived the competitive climb to the very top of the training pyramid, he transferred to Nashville, where he became the first surgical chief resident at the new Vanderbilt University Hospital.

During the fifteen years following his training, Blalock distinguished himself as a researcher in problems related to the circulation. In particular, he accomplished what was hailed as landmark work in the field of shock, proving that the common denominator in this poorly understood complication of so many diseases is a decrease in the volume of blood that is available to the circulation. It was from this major contribution that physicians came to recognize the importance of replacing the volume of blood lost from surgical hemorrhage or trauma; the effective use of blood and plasma transfusions during World War II was a direct outcome of

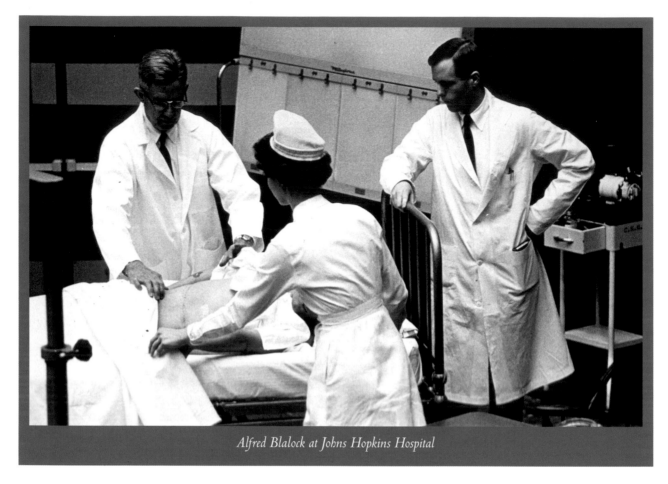
Alfred Blalock at Johns Hopkins Hospital

Blalock's research. It is also correct to state that Alfred Blalock's methods of laboratory investigation and the far-reaching consequences of his experimental findings laid the groundwork for most subsequent investigations into problems of circulatory dynamics.

It was natural that Blalock's field of interest should lead him into studies of the functioning of the heart and great vessels. The physiology of the heart and lungs was coming under increasing scrutiny at a number of major medical centers in the 1930s, with the result that many advances were being made in the rapidly rising specialty of thoracic surgery. Like other investigators, Blalock devised methods of suturing the ends of blood vessels into each other to form what is called an anastomosis, a weld of one conduit into another. One of the studies he undertook was an investigation into the disordered physiology of pulmonary hypertension, the basic pathophysiology of persistent ductus arteriosus. In order to study the changes produced in the lungs by pulmonary hypertension, he had devised an experimental model in the dog, by creating an anastomosis from the major vessel of the foreleg, the subclavian artery, directly into the pulmonary artery. This man-made ductus carried blood at high pressure directly into the vessels of the lungs. It was a masterpiece of experimental plumbing.

In every one of Blalock's researches, he had been aided by a most remarkable assistant. "Aided" is hardly the right word. The fact is that virtually all technical aspects of the investigations were carried out by Vivian Thomas, who in 1930 had come to work in the Vanderbilt laboratory at the age of nineteen, having been forced by lack of funds to abandon his plans to attend Tennessee State College. Soon after meeting him, Blalock recognized that the tall, slender young black man was gifted with the hands of a master technician and the perceptive instincts of a born researcher. Unpretentious, intelligent, and quick to learn, Thomas soon became more of an associate than an assistant. Over the eleven years he worked with Alfred Blalock at Vanderbilt, it was he who solved many of the problems of experimental design and it was he who often suggested the next step in an investigation.

These were the proven problem-solvers to whom Helen Taussig came with her plan. She arranged to meet with them in their surgical research laboratory one morning in the autumn of 1943. Taussig has been described by those who knew her in those days as a tall, slim, attractive woman whose rimless spectacles and midline-parted, bunned-in-the-back hairdo made her look more like America's image of a warmhearted schoolteacher than like the world's foremost pediatric cardiologist. Speaking in the unique manner that was the product of her residual Boston accent and the slight monotone of the hearing-impaired, she described the disabilities of her cyanotic babies and her helplessness in the face of them. Blalock, as always unfailingly courteous, listened with interest to her, interrupting from time to time to ask for clarification of some point,

in that disarmingly casual drawl with which he customarily clothed his most forceful sentences and probing questions.

Thomas listened too, but much of what he heard was too confusing to digest all at one time. Although he had by then learned more about shock and the cardiovascular system than all but a few physicians, the details of Taussig's presentation left him with a jumbled picture of a problem which, as he would put it in his autobiography, "defies verbal description except in highly technical terms." It took several visits to Taussig's collection of defective hearts in the pathology building before he understood the full magnitude of what he and Blalock had been asked to undertake.

Helen Taussig had thrown down a kind of scientific gauntlet to the two men. Blalock had looked it over, thought about it, and perceived where the answer lay. It seemed clear to him that it was his own man-made ductus arteriosus, that "masterpiece of experimental plumbing" which he had devised years earlier to study pulmonary hypertension, that would provide the proper piece of pipe to bring more blood to the lungs of cyanotic children.

The problem of working out the technical details of the proposed operation was handed over to Vivian Thomas. He did one experiment after another, until he perfected the method of creating an anastomosis that diverted the blood from the subclavian to the pulmonary artery. Since the subclavian artery is the main nourishing vessel to the arm, he had to satisfy himself that no disability would result from such a diversion. He accomplished this in the course of operating on some two hundred dogs. Blood was partially shunted into the lungs by passing from the aorta to the subclavian as the artificial ductus into the pulmonary artery. Whether or not such an increase of blood flow to the lungs would sufficiently help a cyanotic child would have to await the operation's first trial on a real patient.

That real patient presented herself almost before the surgical team was ready for her. Over the course of the year of experimentation, several of Taussig's young charges had undergone a steady deterioration. One of them, eleven-month-old Eileen Saxon, had become so blue that she could not live outside an oxygen tent. Taussig asked Blalock if he was willing to take her on as his first patient. He gave the straightforward reply of a surgeon used to great risks: "Yes, that's the type of child on whom you should try. You don't do a new operation on a *good* risk; you do a new operation on a patient who has no hope of survival without it." He told Thomas to have all of his special laboratory instruments and suture materials ready for an operation within the next two weeks.

At that point, Blalock had not done a single experiment on a dog. He had assisted Thomas on a few, and planned to do a few on his own, but Eileen's condition worsened rapidly over the course of the next several days; there was no time for the luxury of a preliminary run in the animal lab. It really made no difference. Blalock knew what had

> *Alfred Blalock's methods of laboratory investigation and the far-reaching consequences of his experimental findings laid the groundwork for most subsequent investigations into problems of circulatory dynamics.*

to be done and he had all of the surgical skill to do it. If the procedure on Eileen Saxon failed, it would not be for want of expert operating.

Several of the members of the team that assembled in the operating room on the morning of November 29, 1944, have recorded their alarmed impressions on first seeing the wizened nine-and-one-half-pound blue-gray bundle of breathlessness that was gingerly lifted from her crib and placed on the table by Dr. Taussig and her associates. It seemed impossible that grown men could reach into the open chest of such a tiny birdlike creature, isolate her fragile little blood vessels, and sew them into each other. That they could so much as consider attempting such a feat of manual dexterity was due to a combination of self-confidence, extraordinary technical skill, and unbounded faith in their own good luck. Blalock's good luck that morning began with his assistants, both of whom were destined to become major contributors to the art of clinical surgery. Between the two of them they had four of the most facile hands that have ever worked in an American operating room: the first assistant was William Longmire, the surgical chief resident; the second was an intern named Denton Cooley. Such helpers can make even the best surgeon look better.

As the preliminary steps began for the induction of anesthesia, Blalock sent word that Vivian Thomas was to come to the operating room. When he arrived, the imperturbable technician stationed himself on a stool behind the professor, but not near enough for Blalock. He was told to pull up even closer, until his long, rangy body was leaning over close enough to the operative field that he was able to see every detail as well as could the surgical team. His presence was like an amulet to the surgeon, but it was more. Several times during the sewing of the anastomosis, Blalock asked Thomas if he was putting the stitches close enough together; several times, Thomas had to point out that a suture was aimed in the wrong direction. With his own skill and judgment, the meticulous assistance of Longmire and Cooley, and the help of the knowledgeable Thomas, Blalock built his first human ductus that morning, while Helen Taussig looked on with a sense of wondrous fulfillment.

Postoperatively, Taussig and her cardiology fellow, Dr. Ruth Whittemore, stayed with their little patient in her room on the ward, monitoring her constantly by every criterion they knew. The blood flow to her arm was satisfactory, she was somewhat less cyanotic than before, and she had survived an operation that many had thought might kill her. The first night was very difficult, and the second only a little better. Ruth Whittemore recently told me, "I slept on a stretcher by her bed for two nights. I wasn't going to let that child die!" Again and again she had to insert a needle into Eileen's chest to draw off constantly reaccumulating air, finally leaving it in place attached to a suction device. The baby slowly improved. Over the succeeding days she became gradually less blue. By the end of the second postoperative week, it was clear that she would recover. When the medical writer Jürgen Thorwald interviewed her mother in 1970, she told him, "When I was allowed to see Eileen for the first time, it was like a mira-

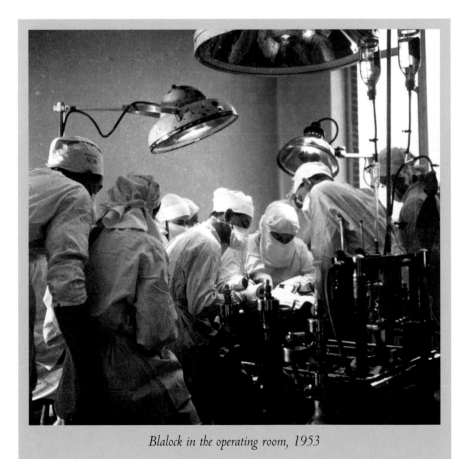

Blalock in the operating room, 1953

cle. . . . I'd never seen her with such a pink color, just like other children. She still turned blue when she kicked her feet hard. But otherwise she looked like a normal child. I was beside myself with happiness."

Dr. Taussig waited until she was sure that Eileen's happy outcome would last, and then she chose another candidate to present to her surgical team. At less than ten pounds, Eileen had been smaller than most of the dogs upon which Vivian Thomas had operated, but the next children were older and in better general condition. Barbara Rosenthal was twelve when she had her operation on February 3, 1945. A week later, on February 10, a six-year-old boy named Marvin Mason underwent the shunting. The second child was more immediately and completely relieved of her cyanosis than had been the first, and the third had an even better result than the second.

The achievement of the Hopkins group could not be kept a secret. Pressured by newspapers and radio stations, the hospital authorities gave in and allowed access to their suddenly famous team. Blalock and Taussig became reluctant but cooperative media stars. No one understood better than they the necessity of broadcasting some hope to the parents of children crippled by cyanotic heart disease. It was not only for the encouragement of victims of tetralogy of Fallot that they agreed to interviews and publicity, but to let the world know that help for other forms of cardiac problems might be just over the horizon.

By November 1, 1945, fifty-five patients had undergone the new operation. By December 30, 1950, Blalock and his associates had put an artificial ductus into 1,037. The mortality rate, originally 20 percent, had dropped to less than 5 percent. Predictably, Helen Taussig's Pediatric Cardiac Clinic became flooded with children from all over the United States and all over the world. Only about a third of the children were considered proper candidates for the operation in those first few years, but every one of the others benefited by the counsel of Helen Taussig and her team of young trainees. Ruth Whittemore, who a decade later at the Yale–New Haven Hospital taught me what little I know about congenital heart disease, was her first fellow. She described those exciting early days as they were seen through the eyes of a young physician in the presence of a master clinical scientist and a master teacher who was also a Hippocratic healer, not only of the whole patient but of his entire family:

In the years 1945–47, after Dr. Taussig's idea of creating an artificial patent ductus to help blue babies became known, her clinic was engulfed by the press, and besieged by letters from parents, referrals from doctors and requests from doctors to visit. Many families arrived without prior notice. The limited space and staff suddenly were overwhelmed by the onslaught. We were still responsible for many children with rheumatic heart disease and we had to adjust quickly to all the needs of each patient and the family. Dr. Taussig organized her activities in such a way that somehow we met the demands as needed. We also served as hosts to scores of well-known physicians who arrived from all over the world, many of whom attached themselves to us throughout our daily activity.

The learning experience was intense. Dr. Taussig, the cardiology fellows, and the cardiac surgeons learned day-by-day and applied this knowledge to the next group *of patients. . . . During these years of rapidly changing developments, Dr. Taussig realized that for this kind of work to spread to as many children as needed, training of pediatricans in cardiology and support of centers to develop in other parts of the country were essential. She met with leaders of the Children's Bureau and enlisted their support to spread the knowledge and care to other geographic areas.*

Dr. Taussig was fond of referring to her patients as her little crossword puzzles. With her rapidly increasing ability to comprehend each enigmatic symptom, she was eager to pass on her new insights to her fellows. They became as skillful at physical and fluoroscopic examination as she was, and equally adept at interpreting the various forms of laboratory data that they were constantly adding to their diagnostic bag of tricks. Dr. Whittemore remembers what she calls Taussig's impressive "ability to think things out, to solve puzzles." She taught more by example than by precept; she knew just what questions to ask herself and just how to use the answers to fill in the empty spaces in the crossword diagram. "She saw the needs and she pondered the solutions to the problems, discussed them with us, and when she was sure she was right, she acted. She sought help from any source that she thought could provide a complete picture pro and con. Then, persistently and persuasively, she carried out her convictions to the betterment of medical science and mankind."

It was not only pediatric cardiology that Helen Taussig was teaching her fellows. She bore witness to the comfort that a healer can bring to a family beset by illness. Everyone who has written personal reminiscences of her recalls her warmth, her compassion, and her consideration of each person around her. If Ruth Whittemore is an example of her teachings, all of those reminiscences are correct. Her teacher never found it necessary to put a clinical distance between herself and the people for whose lives she had accepted responsibility. Neither did Dr. Whittemore. Sitting with me in her office in February of 1987, the Yale cardiologist described the case of a cyanotic boy with tetralogy of Fallot who had survived the brutalities of the Japanese occupation of the Philippines and been taken directly to Hopkins upon his arrival with the first boatload of American returnees on the USS *Gripsholm*. The boy's father had been killed, but his mother had somehow gotten him through the years of privation and then brought him to Dr. Taussig. He was undernourished and exhausted, but he wanted desperately to have his operation. The cardiologists and the surgeons felt that it would be impossible to improve his nutrition until his blood was better oxygenated, and so they decided to go ahead in spite of the great hazard presented by his deteriorated strength. It was a difficult decision, but once all the factors were weighed, there seemed to be no choice. The boy went optimistically to the operating room, but the stress of surgery was too much for his emaciated body to endure—he died a few days later. On that quiet winter afternoon forty years afterward, as Ruth Whittemore recounted the details of his death, she relived her feelings of grief and frustration: "Maybe we did the wrong thing, maybe we should have tried to build him up before operating." Her eyes slowly filled with tears, as though she were speaking of the events of yesterday.

Helen Taussig's personal light became a beacon not only for patients but for pediatricians who wanted to learn about the new field of children's cardiology. As the first person to describe the clinical picture of the various forms of congenital heart disease, she knew more about the abstruse details of caring for these patients than anyone else in the world. She had three fellows in training the second year, and more and more applications every year thereafter.

To many physicians, it must have seemed strange that anyone would want to confine his practice to a field so seemingly small and overspe-cialized as pediatric cardiology, but to those who had some familiarity with its founder's work, the specialty was anything but confining. American and foreign fellows flocked to Hopkins. As had been the case with William Halsted's program in surgery, Taussig trainees spread themselves all over the United States and established pro-grams of their own, so that within two decades the country was supplied with an abundance of highly qualified products of the teachings of the first pediatric cardiologist. They included, besides Ruth Whittemore in New Haven, Robert Ziegler in Detroit, Gilbert Blount in Colorado, Edward

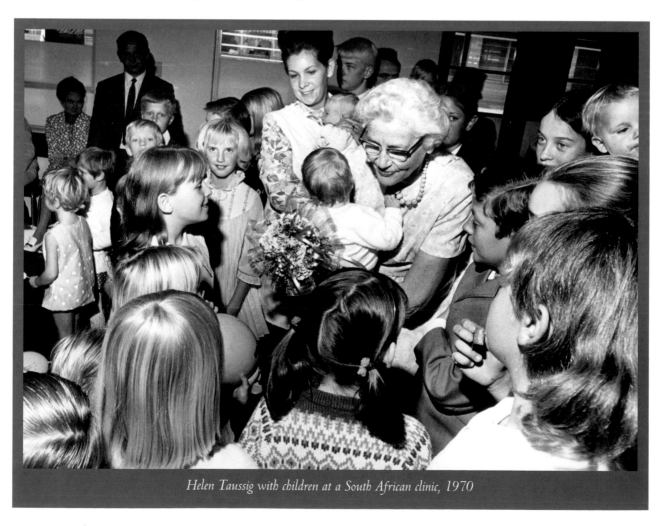

Helen Taussig with children at a South African clinic, 1970

Lambert in Buffalo, Daniel McNamara in Houston, James Manning in Rochester, and Mary Allen Engle in New York. Beginning in 1950, Dr. Taussig held the first of a long series of reunions with her fellows. Starting with a lawn party at her home, these biennial get-togethers became a major academic event, as the world's leading pediatric cardiologists assembled to honor their teacher and share their experiences.

I have always admired the physicians who treat the hearts of children, not only for their skills but for their humanity as well. More, I think, than any other of the burgeoning subcompartments into which the Art is now divided, the whole structure of pediatric cardiology is intertwined with the fabric of its patients' lives; it is an exemplar for those who would be real doctors, whether they have been trained to be nephrologists, microvascular surgeons, interventional radiologists, or members of any of the other splinter-groups of modern healing. Its ranks are filled with men and women whose relationships with their patients and their patients' families are proof that it is possible, while seeming to be the doctor for a single organ or a single disease, to be the doctor in fact for a human being who is sick.

Make no mistake—in this sense there are some Helen Taussigs and Taussig disciples in every branch of medicine; they are highly skilled superspecialists who understand as a matter of everyday experience that there need be no inconsistency between the technocratic methods of modern medicine and the care of our sick brothers and sisters. Of course, there is that about disabled children that calls forth compassion in even the most detached clinician, but it takes more than that fact to account for the universality of caring among pediatric cardiologists. I am sure, by way of explaining it, that many of those who practice the specialty were attracted to it in the first place because they recognized an atmosphere among its fellows that bespeaks the concern of whole human beings for whole human beings. This was not something that Helen Taussig had to teach her disciples; most of them came to her, it seems to me, because they already had it in good measure. It flourished under her care.

In 1947, Dr. Taussig published the first textbook in the specialty she had founded. A project gotten under way ten years earlier reached fruition with the appearance of a beautifully illustrated volume whose publication could not have come at a more propitious moment. With increasing attention being turned toward the diagnosis and treatment of inborn cardiac diseases, *Congenital Malformations of the Heart* became the foundation upon which further studies could be done. Physicians eager to understand the complicated anomalies whose treatment was thrust upon them found the book's straightforward descriptive style invaluable in comprehending the complexities of disordered blood flow. George Saxon, a Houston pediatrician with no formal training in cardiology who found himself considered his area's authority on congenital hearts prior to the arrival of Daniel McNamara, reminisced that "in those days, I held cardiac clinic with a stethoscope in one hand and Dr. Taussig's book in the other." So rapidly did her specialty expand that the book's second edition in 1960 required two volumes, each of more than a thousand pages.

As the number of successful operations increased, the mortality rate continued to drop and the long-term results gave even more justification for what had come to be known as the Blalock-Taussig shunt. Helen Taussig, by then a prominent national figure, was called upon for all manner of responsibilities. Among them was a defense of the use of animals for experimentation. In 1949, antivivisectionist groups in Baltimore became particularly strident in their attacks on the laboratory personnel at Hopkins and the University of Maryland. They not only prevented the schools from using stray dogs found in the city, they forced the arrest of vendors bringing in animals purchased from neighboring states. The medical-school authorities brought the problem to the Baltimore City Council, which then held a series of hearings. Although many prominent spokesmen defended animal experimentation, the highlight of the hearings was the dramatic performance of Helen Taussig. She brought into the hearing room a parade of smiling pink-cheeked former blue babies who had been the ultimate beneficiaries of Vivian Thomas' laboratory work. Many of them were accompanied by their own pet dogs. Next day, the Baltimore newspapers were filled with the story and accompanying photographs. When an antivivisection bill came to a referendum at the next municipal election, it was defeated by a majority of more than four to one.

The cooperative efforts of Blalock and Taussig did not end with the successful launching of the shunt operation. In order to handle the large patient load, they developed a system of dividing the responsibilities for evaluation, intraoperative and postoperative management, and long-term follow-up that became the model not only for most cardiac care centers but also for interdisciplinary treatment in other specialties. The team approach that is today so commonly used in the manage-

ment of many diseases arose out of the pediatric cardiac program at Hopkins.

The relationship between the kind of person who becomes a surgeon and the kind of person who becomes a pediatrician cannot be expected always to run a course of exquisite smoothness, especially if one of them is an accomplished, determined man and the other is an accomplished, determined woman. Based upon what witnesses report, it seems that the rapport between Alfred Blalock and Helen Taussig was better than is seen in most such relationships, but it was not by any means perfect. Although the model of a courtly southern gentleman, Blalock was not always an easy man to deal with. In the words of one of his residents, Mark Ravitch, "He was sure of his prerogatives and jealous of them; he saw to it that they were not encroached upon, and this was so clear that attempts were seldom made. He never forgot—nor really forgave—a slight or an injury. If he was angered his response was likely to be delayed and to be in actions and attitudes rather than in words." He was certainly not a man to cross, and Taussig seldom did cross him. In spite of his surgical skills, he was a paradoxical combination of demanding and dependent in the operating room, sometimes whining his momentary insecurities to whoever was within earshot. Things were often tense during those early blue-baby operations, and Taussig let herself be just deferential enough to keep the peace. In general, they did get along well, though, and made more than one journey together to demonstrate their procedure and its results. One of these was a visit to England in 1947, described by the Guy's Hospital surgeon

Russell Brock in a paper written about Blalock in 1965, a year after his death:

He and Helen Taussig gave a combined lecture in the Great Hall of the British Medical Association; the huge hall was packed. Dr. Taussig delivered her address impeccably and was followed by Dr. Blalock who presented his surgical contribution with his characteristic, apparently casual, drawl but really a forceful and incisive presentation of his brilliant and impressive results. The silence of the audience betokened their rapt attention and appreciation. The hall was quite dark for projection of his slides which had been illustrating patients before and after operation, when suddenly a long searchlight beam traversed the whole length of the hall and unerringly picked out on the platform a Guy's nursing sister, dressed in her attractive blue uniform, sitting on a chair and holding a small cherub-like girl of 2½ years with a halo of blonde curly hair and looking pink and well; she had been operated on at Guy's by Blalock a week earlier. The effect was dramatic and theatrical and the applause from the audience was tumultuous. It was a Madonna-like tableau, a perfect climax to an impressive lecture on an epoch-making contribution and left nothing more to be said by the lecturer. No audience could fail to have been convinced or satisfied by this summation and no one there could possibly forget it.

Episodes such as these, combined with the impressive results of the operation, encour-

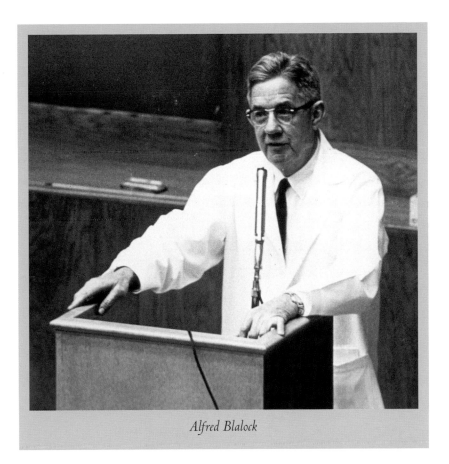

Alfred Blalock

aged other surgeons in the United States and Europe, aided by their newly trained pediatric cardiologists, to attempt the Blalock-Taussig shunt. Moreover, several centers began to experiment not only with alternative ways to accomplish the same objectives, but with more direct operations on the heart itself, for a variety of congenital and acquired conditions. With the burgeoning understanding of cardiac physiology that came out of Baltimore and the units created of its inspiration, it became feasible to correct other heart diseases that had been previously thought incurable. In the late 1940s and early 1950s one advance after another was made in diagnostic methods, supportive measures, and the technical aspects of cardiac surgery. Those were the years in which that specialty was born.

Throughout the 1950s, Helen Taussig pursued a hectic course of teaching, research, and caring for her young patients. She was frequently called upon to serve on national or international committees, to advise federal commissions, or to help in the organization of new programs. In 1959, she became Professor of Pediatrics at Hopkins. She was by that time certainly the best-known and most highly regarded woman physician in the world.

She was interested in everything that involved the well-being of children. When the issue required it, she could be militant in her relentless determination that every child should benefit from the knowledge that medical science was rapidly making ever more available in the middle decades of the twentieth century. It was her persevering campaign in the name of child welfare that led her into the second great achievement of her life, her role in the successful effort to ban Thalidomide from the American market. As in her blue-baby contribution, she was teamed once again with another physician of formidable talents, Frances Kelsey.

In the late 1950s, the West German firm of Chemie Grünenthal put on the European market a new sedative called Contergan. Laboratory testing had shown the drug to be so safe that it could be dispensed without a doctor's prescription. Because of its gentleness, its apparent lack of side effects, and its modest price, it became enormously popular, being sold not only across the counter to individuals, but also to hospitals and mental institutions. Its effectiveness in combating the nausea of pregnancy made it particularly appealing to expectant mothers both as an antiemetic and as a sleeping potion. Under various names, the drug was widely sold in Canada, Great Britain, Portugal, Australia, and New Zealand. In September of 1960, the William S. Merrell Company filed a New Drug Application with the Food and Drug Administration for permission to sell it in the United States under the name Thalidomide.

Dr. Kelsey, who had both a medical degree and a Ph.D. in pharmacology, was skeptical about the application from the first. What aroused her suspicion was the nature of the supporting documents submitted by Merrell; they read more like testimonials than objective scientific reports. "The claims were just too glowing—too good to be true," she would later write. The New Drug Application was refused until better evidence could be presented by the company. Further clinical testing was begun in a limited American market.

While all of this was going on, communications began to appear in German medical journals about disturbances of sensation and muscle strength in long-term users of the drug. In April of 1961, the West German authorities ordered that Contergan be available by prescription only; the identification of neurological symptoms alerted Kelsey to a concern with possible effects on the fetuses of pregnant women. Her concern would prove to be well founded—already, reports were coming in from German physicians of an alarming and inexplicable increase in the numbers of infants being born with a hitherto rare congenital defect called phocomelia. Most of these children had defective or absent forearm bones, and at least half of them had similar abnormalities in their legs. In the most extreme cases, babies were being born with little rudiments of hands and feet arising from extremities that were no more than stubs. There were often associated problems, such as a missing ear or paralysis of the face. It was a horribly crippling anomaly.

No one could guess at the cause until a study by one of the German physicians provided evidence that 50 percent of the affected children had been born to mothers who had used Contergan during pregnancy. In November of 1961, Grünenthal withdrew it from the market. The companies manufacturing it in England, Australia, and Canada soon followed suit.

Dr. Taussig had been unaware of the FDA's involvement with the drug until January of 1962. She was visited at that point by a German alumnus of her training program, who told her, over Sunday dinner, about phocomelia and its as yet unproved relationship to Contergan. In typical Taussig fashion, she decided to find out for herself. Arriving in Germany on February I, 1962, she spent six weeks visiting major clinics to examine infants with the abnormality and question mothers and doctors. One of the bits of evidence that most impressed her was the complete absence of phocomelia among the newborn infants of American soldiers stationed in Germany, except for one case—a child whose mother had gone off the post, where the drug was prohibited, and bought it at a local pharmacy.

Although Taussig undertook the quest on her own, Dr. Kelsey soon learned that one of America's foremost authorities on congenital disease was carrying out a thorough evaluation of Contergan. She stalled Merrell's New Drug Application until Taussig returned to join forces with her. On April II, the pediatrician presented her findings at a national meeting of the American College of Physicians. On May 24, she testified before the Kefauver Committee. She brought graphic and horrifying evidence in the form of photographs of some of the crippled German children. On the following day, her brief editorial on the subject appeared in *Science,* the journal of the American Association for the Advancement of Science.

Although Thalidomide had been withdrawn from American testing in March of 1961, more than two hundred women had already used it. Not only that, but the drug company could not account for two of the five tons of the medication that had been manufactured for investigative purposes, and it was therefore unknown how much of it still remained in the hands of physicians to whom it had been sent for testing. Taussig's testimony and her editorial substantiated Frances Kelsey's objections to the Merrell New Drug Application. Thalidomide was permanently rejected, and Merrell was castigated by the FDA for making false assertions about its safety.

The outcome of the two doctors' successful campaign was a new set of much more stringent drug-testing regulations, which went into effect in February 1963. President Kennedy awarded the Gold Medal for Distinguished Federal Service to Kelsey, and appointed her director of the FDA division created by the new regulations to oversee clinical testing of new drugs. Taussig's reward came from Germany—the hospital of the University of Göttingen named its outpatient clinic for her.

The Thalidomide episode involved Dr. Taussig in another controversy at the same time, concerning the right of a woman to have her pregnancy terminated. She had long felt that America's abortion laws, as they stood on the books in the 1960s, were archaic and unfair, often resulting in tragic burdens not only on women, but on society as well. To someone who had spent her life in the salvaging of children grievously damaged by congenital heart disease, there was no justification for forcing an unwilling mother to give birth to a baby known to be malformed, if there was some safe way to prevent it. She had been witness to the havoc that the birth of such a child often wreaks on siblings, parents, and the entire family structure; she knew better than most the enormous resources required for social agencies to deal with the long-range effects of such problems; she had held the hand of many a troubled youngster whose life would never be normal.

The entire matter was brought dramatically to public attention by the case of Sherry Finkbine, a pregnant American woman who had taken Distavil, the British version of Contergan, during pregnancy. There being a strong likelihood that Mrs. Finkbine was carrying a defective embryo, she was seeking a legal abortion, and being refused by every source she turned to.

Taussig was incensed by what she considered the callous attitude of the authorities. Her argument was not with those whose religious beliefs prohibit abortion for themselves, but with those who impose their views on everyone else. She did not concern herself about the ancient philosophical dilemma of life's originating instant—her only thought was for the misery of families. Her life's experiences had taught her that aborting a defective embryo is aborting a potential tragedy.

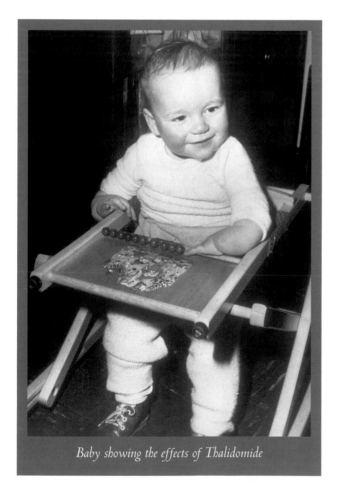

Baby showing the effects of Thalidomide

She did a great deal of testifying in favor of liberalizing abortion laws, but this time her efforts were in vain. When all of Sherry Finkbine's requests were refused, the young woman was forced by the reality of her situation to go to Scandinavia, where she was aborted of a malformed conceptus. In 1981, years after state laws outlawing abortion had been overturned by the U.S. Supreme Court, Taussig was moved by the strident clamors of some of abortion's opponents to tell an interviewer, in her usual forthright fashion:

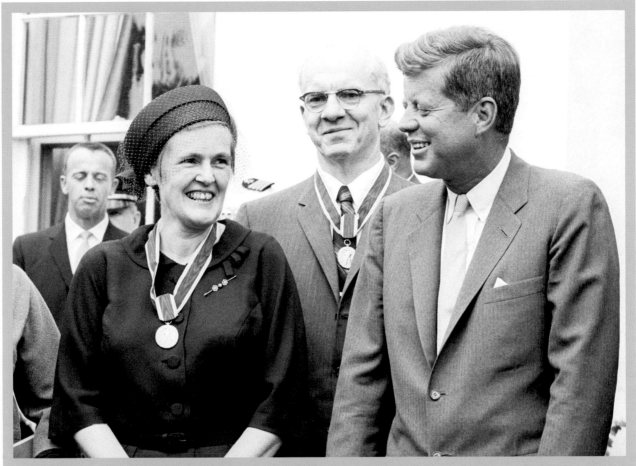

President John F. Kennedy stands with Dr. Frances Kelsey, the medical officer who prevented the sale of the birth-defect-causing drug Thalidomide in the United States.

We are still fighting the Right to Life group, who are so completely convinced that life is sacred from the moment of conception till birth. As far as I can see, after birth they don't care a hang what happens to the child or what sort of a child is born. They take no more care until the person is dying and then they absolve him from sin.

In July of 1963, Dr. Taussig retired as Physician-in-Charge of Harriet Lane's Pediatric Cardiac Clinic. Her retirement did not change a thing. She continued her research so effectively that forty-one of her one hundred major publications were written after that date. When the National Foundation of the March of Dimes established a fellowship for scientists at retirement, she was its first recipient. She used the forty thousand dollars to do a long-term follow-up of the children and adults who had undergone the Blalock-Taussig shunt between 1945 and 1950. It was characteristic of her perspicacity and the devotion her patients and their families felt for her that she was able to obtain a follow-up that was 93 percent complete for ten years, and 88 percent for fifteen years. She personally saw every surviving patient that she could physically get to. The resultant accumulated information was worth more than any mere dispassionate collection of data. It represented a uniquely gratifying report from a unique alumni association, almost all of whose members would have been dead were it not for Helen Taussig, Alfred Blalock, and Vivian Thomas.

Of the 779 patients for whom data were obtained, 685 had survived the postoperative period of two months, for an overall mortality rate of less than 12 percent. At the beginning of the fifteenth postoperative year, 441 of those 685 were still alive. The early results of operation showed 81 percent excellent or good outcomes, 7 percent judged to be fair, and the remainder unimproved or dead. A follow-up study five years later found that only another twenty-four patients had died. By that time, 1975, cardiac surgery had improved to the point where 227 of the survivors had undergone a complete correction of the tetralogy. The Blalock-Taussig shunt was, after all, only a way of getting more blood to the lungs. Once open-heart surgery came into being, it was possible to repair the intracardiac defects directly, by opening up the tight pulmonary outflow tract and closing the hole in the septum.

There was a justifiably proud note at the conclusion of the abstact to the 1975 paper:

Approximately 250 patients have married; 161 have one or more children. Thirty-five percent have graduated from college and 68.7% are earning substantial incomes. The high scholastic achievement of many of these patients is strong evidence that low oxygen saturation of arterial blood is not a prime cause of mental retardation.

The occupations of the patients indicate that the quality of their lives is extremely good and that a cardiac handicap in childhood does not preclude success in adult life. Approximately 69% of these patients have repaid in taxes the cost to society of their rehabilitation.

The Blalock-Taussig shunt had proved to be everything its originators hoped. It not only saved those patients who survived its relatively low mortality, but it gave most of them a quality of life that was comparable to that of a normal individual. Many of the children were tided over until the next era of cardiac surgery dawned, the era of complete correction of congenital heart defects by a direct repair using open-heart techniques.

Although she was seventy-seven years old, the 1975 paper did not end Helen Taussig's research. Even after she left Baltimore a few years later to live in the retirement community of Crosslands, near Philadelphia, she continued her study of congenital heart disease. Her interests turned toward an attempt to discover the basic embryological causes of the defects, and she began a study of the hearts of birds. She conceived the idea that such anomalies are due not to errors that occur in the development of the embryo *per se*, but rather to retention of part of the gene pool inherited from earlier periods in the evolution of the species. In other words, she thought that every anomaly might be a throwback to a more primitive pattern of animal life. Although this was obviously a proposition that would be difficult to prove, she was not deterred in her resolve by the fact that she was well past eighty when she began to work on it. In pursuing her theory, she renewed a friendship of many years past with my own retired (about as retired as she was) Professor of Anatomy, Thomas Forbes. As Tom Forbes showed me their exchange of letters of late 1981, he remarked that he couldn't help thinking of Helen Taussig still as the enthusiastic young Hopkins pediatrician who had asked for a pencil one evening after dinner at the Forbes home in the early 1940s and used it to draw the proposed Blalock-Taussig shunt on the only good linen tablecloth owned by the impecunious and very junior anatomy instructor's wife, Helen. Helen Forbes in later years would tell her husband how much she regretted having washed that memorable diagram away.

At an age when most people would settle for tea, slippers, and privacy, Dr. Taussig remained active not only in researching her new theory, but in the community affairs of Crosslands as well. She made new friends and kept up her writing and her interests in social causes. On May 21, 1986, she packed up several of her fellow Crosslands residents and drove them to the polls to vote in a primary election. As she was backing out of the driveway of the polling place, her car was hit broadside by another vehicle. The only casualty of the collision was Helen Taussig, instantly killed three days before her eighty-eighth birthday.

Helen Taussig's name will forever be linked with that of her coauthor in one of the greatest of the many great medical undertakings of our time. They shared a vision, and each of them was blessed with the talent to make that vision a reality. Both of them did other remarkable things as well, during unusually productive careers, particularly in the training of young physicians. But in one category of those unspoken messages that each left to his professional prog-

eny, there was a far-reaching difference between them: they had opposite concepts of a doctor's relation to his patients. It was not that Alfred Blalock was disagreeable with his patients or inconsiderate of their distress, for he certainly was neither—he could never be unkind to those who came to him for help. But he was a surgeon of his time. Mark Ravitch described a whole profession when he wrote of Blalock: "In spite of his cordiality and courtesy he maintained a constant awareness of himself and his position." Blalock's priorities were not those of Helen Taussig. "In general he seemed to avoid emotional involvement with his patients' course, and one had the impression that when he was most concerned and agitated about patients and most demanding of his house staff, it was the successful outcome of the procedure that concerned him most intensely."

That was not Helen Taussig's way. She saw the successful outcome of her treatment as only one step in the lives of the children entrusted to her care and the restoration of tranquillity to their families. The interplay of emotions was to her a part of the therapeutic process by which the physician and the patient ease each other's pain by entering into each other's lives. A dispassionate analysis of a disease process does not mean that there must be no empathy; objectivity in the choice of a risky course of treatment does not mean that there must be no tears if it fails; Helen Taussig did not hold back. She gave something of herself to every one of her young wards. She was their physician, she was their source of hope, and she was not afraid to be their friend. That was her conception of what it means to be a doctor.

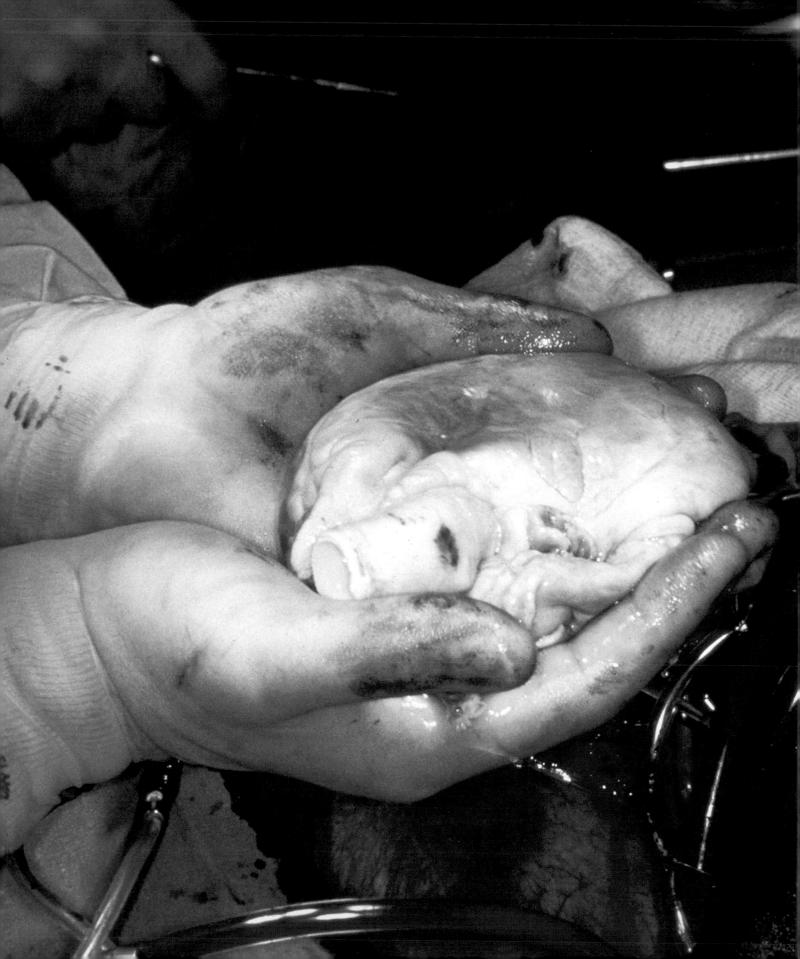

15

NEW HEARTS FOR OLD

The Story of Transplantation

May God keep in His home the soul of the young man whose heart makes my life possible. May He also console the family of the donor by allowing them to know that a legacy of life was left by their son.
—Raymond Edwards, April 9, 1986,
from a letter written to the staff of the
Yale-New Haven Hospital, one month
following his cardiac transplant

A clinical case history of the late twentieth century:

At ten o'clock in the evening of August 20, 1975, a forty-two-year-old meteorologist for the National Weather Service came to the emergency room of Connecticut's 120-bed Milford Hospital, complaining of nausea, loss of appetite, and abdominal pain. The symptoms had begun two days before with a generalized ache, first around the navel, and then gradually shifting its focus to the right lower quadrant. The patient had vomited once, on the first day of symptoms. As he walked from the sign-in desk to an admitting room, it was apparent to the nurse who accompanied him that he was limping just a bit, in such a manner as to bear his weight chiefly on his left leg. The examining physician noted extreme tenderness when he pressed his palpating hand down into the symptomatic area. The overlying muscles were unyielding and rigid, and the abdomen was moderately distended. A gloved finger inserted into the patient's rectum elicited considerable discomfort when its tip probed high up on the right side. The physician made a diagnosis of appendicitis, and called for a surgical consultation.

When the surgeon arrived half an hour later, he noted that the patient was so dehydrated that his speech was a bit thickened by the dryness of his tongue. Because every movement caused pain, he had chosen to lie immobile on his right side with his knees drawn up to his belly. By this time the blood tests ordered by the admitting nurse had been completed, and they revealed a marked elevation of the white count and an increase in the percentage of polymorphonuclear leucocytes, signifying the presence of a severe inflammation. The levels of hemoglobin and the major chemical constituents of the blood were normal. A chest X-ray was likewise normal. The electrocardiogram demonstrated some nonspecific changes in one of the waves, but was otherwise unremarkable.

The surgeon confirmed the diagnosis of the emergency-room physician. After being told the risks and benefits of the proposed surgery, the patient signed what the legal profession calls an informed consent. His abdomen was shaved, and he was wheeled into the operating room.

The operation began approximately two hours after the patient arrived in the emergency room. Following the induction of general anesthesia, a short incision was made in the right lower quadrant, the underlying muscles were spread apart, and the abdominal cavity was opened. A collection of foul-smelling serum and pus burst forth through the incision, of exactly the same kind found by Giovanni Morgagni in the abdomen of the old man of Bologna two and a half centuries earlier. The surgeon delivered the base of the cecum into the field, bringing with it a gangrenous, ruptured appendix.

The appendix was removed, a drain was inserted into the place where it had lain, and the wound was closed. After two hours of recovery, the patient was transferred back to his room. Other than a course of antibiotics and a few doses of Demerol during the first forty-eight post-operative hours, no medication was used. Recovery, after a few feverish, uncomfortable days, was without untoward event. The patient went home a week later. Before long, he was back at work trying to predict the weather, and his ruptured appendix was a memory. All of the costs of his illness were paid by a government-subsidized insurance policy.

That forty-two-year-old man was Raymond Edwards. Because the surgeon who operated on him was a friend of mine, I happened to meet him a few days after the events that have just been described. I didn't see Ray again until eleven years later, when, in chance conversation with another surgical friend, I found out that he was once more recovering from an operation, this one of far greater magnitude than an appendectomy. He was in the Cardiac Intensive Care Unit of the Yale–New Haven Hospital, two days after a successful heart transplant.

In the two and a half centuries since Morgagni had dissected the pus-filled corpse of the old man of Bologna, the great evolution of scientific medicine had taken place. First, it was established that every symptom has a specific anatomical seat of origin, whose location can be traced. The symptom, thought by Morgagni to be "the cry of the suffering organ," was later found to be just as likely the cry of the suffering tissue, or, still later, the cell or molecular structure. Meanwhile, various types of symptoms were differentiated from each other, categorized, and found to occur associated with each other in groups predictable enough to allow for the recognition and classification of distinct disease entities. The rapid development of the art of physical examination in the early nineteenth century made it possible to predict in the living the changes that would be found at postmortem study of the dead. By midcentury, physicians had become quite skillful at diagnosing diseases with their senses and their stethoscopes. Soon afterward, an increasing comprehension of the mysteries of physiology brought an appreciation of not only the physical derangements associated with sickness but the chemical ones as well.

Medical science would not be able to solve the problem of treatment until it solved the problem of primary causes. Morgagni had begun the search for the discoverable *effects* of the disease process. He was careful to point out that he could offer no information about the primary stimulus that produces those effects. What is it that causes a lung to develop pneumonia, and why does a liver become cirrhotic? What produces the shale that coats the inside of an aging blood vessel in layers so thick that it becomes occluded, destroying the tissue it is supposed to nourish? Why do the valves of the heart become thickened and lose their elasticity, and why do the convoluted gyri of the brain sometimes flatten out? What initiates the process of tumor growth, or of heart failure? Why does a kidney lose its ability to filter impurities? What makes the blood sugar rise in diabetes?

In keeping with a reductionist, coning-down approach to disease, it seemed only logical that there should also be some discoverable reductionistic solution to the question of the primary *cause* of each malady as well. If a disease proved itself to be a distinct pathophysiological entity, why should it be straining the bounds of probability for it to have a distinct and specific initiating agent? When Pasteur and Koch, with the help of Lister, discovered the origins of certain ailments in particular pathogenic bacteria, scientific medicine seemed about to fulfill its expectation: each disease has its own separate etiology. If a distinct unitary cause could be found for every ill of mankind, specificity of therapy would be just around the corner. Indeed, the germ concept became the model for a hundred years of medical research. To find the underlying initiating cause of every single malady was henceforth the business of the researcher. Mod-

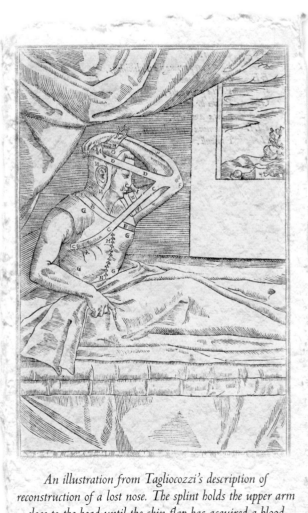

An illustration from Tagliocozzi's description of reconstruction of a lost nose. The splint holds the upper arm close to the head until the skin flap has acquired a blood supply from the vessels of the face.

ern medical investigation has been based, to a large extent, on the proposition that the cause of any specific disease is unitary, and discoverable in the laboratory.

The reductionist approach is empirical. It eschews rationalistic thinking and avoids the pitfalls of speculation unsupported by observation and experiment. Just as it denies that sickness is caused by generalized imbalances of the various internal and external stabilizing mechanisms of man and nature, it also denies that health can be restored by readjusting that unproved balance. It directs its *diagnosis* to objectively verifiable phenomena; it directs its *therapy* to methods whose results are measurable. This is the philosophy of single causes; it is the antithesis of Hippocratic holism; it is the means by which virtually every advance of modern scientific medicine has been made; it is the reason that Raymond Edwards, unlike the old man of Bologna, underwent a rapid diagnosis, an expeditious pathophysiologically based form of therapy, and had a smooth recovery. It is also the reason that the same Raymond Edwards, eleven years later, could have his failing heart replaced by the healthy cardiac apparatus of a seventeen-year-old youth. The transplantation of organs epitomizes the accomplishments of reductionism. For all that, however, there is about it just a little hint that things are about to change.

Even as it represents the acme of the attainments of modern laboratory science, the new field of transplantation is turning our thoughts back again to matters that traditionally have belonged to the realm of the philosophers. The same investigators who contemplate the nature of a strand of DNA must now contemplate the essence of what it means to be human. The electron-microscopist and the tissue-typer are looking, these days, into the nature of man's individuality and perhaps his very soul—his or her personhood, as today's wordsmiths would put it. When the molecular biologists speak in terms of an organism's recognition of *self*, of the rejection of what is *foreign*, and of the acquiring of *tolerance*, the words they use convey the moral and philosophical implications of their work. Their reductionism is carrying them willy-nilly forward into a vision of the healer's art that is as holistic as it is scientific. Their work is forcing us to think of an entire patient, indeed an entire world of patients, and of influences that act not only on their diseases, but upon the tools of healing by which they can be made well.

In giving Ray Edwards a new heart, his surgeons brought to a focus a process of development that began in Greece four centuries before Christ. Starting as a series of speculations, that process did not achieve its greatest manifest success until it cast off the old ideas about humors and imbalances, and invited science to be its handmaiden. For a century we did not question the assumption that all the causes and all the cures of all disease can be discovered in the laboratories of our research institutes and medical schools. We have called medicine an art while we have really thought of it as a science. In science we sought the solution to every problem.

Well, healing *is*, after all, an art. It is in his judgment, his wisdom, and his search for the meaning of humanness that a physician can be a healer, as much as it is in his scientific capabilities. By raising issues that are moral, religious, social, legal, economic, and who knows what else, the very new field of transplantation is showing itself to be the central coming-together place for the various ingredients of the very old field of medicine. It has served also as the meeting ground on which science comes together with the society from which it must draw its support.

The technoscience of today's reductionist research is changing something else as well. That something else is our old friend the theory of primary causes. We are beginning, just barely beginning, to look at disease as the outcome not of one precise agency, but of the concatenation of a group of factors acting together to produce a synergism of etiology. Why does one man smoke two packs of cigarettes a day and never develop lung cancer, while his neighbor does the same and dies of malignancy in his fifties? Why, in the Middle Ages, did not everyone come down with the plague who was exposed to it? Why did the heart of Ray Edwards fail when millions of people must have been exposed to the virus that gave him his cardiomyopathy? The answers are not to be found in the theory of primary causes, but rather in a new approach to biomedical theory, a new paradigm, as some have called it.

There are phenomena that clinicians see every day and yet have no explanation for; they seem to fall outside of the one-disease, one-cause model of medicine. For example, a patient who is optimis-

> *By raising issues that are moral, religious, social, legal, economic, and who knows what else, the very new field of transplantation is showing itself to be the central coming-together place for the various ingredients of the very old field of medicine.*

tic often does better than one with a gloomy outlook—we all know that, but none of us yet understands the mechanism. We also know that not all patients benefit from therapy that is based on our theory of unitary causes. If 10 percent of the sick don't get well in spite of theoretically ideal treatment, there must be something about them that makes them different from the vast majority of their fellows. The nature of illness may be quite a different thing than was supposed a hundred years ago when the bacteriologists got us started on our present pattern by providing proof of the long-held suspicion that single causes do exist. It is time to turn our thoughts to a new model, in which such considerations as psychological and environmental studies share the stage with immunology and genetics and the bacteriology laboratory. It is in this direction that the next image of medicine will be found. When we arrive at it, we will have fulfilled the expections of both our Hippocratic forebears and their Cnidian counterparts. In the melding of their two philosophies lies the future of healing.

The story of Ray Edwards' heart transplant begins in classical antiquity. It begins, in fact, with a myth. The myth has been the source of a word in western languages that can be used to express not

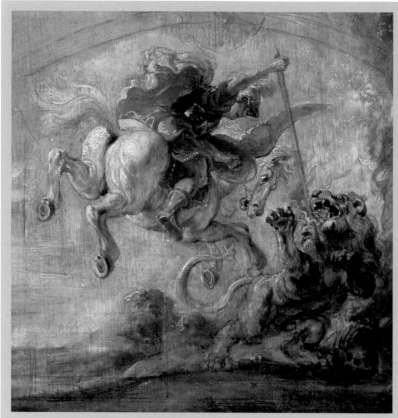
Bellerophon on Pegasus piercing the Chimaira with a lance

of being impossible to achieve. The adjective "chimerical" is defined in *Webster's Unabridged Dictionary* as "imaginary; fanciful; fantastic; wildly or vainly conceived; that has or can have no existence except in the imagination."

By solving the riddle of transplantation, scientists have verified the concept of the chimera in the first sense of its definition, and debunked it in its second. The chimera has proved not to be chimerical after all. The first laboratory-created chimerae were organisms in which the tissues or cells of a donor animal were introduced into a recipient while both partners to the transaction were still in an innocently embryonic stage of development. So far have matters progressed since those early

only what transplantation is, but also what it is not. In the *Iliad,* Homer tells of Bellerophon, an intrepid slayer of monsters who was enjoined by the lord of Lykia to kill the god-created Chimaira. Bellerophon was sent off on the winged horse Pegasus with orders "to kill the Chimaira that none might approach; a thing of immortal make, not human, lion-fronted and snake behind, a goat in the middle, and snorting out the breath of the terrible flame of bright fire." The word "chimera" entered the English language in two forms, the first of which refers to a creature made, like the Chimaira, of the parts of several different individuals or species. The second form is used to signify an idea which is, also like the Chimaira, fanciful and absurd, in the sense

experiments with simple zoological forms of life that we are now witness to the grafting of fully formed complex organs from one adult human being to another. We are living in an era in which transplantations are commonly done of kidneys, livers, and hearts, and we will soon be hearing that the pancreas and the intestine are also being successfully grafted, not to mention tissue from the brain itself. There may yet come a day when only whole-brain transplants continue to defy our med-tech explorers, and perhaps not even that feat will elude their ingenuity and nimble fingers.

The process by which the "vainly conceived" notion of the chimera has been transformed into an everyday reality did not get underway until after the Vesalian reawakening of medicine. If we ignore the pious legends of medieval saints and oriental sages who are said to have exchanged various body parts of some of their patients, we can travel swiftly through three millennia, from the thirteenth century B.C. to the sixteenth century A.D., when we encounter Gaspari Tagliocozzi, a surgeon who was also Professor of Anatomy and Professor of Medicine at the University of Bologna. After Tagliocozzi's death in 1599, the city fathers commissioned a statue in his memory, which they placed in the university's anatomy theatre. To signify the deceased's most lasting contribution, he is depicted holding in his hand a human nose. For Tagliocozzi had developed a technique of reconstructing that essential olfactory appendage onto those who, for one reason or another, were noseless. In an era during which nasal amputation was a common form of punishment, both legal and felonious, such a man was indeed a valued citizen.

The technique of Tagliocozzi's operation need not concern us; it is sufficient to say that it involved swinging what we today call a pedicle flap to the face, of skin which remained connected to the upper arm. The arm was then immobilized in place for twelve days by a specially constructed splint, to allow the graft to seal itself into position. Following this interval, the graft was cut free from the limb, and the new nose gradually worked into proper shape by a series of minor procedures. The method had a high rate of success, and was applicable as well to the reconstruction of lips and ears. For a variety of reasons, it fell from favor in Europe, although nose restoration is said to have enjoyed great popularity among certain practitioners in India during the eighteenth and nineteenth centuries.

What is important about Tagliocozzi is not so much his technical innovation as the insight he had about the distinctiveness of each person's flesh from that of all other individuals. He gave considerable thought to the question of using skin from a donor, and at last rejected the idea, primarily because of the impossibility of keeping two persons bound together for the requisite period of twelve or more days. But he had another reason, which expresses in a few simple sentences the essential mystery of transplantation:

The singular character of the individual entirely dissuades us from attempting this work on another person. For such is the force and power of individuality, that if anyone should believe that he could accelerate and increase the beauty of union, nay more, achieve even the least part of the operation, we consider him plainly superstitious and badly grounded in the physical sciences.

It was "the force and power of individuality" that stood in the way of the predictably successful transplantation of tissues from one adult human being into another. Tagliocozzi, although he has left no written record of it, must have tried grafting skin obtained from donors, and seen his efforts fail every time. Somehow he came to the realization that the human body has a way of recognizing tissues that are part of itself, and casting out tissues that are not. "Bone of my bones, flesh of my flesh," taken in the literal sense, is acceptable for transplantation. Anything else is recognized as foreign, and rejected. Only Adam and Eve and identical twins would be found to qualify.

The story of transplantation becomes, therefore, the story of our evolving comprehension that the cells of each of us harbor within them something that is theirs alone, which gives them their unique, unchanging character. For want of a better term, we may as well call that something by the name of "selfness." Once the existence of selfness was appreciated by science, it became necessary to hunt down its ingredients—what is the specific quality that a cell shares with all of its mates that makes it so singularly a part of one individual and foreign to all others? What is the mechanism by which an animal recognizes cells that come from another animal, and what is the mechanism by which it casts them out, destroying them as invading undesirables? And, having discovered the nature of these mechanisms, how may they be overcome? How can a potential recipient be made less xenophobic, less destructive of protoplasm from a donor? In other words, how can one person be made more tolerant of the transplanted tissues of another?

We have here a long list of questions, and there are even a few more that will come up as the narrative proceeds. The list of those who have attempted to answer them is a thousand times as long as the number of questions itself. Even the naming of only the major contributors would be too lengthy for clarity of description. So this chapter deals not with a single researcher, but with the biomedical science of the late twentieth century, an effort not so much of individuals as of great teams of talented explorers. Today's and tomorrow's transplantation studies are part of an international campaign by many investigators cooperating and competing. The studies involve Nobel laureates and forgotten graduate students, the purest of investigations in millipore science and the pragmatic urgencies of the bedside, as well as the secret personal strivings of each of us for immortality, whether of our names or of our bodies themselves. On the list, and properly so, are some of the great moral questions of our society. For physicians, the questions ultimately find their focus with our patients, who, like Ray Edwards, have come to us because they seek health and sometimes a legacy of life.

From time to time, a physician did manage to transfer some bit of tissue from one individual to another. These experiments seem to have succeeded only on infrequent occasions, and even more rarely when the host was human. To illustrate one of those rare occasions on which a graft is said to have succeeded in spite of the overwhelming odds, there is the story related by Winston Churchill in his *My Early Life*. It took place during the Sudanese war in 1898, and details his donation of a swatch of skin to a wounded comrade-in-arms:

> *The story of transplantation becomes, therefore, the story of our evolving comprehension that the cells of each of us harbor within them something that is theirs alone, which gives them their unique, unchanging character.*

Molyneux had been rescued from certain slaughter by the heroism of one of his troopers. He was now proceeding to England in charge of a hospital nurse. I decided to keep him company. While we were talking, the doctor came in to dress his wound. It was a horrible gash, and the doctor was anxious that it be skinned over as soon as possible. He said something in a low tone to the nurse, who bared her arm. They retired to a corner, where he began to cut a piece of skin off her to transfer to Molyneux's wound. The poor nurse blanched, and the doctor turned upon me. He was a great raw-boned Irishman. "Oi'll have to take it off you," he said. There was no escape, and as I rolled up my sleeve he asked genially, "Ye've heard of a man being flayed aloive? Well this is what it feels loike." He then proceeded to cut a piece of skin and some flesh about the size of a shilling from the inside of my forearm. My sensations as he sawed the razor slowly to and fro fully justified his description of the ordeal. However, I managed to hold out until he had cut a beautiful piece of skin with a thin layer of flesh attached to it. This precious fragment was then grafted on to my friend's wound. It remains there to this day and did him lasting good in many ways. I for my part keep the scar as a souvenir.

This anecdote can be looked at in any of three possible ways: it may be entirely true, in which case it represents one of those extremely rare examples of a successful graft in an unprepared host; or what Churchill considered to be a successful graft was simply his rejected and mummified donation acting as a covering on the luck-struck Molyneux's arm until the recipient's own skin grew in from the edges of this relatively small area; or finally, there is always the possibility that the whole story is apocryphal. Molyneux never chose to publish his own version of the events, nor did the "great raw-boned Irishman" who actually

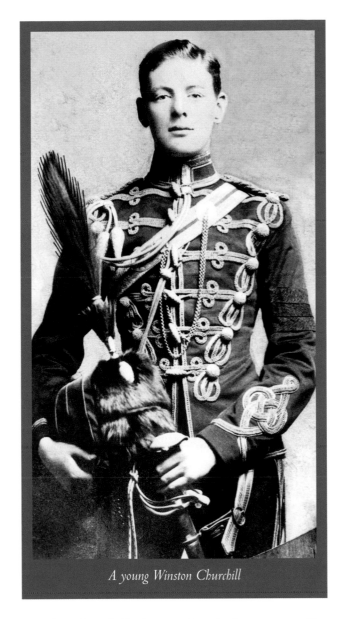

A young Winston Churchill

did the Churchill-flaying. Caught between reality and the charity due the memory of a great man, I choose the second possibility as the best explanation for this miracle of the surgeon's art.

As the result of the work of several nineteenth-century researchers, it gradually came to be appreciated that autografts (tissue from the same animal), allografts (tissue from an animal of the same species), and xenografts (tissue from a different species) each behave in totally different ways when transferred from an experimental donor to a recipient. In the first two decades of the twentieth century, several perceptive researchers began to consider that the virtually universal failure of allografts was due to some as yet unfathomable process of immunity. In their foresighted formulation, grafts were rejected because the recipient's body was immune to them in the same way as it might be immune to any other foreign material. Not only that, but immunity was found to be highly specific for the particular donor who contributed the foreign tissue. There began to be discovered some clear experimental intimation that each organism has a distinctive self, which the distinctive self of a recipient recognizes as foreign, and therefore sets up an immune reaction against. As in other immune reactions, the foreign material carries substances called antigens, which are specific to itself only. When the host detects such a foreign antigen, it produces an antagonist to it, which is like the antibody that combats invading bacteria or viruses. The antigens in a virus cause the patient to make antibodies that combat the microbes by becoming involved in the process by which they are destroyed. In the same way, the tissue antigens of the transplanted graft start off a cascade of events that result in the production of killer cells which attack it.

The process of graft rejection was gradually recognized as a process similar to an antibody-antigen reaction. Quite simply, the host recognizes the foreignness of the grafted tissue and produces killer cells against it, which help to destroy it. From the observations of several investigators of various nationalities, it became clear that each individual has his own very specific kind of antigens,

as specific in fact as his fingerprints. The transplantation immune-response theory achieved its final verification in 1944, when a young Oxford zoologist named Peter Medawar designed an experiment proving beyond doubt that repeated grafting from the same donor results in acceleration of the rejection reaction. Following this, he began a series of brilliantly conceived researches that have formed the basis of much of the modern investigation into transplantation biology and the phenomena of rejection and tolerance.

This, then, is the mechanism of recognition and of rejection all in one. The fluids and cells of the host recognize the donor's antigens as being not their own and create the substances that lead to destruction of the foreign graft. Further attempts at grafting increase the ferocity of the casting-out process.

Once the nature of rejection was established, the hunt began to find methods of typing the tissue antigens in the same way that blood-group antigens are typed. The analogy between blood and other tissues is clear—a blood transfusion is, after all, only a type of transplant, but it is a transplant of a material whose major antigens are shared by large proportions of the population, making transfusion relatively safe. The antigens involved in organ transplantation, however, are far more varied. Nevertheless, they too can be divided, fortunately, into those which are major and those which are far less significant. The search for the major transplantation antigens began in the late 1940s, and by the early 1950s it was possible to carry out a primitive kind of tissue-typing, analogous to the way in which a pint of blood is typed and cross-matched to a potential recipient.

Over the succeeding three decades, tissue-typing improved to the point where it now shows promise as a potentially useful tool in matching up a proposed organ donor with a host. Even its name has been changed—it is called histocompatibility testing. It is now known that there are specific areas on the sixth chromosome of each cell in our bodies which carry all of the known major histocompatibility antigens. Methods have been devised to test for the presence of the strongest of these histocompatibility antigens, or transplant antigens. Depending on the degree of similarity between donor and recipient, the result of the testing is classified as an A, B, C, or D match. It would complete a symmetrical scientific saga if I could tell you that an A match means perfect compatibility, but it most assuredly does not, since so many other minor antigens are involved in the outcome. At the present time, histocompatibility testing can only serve as a useful guide for transplantation. With further development, it is not beyond the range of possibility that it will one day be a much more reliable method of matching a recipient with a donor.

With tissue-typing being such a chancy affair, it cannot be depended upon as a method of avoiding rejection of an allograft. There remain two other logical avenues: either make the immune system of the host more tolerant to the transplantation antigens of the donor, or make the donor tissue itself less menacing. The latter approach

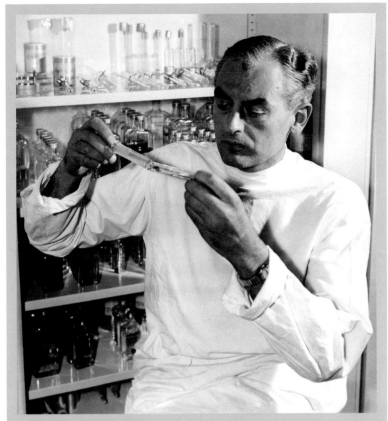

Sir Peter Medawar, winner of the 1960 Nobel Prize for his pioneer studies of the human immune system

has not yet met with significant success. The former, however, the achieving of acquired tolerance, has fared so well in the laboratory that it has proved to be a practical basis upon which to carry out continuing research. It is, in fact, the principle upon which present-day transplantation techniques have been developed.

Ideally, we will one day have methods by which an optimal cross-match of donor with recipient will be possible. When we can accomplish this, it might be combined with the use of injections of an appropriate serum into the host (or some other specific method of manipulating the immune system) so that an acquired tolerance to the donor antigens, both major and minor, is quickly built up in order to combat any residual incompatibility. Allografting could then be carried out in relative safety. There have already been several Nobel Prizes awarded for such studies, which have elucidated not only the basis of rejection, but the basis of tolerance as well. Macfarlane Burnet and Peter Medawar are probably the best known of the investigators who have clarified the earlier obscurity in which the basic nature of these mechanisms was hidden for so long.

Until science has achieved its goal of perfect immunological tolerance, less satisfactory methods will have to suffice, in order that donor tissue may be transplanted without rejection. The only situation in which there is no immunologic problem is the one in which donor and recipient are identical twins, since, coming from the same egg, they have the same antigens. The immune mechanisms of one twin do not consider the antigens of the other to be foreign, because they are the same as his own. Indeed, the first long-term successful kidney transplant was accomplished between such twins at Boston's Peter Bent Brigham Hospital in 1954. Many more have been done since.

Because specific methods are not yet available, transplantation teams have had to rely on general approaches toward suppressing the entire immune mechanism of the host. If a recipient's ability to form effective immune defenses is inhibited, he will be less able to fight off the antigens of donor tissue. The trouble is, of course, that there is no way to limit the inhibition to affecting only those defenses directed against the transplant itself; suppressing the immune system compromises its ability to fight *any* substance which is foreign, including bacteria, viruses, and other more unusual invading agents. The price paid for immunosuppression is infection.

Caught 'twixt the Scylla of sepsis and the Charybdis of rejection, transplant physicians have become consummate high-wire artists. The delicate balance between the two perils has been very difficult to achieve, and is easily upset by the most minimal change in circumstances. To prevent tipping the patient over into the whirlpool of rejection, the clinician has an array of immunosuppressive drugs; to keep the compromised host from falling into the grasping arms of the monster infection, there is an

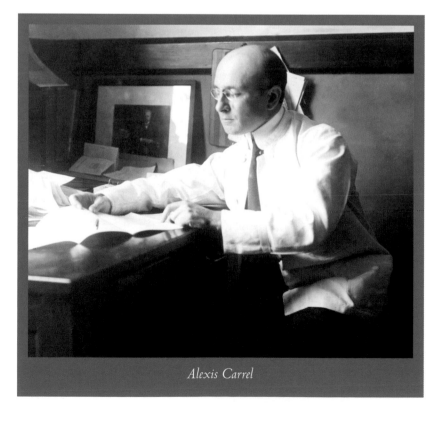

Alexis Carrel

even more impressive armamentarium of antibiotics and aseptic technologies. Treading warily the tightly strung wire, carrying some of each set of nostrums in either hand, is the transplant surgeon, the patient perched precariously on his back. Of course, the surgeon is not alone, but is being cheered on by the counsel of an audience of advisers: the immunologists, the geneticists, the pharmacologists, and the internists. An unexpected shout, or one which is too vociferous, from one or another group may topple him to failure. On high and always teetering, the transplanter is the most visible doctor in the hospital, and the most vulnerable—himself a chimera, in equal parts a hero and a goat, seeming now like the one, now like the other.

When immunosuppression reached a stage of development where it was of practical use, the era of clinical organ transplantation began. The surgeons, of course, had been at work long before the scientists, transplanting structures back and forth in the laboratory between species and individuals as though the only thing that mattered was technical proficiency. They began in the earliest years of the twentieth century. Between 1904 and 1910, the pioneering Alexis Carrel, himself a transplant from France to Chicago, carried out a series of experiments with his associate Charles Guthrie, in which kidneys, hearts, and other organs were grafted. It was during this period that he developed the method of blood-vessel anastomosis that became the basis of the standard technique that has been used by surgeons ever since. For this, he was awarded the Nobel Prize in 1912. Although his ultimate aim was to use his operation to treat patients with kidney failure, he soon realized that such a clinical application would be impossible until the basic biological problem of rejection had been solved. In a 1914 letter to the Swiss surgeon Theodor Kocher, he wrote:

On high and always teetering, the transplanter is the most visible doctor in the hospital, and the most vulnerable—himself a chimera, in equal parts a hero and a goat, seeming now like the one, now like the other.

Concerning homoplastic transplantation [allografts] of organs such as the kidney, I have never found positive results to persist . . . whereas in autoplastic transplantation [autografts] the result was always positive. The biological side of the question has to be investigated very much more and we must find out by what means to prevent the reaction of the organism against a new organ.

Actually, Carrel's associate, Guthrie, had provided a clue to the "biological side of the question" two years earlier, when he wrote:

No one, though many experiments have been reported, has yet succeeded in keeping an animal alive for any great length of time which carried the kidney or kidneys

*of another animal after its own kidneys were removed. .
. . The outlook is by no means hopeless and the principles
of immunity, which yield such brilliant results in many
other fields, would seem to be worthy of being tested in
this case.*

As the biological basis of rejection was being elucidated, efforts continued to graft tissues and organs between unrelated individuals. Although uniformly unsuccessful, these experiments did have the merit of contributing to an understanding of how best to overcome the strictly technical problems of plugging one person's organs into another person's circulation. Almost always, the surgery was done in the laboratory, but every once in a very great while a desperate clinician with a desperate patient tried to scale the impossible mountain with a human kidney transplant, always in vain.

Well, almost always. In 1947, three enterprising young Harvard surgeons, Charles Hufnagel, David Hume, and Ernest Landsteiner (the latter two were residents in training), implanted a fresh cadaver kidney into the upper forearm of a young woman near death of acute shutdown of her kidney tubules. Because the recipient was barely clinging to life, it was decided not to attempt to bring her to the operating suite. Using strict asepsis, the dead donor's kidney was brought to a small end room on one of the Peter Bent Brigham Hospital wards, and transplanted by the light of two small gooseneck study lamps. It began to function immediately, with clear drops of urine gradually filling a bowl held under its exit duct, the ureter. The organ survived only a few days before being rejected, but during those few days it functioned well enough to clear the patient's blood of so much of its impurity that she went

from near-coma to becoming alert, as she recovered from her terminal uremia. Fortunately, her own non-functioning kidneys still had in them the ability to reverse their downhill course, and the short period during which her donor organ tided her over was all that she needed. Two days after the removal of the rejected transplant, she began to make urine on her own, stepped back from the precipice of death, and went on to regain her health uneventfully.

Meantime, Peter Medawar and others had made great strides in tracking down the underlying theoretical framework of transplant immunology. In the issue of *Nature* for October 3, 1953, Medawar and two colleagues described a series of experiments in which they had produced what they called "actively acquired tolerance," by inoculating mouse cells into another mouse while it was still in utero and therefore had not yet developed its immunologic defenses. The cells survived, and their antigens became recognized by the maturing animal as being part of itself. Accordingly, for the rest of the recipient's life, skin from that same donor mouse could be transplanted with impunity to the other animal. The principle underlying the experiments was expressed in the second sentence of that landmark paper: "Mammals and birds never develop, or develop to only a limited degree, the power to react immunologically against foreign homologous tissue cells to which they have been exposed sufficiently early in foetal life."

The significance of Medawar's work lay in its having demonstrated, albeit in a laboratory setting far removed from any clinical implications, that it was possible to pierce the hitherto impenetrable barrier that had prevented successful allografting. As important as the paper was in its purely scientific sense, it was even more important as an exciting stimulus to other researchers. Not only in the laboratories but in the hospitals as well, a new optimism developed that the solution to the problems of graft rejection might be within reach, using a formulation that was consonant with the schemes of Nature herself. Shortly thereafter, an event occurred in Boston that catalyzed the excitement to an even higher pitch: another group of surgeons at the Peter Bent Brigham Hospital successfully transplanted a kidney from one member of a pair of identical twins to the other.

Of course, such a success had no bearing on the question of immunologic tolerance, since each identical twin has exactly the same genetic structure and therefore exactly the same transplant antigens as does his brother. Nevertheless, it was a clinical accomplishment of the greatest magnitude, demonstrating that the surgical techniques had been perfected, and all that was needed was a workable solution to the problems of allograft rejection.

The first clinical attempt at such a solution was, in retrospect, more like a flamethrower than a well-directed arrow. Instead of hitting the bull's-eye, it very nearly destroyed the entire tar-

Karl Landsteiner

get. Several patients, in Boston and in Paris, were given X-ray treatment to the entire body, based on prior demonstration in the laboratory that the immune system might be suppressed by such a gross burning insult to its integrity. The results proved to be too unpredictable and too dangerous to justify continuation of the work. Some of the patients became so immune-suppressed that they required bone-marrow transplants in an attempt to help them ward off the overwhelming infections to which the scorching made them susceptible. There was only one survivor among the twelve irradiated patients who received kidney allografts at the Peter Bent Brigham Hospital between 1958 and 1962.

While the clinical attempts at whole-body irradiation were being carried out, basic science laboratories were abuzz with attempts to develop a drug that could accomplish the same objective more safely. Since it would obviously be a long time before Medawar's concepts of active acquired tolerance might result in a useful patient-directed reality, pharmacologic suppression of the immune system was the logical avenue in which to go shopping. Again, it was in the form of an article in *Nature* that the news came that such a thing might be practicable: on June 13, 1959, Robert Schwartz and William Damashek of the Tufts Medical School reported that they had reduced the rejection process in rabbits by the daily injection of an antimetabolic agent called 6-mercaptopurine. This drug, although it modified the patient's immune response, did not suppress it so deeply and universally as did irradiation. The authors made a striking point that was greeted with hopeful enthusiasm by every researcher who had even the most peripheral interest in transplantation: "In the drug-treated animals it is apparent that although antibody production in general is not blocked, a gross dysfunction of the information-storing device has occurred." In other words, the process of recognition of foreignness was being affected by the drug. In the conclusion of the paper, the researches were linked to those of Medawar: "In any event, these experiments indicate that the term 'acquired immunologic tolerance' previously used only for the response of the immature animals needs to be broadened to include drug-induced tolerance."

The great race was on, to develop, both in the laboratory and clinically, the proper drugs for immunosuppression and the proper criteria for their use. Roy Calne, a young English surgeon, began

experimenting with 6-mercaptopurine in dogs, and things went well. He was awarded a fellowship to continue his work at the Harvard Medical School, and set up shop in the laboratories of the Peter Bent Brigham Hospital in July 1960, under the general direction of the guiding spirit behind all the Brigham transplant work, Dr. Francis D. Moore, successor to Harvey Cushing and Elliot Cutler as chief of surgery. Working with one of the surgeons who had done the original twin transplant, Joseph Murray, Calne prepared the protocols for the first attempts to transplant a kidney into a drug-suppressed patient. First using 6-mercaptopurine and then a closely related compound called azathioprine, the Brigham team achieved success. Before long, safe and effective methods of kidney transplantation had been developed in enough American and European centers that the procedure became practical for increasing numbers of recipients. With use of an artificial kidney machine to clear the blood of impurities, patients were enabled to wait until a proper donor was available, and then to undergo the procedure.

As might be expected, the results of identical-twin transplants have always been excellent, followed by those between close relatives, in whom histocompatibility testing showed that antigenic differences were less significant. But for the majority of recipients, the donor has been a young person who has just been pronounced dead. With proper matching and careful management of immunosuppression, the so-called cadaver kidney has an excellent probability of implanting successfully. Major transplant centers now report 95–100 percent success rates in transplanting kidneys between identical twins, and two-year figures for both related and cadaver donors of better than 80 percent. Although some of the continuing improvement is related to the ever-increasing sophistication of histocompatibility testing, most of it is due to more skillful management of immunosuppression, which has led to a general policy of attempting to decrease its intensity to the minimum required for each patient. The result has been lower infection rates, apparently without any increase in the frequency of rejection.

There have been two other major factors in the present optimistic outlook for most transplant patients: the use of steroids and the development of cyclosporine, an agent derived from a fungus, and found quite serendipitously when its discoverer dug up a sample of earth while on a recreational camping trip in Norway. The steroids, cortisone compounds produced by the outer portion, or cortex, of the adrenal gland, have long been known

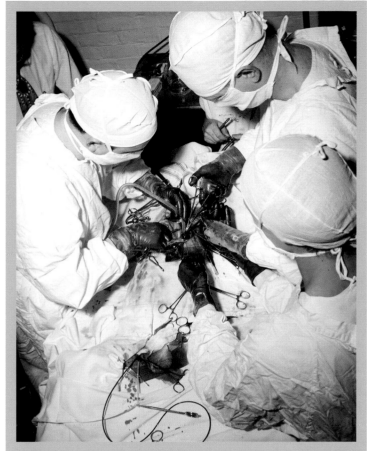

A 1950 operation on a dog to insert a mechanical heart and lung

to have an immunosuppressive action, but one that is not effective enough by itself to prevent rejection. When steroids are combined with azathioprine, however, the immunosuppressive effect of each is enhanced by the other. Moreover, if an organ is suddenly threatened by rejection during the postoperative weeks or months, a brief period of increased steroid dose will often prevent the catastrophe from occurring.

Cyclosporine, first noted in 1974 to have immunosuppressive qualities, has been in general use since 1983, and has rapidly become the major drug utilized in transplantation. Unlike azathioprine, it does not depress the activity of bone mar-

row, and is therefore much less likely to leave the patient exposed to the danger of sepsis. Moreover, it seems to have less of a depressive effect on those immune responses that are important in preventing bacterial and viral infections. Because of the decreased incidence of sepsis, patient survival in all types of transplantation has been improved by this gift from the fungus world. In fact, it is fair to say that the introduction of cyclosporine has resulted in such a revolution in the techniques of safe immunosuppression that only 10 percent of kidney grafts are today lost because of rejection.

No major pharmacological agent is without major side effects, but those of cyclosporine have proved to be more manageable than those of the others. Not only that, but its use tends also to decrease the required dose of steroid, so that the side effects of this agent as well are lessened. In addition to its other virtues, cyclosporine has made histocompatibility testing a less crucial determinant of success.

There are other methods of immunosuppression, such as monoclonal antibodies, and the use of antilymphocyte and antithymocyte globulins, which have limited clinical usefulness at present, but which do hold out some hope of greater effec-

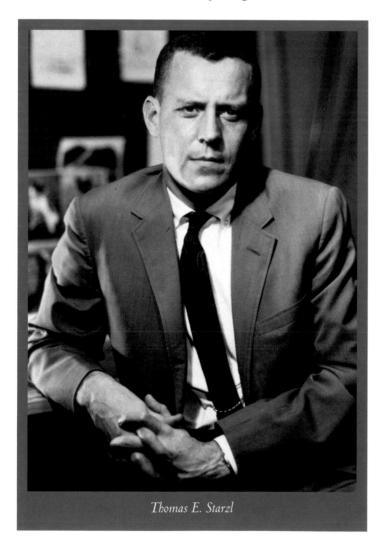

Thomas E. Starzl

tiveness in the future, primarily because they are based on theoretical principles that will be promising areas for ongoing research for years to come. Not entirely surprisingly, blood transfusions seem to suppress immunity to allografts, although the underlying mechanism is still a bit of a riddle. Being allografts themselves, and being incompatible in minor ways with the recipient, it may be that preoperative blood transfusions act in some way to prepare the host's immune mechanisms for the eventual "big graft" by increasing certain blood constituents that suppress rejection. All of this is too new just now, and just a little too abstruse, to require anything beyond mere mention.

The transplantation of kidneys has been the prototype for the transplantation of all other organs. So convinced was the University of Colorado's Dr. Thomas Starzl of the potential for successful allografting of the liver that he refused to become discouraged even after his first five patients died within three weeks of the operation in 1963. Finally, in 1967, the operation succeeded in a one-and-a-half-year-old girl with a malignant liver tumor. She lived for thirteen months, and when she finally succumbed, it was not due to rejection or sepsis, but to recurrent cancer. Each of Starzl's next eight patients survived for periods of between two and thirty months. The operation was thereby proved to be feasible. Although a number of other centers later took up the work of liver transplantation, Dr. Starzl, now at the University of Pittsburgh, continues to be the world's leader in that field. The liver is a much more complicated organ than either kidney or heart, yet liver allografts now have a survival rate at one year of 75 percent for children and 60 percent for adults. Histocompatibility testing does not play a major role in liver transplantation. Suitable cadaver donors are so difficult to acquire that it has been necessary to make use of almost any liver that seems close enough in size.

"Almost any liver that seems close enough in size." Think about that for a moment. It flies in the face of everything that seemingly led up to it, and of any claim made by the transplanters that they are scientists. Of what benefit the extraordinary research accomplishments of the Medawars and Burnets, and of what significance the cavalcade of chapters in this book that describe the gradual entry of science into medicine? When all is said and done, here we are transplanting livers, and hearts too, protected primarily by a drug serendipitously discovered (unearthed, literally) from an obscure Scandinavian fungus, a drug whose real action is still so elusive that it evades our best attempts to understand it. We use cyclosporine because it works—explanations can come later. This is one of those many situations where the boys and girls in the lab have to play catch-up with their fellows on the hospital wards, instead of telling them, in true scientific fashion, how to do their work. Their explanations are drifting in, but the clinicians will remain way out in front for some time yet to come.

Of all the clumsy constructions that are part of the florid verbiage used in legal formalities, a candidate for the least felicitous is that painful phrase "purports and holds himself out to be," when it is used against a craftsman or professional person being sued for an unfortunate outcome of his efforts. With those cruel words, the recipient of a subpoena is informed that, contrary to the evidence of his entire career, he is not actually a skilled member of his guild but only someone who lays claim to that honored position. I have seen the most self-confident of surgeons figuratively cringe when they speak about the effect of seeing this kind of terminology leap up at them from the closely typed lines of hyperbolic prose composed by some zealous attorney. Why then, if it is so painful to think about, do I bring up the purporting and holding out in a section of this book that deals with one of the greatest triumphs of the physician's art?

My purpose is to remind all of us, doctors and laymen alike, that even in this most scientific age of medicine, there is indeed an underlying layer of delusion, even if it is primarily a deluding of ourselves that is at work. As physicians, we certainly do purport—not only do we purport to be healers, but we purport also to use in our healing the most modern of the methods of medical science. Most of the time, we are exactly what we present ourselves to be—but not always. On occasion, we are as guilty as the standard subpoena would have us. We hold ourselves out to be something that we are really not. We are, after all, not really scientists. We have discovered, as our herb-dosing forebears did in similar situations, the empirical fact that a drug named cyclosporine has such an effect on the immune system that it allows us to transplant organs from one person to another. By trial and error, almost by happenstance, we have fallen on a wonder fungus whose real action is an enigma. Although our laboratories come daily closer to some biological explication, the urgencies of patient care have demanded a clinical launch before all the basic mechanisms are clarified. Out goes histocompatibility testing, out goes acquired tolerance, out go all of the truly scientific precedents to this supposedly (and purportedly) most scientific moment in our history. No one would presume to argue that the introduction of cyclosporine is science at work. It is not science—the introduction of cyclosporine is an example of the art of medicine. If the thing works, and it does not violate the dictum of *primum non nocere*, we should damn well use it and let the scientific proof come later. Here we are dealing with the eternal conflict between the scientist and the healer. As long as medicine remains an art, as it forever must, that conflict will always be resolved in favor of the healer.

I am one of those who believe that the term "medical science" has in it the makings of an oxymoron. In the sixteenth and seventeenth centuries, science began to enter the consciousness of the healers. Except in a theoretical sense, it could not be applied to the diagnosis of disease until the early nineteenth century, or to its treatment until fifty years later. Since then, the science of human biology has left off being a handmaiden—it has become the greatest partner that medicine will ever have. But the two allies must not be confused with each other. The healing of the sick remains an art, and it requires a spectrum of skills that range in rigor from those that deal with the cellule to those that deal with the psyche. Sometimes it includes even a bit of well-intentioned subterfuge. As long as judgment, clinical intuition, and bedside decision-making are major components in the treatment of sick people, all hail to the art of medicine. And all hail, also, to those two most

unscientific of the physician's resources: listening to the patient, and caring about him.

Judgment, clinical intuition, decision-making—the taste and the smell, if you will, of a patient, his needs, the surroundings of his disease, and the pathophysiology of the process that has brought him to the doctor—these are the real ingredients of the art of cardiac transplantation. Science brought us to the point where we dared to think about such a chimerical fantasy, and even gave us the technical means to make it possible. The ultimate step and the ultimate success by which the chimera became a reality was, however, the product of a strictly clinical sense of what is right, of exactly what it is that this particular patient, at this particular stage of his disease, needs at this particular time. It involves also an informed guess about what will happen if he does not get it.

This particular patient, the one I want to tell about, is Ray Edwards, and his particular time was March 10, 1986. He was the beneficiary of eight decades of laboratory research and almost twenty years of clinical studies, which had resulted in perfection of the surgical methods and recent rapid progress in the prevention of rejection. Alexis Carrel and Charles Guthrie got things started in 1905 when they transplanted a puppy's heart into the neck of a large adult dog, and saw it beat normally for two hours. A long series of studies were undertaken by a number of investigators over the succeeding years, but never with any thought of applying the work in any clinical situation.

The picture changed considerably in 1953, when the heart-lung machine came into use, because it allowed both of those organs to be replaced during the time it takes to repair abnormalities of the major vessels and the atrial and ventricular chambers. There was thus available a piece of equipment that could bypass the heart, and make human cardiac transplantation a real possibility. Using such a machine in the laboratory, Richard Lower and Norman Shumway of Stanford University reported, in the early 1960s, a series of successes in attempting to transplant dog hearts. Although every one of the survivors rejected its new heart within a few weeks of operation, it had been established that good cardiac function took place even though all nerves to the heart had been cut. With the technical and physiological problems solved, Lower and Shumway continued their work to establish mechanisms by which rejection might be prevented, primarily doing research with histocompatibility testing, as well as the use of azathioprine and steroids.

> *The healing of the sick remains an art, and it requires a spectrum of skills that range in rigor from those that deal with the cellule to those that deal with the psyche.*

This is where things stood on December 3, 1967, when Dr. Christiaan Barnard astounded and delighted the world by performing the first transplant of a human heart on a patient named Louis Washkansky at the Groote Schuur Hospital in Capetown, South Africa. Much more astounded than the rest of the world, and a great deal less delighted, were Shumway, Lower, and the others of the several researchers who had been struggling in the laboratory to solve the problems of rejection. They knew that methods of testing for tissue compatibility were still unsatisfactory,

and they feared that surgeons all over the world might rush to duplicate Barnard's premature feat. Their greatest concerns proved to be well founded. Three days later, a surgeon in Brooklyn transplanted a heart into a seventeen-day-old boy, who died a few hours later. Louis Washkansky himself died on December 21, the day before Barnard left for a six-day tour of the United States, during which he was lionized as a hero of medicine. Mayor John Lindsay was on hand to greet him on his arrival in New York, and President Lyndon Johnson entertained him in that unique style that is only to be experienced on the ranch of a Texas millionaire.

Barnard, who had learned about transplantation by working with Shumway, captured the imagination of America and Europe like a latter-day Lindbergh. He became an instant media star. Having already chosen his second patient, he flew back to Capetown on December 30, thereby providing an opportunity for a London newspaper to sell out its editions with the dramatic headline "Barnard Flying to Next Heart Operation." On January 2, Philip Blaiberg got a new heart. He was recovering smoothly on January 10, when the Brooklyn surgeon tried again. His patient died eight hours later. Blaiberg lived nineteen months, long enough to join his surgeon in the ranks of celebrity—even Liberace visited him in the hospital.

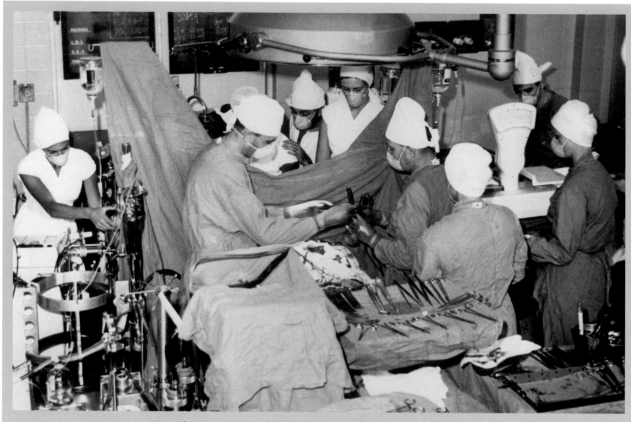

Dr. Christiaan Barnard's surgical team performing open heart surgery

The pressure was on, and even the cautious Shumway could not resist it for long. On January 6, 1968, he operated on his first cardiac-transplant patient, who lived for fifteen days afterward. With the highly regarded Stanford professor having entered the lists, a certain legitimacy was conferred on the cardiac extravaganza; more and more surgeons rushed off to the races. Reports of similar operations came in from England, Brazil, Argentina, France, Canada, and several centers in the United States. Finally even Richard Lower, by then at the Medical College of Virginia, succumbed to transplant fever. Still as worried as Shumway about not having solved the immunity puzzle, he operated on his first patient on May 25. In the previous

month alone, thirteen people had undergone heart transplantation in hospitals throughout the world. Lower's patient lived six days. In the fifteen months following the operation on Louis Washkansky, 118 operations were done, in eighteen different countries. The great majority of the patients died within weeks or months.

Finally, the surgeons who had unripely rushed in with too much hope and too little restraint had to face the reality that it was still too early. The figure of ninety-nine transplants in 1968 dropped to forty-eight in 1969, seventeen in 1970, and only nine in 1971. Fifty-six of the world's fifty-eight heart-transplant teams closed up shop and returned to regular cardiac surgery. Barnard persisted, and so did Shumway. At Stanford, Shumway's became the only ongoing program in America, because his laboratory science was at such a high level that it could keep pace with his clinical surgery. Even in August 1970, he maintained enough faith to make a guardedly optimistic comment in an issue of *California Medicine:* "At this point we believe cardiac transplantation remains within the realm of clinical investigation."

Quietly and without fanfare, the Stanford group continued its work. As their methods improved, so did their clinical results. Encouraged by Shumway's reports, other teams gradually began to take heart, in a manner of speaking. Slowly, the long moratorium on cardiac transplantation began to come to an end. In 1984, twenty-nine centers in the United States performed approximately three hundred transplants. At the time of this writing, there are about one hundred American teams operating. Survival is now not only satisfactory, it is downright astounding. Seventy-five percent of these otherwise hopeless patients are alive at one year postoperatively, 65 percent at three years, and almost 60 percent at five years. There is every reason to believe that these figures, as remarkable as they are, will continue to improve.

In order to be considered a candidate for a cardiac transplant, a patient must be in such an advanced state of disease that life expectancy is estimated at no more than a few months. This is designated as Class IV in a categorization established by the New York Heart Association some years ago; it signifies end-stage failure of the heart muscle. The majority of such patients have severe coronary artery disease, and have lost a great deal of function in the ventricles as a result of multiple occlusions of these vessels. Another major group consists of those people who present with progressive deterioration of the heart muscle of undetermined cause, a condition termed idiopathic cardiomyopathy. Although it is often attributed to some preceding viral infection, the underlying basis of cardiomyopathy in any individual is usually difficult to pin down.

It was such a cardiomyopathy, thought to be viral in origin, that first brought Ray Edwards to a cardiologist. For no apparent reason, he began to find himself, in the autumn of 1975, to be increasingly tired and short of breath. Finally, in January of 1976, when he was unable to go on, he

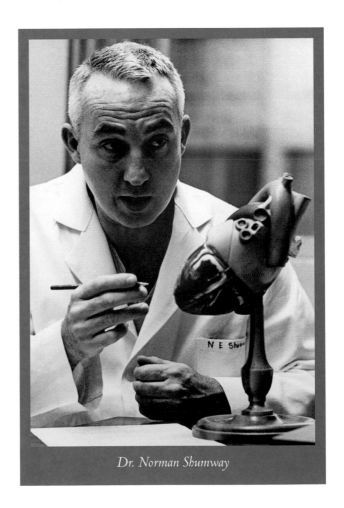

Dr. Norman Shumway

went to the emergency room of the Milford Hospital, only to be told that he was suffering from what the duty physician called "a classical case of hypoglycemia." Fortunately, he was given the name of an internist, Dr. Henri Coppes, in order to arrange for a proper workup of his symptoms. When Ray went to his appointment with the internist the following day, he had so much difficulty breathing that he could barely make his way from the parking lot to the office. Dr. Coppes immediately recognized the severity of the cardiac failure presented by his new patient, hospitalized him, and with consultation from a cardiologist, got him out of immediate danger.

Thus began a program of support for a heart that was trying desperately to fail. At first, Dr. Coppes was able to keep his patient in some reasonable semblance of health, but the situation finally began to deteriorate rapidly in 1983. Seeking further help, Coppes arranged for Ray to seek consultation with Dr. Lawrence Cohen, who carries with modesty and a sense of humor the splendiferous title of Ebenezer K. Hunt Professor of Medicine at Yale. By careful titration of medications, Dr. Cohen was able to bring about some improvement, but not enough to make him optimistic about the future. Ray's state of mind was not helped by a transient mild stroke he suffered in June of 1985, manifested by slurred speech. His heart rate had dropped from a normal of seventy-two down to twenty-eight beats per minute—a pacemaker was inserted to bring it back up to normal so that the output of the ventricles might be improved.

Dr. Cohen had first begun to consider heart transplantation for Ray as early as mid-1984. As his condition worsened, this possibility loomed ever larger. A cardiac catheterization and nuclear scans were done in October 1985, and the results were so discouraging that there seemed no other way to turn. With each beat, Ray's massively dilated left ventricle was ejecting only 15 percent of the blood within it. With such an ineffectual pump, it was only a matter of months before intractable failure would supervene. By the time of the catheterization, Ray was taking an array of medications that represented pharmacology's final offensive against the onrushing inevitability of his death.

On January 9, 1986, Ray met with the Yale–New Haven Hospital transplant team of surgeons, nurses, and technicians. The team's director, Dr. Alexander Geha, described the sequence of events that would lead up to the proposed operation, and those that were likely to follow it. Even were Ray Edwards a less stoic Connecticut Yankee than he is, his decision would have been the same. Taking as deep a breath as his congested lungs allowed him, he told Dr. Geha to start the countdown.

The following weeks were difficult ones for Monica and Ray Edwards. Even the meticulous manipulation of medications by Dr. Cohen did not slow the insidious decline of Ray's heart muscle. The threat of a sudden complete collapse loomed like death itself over each day of that long dreary waiting period for a suitable donor. Finally, after two months of restless anxiety, the call came. On the evening of March 9, 1986, Monica packed Ray's small bag, helped him into their Dodge, and drove the fifteen-mile distance to New Haven.

In another New England city, a second couple was also facing a tragedy, of quite a different sort. Unlike Ray Edwards, there was no possible miracle in store for them. On the night of March 6, their seventeen-year-old son had been brought mortally injured to a local hospital, following an automobile accident. His chest was crushed in the collision, but his robust, healthy heart had not been damaged. It beat still, with the vivacity of youth, belying the ruined body that enclosed it. As gently as possible, the attending physicians told the boy's parents that he was brain-dead.

With what a mixture of courage and altruism and love must that grieving couple have made their decision. Left without hope, they had yet faith and charity. They asked that their son's heart and kidneys be transplanted into the bodies of three anonymous people who could not live without them.

Early on the morning of March 10, Dr. John Elefteriades, accompanied by one of the Yale surgical residents, arrived by helicopter from New Haven in that small New England city where the donor waited, his life having been snuffed out, in the eyes of the law, at the moment of impact four days before, but his strong young heart still beating as though in expectation of some form of reprieve. The boy was taken to the hospital's operating room with all of his mechanical life-support systems intact. Dr. Elefteriades and his assistant made an incision through the middle of the breastbone and harvested the living heart.

Here there is no choice but to pause—that word, "harvest." The transplanters use it so freely, but the rest of us have to stop and think about it every now and then. Perhaps you have never seen it used in such a sense. The word implies that the earth is yielding up its treasures to nourish mankind; it implies the performance of a worshipful act, the receiving of one of the benisons of a fructified soil; it implies a gift of God's abundance; it implies nourishment and life. The heart of an unknown youth was a golden harvest for Raymond Edwards.

Elefteriades (another pause—the name itself conjures up the image of a grove of olive or eucalyptus trees on the island of Cos, and a philosopher-physician poulticing the wounds of his patient with the sweet balm of healing), gently cradling the container in which lay the stilled heart in its bath of iced saline solution, was driven swiftly back to the helicopter and airlifted to a landing pad near the sprawling campus of the Yale–New Haven Hospital. The short remaining distance of the journey was negotiated behind the screaming sirens of a police cruiser.

Ray Edwards was by this time anesthetized and connected to the heart-lung machine. As soon as Dr. Geha was notified that the helicopter had landed in New Haven, he started the bypass and began cutting away the flaccid bag of diseased cardiac muscle from his patient's chest. When Ray's pitiful excuse for a heart had been excised, its place was taken by the donor organ, which was then rapidly sewn into the proper vascular connections. As

The threat of a sudden complete collapse loomed like death itself over each day of that long dreary waiting period for a suitable donor.

soon as all the suture lines were securely in position, the clamps that still separated Ray from his donor organ were removed, and a perfect, spontaneous beat started up instantly. The exhilaration of the operating team was just a bit premature, however, because a dysrhythmic fibrillating motion soon turned the heart muscle into a quivering mass of detumescent flesh. The surgeon immediately administered one quick burst of electric stimulation from the defibrillator, and the transplant resumed its proud, thrusting pulsation, becoming promptly a dynamic part of the still unaware patient whose sleeping body was preparing itself to become its welcoming new home. That single shock brought Ray Edwards back to life. An hour later, he was in the Cardiac Intensive Care Unit, gradually awakening to the realization that he and the heart of his young benefactor had begun their journey together, to a new vitality.

When I visited Ray two days after his transplant, he looked better than he had two days after his appendectomy. We chatted briefly in the euphoric haze that permeated the whole atmosphere of that place. Another patient had undergone the same procedure several days earlier, and he too was doing well. Both men were being given azathioprine, cyclosporine, steroids, and antibiotics. Neither of them had a single hitch in his

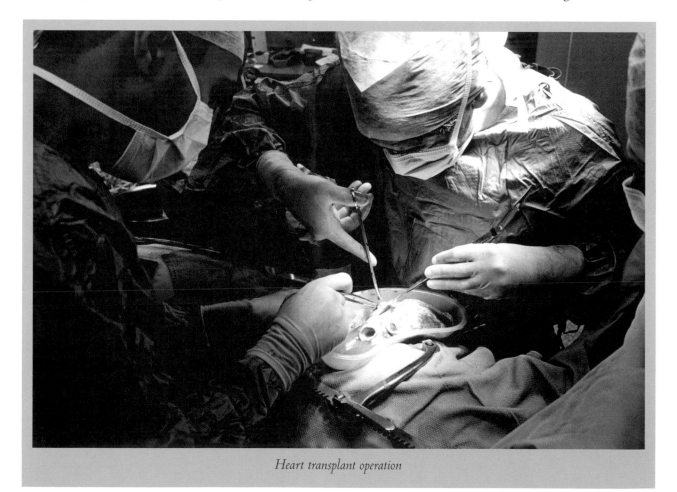

Heart transplant operation

uncomplicated recovery. In the familiar words so often used by the residents, "They didn't turn a hair!"

I have kept close track of Ray since then. He has had a few minor episodes of impending rejection, identifiable only by biopsy of the heart muscle. This procedure is not as bad as it sounds. Under local anesthesia, a long flexible wirelike probe called a bioptome is inserted into a neck vein and then passed down into the right ventricle. At its tip are two fine jaws that can be closed by the operating surgeon in such a way as to snip off little bits of heart muscle for microscopic examination. Ray's rejection episodes were so insignificant that they would have gone undetected were it not for the biopsies, which are done at routine intervals. Repeat studies, in each case after a period of increased steroid dosage, were always normal.

Meanwhile, Ray has found himself not only a new heart but a completely new occupation as well. His love for meteorology had begun to be muddied by the burden of administrative duties associated with his position as chief of the local weather station. He has now gone back to school. He is learning medical technology, with the same curiosity and determination that he brought to his previous studies, first of meteorology and then of the literature of cardiac transplantation.

Until he became too sick to continue, Ray had always been a devoted climber of the tree-covered peaks and summits that make up the low mountain ranges of New England. Among his favorite hills was Mt. Monadnock, in the southwest corner of New Hampshire, whose steep winding trails present a formidable challenge to the most hearty of hearts and most sturdy of legs. On October 4, 1986, with a light pack on his shoulders,

Ray was back at it, scrambling up the sides of the 3,165-foot Monadnock barely six months after being given the legacy of life by the young man who is never out of his prayers.

Ray Edwards was one of approximately one thousand Americans to undergo cardiac transplantation in 1986. Although there are estimated to be more than twenty thousand hearts potentially available each year and nineteen hundred patients who may be candidates for a transplant, there is not yet a sufficient national effort to ensure that each possible donor heart is used. At least a third of patients with end-stage disease die while awaiting a suitable heart. Through the North American Transplant Coordinators Organization and regional retrieval programs, mechanisms have been set up for speedy identification and transport of organs from one part of the country to another, but the major difficulty has remained a personal one. Too few American families have yet begun to think of transplantation as anything other than a newsworthy example of medical frontiers-manship at its most dramatic. What will be required for the future is a national sense of personal involvement, of a kind of imminence of the possibility that any of us, at any time, may need to decide that the last charity of someone we love may give life to another.

What is also needed is a confrontation with personal mortality, so that more of us will volunteer to be donors should death strike suddenly. In 1985, in spite of national acceptance of the Uniform Anatomical Gift Act, a donor card was carried by fewer than 4 percent of those people whose organs were transplanted after death. When we add to this the fact that fewer than 30 percent of the hearts transplanted in 1986 became available as the result of a specific offer by a family, it becomes clear that more of us need to think long and hard about the gift of life. It has been estimated that under present circumstances no more than fifteen hundred hearts will ever be available in the United States in any given year. Until the day when the concept of a permanent, totally implantable artificial heart becomes a reality, transplantation will remain the only way.

The mere discussion of organ donations reveals an entire new realm of medicine's future. Healing is becoming less and less a transaction between a doctor and his patient; more and more it is an expression of an entire society and its values. The technology of medical care is too expensive, it touches on too many areas of concern to every citizen, for it to exist any longer free of influence by everything that goes on in the world around it. A third-world dictator shouts a few anti-American imprecations, and our government spends enough money moving warships to pay a year's rent on every federally funded pediatric cardiology clinic in the nation. Or, more specifically related to the Ray Edwardses of America, the Department of Health and Human Services has estimated that the costs of cardiac transplant procedures will be at least $150 million per year even if only the minimal number of donors become available; if a suitable heart could be found for every patient who might benefit from

it, costs could reach $4.4 billion. Funding is finite, as much as we might wish it otherwise. Of the many medical neologisms in every doctor's recently memorized socioeconomic lexicon, among the most obnoxious, and yet one of the most imperative, is the term "cost-effective." The well-known need to get value for money is now being applied to decision-making at the bedside of every patient in the western world. If we spend the $4.4 billion for a group of primarily older patients with failing hearts, we won't be able to pay the rent on all those cardiac clinics, nor can we fund all of the necessary research for the treatment of childhood cancers. It is not the doctor who will decide, nor should he; it is society.

Society has even had to decide how to define the word "death." No longer is the heartbeat the ultimate clinical sign. When the healers began to need more hearts and livers for transplantation, they developed a new criterion, the cessation of the activity of the brain. They turned to society for sanction, and it was not long in coming. The ministers of the cloth and the ministers of the crown considered and concurred—it is both ethical and legal to remove organs from those who cannot return from inanimate hopelessness. The principle was thus established: the living have a moral claim on the bodies of the dead.

> *Fewer than 30 percent of the hearts transplanted in 1986 became available as the result of a specific offer by a family; it becomes clear that more of us need to think long and hard about the gift of life.*

Diagnostic studies that until recently were thought to be basic to the proper investigation of every disease process are now being reevaluated on a case-by-case basis, and very often discarded from the clinical arsenal. In the 1960s, it was considered poor medicine not to do a gastrointestinal X-ray series for each patient with gallstones; it is now considered poor medicine if we waste money on such a study, since it has been shown not to be cost-effective. There is beginning to creep into the bibliographical section of some of our most prominent clinicians' curricula vitae a sprinkling of recently written papers on the economic and social aspects of healing. Our leading journals are plentifully punctuated with editorials on such matters as efficient bed utilization and inefficient use of resources.

There is a paradox in paradise. The compulsively thorough workup learned during residency training two or three decades ago by a physician who is today at the height of his clinical abilities is now the mark of a shotgun doctor, who is called unmindful of costs and too little reliant on his bedside judgment. Those few collateral laboratory tests, that extra day in the hospital "just to be sure," are an unaffordable luxury. It would be nice if we could demonstrate that some money has been saved in this way, but any savings are so deeply buried in the expenses of staggeringly complicated new diagnostic and therapeutic modalities that no one seems to be able to prove anything with certainty, except, of course, that we are able to heal more people than ever before. The only demonstrable certainty, in fact, is societal involvement. Whether in finances, in ethics, or in laws, the voice of the people will be, must be, heard.

For example, who is to say whether a given person should be persuaded to provide a kidney for transplantation into his uremic brother? The principle of *primum non nocere* applies to the care of the sick, but this potential donor is not a patient. Harm *is* done by exposing him to a major operation and then leaving him afterward with one kidney. Though it may have no lasting effect on his health, it is harm nevertheless. Theologians, and ethicists, and lawyers have judged that it is permissible, in the interests of the greater good. They articulate the values of society.

In the example of the kidney donor, society functions as an adviser to the physician, even as an advocate. There are situations in which it must function as an adversary. To the Hippocratic physician, nothing and no one was more important than his patient; this has always been a guiding principle of clinical medicine. Other patients, future patients, and the rest of mankind have been secondary considerations when a doctor is making decisions at the bedside of the sick. That day too is past. Limitations on resources are only part of the reason for the change of attitude. New methods of treatment are constantly appearing on the clinical scene, and they need evaluation, particularly in the case of scourges such as cancer and infectious disease. It is necessary to enter large numbers of patients in statistical studies in which treatment modalities are tested against other treatment modalities and against no treatment at all. These are called randomized prospective trials, which means that patients are chosen for one or the other of the proposed treatments without regard to any criteria except the order in which they happen to come into the study. If the treatment being tested is a drug, the research protocol must be double-blind, in the sense that neither investigators nor subjects know which of the various drugs any individual patient is getting.

For a prospective randomized double-blind study to have any value, every involved doctor must be disinterested in the outcome. And yet, it is virtually impossible for any physician not to have a preconceived notion about how the study will turn out. The very nature of such a research effort means, therefore, that the participating doctors are abandoning each individual patient to a therapeutic choice based on chance, where there is only a 50, 33 , 25, or smaller percent possibility that he will receive the medicine or surgery that the physician deems to be best for the particular way in which he manifests his disease process.

This is a new wrinkle to an old dilemma that people have faced ever more often since some of us first became entrusted with caring for the health of others of us: there is sometimes a conflict between what is best for the individual patient I see in my office today and what is best, in the long run, for the greatest number over the greatest period of time. In the past, the conflict was always resolved in favor of the individual and the immediate; increasingly, there is scientific and societal pressure to resolve it in favor of the prospective good of humankind. Now that the dilemma has been acknowledged and enunciated, we will forever after carry it with us into the decision-making process for every one of our patients.

That dilemma may soon manifest itself in a form that will mightily test the still tenuous structure that biomedicine, ethics, law, and finance are struggling to create. When (not if, but when) the massive effort against AIDS results in what appears to be an effective vaccine or an undeniably promising form of treatment, what will society do, and what will its most involved elements demand? Will members of high-risk groups, will their families, will the rest of us, sit still for randomized prospective double-blind studies while victims continue to suffer and die? The inevitable solution to such a quandary will be acclaimed with joy and greeted with thanksgiving by the very researchers whose long-range efforts it most disrupts, even though that solution may result in precedents that threaten the methodologies of science and perhaps even the health of patients yet unborn who will have diseases yet unknown. The detachment of laboratory scientists will be strained to the breaking point, and it will, predictably, break. This is as it should be. It will confirm our values as a society of human beings; it will confirm the Hippocratic values of medicine.

Philosophers and congressmen, ethicists and accountants, corporate executives and hospital administrators, theologians and actuaries, patients'-rights advocates and lawyers—all have something to say about the uses of the Art and its science, and should. The task of bringing the rich fruits of medical progress to the citizens of our country is not a burden that can be carried very far by the healers alone. Though physicians were at first skeptical of the intrusions of social, economic, and political institutions into an arena that we have always considered our own, we recognize that this too is past. We need all the help we can get.

Still, for all of the transformations wrought by the masterful new engines of medicine and by their multitudinous varieties of fuel, there is one singular ingredient of the art of healing that should not be allowed to vanish. That ingredient, so basic and so changeless, is a relationship; it takes place in the quiet surroundings of the sickroom or in the doctor's office. There occurs in those protected places a transaction which, in a most fundamental way, is an act of giving, and it has to do with such elemental things that pass between two people as listening, and touching, and talking. Whether it culminates in the transplantation of an organ or the transmission of a few encouraging words, it is something that I have never been able to approach with anything but awe, because the experience of healing is a joining between doctor and patient in which one human being is privileged to help another. It has brought blessedness to my life.

ACKNOWLEDGMENTS

Tatooed onto the surface of my psyche is a pedagogical motto that was thundered at me and my college-biology classmates four decades ago: in order to receive a proper grade, the answer to every examination essay-question must fulfill the five criteria of being clear, consecutive, concise, complete, and correct; anything less would be considered defective. Delivered by a crusty, nematode-loving misanthrope who had only disdain for those of us who cared about mammals (or, heaven forbid, planned careers in clinical medicine), that ringing admonition has echoed in my thoughts ever since, on each new occasion of putting thoughts to paper. I have treated Professor Horace Wesley Stunkard's dictum like an article of religious faith, perhaps to assuage my guilt at letting him down when I rejected the laboratory in favor of the clinic. More likely, though, I remember his alliterative adjectives because they add up to sound advice.

With Stunkard in mind, I ran the sundry chapters of this volume through a gauntlet of readers. A book, of course, is not an exam essay, and it is impossible (and surely not even desirable) to make it complete. To replace that one *c*, I added two others: cohesive and consistent. If the reader finds that the Stunkardian criteria have been met, it is to the credit of those colleagues and friends who were willing to take potshots at this book during the course of its writing; if there are deficiencies, it is only because I have sometimes not heeded their counsel. It is not enough to list names in acknowledgment; what follows is meant as a tribute, not only in gratitude for the contributions of my gauntlet-gang, but also for their skillful pummeling.

My wife, Sarah Peterson, has always been my first editor, and my toughest. Her specialty is the recognition of rambling and the discouragement of drift. Fortunate indeed is the author whose initial manuscript-surveyer knows exactly what he is trying to say, and insists that he get on with it. I would like to write much more about the contributions of this particular editor, but she would make me delete it, on the ground that it sounds sentimental and sappy.

After the scrutiny of Sarah, certain chapters were sent off to colleagues who are especially knowledgeable about some particular topic or period. Every one of those essays was returned with comments or suggestions that were extremely helpful. In alphabetical order, I am in debt to: Raymond Edwards, Marc Lorber, Robert Massey, Jeremy Norman, John Harley Warner, and Ruth Whittemore.

I am particularly grateful to four other friends for applying their critical faculties to the entire volume. They are, respectively, a teacher of literacy, a medical historian, a biomedical scientist, and the director of a library of medical history: Joan Behar, Thomas Forbes, Ion Gresser, and Ferenc Gyorgyey. To Ferenc, a special tribute: without our countless hours of discussion, his vast knowledge of the medical-historical literature, and the generosity with which he made available the treasures of his unique library, this book would have died a-borning; without the inspiration of his friendship, the project would never have been conceived—Köszönöm kedves barátom!

I began to write a series of medical biographies at the suggestion of Leslie B. Adams, Jr., approximately five years ago. His Classics of Medicine Library published a group of some fifteen of my monographs and my book, *The Origins of Anesthesia*. It is characteristic of the support he has always given to my endeavors that he and his house, Gryphon Editions (now a subsidiary of Macmillan), have kindly allowed me to use considerable material from some of those publications. Sections of the chapters dealing with the following individuals first appeared in essays that I wrote for Les Adams: Hippocrates, Paré, Morgagni, Hunter, and Halsted, as well as the chapter on anesthesia.

Much of the material on Ignac Semmelweis is taken from my essay in *The Journal of the History of Medicine and Allied Sciences*, published in 1979. The Lister chapter was presented in part as the 32nd Annual Samuel C. Harvey Lecture in the History of Surgery, at Yale, in 1987.

I have made two new friends during the several years of this book's gestation:

Robert Gottlieb had faith in the project from the beginning and made himself the captain of my cheering section; he fueled the engines of my enthusiasm with his warmth and intellect. When he left Knopf, he did not leave me.

And finally, there is Corona Machemer. Although she picked up the manuscript in midstream, she has treated it with the care of a devoted parent. She is a marvelously skilled lover of the English language who understands what I have wanted to do in this book. After thirty years as a surgeon, I thought I knew something about tender care, until she entered the life of *Doctors* and began to share her insights with me. When Bob Gottlieb took his sneakers and blue pencil off to *The New Yorker*, he assured me that he had found "the absolutely perfect editor" to replace him. To that encomium, I can only add, "Yes, and amen."

S. B. N.

BIBLIOGRAPHY

1 THE TOTEM OF MEDICINE: HIPPOCRATES

Adams, F. *The Genuine Works of Hippocrates.* London: New Sydenham Society, 1849. (Birmingham: Classics of Medicine Lib., 1985.)

Ader, R., ed. *Psychoneuroimmunology.* New York: Academic Press, 1981.

Amundsen, D. W. "History of Medical Ethics: Ancient Greece and Rome." In W. T. Reich, *Encyclopedia of Bioethics,* vol. 3. New York: Free Press, 1978.

Carrick, P. *Medical Ethics in Antiquity.* Dordrecht, Netherlands: D. Reidel, 1985.

Chance, B. "On Hippocrates and the Aphorisms." *Ann. Med. Hist.* 2 (N.S.):31–46 (1930).

Coar, T. *The Aphorisms of Hippocrates.* London: Valpy, 1822. (Birmingham: Classics of Medicine Lib., 1982.)

Drabkin, M. "A Select Bibliography of Greek and Roman Medicine." *Bull. Hist. Med.* 11:399–408 (1942).

Edelstein, L. *Ancient Medicine.* Baltimore: Johns Hopkins Univ. Press, 1967.

Galhos, F. N., and Ariyan, S. "Hippocrates, the True Father of Hand Surgery." *Surg. Gyn. Obst.* 160:178–184 (1985).

Galdston, I. "The Decline and Resurgence of Hippocratic Medicine." *Bull. N.Y. Acad. Med.* 44:1237–1256 (1968).

Hudson, R. P. *Disease and Its Control: The Shaping of Modern Thought.* Westport, Conn.: Greenwood Praeger, 1987.

Jones, W. H. S. *The Works of Hippocrates.* Cambridge: Harvard Univ. Press, 1957.

Littré, P. E. *Oeuvres Complètes d'Hippocrate.* 10 vols. Paris: J. B. Bailliere, 1861.

Lund, F. B. "The Life and Writings of Hippocrates." *Bost. Med. Surg. J.* 191:1009–1014 (1924).

Michler, M. "Medical Ethics in Hippocratic Bone Surgery." *Bull. Hist. Med.* 42:297–311 (1968).

Miller, G. "'Airs, Waters and Places' in History." *J. Hist. Med.* 17:129–140 (1962).

Moon, R. O. *Hippocrates and His Successors in Relation to the Philosophy of Their Time.* London: Longmans, Green, 1923.

Richards, D. W. "Hippocrates of Ostia." *J.A.M.A.* 204:1049–1056 (1968).

Sigerist, H. E. "On Hippocrates." *Bull. Johns Hopkins Inst. Hist. Med.* 2:190–214 (1934).

———. "Hippocrates and the Collection of Hippocratic Writings," *A History of Medicine,* vol. 2. New York: Oxford Univ. Press, 1961.

Singer, C. "The Father of Medicine." *Times Lit. Supp.,* April 3, 1924, 197–198.

Temkin, O. "Greek Medicine as Science and Craft," *The Double Face of Janus.* Baltimore: Johns Hopkins Press, 1977.

Thomas, L. "Your Very Good Health," in *The Lives of a Cell.* New York: Viking Press, 1984, pp. 81–86.

Veatch, R. M. *A Theory of Medical Ethics.* New York: Basic Books, 1981.

2 THE PARADOX OF PERGAMON: GALEN

Brain, P. "Galen on the Ideal of the Physician." *S. Afr. Med. J.* 25(II):936–938 (1977).

———. *Galen on Bloodletting: A Study of the Origins, Development and Validity of His Opinions, with a Translation of the Three Works.* New York: Cambridge Univ. Press, 1986.

King, L. S. *Medical Thinking.* Princeton: Princeton Univ. Press, 1982.

Kudlein, F. "The Third Century A.D.—A Blank Spot in the History of Medicine?" In L. G. Stevenson and R. F. Multhauf, *Medicine, Science, and Culture.* Baltimore: Johns Hopkins Press, 1968.

Leiber, E. "Galen: Physician as Philosopher; Maimonides: Philosopher as Physician." *Bull. Hist. Med.* 53:268–285 (1979).

May, M. T. *Galen on the Usefulness of the Parts of the Body.* Ithaca, N.Y.: Cornell Univ. Press, 1968.

Moon, R. O. "The Relation of Galen to the Philosophy of His Time." *Brit. Med. J.* 4:1449–1451 (1908).

Nutton, V. *Karl Gottlob Kühn and His Edition of the Works of Galen.* Oxford: Oxford Microform Pub., 1976.

———. "Galen in the Eyes of His Contemporaries." *Bull. Hist. Med.* 58:315–324 (1984).

Payne, J. F. *Harvey and Galen.* London: Henry Frowde, 1897.

Prendergast, J. S. "Galen's View of the Vascular System in Relation to That of Harvey." *Proc. Roy. Soc. Med.* 23:1839–1847 (1928).

———. "The Background of Galen's Life and Activities and Its Influence on His Achievements." *Proc. Roy. Soc. Med.* 21:1131–1148 (1930).

Price, D. deS. "The Development and Structure of the Biomedical Literature." In K. S. Warren, ed., *Coping With the Biomedical Literature.* New York: Praeger, 1981.

Riese, W. "The Structure of Galen's Diagnostic Reasoning." *Bull. N.Y. Acad. Med.* 44:778–791 (1968).

Sarton, G. *Galen of Pergamon.* Lawrence: Univ. of Kansas Press, 1954.

Siegal, R. E. *Galen's System of Physiology and Medicine.* Basel: S. Karger, 1968.

Singer, C. *Greek Biology and Greek Medicine.* Oxford: Clarendon Press, 1922.

———. *The Evolution of Anatomy.* New York: Knopf, 1925.

———. *Galen and Anatomical Procedures.* London: Geoffrey Cumberlege, 1956.

Slater, P. E. Letter to the editor. *N. Eng. J. Med.* 313:455 (1985).

Smith, W. O. *The Hippocratic Tradition.* Ithaca, N.Y.: Cornell Univ. Press, 1979.

Temkin, O. *Galenism: Rise and Decline of a Medical Philosophy.* Ithaca, N.Y.: Cornell Univ. Press, 1973.

———. "On Galen's Pneumatology," *The Double Face of Janus.* Baltimore: Johns Hopkins Press, 1977.

Toledo-Pereyra, L. H. "Galen's Contribution to Surgery." *J. Hist. Med.* 28:357–375 (1973).

Walsh, J. "Galen's Discovery and Promulgation of the Function of the Recurrent Laryngeal Nerves." *Ann. Med. Hist.* 8:176–184 (1926).

———. "Galen Clashes with the Medical Sects at Rome." *Med. Life* 35:408–443 (1928).

———. "Galen's Writings and Influences Inspiring Them." *Ann. Med. Hist.* 6(N.S.):1–30, 143–149 (1934); 7(N.S.):428–437, 570–589 (1935); 8(N.S.):65–90 (1936); 9(N.S.):34–51 (1937).

Walzer, R. *Galen on Jews and Christians.* London: Oxford Univ. Press, 1949.

Wilson, L. G. "Erasistratus, Galen, and the Pneuma." *Bull. Hist. Med.* 33:293–314 (1959).

3 THE REAWAKENING: ANDREAS VESALIUS AND THE RENAISSANCE OF MEDICINE

Castiglione, A. "Three Pathfinders of Science in the Renaissance." *Bull. Med. Lib. Ass.* 31:203–207 (1943).

Chastel, A. "Treatise on Painting." In L. Reti, *The Unknown Leonardo.* New York: McGraw-Hill, 1974.

Cushing, H. *A Biobibliography of Andreas Vesalius.* 2nd ed. London: Archon, 1962.

Edelstein, L. "Andreas Vesalius, the Humanist." *Bull. Hist. Med.* 14:547–561 (1943).

Fisch, M. H. "Vesalius and His Book." *Bull. Med. Lib. Ass.* 31:208–221 (1943).

Garrison, F. H. "In Defense of Vesalius." *Bull. Soc. Med. Hist. Chicago* 4:47–65 (1916).

Hoolihan, C. "The Transmission of Greek Medical Literature from Antiquity to the Renaissance." *Med. Heritage* 2:430–442 (1985).

Jones, T. "The Artists of Vesalius' Fabrica." *Bull. Med. Lib. Ass.* 31:222–227 (1943).

Keele, K. D. "Leonardo da Vinci's Influence on Renaissance Anatomy." *Med. Hist.* 8:360–370 (1964).

Klebs, A. C. "Leonardo da Vinci and His Anatomical Studies." *Bull. Soc. Hist. Med. Chicago* 4:66–83 (1916).

Lambert, S. W., Wiegand, W., and Ivins, W. M. *Three Vesalian Essays.* New York: Macmillan, 1952.

O'Malley, C. D. *Andreas Vesalius of Brussels.* Berkeley: Univ. of Cal. Press, 1964.

———. "Andreas Vesalius (1514–1564), In Memoriam." *Med. Hist.* 8:299–308 (1964).

———, and Saunders, J. B. de C. M. *Leonardo da Vinci on the Human Body.* New York: Henry Schuman, 1952.

Petrucelli, R. J. "Giorgio Vasari's Attribution of the Vesalian Illustrations to Jan Stephan of Calcar: A Further Examination." *Bull. Hist. Med.* 45:29–37 (1971).

Roth, M. *Andreas Vesalius Bruxellensis*. Berlin: Georg Reimer, 1892.

Saunders, J. B. de C. M., and O'Malley, C. D. *The Illustrations from the Works of Andreas Vesalius of Brussels*. Cleveland: World, 1950.

Schultz, B. *Art and Anatomy in Renaissance Italy*. Ann Arbor: UMI Research Press, 1982.

Sigerist, H. E. "Commemorating Andreas Vesalius." *Bull. Hist. Med.* 14:541–546 (1943).

Singer, C. *The Evolution of Anatomy*. New York: Knopf, 1925.

Streeter, E. C. "Vesalius at Paris." *Yale J. Biol. Med.* 16:121–128 (1943).

Vesalius, A. *The Epitome of His Book on the Fabric of the Human Body*. Trans. by L. R. Lind. New York: Macmillian, 1949.

Washburn, W. H. "Galen, Vesalius, Da Vinci—Anatomists. *Bull. Soc. Med. Hist. Chicago* 4:1–17 (1916).

Zilboorg, G. "Psychological Sidelights on Andreas Vesalius." *Bull. Hist. Med.* 14:562–575 (1943).

4   THE GENTLE SURGEON: AMBROISE PARÉ

Anson, B. J. "The Ear and the Eye in the *Collected Works of Ambroise Paré*, Renaissance Surgeon to Four Kings of France." *Trans. Am. Acad. Ophthal. Otol.* 74:249–277 (1970).

Doe, J. *A Bibliography of the Works of Ambroise Paré*. Chicago: Univ. of Chicago Press, 1937.

Garrison, F. H. *An Introduction to the History of Medicine*. 4th ed. Philadelphia: Saunders, 1929.

Gibson, T. "The Prostheses of Ambroise Paré." *Brit. J. Plast. Surg.* 8: 3–8 (1955).

Hamby, W. B., ed. The Case Reports and Autopsy Records of Ambroise Paré. Springfield: Charles C. Thomas, 1960.

——. *Ambroise Paré, Surgeon of the Renaissance*. St. Louis: Warren H. Green, 1967.

Hill, B. H. "Ambroise Paré: Sawbones or Scientist." *J. Hist. Med.* 15: 45–58 (1960).

Malgaigne, J. F. *Surgery and Ambroise Paré*. Trans. by W. B. Hamby. Norman: Univ. of Oklahoma Press, 1965.

Packard, F. R. *Life and Times of Ambroise Paré*. New York: Paul B. Hoeber, 1921.

Paré, A. *The Workes of That Famous Chirurgeon Ambrose Parey*. Trans. by T. Johnson. London: Cotes and Young, 1634.

——. *The Apologie and Treatise*. Trans. by G. Keynes. London: Falcon Educational Books, 1951. (Birmingham: Classics of Medicine Lib., 1984.)

——. *Ten Books of Surgery with the Magazine of Instruments Necessary for It*. Trans. by R. W. Linker and N. Womack. Athens: Univ. of Georgia Press, 1969.

Sigerist, H. E. "Ambroise Paré's Onion Treatment of Burns." *Bull. Hist. Med.* 15:143–149 (1944).

Singer, D. W. *Selections from the Works of Ambroise Paré*. London: John Bale Sons and Danielsson, 1924.

Wangensteen, O. H., Wangensteen, S. D., and Klinger, C. F. "Wound Management of Ambroise Paré and Dominique Larrey, Great French Military Surgeons of the 16th and 19th Centuries." *Bull. Hist. Med.* 46:207–234 (1972).

5   "NATURE HERSELF MUST BE OUR ADVISOR": WILLIAM HARVEY'S DISCOVERY OF THE CIRCULATION OF THE BLOOD

Bylebyl, J. "The Growth of Harvey's *De Motu Cordis*." *Bull. Hist. Med.* 47:427–470 (1973).

——. "William Harvey, a Conventional Medical Revolutionary." *J.A.M.A.* 239:1295–1298 (1978).

——. *William Harvey and His Age: The Professional and Social Context of the Discovery of the Circulation*. Baltimore: Johns Hopkins Press, 1979.

Cohen, B. "The Germ of an Idea, or, What Put Harvey on the Scent?" *J. Hist. Med.* 12:102–105 (1957).

Comroe, J. H. "Harvey's 1651 Perfusion of the Pulmonary Circulation of Man." *Circulation* 65:1–3 (1982).

Franklin, K. J. "On Translating Harvey." *J. Hist. Med.* 12:114–119 (1957).

——. *William Harvey, Englishman*. London: MacGibbon and Kee, 1961.

Fulton, J. F. *Michael Servetus, Humanist and Martyr*. New York: Herbert Reichner, 1953.

Graham, P. W. "Harvey's *De Motu Cordis*: The Rhetoric of Science." *J. Hist. Med.* 33:469–476 (1977).

Harvey, W. *Anatomical Studies on the Motion of the Heart and Blood*. Trans. by Chauncey D. Leake. Springfield: Charles C. Thomas, 1931.

——. *Anatomical Studies on the Motion of the Heart and Blood*. Trans. by G. Keynes. Birmingham: Classics of Medicine Lib., 1978.

Herringham, W. *Circumstances in the Life and Times of William Harvey*. Oxford Univ. Press, 1929.

Jones, A. M. "Dogma and Experiment in Harvey's Time." *Brit. Ht. J.* 19:448–456 (1957).

Keele, K. D. "William Harvey: The Man and the College of Physicians." *Med. Hist.* 1:265–278 (1957).

——. *William Harvey, the Man, the Physician, and the Scientist*. London: Thos. Nelson & Sons, 1965.

Keynes, G. L. *The Personality of William Harvey*. Cambridge: Cambridge Univ. Press, 1949.

——. *The Life of William Harvey*. Oxford: Oxford Univ. Press, 1966.

O'Malley, C. D. *Michael Servetus*. Philadelphia: Am. Phil. Soc., 1953.

Osler, W. *The Growth of Truth as Illustrated in the Discovery of the Circulation of the Blood*. Harveian Oration, 1906. London: Henry Frowde, 1906.

Pagel, W. "The Philosophy of Circles—Cesalpino-Harvey." *J. Hist. Med.* 12:140–157 (1957).

——. *William Harvey's Biological Ideas: Selected Aspects and Historical Background*. New York: Hafner, 1967.

Payne, L. M. "Sir Charles Scarburgh's Harveian Oration, 1662." *J. Hist. Med.* 12:158–164 (1957).

Pickering, G. "William Harvey, Physician and Scientist." *Brit. Med. J.* 2:1615–1619 (1964).

Power, D. *William Harvey*. New York: Longmans, Green, 1897.

Sigerist, H. E. "William Harvey's Position in the History of European Thought." In F. Marti-Ibañez, ed., *Henry E. Sigerist on the History of Medicine*. MD Publications, 1960.

Whitteridge, G. *William Harvey and the Circulation of the Blood*. London: MacDonald, 1971.

Zeman, F. D. "The Old Age of William Harvey." *Arch. Int. Med.* 111: 829–834 (1963).

6   THE NEW MEDICINE: THE ANATOMICAL CONCEPT OF GIOVANNI MORGAGNI

Bell, W. J. *John Morgan, Continental Doctor*. Philadelphia: Univ. of Pa. Press, 1965.

Castiglioni, A. "G. B. Morgagni and the Anatomico-Pathological Conception of the Clinic." *Proc. Roy. Soc. Med.* 28:375–378 (1934).

Gairdner, W. T. "The Progress of Pathology." *Brit. Med. J.* 2:515–517 (1874).

Jarcho, S. "Giovanni Battista Morgagni: His Interests, Ideas, and Achievements." *Bull. Hist. Med.* 22:503–527 (1948).

——. "Morgagni and Auenbrugger in the Retrospect of Two Hundred Years." *Bull. Hist. Med.* 35:489–496 (1961).

——. *The Clinical Consultations of Giambattista Morgagni*. Boston: Francis A. Countway Lib. of Med., 1984.

Klemperer, P. "Pathologic Anatomy at the End of the Eighteenth Century." *J. Mt. Sinai Hosp.* 24:589–603 (1957).

——. "The Pathology of Morgagni and Virchow." *Bull. Hist. Med.* 32:24–38 (1958).

——. "Morbid Anatomy Before and After Morgagni." *Bull. N. Y. Acad. Med.* 37:741–760 (1961).

Morgagni, G. B. *The Seats and Causes of Diseases Investigated by Anatomy*. Trans. by B. Alexander. London: Millar and Cadell, 1769. (Birmingham: Classics of Medicine Lib., 1983.)

Morgan, J. *The Journal of Dr. John Morgan*. Philadelphia: Lippincott, 1907.

Nuland, S. B. *Giovanni Morgagni and the New Medicine*. Birmingham: Classics of Medicine Lib., 1983.

Pottle, F. A. *James Boswell, The Earlier Years: 1740–1769*. New York: McGraw-Hill, 1966.

Steven, J. L. *Morgagni to Virchow: An Epoch in the History of Medicine*. Glasgow: Alexander MacDougall, 1905.

Tedeschi, C. G. "Giovanni Battista Morgagni, the Founder of Pathologic Anatomy." *Boston Med. Quart.* 12:112–125 (1961).

——. The Pathology of Bonet and Morgagni: A Historical Introduction to the Autopsy." *Hum. Path.* 5:601–603 (1974).

Virchow, R. "Morgagni and the Anatomic Concept." Translation. *Bull. Hist. Med.* 7:975–990 (1939).

Yonace, A. H. "Morgagni's Letters." *J. Roy. Soc. Med.* 73:145–149 (1980).

7 "WHY THE LEAVES CHANGED COLOR IN THE AUTUMN": SURGERY, SCIENCE, AND JOHN HUNTER

Adams, J. *Memoirs of the Life and Doctrines of the Late John Hunter, Esq.* London: J. Callow & J. Hunter, 1818.

Austin, F., and Jones, B. "William Clift: The Surgeon's Apprentice." *Ann. Roy. Coll. Surg.* 60:261–265 (1978).

Beekman, F. "The Self-Education of Young John Hunter." *J. Hist. Med.* 6:506–515 (1951).

Brain, R. "The Neurology of John Hunter's Last Illness." *Brit. Med. J.* 2:1371–1373 (1952).

Cushing, H. W., and others. "Exercises in Celebration of the Bicentenary of the Birth of John Hunter." *New Eng. J. Med.* 200:810–823 (1929).

Dempster, W. J. "Towards a New Understanding of John Hunter." *Lancet* 1:316–318 (1978).

Dobson, J. *William Clift.* London: Heinemann, 1954.

——. "John Hunter's Artists." *Med. Biol. Illustr.* 9:138–143 (1959).

——. "John Hunter's Views on Cancer." *Ann. Roy. Coll. Surg.* 25:176–181 (1959).

——. "The Training of a Surgeon." *Ann. Roy. Coll. Surg.* 34:1–36 (1964).

——. *John Hunter.* Edinburgh: E. & S. Livingstone, 1969.

Foot, J. *The Life of John Hunter.* London: T. Becket, 1794.

Forbes, T. R. "Testis Transplantations Performed by John Hunter." *Endocrinology* 41:329–331 (1947).

——. "John Hunter as Expert Witness." *Trans. and Stud. Coll. Phys. Phila.* (Ser. V) 2:75–80 (1980).

Gask, G. E. "John Hunter in the Campaign in Portugal." *Brit. J. Surg.* 24:640–668 (1937).

Gloyne, S. R. *John Hunter.* London: E. & S. Livingstone, 1950.

Gross, S. D. *John Hunter and His Pupils.* Philadelphia: Presley Blakiston, 1881.

Hamilton, H. W. "William Combe and John Hunter's Essay on the Teeth." *J. Hist. Med.* 14:169–178 (1959).

Holmes, T. *Introductory Address, Centenary of John Hunter's Death.* London: Adlard & Son, 1893.

Hunter, I. "Syphilis in the Illness of John Hunter." *J. Hist. Med.* 8:249–262 (1953).

Hunter, J. *A Treatise on the Blood, Inflammation and Gunshot Wounds.* London: George Nicol, 1794. (Birmingham: Classics of Medicine Lib., 1982.)

Jarcho, S. "John Hunter on Inflammation." *Am. J. Cardiol.* 26:615–618 (1970).

Jones, F. W. "John Hunter and the Medical Student." *St. George's Hosp. Gaz.* 37:1–8 (1951).

——. "John Hunter as a Geologist." *Ann. Roy. Coll. Surg.* 12:219–245 (1953).

Keith, A. "The Portraits and Personality of John Hunter." *Brit. Med. J.* 1:205–209 (1928).

Le Fanu, W. R. "John Hunter's Letters." *Bull. Med. Lib. Ass.* 33:449–454 (1945).

Lewis, G. P. "Inflammation with Emphasis on its Mediation." *Ann. Roy. Coll. Surg.* 60:192–201 (1978).

Livesley, B. "The Spasms of John Hunter: A New Interpretation." *Med. Hist.* 17:70–75 (1973).

Makins, G. H. "Influence Exerted by the Military Experience of John Hunter on Himself and the Military Surgeon of Today." *Lancet* 1:249–254 (1917).

Mather, G. R. *Two Great Scotsmen: The Brothers William and John Hunter.* Glasgow: James Maclehose & Sons, 1893.

Nuland, S. B. *Nature's High Priest, John Hunter.* Birmingham: Classics of Surgery Lib., 1985.

Oppenheimer, J. L. "Everard Home and the Destruction of the John Hunter Manuscripts," *New Aspects of John and William Hunter.* New York: Henry Schuman, 1946.

Ottley, D. *The Life of John Hunter, F.R.S.* Philadelphia: Haswell, Barrington & Haswell, 1841.

Paget, S. *John Hunter, Man of Science and Surgeon.* London: T. Fisher Unwin, 1897.

Poynter, F. N. L. "Hunter, Spallanzani, and the History of Artificial Insemination." In L. G. Stevenson and R. P. Multhauf, *Medicine, Science, & Culture.* Baltimore: Johns Hopkins Press, 1968.

Qvist, G. "John Hunter's Alleged Syphilis." *Ann. Roy. Coll. Surg.* 59: 205–209 (1977).

——. *John Hunter, 1728–1793.* London: Heinemann, 1981.

Schwartz, L. L. "John Hunter and the Physiological Basis of Dental Practice." *J. Am. Coll. Dent.* 20:160–170 (1953).

Stevenson, L. G. "The Elder Spence, William Combe, and John Hunter: Sidelights on Eighteenth Century Dentistry and Hunter's Natural History of the Human Teeth." *J. Hist. Med.* 10:182–196 (1955).

Taylor, T. *Leicester Square, Its Associations and Its Worthies.* London: Bickers & Son, 1874.

Viets, H. "A Note on John Hunter at Oxford." *Bost. Med. Surg. J.* 182:545–547 (1920).

Weimerskirch, P. J., and Richter, G. W. "Hunter and Venereal Disease." *Lancet* 1:503–504 (1979).

8 "WITHOUT DIAGNOSIS THERE IS NO RATIONAL TREATMENT": RENÉ LAENNEC, INVENTOR OF THE STETHOSCOPE

Ackerknecht, E. H. "Elisha Bartlett and the Philosophy of the Paris Clinical School." *Bull. Hist. Med.* 24:43–60 (1950).

——. *Medicine at the Paris Hospital, 1794–1848.* Baltimore: Johns Hopkins Press, 1967.

Alcock, J. R. *Medical Guide to Paris—A Description of the Principal Hospitals of Paris.* London: Burgess & Hill, 1828.

Bedford, E. "Cardiology in the Days of Laennec." *Brit. Ht. J.* 34:1193–1198 (1972).

Bishop, P. J. "Evolution of the Stethoscope." *J. Roy. Soc. Med.* 73:448–456 (1980).

——. "Reception of the Stethoscope and Laennec's Book." *Thorax* 36:487–492 (1981).

Cawadias, A. P. "Corvisart and His Role in the History of Clinical Science and of the Art of Medicine." In E. A. Underwood, ed., *Science Medicine and History,* vol. 2. London: Oxford Univ. Press, 1953.

Corvisart, J. N. *An Essay on the Organic Diseases and Lesions of the Heart and Great Vessels.* Trans. by J. Gates. Boston, 1812. (Includes Auenbrugger's On Percussion of the Chest, 1761.)

Coues, W. P. "Laennec, the Man—1781–1826." *Boston Med. Surg. J.* 195:208–217 (1926).

Fessel, W. J. "The Nature of Illness and Diagnosis." *Am. J. Med.* 75:555–560 (1983).

Hale-White, W. *Selected Passages from De l'Auscultation Médiate, with a Biography.* London: John Bale, Sons & Danielsson, 1923.

Hooke, R. "The Method of Improving Natural Philosophy," *The Posthumous Works of Robert Hooke,* ed. by Richard Waller. London: Samuel Smith and Richard Walford, 1705. (Sources of Science Series, No. 73, London, Johnson Reprint Co.)

Jarcho, S. "Auenbrugger, Laennec, and John Keats." *Med. Hist.* 5:167–172 (1961).

——. "An Early Review of Laennec's Treatise." *Am. J. Cardiol.* 9:962–969 (1961).

Jones, R. M. *The Parisian Education of an American Surgeon.* Philadelphia: Am. Phil. Soc., 1978.

Keele, K. D. *The Evolution of Clinical Methods in Medicine.* Springfield: Charles C. Thomas, 1963.

Kervran, R. *Laennec, His Life and Times.* Oxford: Pergamon, 1960.

Laennec, R. T. H. *A Treatise on Diseases of the Chest.* Trans. by J. Forbes. London: Underwood, 1821. (Birmingham: Classics of Medicine Lib., 1979.)

Lee, E. *Observations on the Principal Medical Institutions and Practice of France, Italy and Germany.* Philadelphia: Haswell, Barrington, & Haswell, 1837.

Le Fanu, W. R. "Laennec and Matthew Baillie." *Ann. Roy. Coll. Surg.* 36:67–68 (1965).

Mann, R. J., and Mann, F. D. "Laennec as a Critical Pathologist." *J. Hist. Med.* 36:446–454 (1981).

Maulitz, R. C. "Channel Crossing: The Lure of French Pathology for English Medical Students, 1816–1836." *Bull. Hist. Med.* 55:475–496 (1981).

——. *Morbid Appearances, The Anatomy of Pathology in the Early Nineteenth Century.* New York: Cambridge Univ. Press, 1987.

Norwood, W. F. "Medical Education and the Rise of Hospitals." *J.A.M.A.* 186:1008–1012 (1963).

Osler, W. "The Young Laennec." *Can. Med. Ass. J.* 3:137–141 (1913).

Reiser, S. J. *Medicine and the Reign of Technology.* Cambridge: Cambridge Univ. Press, 1978.

Sakula, A. "Laennec's Influence on Some British Physicians in the Nineteenth Century." *J. Roy. Soc. Med.* 74:759–767 (1981).

Segall, H. N. "Cardiovascular Sounds and the Stethoscope, 1816–2016." *Canad. Med. Ass. J.* 88:308–318 (1963).

Stewart, F. C. *The Hospitals and Surgeons of Paris.* New York: J. & H. G. Langley, 1843.

Thayer, W. S. "On Some Unpublished Letters of Laennec." *Johns Hopkins Hosp. Bull.* 31:425–435 (1920).

Webb, G. B. "René Théophile Hyacinthe Laennec." *Ann. Med. Hist.* 9:27–59 (1927).

——. *René Théophile Hyacinthe Laennec: A Memoir.* New York: Paul B. Hoeber, 1928.

9 THE GERM THEORY BEFORE GERMS: THE ENIGMA OF IGNAC SEMMELWEIS

Benedek, I. *Ignaz Philipp Semmelweis, 1818–1865.* Vienna: Böhlau, 1983.

Billroth, T. *The Medical Sciences in the German Universities.* New York: Macmillan, 1924.

Carter, K. C., ed. *Ignac Semmelweis: The Etiology, Concept, and Prophylaxis of Childbed Fever.* Madison: Univ. of Wisconsin Press, 1983.

Gortvay, G., and Zoltàn, I. *Semmelweis, His Life and Work.* Budapest: Hungarian Acad. Sci., 1968.

Gyorgyey, F. A. "Puerperal Fever 1847–1861." M.S. thesis. Yale Univ., 1968.

Haranghy, L., Nyiro, G., Regoly-Merei, G., and Hüttel, T. *Die Krankheit von Semmelweis.* Budapest: Medicina Verlag, 1965.

Holmes, O. W. "The Contagiousness of Puerperal Fever," *Medical Essays.* Boston: Houghton, Mifflin, 1895.

Klemperer, P. "Notes on Carl von Rokitansky's Autobiography and Inaugural Address." *Bull. Hist. Med.* 35:374–380 (1961).

Lesky, E. *The Vienna Medical School of the 19th Century.* Baltimore: Johns Hopkins Press, 1976.

Menne, F. R. "Carl Rokitansky the Pathologist." *Ann. Med. Hist.* 7:379–386 (1925).

Nuland, S. B. "The Enigma of Semmelweis: An Interpretation." *J. Hist. Med.* 34:255–272 (1979).

Semmelweiss, I. P. *The Etiology, the Concept and the Prophylaxis of Childbed Fever.* Trans. by F. P. Murphy. Birmingham: Classics of Medicine Lib., 1981. (Includes *The Open Letters*, trans. by S. B. Nuland and F. A. Gyorgyey.)

Silló-Seidl, G. *Die Affaire Semmelweis.* Vienna: Herold Verlag, 1985.

Sinclair, W. *Semmelweis—His Life and His Doctrine.* Manchester, 1909.

Slaughter, F. G. *Immortal Magyar.* New York: Schuman, 1950.

10 SURGERY WITHOUT PAIN: THE ORIGINS OF GENERAL ANESTHESIA

Bigelow, H. J. "Insensibility During Surgical Operations Produced by Inhalation." *Boston Med. Surg. J.* 35:309–317 (1846).

Carmichael, E. B. "Crawford Williamson Long—Discoverer of Surgical Anesthesia." *J. Med. Ass. Ala.* 36:843–857 (1967).

Cartwright, F. F. "Humphry Davy's Contribution to Anesthesia." *Proc. Roy. Soc. Med.* 43:571–578 (1950).

——. *The English Pioneers of Anesthesia (Beddoes, Davy and Hickman).* Bristol: Wright, 1952.

Cole, F. *Milestones in Anesthesia: Readings in the Development of Surgical Anesthesia, 1665–1940.* Lincoln: Univ. of Nebraska, 1965.

Duncum, B. M. *The Development of Inhalation Anesthesia.* London: Oxford Univ. Press, 1947.

Elliotson, J. *Numerous Cases of Surgical Operations Without Pain in the Mesmeric State.* London: H. Bailliere, 1843.

Ellis, E. S. *Ancient Anodynes.* London: Heinemann, 1946.

Ellis, R. H. "The Introduction of Ether Anaesthesia to Great Britain. 1: How the News Was Carried from Boston, Massachusetts, to Gower Street, London." *Anaesthesia* 31:766–777 (1976).

——. "The Introduction of Ether Anaesthesia to Great Britain. 2: A Biographical Sketch of Dr. Francis Boott." *Anaesthesia* 32:197–208 (1977).

Esdaile, J. *Mesmerism in India.* London: Longman, Brown, Green & Longmans, 1846.

Faulconer, A., and Keys, E. *Foundations of Anesthesiology.* Springfield: Charles C. Thomas, 1965.

Greene, N. M. "A Consideration of Factors in the Discovery of Anesthesia and Their Effects on Its Development." *Anesthesiology* 35:515–522 (1971).

——. "Anesthesia and the Development of Surgery." *Anesth. Analg.* 58:5–12 (1979).

Hickman, H. H. *A Letter on Suspended Animation Addressed to T. A. Knight, Esq.* Ironbridge: W. Smith, 1824.

Jackson, C. T. "Etherization of Animals and of Man." *Trans. Am. Inst. City of N.Y. for 1851,* Albany, 167–173, 1852.

Keys, T. E. *The History of Surgical Anesthesia.* New York: Henry Schuman, 1945.

——. "The Early Pneumatic Chemists and Physicians—Their Influence on the Development of Surgical Anesthesia." *Anesthesiology* 30:447–462 (1969).

Long, C. W. "An Account of the First Use of Sulphuric Ether by Inhalation as an Anesthetic in Surgical Operations." *South. Med. Surg. J.* 5:705–713 (1849).

Miller, A. H. "The Origin of the Word 'Anesthesia.'" *Boston Med. Surg. J.* 197:1218–1222 (1927).

Morton, W. T. G. *Remarks on the Proper Mode of Administering Sulfuric Ether by Inhalation.* Boston: Dutton & Wentworth, 1847.

Nuland, S. B. *The Origins of Anesthesia.* Birmingham: Classics of Medicine Lib., 1983.

Raper, H. R. "A Review of the Crawford W. Long Centennial Anniversary Celebration." *J. Am. Coll. Dent.* 10:137–154 (1943).

——. *Man Against Pain.* New York: Prentice-Hall, 1945.

Robinson, V. *Victory Over Pain: A History of Anesthesia.* New York: Henry Schuman, 1946.

Rosen, G. "Mesmerism and Surgery." *J. Hist. Med.* 1:527–550 (1946).

Singer, C. *Greek Biology and Greek Medicine.* London: Oxford Univ. Press, 1922.

Smith, W. D. "A History of Nitrous Oxide and Oxygen Anaesthesia: The Discovery of Nitrous Oxide and Oxygen." *Brit. J. Anaesth.* 44:297–304 (1972).

——. "A History of Nitrous Oxide and Oxygen Anaesthesia: Henry Hill Hickman in His Time." *Brit. J. Anaesth.* 50:519–530, 623–627, 853–861 (1978).

Stevenson, L. G. "Suspended Animation in the History of Anesthesia." *Bull. Hist. Med.* 49:482–511 (1975).

Tallmadge, G. K. "Some Anesthetics of Antiquity." *J. Hist. Med.* 1:515–520 (1946).

Taylor, F. L. *C. W. Long and Ether Anesthesia.* New York: Paul B. Hoeber, 1928.

Viets, H. R. "The Earliest Printed References in Newspapers and Journals to the First Public Demonstration of Ether Anesthesia in 1846." *J. Hist. Med.* 4:149–169 (1949).

Warren, J. C. "Inhalation of Ethereal Vapor for the Prevention of Pain in Surgical Operations." *Boston Med. Surg. J.* 35:375–379 (1846).

——. "The Influence of Anesthesia on the Surgery of the Nineteenth Century." *Trans. Am. Surg. Ass.* 15:1–25 (1897). (Boston: Merrymount Press, 1906.)

Welch, W. H. "The Influence of Anesthesia Upon Medical Science." *Boston Med. Surg. J.* 135:401–403 (1896).

——. "A Consideration of the Introduction of Surgical Anesthesia." *Boston Med. Surg. J.* 159:599–604 (1908).

Wells, H. *A History of the Discovery of the Application of Nitrous Oxide Gas, Ether and Other Vapors to Surgical Operations.* Hartford: J. Gaylord Wells, 1847.

Young, H. H. "Crawford W. Long: The Pioneer in Ether Anesthesia." *Bull. Hist. Med.* 12:191–225 (1942).

Youngson, A. J. *The Scientific Revolution in Victorian Medicine.* New York: Holmes & Meier, 1979.

11 THE FUNDAMENTAL UNIT OF LIFE: SICK CELLS, MICROSCOPES, AND RUDOLF VIRCHOW

Ackerknecht, E. H. *Rudolf Virchow—Doctor, Statesman, Anthropologist.* Madison: Univ. of Wisconsin Press, 1953.

Bamforth, J., and Osborn, G. R. "Diagnosis from Cells." *J. Clin. Path.* 11:473–482 (1958).

Craig, G. A. *Germany, 1866–1945.* New York: Oxford Univ. Press, 1978.

Gardner, L. J. "Doctors Afield—Rudolf Virchow." *New Eng. J. Med.* 252:587–589 (1955).

Goldman, L. "War and Science—Rudolf Virchow." *Ann. Med. Hist.* (N.S.) 8:558–561 (1936).

Holmes, F. L. "The Milieu Intérieur and the Cell Theory." *Bull. Hist. Med.* 37:315–335 (1963).

Krumbhaar, E. B. "The Centenary of the Cell Doctrine." *Ann. Med. Hist.* (3S) 1:427–437 (1939).

Long, E. R. *A History of Pathology.* New York: Dover, 1965.

Mann, G. *The History of Germany Since 1789.* New York: Praeger, 1968.

McFarland, J. "Personal Reminiscences of Virchow." *Phila. Med. J.* Sept. 13, 1902, 361–362.

Mendelsohn, E. "Cell Theory and the Development of General Physiology." *Archives Internationales d'Histoire des Sciences* 16:419–429 (1963).

Osler, W. "Rudolf Virchow: The Man and the Student." *Boston Med. Surg. J.* 125:425–427 (1891).

Pagel, W. "The Speculative Basis of Modern Pathology." *Bull. Hist. Med.* 18:1–43 (1945).

Plaut, A. "Rudolf Virchow and Today's Physicians and Scientists." *Bull. Hist. Med.,* 27:236–251, 1953.

Pridan, D. "Rudolf Virchow and Social Medicine in Historical Perspective." *Med. Hist.* 8:274–278 (1964).

Rather, L. J. "Rudolf Virchow and Scientific Medicine." *Arch. Int. Med.* 100:1007–1014 (1957).

———. "Harvey, Virchow, Bernard, and the Methodology of Science." In R. Virchow, *Disease, Life, and Man.* Trans. by L. J. Rather. Palo Alto: Stanford Univ. Press, 1958.

———. "Rudolf Virchow's Views on Pathology, Pathological Anatomy, and Cellular Pathology." *Arch. Path.* 82:197–204 (1966).

———. *The Genesis of Cancer: A Study in the History of Ideas.* Baltimore: Johns Hopkins Press, 1978.

Rosen, G., and Caspari-Rosen, B. *400 Years of a Doctor's Life.* New York: Henry Schuman, 1947.

Schleich, C. L. *Those Were Good Days!* London: Allen & Unwin, 1935.

Schlumberger, H. G. "Rudolf Virchow, Revolutionist." *Ann. Med. Hist.* (3S) 4:147–153 (1942).

———. "Rudolf Virchow and the Franco-Prussian War." *Ann. Med. Hist.* (3S) 4:253–267 (1942).

Semon, F. "The Celebration of Rudolf Virchow's 80th Birthday: A Personal Impression." *Brit. Med. J.,* Oct. 19, 1901.

———. "Some Personal Reminiscences of Rudolf Virchow." *Brit. Med. J.,* Sept. 13, 1902, 800–802.

Virchow, R. *Cellular Pathology.* Trans. from 2nd ed. by F. Chance. London: John Churchill, 1860.

———. *Collected Essays on Public Health and Epidemiology.* Trans. by L. J. Rather from 1879 edition (Berlin: August Hirschwald). Canton, Mass.: Science Hist. Pub., 1985.

Welch, W. H. "Rudolf Virchow, Pathologist." *Boston Med. Surg. J.* 125:453–457 (1891).

Wilson, J. W. "Virchow's Contribution to the Cell Theory." *J. Hist. Med.* 2:163–178 (1947).

12 "To Tend the Fleshly Tabernacle of the Immortal Spirit": Joseph Lister's Antiseptic Surgery

Brinton, H. H. *Friends for 300 Years.* Philadelphia: Pendle Hill Publications, 1965.

Bullock, W. "Lister as a Pathologist and Bacteriologist." *Brit. Med J.* 2:654–656 (1927).

Cameron, H. C. *Reminiscences of Lister and of His Work in the Wards of the Glasgow Royal Infirmary, 1860–1869.* Glasgow: Jackson, Wylie, 1927.

Churchill, E. D. "Healing by First Intention and with Suppuration: Studies in the History of Wound Healing." *J. Hist. Med.* 19:193–214 (1964).

Edgar, I. I. "Modern Surgery and Lord Lister." *J. Hist. Med.* 16:145–160 (1961).

Fisher, R. B. *Joseph Lister.* New York: Stein & Day, 1977.

Ford, W. W. "The Bacteriological Work of Joseph Lister." *Scientific Monthly* 26:70–75 (1927).

Garrison, F. H. "Lister in Relation to the Victorian Background." *Bull. N.Y. Acad. Med.* 4:167–172 (1928).

Glenn, W. W. L. "Some Evidence of the Influence of the Development of Aseptic Techniques on Surgical Practice." *Surgery* 43:688–698 (1958).

Godlee, R. J. *Lord Lister.* Oxford: Clarendon, 1924.

Greene, N. M. "Anesthesia and the Development of Surgery (1846–1896)." *Anesth. Analg.* 58:5–12 (1979).

Howie, W. B., and Black, S. A. B. "A Patient's Account of Lister's Care." *J. Hist. Med.* 32:239–251 (1977).

Judd, C. C. W. "The Life and Work of Lister." Lister Prize Essay. *Bull. Johns Hopkins Hosp.* 21:293–304 (1910).

Keen, W. W. "Before and After Lister," *Papers and Addresses.* Philadelphia: Geo. W. Jacobs, 1923.

Kelly, H. A. "Reminiscences in the Development of Gynecology." *J. Conn. State Med. Soc.* 1:459–467 (1937).

King, L. S. "Germ Theory and Its Influence." *J.A.M.A.* 249:794–798 (1983).

Leeson, J. R. *Lister As I Knew Him.* London: Bailliere, Tindall & Cox, 1927.

Linder, F., and Forrest, H. "The Propagation of Lister's Ideas." *Surg. Gyn. Obst.* 127:1081–1086 (1968).

Lister, J. *Introductory Lecture Delivered in the University of Edinburgh, Nov. 8, 1869.* Edinburgh: Edmonstone Douglas, 1869.

———. The Collected Papers of Joseph, Baron Lister. 2 vols. London: Clarendon, 1909.

Little, J. L. "Two Lectures on Lister's Antiseptic Method of Treating Surgical Injuries." In E. C. Seguin, ed., *A Series of American Clinical Lectures.* New York: Putnam, 1878.

Morton, J. J. "The Struggle Against Sepsis." *Yale J. Biol. Med.* 31:397–417 (1959).

Rains, A. H. J. *Joseph Lister and Antisepsis.* Hove: Priory Press, 1977.

Ravitch, M., and McAuley, C. E. "Airborne Contamination of the Operative Wound." *Surg. Gyn. Obst.* 159:177–188 (1984).

Richmond, P. A. "Variants to the Germ Theory of Disease." *J. Hist. Med.* 9:290–303 (1954).

———. "American Attitudes Toward the Germ Theory of Disease (1860–1880)." *J. Hist. Med.* 9:428–454 (1954).

Stewart, G. D. "Lister the Surgeon." *Bull. N.Y. Acad. Med.* 4:159–167 (1928).

Tait, J. "Lister as Physiologist." *Bull. N.Y. Acad. Med.* 4:148–159 (1928).

Tait, L. "The Germ Theory and Advances in Abdominal Surgery." *N. Y. Med. J.,* July 2, 1887, 1–7.

Thomson, St. C. "A House-Surgeon's Memories of Joseph Lister." *Ann. Med. Hist.* 2:93–108 (1919).

Toledo-Pereyra, L. H., and Toledo, M. M. "A Critical Study of Lister's Work on Antiseptic Surgery." *Am. J. Surg.* 131:736–744 (1976).

Treves, F. "The Old Receiving Room," *The Elephant Man and Other Reminiscences.* London: Cassell, 1923.

Turner, A. L. *Joseph, Baron Lister—Centenary Volume, 1827–1927.* Edinburgh, 1927.

Wangensteen, O. H. "Nineteenth Century Wound Management of the Parturient Uterus and Compound Fracture: The Semmelweis-Lister Priority Controversy." *Bull. N.Y. Acad. Med.* 46:565–592 (1970).

———, and Wangensteen, S. D. "Lister, His Books, and Evolvement of His Antiseptic Wound Practices." *Bull. Hist. Med.* 48:100–128 (1974).

Watson Cheyne, W. *Lister and His Achievement.* First Lister Oration. London: Longmans, Green, 1925.

Youngson, A. J. *The Scientific Revolution in Victorian Medicine.* New York: Holmes & Meier, 1979.

Also see:

Boston Med. Surg. J. 95:327–330 and 366–368 (1876) for account of Centennial Medical Congress.

Boston Evening Transcript, March 13, 1912, for interview of J. Collins Warren.

Times of London, Thursday, April 7, 1927, Health and Hygiene Number, Weekly Illustrated Edition.

13 MEDICAL SCIENCE COMES TO AMERICA: WILLIAM STEWART HALSTED OF JOHNS HOPKINS

Barnes, A. C. "A Comment on Historical 'Truth.'" *Persp. Biol. Med.* 21:131–138 (1977).

Becker, W. F. "Pioneers in Thyroid Surgery." *Ann. Surg.* 185:493–504 (1977).

Bloodgood, J. C. "Halsted Thirty-six Years Ago." *Am. J. Surg.* 14:89–148 (1931).

Chesney, A. M. *The Johns Hopkins Hospital and the Johns Hopkins University School of Medicine.* 2 vols. Baltimore: Johns Hopkins Press, 1943.

Colp, R. "Notes on Dr. William S. Halsted." *Bull. N.Y. Acad. Med.* 60:876–887 (1974).

Crowe, S. J. *Halsted of Johns Hopkins.* New York: Charles C. Thomas, 1957.

Cushing, H. W. "William Stewart Halsted, 1852–1922." *Science* 56:1452–1460 (1922).

——. *The Life of Sir William Osler.* 2 vols. Oxford: Clarendon Press, 1925.

Dumont, A. E. "Halsted at Bellevue—1883–1887." *Ann. Surg.* 172:929–935 (1970).

Finney, J. M. T. "A Personal Appreciation of Dr. Halsted." *Johns Hopkins Hosp. Bull.* 36:28–33 (1925).

——. "The Halsted Surgical Clinic." *Bull. Johns Hopkins Hosp.* 52: 106–113 (1933).

Flexner, S., and Flexner, J. T. *William H. Welch and the Heroic Age of American Medicine.* New York: Viking, 1941.

Fulton, J. F. *Harvey Cushing—a Biography.* Springfield: Charles C. Thomas, 1946.

Halsted, W. S. "Practical Comments on the Use and Abuse of Cocaine." *N.Y. Med. J.* 42:294–295 (1885).

——. *Surgical Papers.* 2 vols. Baltimore: Johns Hopkins Press, 1924.

Harvey, A. M. *Adventures in Medical Research: A Century of Discovery at Johns Hopkins.* Baltimore: Johns Hopkins Press, 1974.

——. *Research and Discovery in Medicine: Contributions from Johns Hopkins.* Baltimore: Johns Hopkins Press.

Harvey, S. C. "The Story of Harvey Cushing's Appendix." *Surgery* 32:501–514 (1952).

Henderson, W. O. "The Revival of Football at Yale." *Yale Alumni Weekly*, Jan. 11, 1924, 451.

Heuer, G. J. "Dr. Halsted." *Bull. Johns Hopkins Hosp.* 90:1–105 (1952).

Holman, E. "William Stewart Halsted as Revealed in His Letters." *Stanford Med. Bull.* 10:137–151 (1952).

——, and others. "William Stewart Halsted Centenary." *Surg.* 32:443–550 (1952).

Hughes, E. F. X. "Halsted and American Surgery." *Surg.* 75:169–177 (1974).

Lesky, E. *The Vienna Medical School of the 19th Century.* Baltimore: Johns Hopkins Press, 1976.

Lewison, E. F. "The Surgical Treatment of Breast Cancer: An Historical and Collective Review." *Surg.* 34:904–953 (1953).

Ludmerer, K. M. *Learning to Heal: The Development of American Medical Education.* New York: Basic Books, 1985.

MacCallum, W. G. *William Stewart Halsted, Surgeon.* Baltimore: Johns Hopkins Press, 1930.

McClure, R. D., and Szilagyi, E. "Halsted, Teacher of Surgeons." *Am. J. Surg.* 82:122–131 (1951).

Miller, J. M. "William Stewart Halsted and the Use of the Surgical Rubber Glove." *Surgery* 92:541–543 (1982).

Mitchell, J. F. "The Introduction of Rubber Gloves for Use in Surgical Operations." *Ann. Surg.* 122:902–904 (1945).

Olch, P. D. "William S. Halsted's New York Period, 1874–1886." *Bull. Hist. Med.* 40:495–510 (1966).

——. "William S. Halsted and Local Anesthesia." *Anesth.* 42:479–486 (1975).

Penfield, W. "Halsted of Johns Hopkins." *J.A.M.A.* 210:2214–2218 (1969).

Proskauer, C. "Development and Use of the Rubber Glove in Surgery and Gynecology." *J. Hist. Med.* 13:373–381 (1958).

Ravitch, M. "The Place of the Halsted Radical Mastectomy." *Johns Hopkins Med. J.* 129:202–211 (1974).

——, and Hitzroth, J. M. "The Operations for Inguinal Hernia." *Surgery* 48:439–466, 615–636 (1960).

Reid, M. R. "Dr. Halsted's Friday Clinics." *Johns Hopkins Hosp. Bull.*, 50–59, 1925.

Roosa, D. B. S. "Thomas Alexander McBride—An Account of His Last Illness." *N.Y. Med. J.* 44:365–366 (1886).

Shryock, R. H. "Women in American Medicine." *J. Am. Women's Med. Ass.* 5:371–379 (1950).

Smith, S. "The Comparative Results of Operations in Bellevue Hospital." *Med. Record* 28:427–431 (1885). In G. H. Brieger, *Medical America in the Nineteenth Century.* Baltimore: Johns Hopkins Press, 1972.

Welch, W. H. "In Memoriam—William Stewart Halsted." *Bull. Johns Hopkins Hosp.* 36:34–39 (1925).

14 A TRIUMPH OF TWENTIETH-CENTURY MEDICINE: HELEN TAUSSIG AND THE BLUE-BABY OPERATION

Abbott, M. E., and Weiss, E. "The Diagnosis of Congenital Cardiac Disease." In G. Blumer, *Bedside Diagnosis.* Philadelphia: W. B. Saunders, 1928.

Allen, J. G. "Alfred Blalock and Our Heritage." *Arch. Surg.* 89:929–931 (1964).

Blalock, A., and Taussig, H. B. "The Surgical Treatment of Malformations of the Heart in Which There Is Pulmonary Stenosis or Pulmonary Atresia." *J.A.M.A.* 128:189–202 (1945).

Dietrich, H. J. "Helen Brooke Taussig, 1898–1986." *Trans. and Stud. Coll. Phys. Phila.* 8:265–271 (1986).

Engle, M. E. "Dr. Helen B. Taussig, the Tetralogy of Fallot, and the Growth of Pediatric Cardiac Services in the United States." *Johns Hopkins Med. J.* 140:147–150 (1977).

Field, J. "Medical Education in the United States: Late Nineteenth and Twentieth Centuries." In C. D. O'Malley, *The History of Medical Education.* Berkeley: Univ. of Cal. Press, 1970.

Flexner, A. *An Autobiography.* New York: Simon & Schuster, 1960.

Francis, W. W. "Maude Abbott (1869–1940)." *Bull. Hist. Med.* 10:305–308 (1941).

Goodman, G. "Helen Taussig." M.D. thesis. Yale Univ., 1983.

Harvey, A. M. *Adventures in Medical Research: A Century of Discovery at Johns Hopkins.* Baltimore: Johns Hopkins Press, 1974.

——. "The First Full-Time Academic Department of Pediatrics: The Story of the Harriet Lane Home." *Johns Hopkins Med. J.* 137:27–42 (1975).

——. "Helen Brooke Taussig." *Johns Hopkins Med. J.* 140:137–141 (1977).

——. "A Conversation with Helen Taussig." *Med. Times* 106:28–44 (1978).

Hudson, R. P. "Abraham Flexner in Perspective: American Medical Education 1865–1910." *Bull. Hist. Med.* 46:545–561 (1972).

King, L. *American Medicine Comes of Age—1840–1920.* Chicago: A.M.A., 1984.

MacDermott, H. E. *Maude Abbott: A Memoir.* Toronto: Macmillan, 1941.

Munger, D. B. "Robert Brookings and the Flexner Report." *J. Hist. Med.* 23:356–371 (1968).

Ravitch, M. M. "Alfred Blalock, 1899–1964." In M. M. Ravitch, ed., *The Papers of Alfred Blalock.* Baltimore: Johns Hopkins Press, 1966.

——. "The Contributions of Alfred Blalock to the Science and Practice of Surgery." *Johns Hopkins Med. J.* 140:57–67 (1977).

Taussig, H. B. *Congenital Malformations of the Heart.* New York: Commonwealth Fund, 1947.

——. "Little Choice and a Stimulating Environment." *J. Am. Med. Women's Ass.* 36:43–44 (1981).

——, and others. "Long-Time Observations on the Blalock-Taussig Operation." *Johns Hopkins Med. J.* 129:243–257 (1971).

——. "Long-Time Observations on the Blalock-Taussig Operation VIII. 20 to 28 Year Follow-up on Patients with a Tetralogy of Fallot." *Johns Hopkins Med. J.* 137:13–19 (1975).

Thomas, V. *Pioneering Research in Surgical Shock and Cardiovascular Surgery.* Philadelphia: Univ. of Pa. Press, 1985.

Thorwald, J. *The Patients.* New York: Harcourt, Brace, Jovanovich, 1971.

Wangensteen, O. H. "Reflections on the Blalock Papers." *Bull. Hist. Med.* 42:357–361 (1968).

15 NEW HEARTS FOR OLD: THE STORY OF TRANSPLANTATION

Amos, D. B. "Transplantation Antigens and Immune Mechanisms." In D. C. Sabiston, *Textbook of Surgery*, 13th ed. Philadelphia: Saunders, 1986.

Bahnson, H. T. "Substitute Hearts." *Bull. Am. Coll. Surg.* 72:4–10 (1987).

Baldwin, J. C., and Shumway, N. "Cardiac and Cardiopulmonary Homotransplants." In D. C. Sabiston, *Textbook of Surgery,* 13th ed. Philadelphia: Saunders, 1986.

Barker, C. F., Naj, A., and Perloff, L. J. "Renal Transplantation." In D. C. Sabiston, *Textbook of Surgery,* 13th ed. Philadelphia: Saunders, 1986.

Billingham, R. E., Brent, L., and Medawar, P. B. "Actively Acquired Tolerance of Foreign Cells." *Nature* 172:603–606 (1953).

Bollinger, R. R., and Stickel, D. L. "Historical Aspects of Transplantation." In D. C. Sabiston, *Textbook of Surgery,* 13th ed. Philadelphia: Saunders, 1986.

Bow, L. M., and Schweizer, R. T. "Clinically Relevant Factors in Transplantation Immunology." *Conn. Med.* 50:497–500 (1986).

Burnet, F. M. *The Integrity of the Body: A Discussion of Modern Immunological Ideas.* Cambridge: Harvard Univ. Press, 1962.

Calne, R. Y. "The Rejection of Renal Homografts: Inhibition in Dogs by 6-Mercaptopurine." *Lancet* 1:417–418 (1960).

——. *A Gift of Life: Observations on Organ Transplantation.* New York: Basic Books, 1970.

——. *Liver Transplantation.* London: Grune & Stratton, 1983.

Carrel, A. "Results of the Transplantation of Blood Vessels, Organs and Limbs." *J.A.M.A.* 51:1662–1667 (1908).

——, and Guthrie, C. C. "Functions of a Transplanted Kidney." *Science* 22:473–475 (1905).

——. "Successful Transplantation of Both Kidneys from a Dog into a Bitch with Removal of Both Normal Kidneys from the Latter." *Science* 23:394–395 (1906).

Converse, J. M., and Casson, P. R. "The Historical Background of Transplantation." In F. T. Rapaport and J. Dausset, eds., *Human Transplantation.* New York: Grune & Stratton, 1968.

Dornfeld, L. "Tissue Typing or Histocompatibility Testing Simplified." *Urology* (supp.) 9:49–51 (1977).

Dougherty and others. "Cardiac Transplantation." *Conn. Med.* 50: 429–440 (1986).

Evans, R. "The Heart Transplant Dilemma." *Issues in Science and Technology,* Spring 1986, 91–101.

Evans, R. W., and others. "Donor Availability as the Primary Determinant of the Future of Heart Transplantation." *J.A.M.A.* 255:1892–1898 (1986).

Gibson, T., and Medawar, P. B. "The Fate of Skin Homografts in Man." *J. Anat.* 77:299–310 (1942–43).

Hamburger, J. "Medical Ethics and Organ Transplantation." *J. Am. Med. Women's Ass.* 23:981–984 (1968).

Lower, R. R., Stofer, R. C., and Shumway, N. "Homovital Transplantation of the Heart." *J. Thor. Cardiovasc. Surg.* 41:196–200 (1961).

——, Dong, E., and Shumway, N. "Long-Term Survival of Cardiac Homografts." *Surgery* 58:110–119 (1965).

McCormick, R. A. "Organ Transplantation—Ethical Principles." In W. T. Reich, ed., *Encyc. Bioethics.* New York: Free Press, 1978.

Medawar, P. B. "Tests by Tissue Culture Methods on the Nature of Immunity to Transplanted Skin." *Quart. J. Mic. Sci.* 89:239–252 (1948).

——. *Memoir of a Thinking Radish: An Autobiography.* New York: Oxford Univ. Press, 1986.

Moody, F. D. "Clinical Research in the Era of Cost Containment." *Am. J. Surg.* 153:337–340 (1987).

Moore, F. D. *Transplant: The Give and Take of Tissue Transplantation.* New York: Simon & Schuster, 1972.

——. "Transplantation: A Perspective." *Transplant. Proc.* 12:539–550 (1980).

Morrison, K. E. "Brain Transplantation—Still Fantasy?" *J. Roy. Soc. Med.* 80:441–444 (1987).

Schwartz, R., and Damashek, W. "Drug-Induced Immunological Tolerance." *Nature* 183:1682–1683 (1959).

Smith, H. L. "Heart Transplantation." In W. T. Reich, ed., *Encyc. Bioethics.* New York: Free Press, 1978.

Starzl, T. E. "The Succession from Kidney to Liver Transplantation." *Transplant. Proc.* 13:50–54 (1981).

Thorwald, J. *The Patients.* New York: Harcourt, Brace, Jovanovich, 1971.

Index